European Handbook of Neurological Management

Volume 2

Contents

Introduction, 1

1 Guidance for the preparation of neurological management guidelines by EFNS Scientific Task Forces: revised recommendations 2004, 5

2 Neurostimulation therapy for neuropathic pain, 11

3 Trigeminal neuralgia management, 31

4 Molecular diagnosis of neurogenetic disorders: general issues, Huntington's disease, Parkinson's disease and dystonias, 51

5 Molecular diagnosis of mitochondrial disorders, 61

6 Molecular diagnosis of ataxias and spastic paraplegias, 73

7 Molecular diagnosis of channelopathies, epilepsies, migraine, stroke and dementias, 87

8 Molecular diagnosis of neurogenetic disorders: motoneuron, peripheral nerve and muscle disorders, 97

9 Intravenous immunoglobulin in the treatment of neurological diseases, 111

10 Sleep disorders in neurodegenerative disorders and stroke, 129

11 Management of community-acquired bacterial meningitis, 145

12 Diagnosis and management of European lyme neuroborreliosis, 159

13 Disease-specific cerebrospinal fluid investigations, 175

14 Neuroimaging in the management of motor neuron diseases, 199

15 Management of low-grade gliomas, 213

16 Treatment of tension-type headache, 225

17 Diagnosis, therapy and prevention of Wernicke's encephalopathy, 239

18 Recommendations for the diagnosis and management of spontaneous intracerebral haemorrhage, 253

19 Diagnostic approach to pauci- or asymptomatic hyperCKemia, 279

20 Diagnosis and management of neuromyelitis optica, 287

21 Screening for tumours in paraneoplastic syndromes, 309

22 Treatment of miscellaneous idiopathic headache disorders, 321

23 Treatment of medication overuse headache, 337

Index, 345

Introduction

Nils Erik Gilhus,[1,2] *Michael P. Barnes,*[3] *Michael Brainin*[4,5]

[1]Department of Clinical Medicine, University of Bergen, Norway; [2]Department of Neurology, Haukeland University Hospital, Bergen, Norway; [3]Hunters Moor Neurorehabilitation Ltd, University of Newcastle, England; [4]Center of Clinical Neurosciences, Donau-Universität Krems, Austria; [5]Department of Neurology, Landesclinicum Tulln, Austria

This second volume of the *European Handbook of Neurological Management* represents a step forward for European neurology. The first volume of the Handbook was launched in 2006 and contained all 41 guidelines completed and approved by European Federation of Neurological Societies (EFNS) until then. Since 2006 another 21 guidelines on new therapeutic or diagnostic topics have been accomplished and approved. These new EFNS guidelines have been collected in this volume, and represent the complete compendium of EFNS guidelines 2006–2011.

The reason why guidelines are developed is to improve practice. All guidelines in this book represent relevant clinical topics for neurologists. The topics have been suggested by neurologists through the EFNS Scientist panels because they have felt the need for better practice. To fulfil this aim, it is not sufficient to just complete well-balanced and correct guidelines on relevant topics. The guidelines have also to be implemented. This book is an important way of making them available for neurologists and neurology units. The guidelines have already been published in the *European Journal of Neurology*, or will soon be published there. This Handbook with the guidelines further promotes their use, making them easily available for neurologists at work. Together with the first volume of the European Handbook of Neurological Management (second edition 2010), there are now 62 EFNS guidelines available, covering important areas of neurological practice. Guidelines like these are needed to improve and change clinical routines and to guide patient treatment. Although the guidelines are produced by European neurologists they have global relevance, and should also be useful for non-neurologists treating patients with disorders of the brain, spinal cord, nerves and muscles.

All guidelines in the European Handbook of Neurological Management have been made according to the procedures agreed by EFNS and the EFNS Scientific Committee. The EFNS Scientist panels have been instrumental in proposing topics for guidelines as well as for recruiting leading European experts to produce them. The detailed standards for the collection of scientific data and for the critical evaluation of such data have been included as Chapter 2 in the Handbook.

This second volume of the *European Handbook of Neurological Management* has focused on therapeutic interventions, with less diagnostic guidelines included. This is a much needed development. Neurology and neurological practice have a similar focus on therapy. An increasing number of brain and nervous system disorders are targets for effective therapy. There are often several alternative therapeutic options, or various measures should be combined to obtain an optimal result. Such aspects make guidelines necessary. Furthermore, new therapeutic options can be expensive. Society needs to evaluate costs versus benefit. EFNS guidelines do usually not include the cost aspects of their medical recommendations. Even so these guidelines should be useful also in health planning and as evidence in evaluating cost-benefit, thereby leading to sensible conclusions regarding necessary funding for the treatment of neurological disorders.

Neurogenetic and neuroinflammatory disorders have a prominent place in this second volume of the Handbook, with 10 new guidelines. This reflects the rapidly expanding knowledge of disorders with a genetic dysfunction or with ongoing inflammation. Such new knowledge leads to diagnostic and therapeutic possibilities, summarized and evaluated in the guidelines.

Pain disorders have a separate section in this volume. In addition to being hot topics, the chosen themes for guidelines also reflect the activity of the respective EFNS Scientist panels. Several of the guidelines have been joint projects between EFNS and collaborating organizations. Some have even been co-published, i.e. they have appeared in both European Journal of Neurology and another scientific journal. The guideline paper on 'Treatment of medication overuse headache' has been accepted into this Handbook after a full external revue as all the other guidelines. However, a later and more extensive version of the paper has been planned, and only this planned version will be submitted to a scientific journal. The guideline on 'Management of spontaneous intracerebral haemorrhage' has been produced by the European Stroke Initiative and has been approved by EFNS as well as other neurological organisations. This guideline was originally published in *Cerebravascular Diseases*.

Neurological management of clinical disorders tends to show some variation between countries and geographical regions. A strength of the present Handbook and of the individual guidelines is that they have all been authored by neurologists from most parts of Europe. Thus they combine several traditions and therefore have

a broad spectrum of evaluations and recommendations. The Scientific committee of EFNS and the respective Scientist panels have overseen the process and evaluated the main recommendations given. Independent external expert reviewers have a key role in the EFNS guideline production. As editors we express our sincere thanks to all those reviewers that have been absolutely necessary in improving the guidelines and checking disease-specific evidence classification and recommendations. A few guidelines suggested to EFNS have not been accepted as such because the evidence base was not sufficient to reach scientifically sound recommendations. However, in contrast to some other guideline systems, topics without any excellent controlled studies have been chosen, and recommendations based on less well-controlled studies are included. In our view, such recommendations can be more useful in clinical practice than recommendations where controlled studies have already and without any doubt given the answers.

EFNS intends to continue the production of guidelines on new neurological topics. Guidelines on previously covered topics need to be updated. Recently a new EFNS guideline production group has been formed with the aim to further harmonize the guidelines. This group will support and guide the task forces for each guideline, and also help the scientist panels in their initiating and follow-up regarding guideline production. New systems for formal evaluation of single studies are under way, to ensure that evaluation is consistent and transparent. There is an increasing tendency for guidelines to be used outside the medical profession, which poses new challenges.

Guidelines are useful and widely read because they evaluate present evidence and give recommendations. They express an opinion on which several international experts have agreed. This means that they are more than a review of evidence. Guidelines should be regarded as a practice parameter. The present guidelines have been approved by EFNS, but this does not infer any legal responsibility.

EFNS has as one of its major aims to support and disseminate neurological research and neurological teaching. The organization is a federation of 44 European national neurological societies and 8 associated national member societies. The 24 scientist panels, each with participants from most member countries, represent the scientific backbone of the EFNS. *European Journal of*

Neurology is owned by EFNS. EFNS, its national members, the scientist panels, and the *European Journal of Neurology* have all contributed to the guidelines in this volume of the *European Handbook of Neurological Management*. The main effort has, however, been done by the authors in the task forces. The editors are grateful for their efforts and their distinguished work. We will thank the EFNS office and executive director Lisa Müller for the following up of all task forces. We will also thank Professor Richard Hughes, present president of EFNS, who was the key person in the initiation and early organization of the guideline work within EFNS.

We hope that this Handbook will be used. We hope that the guidelines will be a helpful guide in treating individual patients and in establishing better routines in neurological units. Although the guidelines also illustrate how more and better research is needed, each guideline represents, in our opinion, a step forward for the management of patients with disorders in the brain and nervous system.

CHAPTER 1

Guidance for the preparation of neurological management guidelines by EFNS Scientific Task Forces: revised recommendations 2004*[1]

M. Brainin,[1] M. Barnes,[2] J-C. Baron,[3] N. Gilhus,[4] R. Hughes,[5] K. Selmaj[6] and G. Waldemar[7]

[1]Donauklinikum and Donau-Universität, Maria Gugging, Austria; [2]University of Newcastle and Hunters Moor Regional Neurorehabilitation Ltd, Newcastle upon Tyne, UK; [3]Addenbrooks Hospital, Cambridge, UK; [4]University Bergen, Bergen, Norway; [5]Guy's, King's and St Thomas' School of Medicine, London, UK; [6]Medical University of Lodz, Lodz, Poland; [7]Copenhagen University Hospital, Denmark

Summary

Since the publication of the first EFNS Task Force reports in 1997, a total of 20 evidence-based guidelines for the treatment and management of neurological diseases have been published by the EFNS (www.efns.org/guidelines). In 2001 recommendations for the preparation of neurological guidelines were issued by the EFNS Scientific Committee [1]. These have now been updated and revised. More unified criteria for standards of reporting are set up, which include classes of scientific evidence and predefined levels of recommendation. These criteria, as well as others listed below, should be used for all working groups that aim at recommending treatment, diagnostic procedures or other interventions within the framework of the EFNS.

*Report of the Guideline Standards Subcommittee of the EFNS Scientific Committee.
[1]This guidance was approved by the EFNS Scientific Committee.

The EFNS neurological treatment guidelines/management recommendations on a European scale

Neurological diseases and disability are a primary concern world-wide. In a global survey it was found that out of the leading 10 disabling diseases eight were due to diseases of the brain [2]. For Europe, brain diseases cause a loss of 23% of the years of healthy life and 50% of years lived with disability. Thus 35% of the total burden of disability-adjusted life-years is caused by brain diseases alone [3]. In Europe, both mortality and morbidity due to neurological causes are increasing and the health expenditure for this burden is growing rapidly. In contrast, part of the cost is due to treatments that have become established without scientific evidence. Although the situation varies from country to country, this is the case for many treatments for common diseases such as stroke, migraine and other headaches, parkinsonism and epilepsy, but also for other conditions, including many segments of neurological prevention and neurorehabilitation.

The EFNS has recognized the demands for the development of European standards for the management and treatment of neurological diseases and since 1997 has published some 20 such guidelines. They have been distributed widely on the Web and as printed material. Several have been translated into other European languages for use of national neurological societies. The Task Force applications and practice recommendations published within the framework of the EFNS (www.efns.org) have increased and therefore underwent a critical review. To meet the needs of future Task Forces preparing guidelines, more specific instructions than the previous guidance [1] seemed necessary and this chapter responds to that need.

Aim of guidelines

The aim of an EFNS neurological management guideline is to provide evidence-based guidance for clinical neurologists, other healthcare professionals and healthcare providers about important aspects of management of neurological disease. It provides the view of an expert Task Force appointed by the Scientific Committee of the EFNS. It represents a peer-reviewed statement of minimum desirable standards for the guidance of practice, based on the best available evidence. It is not intended to have legally binding implications in individual cases.

Scientific basis of guidelines

The increasing burden of neurological diseases and disability can only be met by implementing measures of prevention and treatment that are scientifically proven and based on evidence-based criteria. Sets of treatment recommendations and management guidelines have been prepared by the EFNS and also by the American Academy of Neurology (AAN). The critical standards used in both organizations aim to evaluate the scientific evidence according to pre-specified levels of certainty and grade the recommendations according to the strength of available scientific evidence.

This Subcommittee of the EFNS recommends the use of such classes of evidence and grades of recommendations in the way developed by the AAN [4]. They have been applied for a therapeutic measure [5] and for a diagnostic measure [6] within the AAN practice guidelines groups. The definitions and requirements for the classes of evidence and levels of recommendations from the AAN have been adapted and slightly modified (Boxes 1.1–1.4).

Some of the issues under discussion include the question of classifying secondary endpoints from large, randomized, controlled trials as either first- or second-class evidence. The Subcommittee members agree that these secondary endpoints should usually not have the same scientific weight as the primary ones. This becomes relevant when both the primary and secondary endpoints are positive (or negative), implying that they both bear statistically significant results in favour of (or contrary to) the intervention under investigation. To name but

---

Box 1.1 Evidence classification scheme for a therapeutic intervention.

Class I: An adequately powered prospective, randomized, controlled clinical trial with masked outcome assessment in a representative population OR an adequately powered systematic review of prospective randomized controlled clinical trials with masked outcome assessment in representative populations. The following are required:

a. Randomization concealment.

b. Primary outcome(s) is (are) clearly defined.

c. Exclusion/inclusion criteria are clearly defined.

d. Adequate accounting for drop-outs and cross-overs with numbers sufficiently low to have minimal potential for bias.

e. Relevant baseline characteristics are presented and substantially equivalent among treatment groups or there is appropriate statistical adjustment for differences.

Class II: Prospective matched group cohort study in a representative population with masked outcome assessment that meets a–e above *or* a randomized, controlled trial in a representative population that lacks one of the criteria a–e.

Class III: All other controlled trials (including well-defined natural history controls or patients serving as own controls) in a representative population, where outcome assessment is independent of patient treatment.

Class IV: Evidence from uncontrolled studies, case series, case reports or expert opinion.

Box 1.2 Evidence classification scheme for the rating of recommendations for a therapeutic intervention.

Level A rating (established as effective, ineffective, or harmful): requires at least one convincing Class I study or at least two consistent, convincing Class II studies.

Level B rating (probably effective, ineffective, or harmful): requires at least one convincing Class II study or overwhelming Class III evidence.

Level C rating (possibly effective, ineffective, or harmful): requires at least two convincing Class III studies.

Box 1.3 Evidence classification scheme for a diagnostic measure.

Class I: A prospective study of a broad spectrum of persons with the suspected condition, using a gold standard for case definition, where the test is applied in a blinded evaluation, and enabling the assessment of appropriate tests of diagnostic accuracy.

Class II: A prospective study of a narrow spectrum of persons with the suspected condition, or a well-designed retrospective study of a broad spectrum of persons with an established condition (by gold standard) compared to a broad spectrum of controls, where test is applied in a blinded evaluation, and enabling the assessment of appropriate tests of diagnostic accuracy.

Class III: Evidence provided by a retrospective study where either persons with the established condition or controls are of a narrow spectrum, and where test is applied in a blinded evaluation.

Class IV: Any design where test is not applied in blinded evaluation OR evidence provided by expert opinion alone or in descriptive case series (without controls).

Box 1.4 Evidence classification scheme for the rating of recommendations for a diagnostic measure.

Level A rating (established as useful/predictive or not useful/predictive): requires at least one convincing Class I study or at least two consistent, convincing Class II studies.

Level B rating (established as probably useful/predictive or not useful/predictive): requires at least one convincing Class II study or overwhelming Class III evidence.

Level C rating (established as possibly useful/predictive or not useful/predictive): requires at least two convincing Class III studies.

one example: many intervention trials with cardiovascular endpoints (e.g., myocardial infarction) also have a secondary neurological endpoint (e.g., stroke). Assuming that both are positive, this does not imply that the treatment is effective for both cardiac and cerebral endpoints with equal scientific certainty because the inclusion parameters, endpoint definitions and diagnostic work-up regularly differ in precision and in absolute numbers of cases for both endpoints and usually heavily favour the primary one. These issues have not been handled uniformly in the past and therefore these new, extended guidelines have been revised.

One other issue to be discussed within the framework of each Task Force when evaluating scientific evidence refers to important clinical areas for which no high-class evidence is available or likely to become available in the near future. In such cases – which should be marked as exceptional – it may be possible to recommend best practice based on the experience of the guideline development group. An example of such an important area is the problem of recommendations for driving after stroke where it is not easily conceivable to gather a large body of randomized evidence. Such good practice points have been used by the Scottish Intercollegiate Guidelines Network [7] and make the recommendations more useful for health workers [8]. But such good practice points should not imply that they are based on more than class IV evidence, which implies high clinical uncertainty. No impression is intended that a randomized trial to test the intervention can be avoided by assigning such points to a specific recommendation.

Critical review of guidelines

Current methods of developing guidelines have improved from the informal consensus (TOBSAT = the old boys sat at a table, see [9]) and adapted to formal consensus methods, which use a systematic approach to assess the experts' opinion and reach an agreement on recommendation. The evidence-based consensus links its work directly to scientific evidence [10]. According to the AAN, the strength of the 'guideline development process aims at the evidence-based category, with little use for expert opinion' in order to reduce the likelihood of severe bias when relying on informal consensus alone [11]. Consequently, guideline development has also been subjected to systematic evaluation. Following a systematic search, practice guidelines published in peer-reviewed medical literature between 1985 and 1997 were assessed with a 25-item measurement instrument, which included the use of levels of evidence. From 279 guidelines investigated, the mean overall adherence to such levels of evidence was 43% but improved significantly between 1985 and 1997 (36.9% vs. 50.4%; $P < 0.001$) [10]. Grilli *et al.* [9] found similar discrepancies when investigating 431 guidelines between 1988 and 1998. The authors suggest the development of common standards of reporting, similar to the CONSORT statement for reporting the results of clinical trials [12]. A more recent review of guidelines for stroke prevention has shown that there are notable differences on information about panel selection, funding source and consensus methods. Thus it concludes that current stroke prevention guidelines do not provide adequate information to permit assessment of their quality [13].

Guideline recommendations should also include the description of methods used for synthesizing individual judgements. The development of the consensus reached is important but minority statements should also be included when necessary [14]. All critical reviews are recommended to make use of a systematic and formal procedure of establishing guidelines. One recent and major effort was published by a Conference on Guideline Standardization (COGS) which produced a checklist to be used prospectively by developers to enable standardized recommendations [15]. This was achieved by means of a reiterative method (mostly several rounds of balloting by panel experts who gave differing weights to different pieces of scientific evidence). This method has reproducible results and is less likely to be biased by individual opinion. It involves stricter definitions for collecting and synthesizing evidence about potential harms, benefits and patients' preferences, and more effective considerations for implementation. Unfortunately, this COGS method is very laborious. The EFNS guidance proposed here captures the most important elements of the COGS proposals.

In addition to management guidelines, appropriate methods are needed to develop expert consensus on the process of care. Examples include the timely referral for diagnostic procedures (e.g., nerve conduction velocity testing in carpal tunnel syndrome) and measures to improve patient satisfaction [11]. Such process-related guidelines must take patient preferences into account and are no less important than treatment guidelines. Finally, there is evidence that adherence to guidelines improves patient outcome. This has been shown, for example, for post-acute rehabilitation following stroke, indicating that such guidelines can also be used as quality of care indicators [16].

Due to these quality issues the goals and the process of the Task Force work are described in more detail below. These will be reviewed every four years and updated if necessary by the Subcommittee.

Collection of scientific data

1. The Cochrane Library should be consulted by every person or group planning to develop a guideline. For many therapeutic options there is little randomized evidence, and non-randomized studies also have to be considered. Authors of treatment guidelines should liaise with the coordinating editors of the appropriate Cochrane review group and review the list of registered titles of the Cochrane systematic reviews which have not yet been converted into protocols (www.cochrane.no/titles). The EFNS and the AAN have agreed to share their list of practice parameters or management guidelines under preparation.

2. Collection of data from original scientific papers in referee-based scientific journals is the cornerstone for evaluation of scientific evidence. Such papers can be identified from several bibliographic databases. It is important to use specific and sensitive keywords as well as combinations of keywords. One keyword is rarely sufficient. Both older and new scientific papers should be included. It is always necessary to collect the data from the paper itself, not from secondary literature. The full paper should always be read, not only the abstract. Data can be included from papers which have been accepted but not yet published, but not usually before acceptance. In accordance with the Cochrane Library, unpublished data [17] from randomized trials can be used provided they are of high quality. Such exceptions should be explained in the synthesizing evidence section of the report.

3. Collection of papers containing any previous meta-analyses of the same or similar topics should always be undertaken. Such papers are always helpful, but they usually do not give the full and final conclusion for a Task Force.

4. Collection of review/overview papers is done from the same bibliographic databases. Such reviews are usually well known by the experts in the field and may be included in the work of the Task Force. The conclusions of such papers should never be used without independently evaluating the scientific evidence of the papers from the original data.

5. Scientific data from papers published in refereed journals not included in the main databases may be included. As such papers are more difficult to identify, it is not a prerequisite for a Task Force to collect them.

6. Scientific data from non-refereed journals, books or other publications should usually not influence recommendations and conclusions. It is therefore not important to collect them.

7. Previous guideline documents and recommendations should be sought from Medline, EMBASE and other sources, including national and international neurology organizations, patient organizations and national or supranational health-related bodies. Although Task Force conclusions should rely on quality-assured scientific data alone, it is appropriate to discuss previous guidelines and recommendations (which may be registered by the International Network of Agencies for Health Technology Assessment, www.inahta.org).

Recommendations for the process of proposing, planning and writing a guideline

1. Neurological Management Guidelines will be produced by Task Forces appointed by the Scientific Committee.

2. Proposals for Task Forces concerning neurological management should be submitted to the Scientific Committee. The proposal should include the title, objectives, membership, conflict of interests, a short (100–300 words) explanation of why the guideline is needed, already existing guidelines on the same or related topic, search strategy, method for reaching consensus and a time-frame for accomplishment. Task Forces will usually be appointed following a proposal from the chair of a Scientific Panel to the Scientific Committee.

3. The Task Force will consist of a chair and at least six but not usually more than 12 members. No more than two members should usually come from any one country. Conflicts of interest must be declared by members at the time of the formation of the Task Force. The chair should be free from conflicts of interest. If feasible, the group should include a patient advocate (normally an officer

from a European patient organization if the Task Force deals with a clinically relevant topic) and other relevant specialists (e.g., a statistician) and health professionals. If Task Forces have a budget, they must nominate a secretary and treasurer and submit an annual account to the Management Committee.

4. The Task Force will review the available evidence and include within its report the search strategy employed. Where appropriate, the evidence concerning healthcare interventions must be based on a thorough systematic literature search and review. The report should include a structured summary which contains the main conclusions. Irreconcilable differences between group members should be referred to the Scientific Committee through the chair.

5. Existing guidelines prepared by other organizations (including European neurology subspeciality societies, European national neurological societies, non-European neurological societies and other organizations) will be sought and (where appropriate) adopted in part or whole with appropriate acknowledgement and respect for copyright rules.

6. The format of the guidelines will use the style of the *European Journal of Neurology* and follow a template with these sections:

   1. Title. This should read: *EFNS Guideline on ......Report of an EFNS Task Force on ... ...* [title of Task Force, if different from the topic of the guideline]
   2. Structured abstract
   3. Membership of Task Force
   4. Objectives
   5. Background
   6. Search strategy
   7. Method for reaching consensus
   8. Results
   9. Recommendations
   10. Statement of the likely time when the guidelines will need to be updated
   11. Conflicts of interest
   12. References

7. The length of the guideline report should not be more than eight printed pages, including references (4,000 words). Supplementary material may be published on the EFNS website. The authors will be the EFNS Task Force on management/diagnosis/other of condition. The authors will be listed as members of the Task Force, with the chair first and the other authors in alphabetical order.

8. The Task Force should submit the completed guideline for approval to the chair of the Scientific Committee.

9. The Scientific Committee will have the proposed management guideline reviewed by its members, the president of the EFNS and the chairs of any Scientist Panels which might be affected by the guidelines but where not involved in the preparation of them. Additional external peer reviewing may be sought, especially in areas where few neurological experts are available. Within 8 weeks of submission, the chair of the Scientific Committee will advise the chair of the Task Force whether the guidelines have been accepted as the official guidelines of the EFNS or not. If revision is needed, the Task Force will prepare a revised version and submit this to the review process, highlighting the revisions and documenting the responses to each of the referees' comments.

10. Following approval, the management guidelines will be submitted by the chair of the Task Force to the editor(s) of the *European Journal of Neurology* with a view to publication. The editor(s) will have the power to accept or reject the guidelines for publication and may make minor editorial changes.

11. The validity of published guidelines will be reviewed by the chairs of the Task Force and the relevant Scientist Panel at least every 2 years.

12. Guidelines will be published on the EFNS website and in the *European Journal of Neurology*.

13. National societies will be encouraged to translate guidelines for dissemination in their own countries.

References

1. Hughes, RAC, Barnes, MP, Baron, JC, Brainin, M. Guidance for the preparation of neurological management guidelines by EFNS scientific task forces. *Eur J Neurol* 2001; **8**:549–50.
2. Üstün, TB, Rehm, J, Chatterji, S, *et al.* Multiple-informant ranking of the disabling effects of different health conditions in 14 countries. *Lancet* 1999; **354**:111–15.
3. Olesen, J, Leonardi, M. The burden of brain diseases in Europe. *Eur J Neurol* 2003; **10**:471.
4. American Academy of Neurology, Quality Standards Subcommittee. Process for developing practice parameters 1999.
5. Hirtz, D, Berg, A, Bettis, D, *et al.* Practice parameter: treatment of the child with a first unprovoked seizure. Report of the Quality Standards Subcommittee of the American Academy of Neurology and the Practice Committee of the Child Neurology Society. *Neurology* 2003; **60**:166–75.
6. Shevell, M, Ashwal, S, Donley, D, *et al.* Practice parameter: evaluation of the child with global developmental delay. Report of the Quality Standards Subcommittee of the American Academy of Neurology and The Practice Committee of the Child Neurology Society. *Neurology* 2003; **60**:367–80.
7. Scottish Intercollegiate Guidelines Network (SIGN). SIGN Guidelines. An introduction to SIGN methodology for the development of evidence-based clinical guidelines 1999. www.sign.ac.uk/methodology/index.html (accessed 1st July 2011).
8. Scottish Intercollegiate Guidelines Network (SIGN). Management of patients with stroke. A national clinical guideline 2002. Edinburgh. www.sign.ac.uk (accessed 1st July 2011).
9. Grilli, R, Magrini, N, Penna, A, *et al.* Practice guidelines developed by specialty societies: the need for a critical appraisal. *Lancet* 2000; **355**:103–6.
10. Shaneyfelt, TM, Mayo-Smith, MF, Rothwange, J. Are guidelines following guidelines? The methodological quality of clinical practice guidelines in the peer-reviewed medical literature. *JAMA* 1999; **281**:1900–5.
11. Franklin, GM, Zahn, CA. AAN clinical practice guidelines. *Neurology* 2002; **59**: 975–6.
12. Moher, D, Schulz, KF, Altman, DG; The CONSORT Group. The CONSORT statement: revised recommendations for improving the quality of reports of parallel-group randomised trials. *Lancet* 2001; **357**:1191–4.
13. Hart, RG, Bailey, RD. An assessment of guidelines for prevention of ischemic stroke. *Neurology* 2002; **59**:977–82.
14. Black, N, Murphy, M, Lauping, D, *et al.* Consensus developing methods: a review of best practices creating clinical guidelines. *J Health Serv Res Policy* 1999; **4**:236–8.
15. Shiffman, RN, Shekelle, P, Overhage, M, *et al.* Standardized reporting of clinical practice guidelines: a proposal from the Conference on Guideline Standardization. *Ann Intern Med* 2003; **139**:493–8.
16. Duncan, PW, Horner, RD, Reker, DM, *et al.* Adherence to postacute rehabilitation guidelines is associated with functional recovery in stroke. *Stroke* 2002; **33**:167–78.
17. Cochrane Collaboration, www.cochrane.org.
18. Grimshaw, J, Eccles, M, Russell, I. Developing clinically valid practice guidelines. *J Eval Clin Pract* 1995; **1**:37–48.
19. Miller, J, Petrie, J. Development of practice guidelines. *Lancet* 2000; **355**:82–3.
20. Shekelle, PG, Woolf, SH, Eccles, M, Grisham, J. Developing guidelines. *BMJ* 1999; **318**:593–6.

CHAPTER 2

Neurostimulation therapy for neuropathic pain

G. Cruccu,[1,2] T. Z. Aziz,[3] L. Garcia-Larrea,[1,4] P. Hansson,[1,5] T. S. Jensen,[1,6] J.-P. Lefaucheur,[7] B. A. Simpson[8] and R. S. Taylor[9]

[1]EFNS Panel on Neuropathic Pain, Vienna, Austria; [2]La Sapienza University, Rome, Italy; [3]Oxford Functional Neurosurgery, Department of Neurosurgery, Radcliffe Infirmary, Oxford, UK; [4]INSERM 'Central integration of pain' (U879), Bron, University Lyon 1, France; [5]Karolinska University Hospital and Pain Section, Department of Molecular Medicine and Surgery, Karolinska Institute, Stockholm, Sweden; [6]Danish Pain Research Centre, Aarhus University Hospital, Aarhus, Denmark; [7]Henri Mondor Hospital, AP-HP, Créteil, France; [8]University Hospital of Wales, Heath Park, Cardiff, UK; [9]Peninsula Medical School, Universities of Exeter and Plymouth, UK

Background and objectives

Although pharmacological research is making major efforts in the field of neuropathic pain, a considerable number of patients do not achieve sufficient pain relief with medication alone, defined as a sufficient level of pain relief that allows the patient to have an acceptable quality of life. In evidence-based studies on pain it is customary to consider as 'responders' to treatment those patients that report pain relief >50%. On that basis, it would appear from the most recent reviews and the European Federation of Neurological Societies (EFNS) guidelines that only 30–40% of the patients with chronic neuropathic pain achieve that target with pharmacotherapy [1, 2]. However, the 50% rule is being increasingly argued for because in many patients objective markers of satisfactory improvement may coexist with nominal levels of scaled pain relief of much less than 50% [3, 4]. It was therefore proposed that a clinically meaningful reduction of chronic pain in placebo-controlled trials would be a 2-point decrease (i.e., a 30% reduction) on a 0–10 rating scale [5].

Ancillary, harmless treatments, such as physical and psychological therapies, are often used. Although they may help patients to cope, this is often not enough for patients with severe pain. Among the alternatives, a number of previously common surgical lesions aimed at relieving neuropathic pain (e.g., neurotomies) have now been abandoned.

Neurostimulation therapy is increasingly being used either as a substitute for surgical lesions or in addition to the current medical therapy in several conditions, including Parkinson's disease, dystonia, obsessive compulsive disorder and refractory pain, while trials are in progress in other movement and psychiatric disorders, epilepsy and migraine. The neurostimulation techniques proposed for treating pain are: transcutaneous electrical nerve stimulation (TENS), peripheral nerve stimulation (PNS), nerve root stimulation (NRS), spinal cord stimulation (SCS), deep brain stimulation (DBS), epidural motor cortex stimulation (MCS) and repetitive transcranial magnetic stimulation (rTMS). These techniques vary greatly in their degree of invasiveness, stimulated structures and rationale, but they are all adjustable and reversible.

Our Task Force aimed at providing the neurologist with evidence-based recommendations that may help to determine when a patient with neuropathic pain should

European Handbook of Neurological Management: Volume 2, Second Edition. Edited by Nils Erik Gilhus, Michael P. Barnes, Michael Brainin.
© 2012 Blackwell Publishing Ltd. Published 2012 by Blackwell Publishing Ltd.

try a neurostimulation procedure. To provide a better understanding, the results are preceded by a description of the procedure and its supposed rationale.

Search methods

Task Force members were divided into subgroups and assigned the search for specific neurostimulation procedures, with two persons carrying out an independent search for each procedure. A two-stage approach to the relevant literature search was undertaken. First, the Medline, EMBASE and Cochrane databases were searched for systematic reviews, from inception date to May 2006. (Detailed searches are listed online in the Supplementary Material, Appendix 1.) Recent textbooks known to the authors were also examined for relevant references. These reviews and books were used to identify the primary literature. Second, given the search cut-off dates of previous systematic reviews, an update search for primary studies (randomized controlled trials, non-randomized controlled trials, observational comparative studies and case-series) was undertaken. Studies identified in this way were added to the body of evidence for each neurostimulation procedure under each indication heading.

All study designs were included, other than case reports and very small (<8) case-series. In addition, we excluded those multiple-indication case-series without disaggregated reported outcomes. Both reviewers undertook the study selection. For each indication, the number and type of studies were indicated and a summary of efficacy and harm findings given. Where there was more than one systematic review or primary publication on the same series of patients, we took the most comprehensive analysis. The evidence was graded and a recommendation for each indication applied according to the EFNS guidelines [6]. (The full list of references of all the assessed studies can be found in Supplementary Material, Appendix 2.)

Results

Peripheral stimulations (TENS, PNS and NRS)

The common wisdom that rubbing the skin over a painful area relieves pain found scientific support in the gate-control theory proposed by Melzack and Wall [7].

Since then, electrical stimulation for pain relief has spread worldwide. The best known technique is TENS. Surface electrodes are placed over the painful area or the nerve that innervates it and the stimulation is delivered at high frequency and low intensity (below pain threshold), to produce an intense activation of $A\beta$ afferents and to evoke paresthesiae over the painful area. A completely different approach is the use of low-frequency, high-intensity stimuli that do elicit painful sensations (this technique is also called acupuncture-like or, when delivered through needle electrodes, electro-acupuncture). In both cases, stimulation sessions of variable duration (often 20–30 min) are repeated at variable intervals. Because the pain relief is immediate but short-lasting, many patients use a portable stimulator, which can be kept on for hours or switched on during intermittent aggravations. To provide a more stable and efficient stimulation, electrodes can be percutaneously implanted to contact the nerve (usually the main limb nerves but also branches of the trigeminal or occipital nerves) and connected subcutaneously to a stimulation unit (PNS). To cover painful areas that are not accessible from the surface (e.g., pelvic viscera), a lead for SCS can be implanted at the root exit from the spine (NRS) or into Meckel's cave to stimulate the Gasserian ganglion. For all these techniques, when the currents are applied at high frequency and low intensity, the accepted mechanism is that of the homotopical inhibition exerted by large-size afferents on spinothalamic pathways.

Whether this inhibition is exerted mostly on presynaptic terminals or second-order neurons, or involves long-loops, or whether it is more efficacious on lamina I or lamina V neurons, is of no practical consequence. It is important to know that inhibition is strictly homotopical (i.e., the large-fibre input must generate paraesthesiae covering the entire painful area) and that pain relief rapidly declines after stimulation is stopped. The less used low-frequency high-intensity stimulation ('acupuncture-like') is thought to activate the antinociceptive systems through a long-loop; because it is at least partly naloxone-reversible, the analgesic effect is thought to be also mediated by the opioid system [8, 9]. Hence in theory it may also be effective in central pain. Importantly, the peripheral stimulation must be painful, can be heterotopic, and has long-lasting effects. Rather than the diagnosis, the main indications are derived from the therapeutic rationale. In the standard TENS, pain must be confined to a relatively small area or a territory that is innervated by an easily accessible nerve. Another important condition regards the sparing of Aβ-fibre function: patients with severe loss of such fibres (as easily assessed by the TENS-evoked sensation) are unsuitable. Finally, because transcutaneous stimulations are virtually harmless (apart from possible interference with cardiac pacemakers), TENS is often used as an ancillary support to drug or other physical treatments, in many different conditions. In contrast, PNS/NRS have more restricted indications and are used in pharmaco-resistant patients.

Evidence identified

Whereas there are many controlled studies and meta-analyses in nociceptive pains, the search on neuropathic pain yielded disappointing results. We identified one systematic review on outpatient services for chronic pain [10], which analysed 38 RCTs (only two studies dealing with neuropathic pain) and came to the conclusion that the pain-relieving effect of TENS increases with dose (duration of the session × frequency of sessions × total duration).

Our search on TENS in neuropathic pain (Table 2.1) found nine controlled trials (Classes II–IV) which, although not all dealing exclusively with neuropathic pain, allowed us to extract data for about 200 patients with pain of ascertained neuropathic origin. Four studies dealt with painful diabetic neuropathy: one Class II study found very high-frequency stimulation of the lower-limb muscles more efficacious than standard TENS [11]; the others (all Class III) found low-frequency TENS or acupuncture-like more efficacious than sham stimulations [12, 13, 14]. Two Class III studies dealt with peripheral mononeuropathies: both found standard TENS better than placebo [15, 16]. One small RCT in post-herpetic neuralgia (PHN) found conventional TENS to have little effect, while electro-acupuncture was decidedly better [17]. One crossover, small-sample study (Class III) in painful cervical radiculopathy found that standard TENS applied to the cervical back was better than placebo, but a TENS with random frequency variation was superior (Table 2.1) [18].

Regarding PNS, we found six clinical trials (no RCT), in 202 patients with various kinds of peripheral neuropathy or mixed pains. These studies reported an average success rate of 60%.

Regarding NRS, we only found two Class IV studies in patients with pelvic pain or interstitial cystitis (Table 2.1).

Recommendations

We cannot draw any conclusion for PNS and NRS. Even for TENS, it is difficult to come to conclusive recommendations. The total number of patients with ascertained neuropathic pain was only some 200, with diseases, comparators and results varying considerably from study to study. Stimulation parameters also vary considerably between the studies, using different pulse waveforms and a wide range of frequencies, not to mention number and duration of the sessions. In conclusion, standard high-frequency TENS is possibly better than placebo (Level C) though probably worse than acupuncture-like or any other kind of electrical stimulation (Level B).

Spinal cord stimulation

This technique consists of inserting electrodes into the posterior epidural space of the thoracic or cervical spine ipsilateral to the pain (if unilateral) and at an appropriate rostro-caudal level to evoke the topographically appropriate paraesthesiae which are a prerequisite for (but not a guarantee of) success. Catheter or wire electrodes can be inserted percutaneously under local or general anaesthesia; plate (surgical) electrode systems require an open operation but may perform better. Power is supplied by an implanted pulse generator (IPG).

The introduction of SCS followed from the gate-control theory [7] of pain transmission but SCS does not have a simple antinociceptive action. It can modulate the spontaneous and evoked elements of neuropathic pain, including allodynia, it has an anti-ischaemic action, both cardiac and in the periphery, and other autonomic effects including the normalization of the autonomic manifestations of complex regional pain syndromes (CRPS). The relative contributions of local segmental actions in the spinal cord and long-loop effects have not yet been elucidated. It is known that the effect of SCS is mediated by large-myelinated Aβ afferents, whose collaterals ascend in the dorsal columns. Whereas sensory loss because of distal axonopathy or peripheral nerve lesion is not an exclusion criterion, sparing of the dorsal columns is probably necessary [19].

Patient selection is mostly based on diagnosis. It is recognized that SCS may be effective against various

Table 2.1 Summary of efficacy and safety of peripheral stimulations (TENS, PNS, and NRS).

Technique/condition	Available evidence	No. patients	Summary of efficacy	Summary of harms	Comparator	Blind	Random	EFNS class	Comments
TENS/chronic pain	One meta-analysis [10], analysing 38 RCTs; only two on neuropathic pain: Thorsteinsson 1977 and Rutgers 1988 [16, 17]	–	There is no evidence; but it is clear that the effect increases with dose (duration of the session × frequency of sessions × total duration)	Practically nothing	Various	Yes	Yes	I	
TENS/NeP Painful diabetic neuropathy	Reichstein 2005 [11]	25	TENS compared with HF muscle: 25% success with TENS and 69% with HF	Practically nothing	High-frequency muscle stimulation	Yes	Yes	II	Reichstein [11] has no placebo, TENS goes far worse than HF muscle stimulation
Diabetic neuropathy	Forst 2004 [14]	19	LF TENS reduced VAS by 23%, significant difference from placebo	Practically nothing	Placebo	Yes	Yes	III	
Painful diabetic neuropathy	Hamza 2000 [13]	50	Painful PENS reduced VAS by 60%, significant difference from sham, and improved QoL	Practically nothing	Sham		Yes	III	Crossover with an inadequate comparator (needles with no current)
Diabetic neuropathy	Kumar 1997 [12]	35	LF TENS with biphasic stimuli exponentially decaying was significantly better than sham in reducing neuropathic symptoms	Practically nothing	Sham		Yes	III	Sham inadequate and report of improvement of all symptoms.
Traumatic neuropathy	Cheing 2005 [15]	19	Significantly better than placebo	Practically nothing	Placebo	Yes	Yes	II	
Radiculopathy	Bloodworth 2004 [18]	11	Random TENS and TENS on the cervical back were significantly better than placebo, with R-TENS better than TENS	Practically nothing	Placebo and Random-TENS	Yes	Yes	III	Few patients and crossover

Condition	Study	n	Result	Complications	Control			Class	Comments
Mixed pains	CT Tulgar 1991 (internal control)	8	Two did not get sufficient pain relief; one received prolonged pain relief; three went better with 'burst', one with high-rate and one with low-rate modulated TENS	Practically nothing	Four modes of TENS stimulation	Yes	No	IV	Few patients who chose which mode of TENS they preferred
PHN	RCT Rutgers 1988 [17]	few		Practically nothing	Acupuncture	See McQuay et al. 1997 [10]	Yes		
Peripheral neuropathy	RCT Thorsteinsson 1977 [16]	24	Significantly better than placebo	Practically nothing	Placebo	Yes	Yes	III	
PNS/NeP	No meta-analyses, no RCTs			Sometimes need for reoperation	None	No	No	Class IV not enough evidence for any recommendation	Very few and old papers, this technique does not seem to be getting popular
CRPS II	Buschmann 1999	52	Successful in 47						
Peripheral (n)	Nashold 1982	35	Successful in 15						
Post-traumatic	Law 1980	22	Successful in 13						
Mixed/various	Picaza 1977	37	Successful in 18						
Mixed/various	Campbell 1976	33	Successful in 8						
Peripheral (n) radiculopathy, amputation	Picaza 1975	23	Successful in 20						
Totals		202	Successful in 121 (60%)						
NRS/NeP	No meta-analyses, no RCTs			Sometimes need for reoperation	None	No	No	Class IV not enough evidence for any recommendation	
Neuropathic pelvic pain	CT Everaert 2001	26	Successful in 16						
Interstitial cystitis	Whitmore 2003, no control	33	Significant improvement						

TENS, transcutaneous electrical nerve stimulation; LF TENS, low-frequency, high-intensity TENS, also called acupuncture-like; PNS, peripheral nerve stimulation with implanted electrodes; NRS, nerve root stimulation with implanted electrodes; QoL, quality of life; CT, controlled trial; HF, high frequency; PENS, percutaneous electrical nerve stimulation.

ischaemic and specific neuropathic pain syndromes. Additional tests may be useful to confirm SCS indication, such as somatosensory-evoked potentials (SEPs) [19], whereas the response to TENS does not seem to be a reliable guide. Trial stimulation via externalized leads is widely employed as it identifies patients who do not like the sensation from SCS and those in whom appropriate stimulation cannot be achieved. However, this testing is not a guarantee of long-term success in neuropathic pain.

Evidence identified

We identified a number of systematic reviews and meta-analyses [20, 21, 22] and a few narrative but detailed reviews [23, 24, 25]. The majority of systematic reviews, as well as primary studies, to date have focused on patients with failed back surgery syndrome (FBSS) or complex regional pain syndrome (CRPS). Concerning FBSS there are two Class II RCTs, the first showing that SCS is more effective than reoperation [26] and the second that its addition is more effective than conventional medical care alone [27, 28]. In these trials the responders (pain relief >50%) to SCS were 47–48% vs. 9–12% with comparator, at 6–24 months. In the pooled data from case-series in 3,307 FBSS patients, the proportion of responders was 62%. In CRPS type I, results and evidence level are also good, with a single Class II RCT of SCS compared with conventional care alone [29, 30]. In this RCT, SCS reduced the visual analogue scale score by a mean 2.6 cm more than comparator at 6 months and by 1.7 cm at 5 years. In the pooled data from case-series (n = 561) in CRPS I and II, the proportion of responders was 67%. Both RCTs and case-series have also found significant improvement in functional capacity and quality of life.

In a pooled safety analysis of SCS across all indications, the undesired events were mostly dysfunction in the stimulating apparatus: lead migration (13.2%), lead breakage (9.1%) and other minor hardware problems [20]. Also the medical complications were minor and never life-threatening. They were usually solved, like the hardware problems, by removing the device. The overall infection rate was 3.4%.

The effect of SCS has also been studied in many other conditions. We found positive case-series evidence for CRPS II, peripheral nerve injury, diabetic neuropathy, PHN, brachial plexus damage, amputation (stump and phantom pains) and partial spinal cord injury, and negative evidence for central pain of brain origin, nerve root avulsion and complete spinal cord transection. However, all reports are Class IV, thus precluding any firm conclusion. The efficacy and safety outcomes of SCS are detailed by indication in Table 2.2.

Recommendations

We found Level B evidence for the effectiveness of SCS in FBSS and CRPS I. The evidence is also positive for CRPS II, peripheral nerve injury, diabetic neuropathy, PHN, brachial plexus lesion, amputation (stump and phantom pains) and partial spinal cord injury, but still requires confirmatory comparative trials before the use of SCS can be unreservedly recommended in these conditions.

Deep brain stimulation

Deep brain stimulation for the treatment of medically refractory chronic pain preceded the gate-control theory [31]. Deep brain targets in current use include the sensory (ventral posterior) thalamus and periventricular grey matter (PVG) contralaterally to the pain if unilateral, or bilaterally if indicated. Both sites have been targets of analgesic DBS for three decades [32, 33]. After accurate target localization using MRI, stereotactic computerized tomography and brain atlas co-registration as appropriate, an electrode is stereotactically inserted into the subcortical cerebrum under local anaesthesia. The electrodes are connected to a subcutaneous IPG, placed in the chest or abdomen.

The mechanisms by which DBS relieves pain remain unclear. Animal experiments have shown that thalamic stimulation suppressed deafferentation pain, most probably via thalamo-corticofugal descending pathways. Autonomic effects of PVG stimulation are under investigation, and a positive correlation between analgesic efficacy and magnitude of blood pressure reduction has been demonstrated in humans [34]. It is currently believed that stimulation of ventral PVG engages non-opioid-dependent analgesia commensurate with passive coping behaviour, whereas stimulation of dorsal PVG involves opioid-related fight-or-flight analgesia with associated autonomic effects [34]. The effect of frequency – lower frequencies (5–50 Hz) being analgesic and higher frequencies (>70 Hz) pain-provoking – suggests a dynamic

Table 2.2 Summary of efficacy and safety of spinal cord simulation (SCS).

Indication	Volume of evidence (no. trials (no. patients))	EFNS class	Summary of efficacy	Summary of harms	EFNS level	Comments
FBSS	**Systematic review and meta-analysis**	II	**RCTs**	*Most common complications were:*	B	*PROCESS study:*
	Taylor et al. 2005 [21] and Cameron 2004 [20] [1 RCT (60)] (SCS vs. reoperation)		*Pain relief ≥50%:* SCS 9/24 (37.5%) vs. reop. 3/26 (11.5%) (P = 0.475) at 2 years	Lead migration 361/2753 (13.2%)		Trial protocol published [27] First oral presentation at EFIC Istanbul, Sept. 2006
	[1 cohort study (44)]		SCS 24/48 (48%) vs. CMM 4/52 (9%) P < 0.0001 at 6-months	Infection 100/2972 (3.4%)		Final results in press [28]
	[72 case series (2956)]		*Use of opioids:*	Lead breakage 250/2753 (9.1%)		
	New primary studies		SCS 3/23 vs. reop. 11/16 (P = 0.0005) at 2-years	Hardware malfunction 80/2753 (2.9%)		
	[1 RCT (100)] (SCS vs. CMM)		SCS 25/48 (50%) vs. CMM 31/52 (70%) (P = 0.058) at 6 months	Battery failure 35/2107 (1.6%)		
	'PROCESS' Kumar et al. (2005, 2007) [27, 28]		**Case series**	Unwanted stimulation 62753 (2.4%)		
	[6 cases series (361)] Kumar et al. 2006; North et al. 2005 I & ii [26]; Spincemaille et al. (2005); Van Buyten et al. (2003); May et al. (2002)		*Pain relief ≥50%:* 62% (95% CI: 56–72)	'Most complications were not life threatening and could usually be resolved by removing the device'.		
			Disability Pooled results across two case series show significant improvement in ODI following SCS with mean follow-up of 6 months	Overall 43% of patients experience one or more complications		
			Quality of life Pooled results across two case series show significant improvement in SIP following SCS with mean follow-up of 6 months			
Failed neck surgery syndrome	No evidence found			As FBSS		

continued

Table 2.2 continued

Indication	Volume of evidence (no. trials (no. patients))	EFNS class	Summary of efficacy	Summary of harms	EFNS level	Comments
CRPS	**Systematic review/meta-analysis** Taylor et al. (2006) and Cameron (2004) [20, 21] [1RCT (54)] – type I CRPS. Overall [25 cases series (500)] (12 case series type I, eight cases series in type II, five case series in both I and II) **New primary studies** 5-year follow-up on above RCT Kemler et al. (2006) [30] [2 cases series (61)] Kumar et al. (2006); Harke et al. (2005)	Type I: II Type II: IV	**RCT** (at 6 and 12 months and 5-years) *Change in VAS pain:* SCS + physical therapy .4 (SD 2.5) vs. physical therapy: 0.2 (1.6) $P < 0.0001$ at 6-months *Quality of life (EQ-5D):* −2.7 (SD 2.8) vs. 0.4 (1.8) $P < 0.001$ at 6 months **Case-series** *Pain relief ≥50:* 67% (95% CI: 51–74) *Disability:* 3/3 studies showed a significant improve in functional capacity following SCS *Quality of life:* 2/2 studies showed a significant improvement in HRQoL following SCS Some evidence that level of pain relief with SCS in CRPS type II patients >CRPS type I 85% good and excellent at ≥2 years.	As FBSS Overall 33% of patients experience one or more complications	CRPS type I: B CRPS type II; D	
Peripheral nerve injury	One retrospective two-centre mixed case series [n = 152] Lazorthes et al. (1995)	IV		Not disaggregated. Transient paraparesis in 1/692 (whole series)	D	Pain NRS, activity and analgesic drug intake scored
Diabetic neuropathy	One prospective case series (n = 8) Tesfaye et al. (1996); Daousi et al. (2004) One retrospective mixed case series ([n = 14) Kumar et al. (2006)	IV IV	*Pain relief* >50% pain relief in 6/8 at 14 months (6/7: one died at 2 months) >50% relief in 5/6 at 3 years (background and peak pain) >50% relief in 4/4 at 7 years (background pain) >50% relief in 3/4 at 7 years (peak pain) *Exercise tolerance* Increased by 150% in 6/6 *Pain relief* >50% relief in 12/14 'long-term'	Lead migration in 2/8 Superficial infection in 2/8 Skin reaction in 1/8	D	Prospective VAS + McGill. Sep. pain elements. Preservation of large fibre (vibration and joint position) function essential Five outcome measures Third party assessor Follow-up unclear
Other peripheral neuropathy	One retrospective mixed case-series (n = 23) Kim et al. (2001)	IV	*Pain relief* >50% relief in 10/23 (43.5%) at 1 year	Not disaggregated	D	

Condition	Studies	Level	Outcome	Complications	Grade	Comments
Post-herpetic neuralgia	Four retrospective case-series (3 mixed) [10; 28; 8; 4 (50)] Kumar et al. (2006); Harke et al. (2002); Meglio et al. (1989); Sanchez-Ledesma et al. (1989)	IV	*Pain relief* Significant long-term in 38/50 (pooled) Medication stopped in 21/31 Opioids stopped in 18/19	Lead fracture in one Receiver failure in one Leads replaced in three to improve coverage	D	Success varies between series due to variable deafferentation
Intercostal neuralgia	No evidence found relating to this specific diagnosis					
Brachial plexus damage/avulsion	Two retrospective case series (2 mixed) [8; 8 (16)] Simpson et al. (2003) Hood; Siegfried (1984)	IV	*Pain relief* Significant relief in 8/16	Nil, or not disaggregated	D	Different scoring methods Evidence of full avulsion (cf. damage) of specific relevant nerve roots not always given
Amputation pain (phantom and stump)	Three retrospective case-series [25; 9; 61 (95)] Lazorthes et al. (1995); Simpson (1991); Krainick & Thoden (1989); Krainick et al. (1975)	IV	*Phantom pain* Significant relief in 7/14 *Stump pain* Significant relief in 5/9 *Mixed – stump/phantom not specified* Krainick's series: 56% of 61 had >50% relief (early), dropping to 43% (late). Reduced drug intake correlated *Lazorthes:* 60% of 25 good or excellent long-term (≥2 years)	Infection 1.6% Surgical revisions 31%	D	Phantom and stump pains not always distinguished
Facial pain (trigeminopathic) Central pain of spinal cord origin	Insufficient evidence Five retrospective case series (4 mixed) [19; 11; 101; 9; 35 (175)] Kumar et al. (2006); Barolat et al. (1998); Lazorthes et al. (1995); Cioni et al. (1995); Meglio et al. (1989); Tasker et al. (1992)	IV	*Pain relief* a) *cord injury:* 15/62 significant long term pain relief overall incomplete: 11/33 significant relief complete: 0/11 significant relief b) *MS:* long-term pain relief on five outcome measures in 15/19 (Kumar) bowel/ sphincter function improved in 16/28 Gait improved in 15/19 (no details) c) *mixed incl trauma, tumour surgery, viral etc:* 34% good/excellent at ≥2 years (Lazorthes; n = 101). Pain relief, analgesic drug intake and activity	Not stated/not disaggregated in four studies Aseptic meningitis 1/9 Superficial infection 1/9 Electrode dislodgement 1/9	D	Completeness of lesion not always stated Much greater success where clinically incomplete lesion Success correlates with sensory status: the less sensory deficit the better the results
Central pain of brain origin	Two retrospective case series (1 mixed) [45; 10 (55)] Katayama et al. (2001); Simpson (1991) [39]	IV	*Pain relief* Significant in 6/55 >60% reduction in VAS in 3/45	Not stated/not disaggregated	D	

CMM, conventional medical management; ODI, Oswestry Disability Index; SIP, sickness impact profile; VAS, visual analogue scale; HRQoL, health-related quality of life; NRS, numerical rating scale; MS, multiple sclerosis.

model whereby synchronous oscillations modulate pain perception.

As with any implanted technique of neurostimulation for treating pain, patient selection is a major challenge. Trial stimulation via externalized leads can identify those in whom DBS is not efficacious or poorly tolerated [35, 36]. However, successful trial stimulation has not resulted in long-term success for up to half of cases. Contraindications include psychiatric illness, uncorrectable coagulopathy and ventriculomegaly precluding direct electrode passage to the surgical target [37].

Evidence

We identified several reviews and one meta-analysis [37], which concluded that DBS is more effective for nociceptive pain than for neuropathic pain (63% vs. 47% long-term success). In patients with neuropathic pain, moderately higher rates of success were seen in patients with peripheral lesions (phantom limb pain, radiculopathies, plexopathies and neuropathies) [37]. We identified a number of primary studies for 623 patients and a mean success rate of 46% at long term (Table 2.3). However, most studies were Class IV case-series. Among these, two studies (Table 2.4) targeted the somatosensory thalamus or PAG/PVG, using current standards of MRI in target localization and current DBS devices: one study, in 15 patients with central post-stroke pain (CPSP), considered DBS successful (pain relief >30%) in 67% of patients at long term [36]; the other, in 21 patients with various

neuropathic pain conditions, concluded that DBS had low efficacy, with only 24% of patients maintaining long-term benefit (i.e., they were willing to keep using DBS after 5 years), none of these patients having CPSP [38]. Another study, comparing the efficacy of SCS, DBS (targeting the thalamus) and MCS in 45 patients with CPSP, reported DBS success in only 25% of patients [39]. The other studies were more than a decade old and had various targets; their results are summarized by clinical indication in Table 2.5 and by stimulation target in Table 2.6.

Recommendations

There is weak positive evidence for the use of DBS in peripheral neuropathic pain, including pain after amputation and facial pain (expert opinion requiring confirmatory trials). In CPSP, DBS results are equivocal and require further comparative trials.

Motor cortex stimulation

During the past decade MCS has emerged as a promising tool for the treatment of patients with drug-resistant neuropathic pain. The technique consists in implanting epidural electrodes over the motor strip. Electrodes are most commonly introduced through a frontoparietal craniotomy ($40 \times 50\,mm$) over the central area, under general anaesthesia, or through a simple burr hole under local anaesthesia. The craniotomy technique minimizes

Table 2.3 Summary of deep brain stimulation studies.

Study	Type of study	Number of patients implanted	Number successful at long-term follow-up (%)	Follow-up time (months); range (mean)	EFNS class
Richardson & Akil (1977) [33]	Prospective case series	30	18 (60)	1–46	IV
Plotkin (1980)		10	40	36	IV
Shulman et al. (1982)		24	11 (46)	(>24)	IV
Young et al. (1985)		48	35 (73)	2–60 (20)	IV
Hosobuchi (1986)		122	94 (77)	24–168	IV
Levy et al. (1987) [53]		141	42 (12)	24–168 (80)	IV
Siegfried (1987)		89	38 (43)	<24	IV
Gybels et al. (1993)		36	11 (31)	48	IV
Kumar et al. (1997) [12]		68	42 (62)	6–180 (78)	IV
Katayama et al. (2001) [39]		45	11 (25)	N/A	III
Hamani et al. (2006) [38]		21	5 (24)	2–108 (24)	IV
Owen et al. (2006) [35]		34	12 (35)	1–44 (19)	IV

Table 2.4 Summary of efficacy and safety of deep brain stimulation by indication from recent and currently applicable studies.

Indication	Volume of evidence no. trials (no. patients)	EFNS class	Summary of efficacy (%)	Summary of safety
Amputation pain (phantom and stump)	2 (5; 1)	IV	100; 100	No indication of specific complications: four wound infections; two DBS lead fractures; one intra-operative seizure; one postoperative burr hole site erosion
Post-stroke	2 (16; 8)	IV	69; 0	
Facial pain (trigeminopathic)	2 (4; 4)	IV	100; 25	
Cephalalgia not including trigeminopathic facial pain	2 (3; 1)	IV	100; N/A	
Central pain of spinal cord origin	2 (2; 4)	IV	0; 25	
Multiple sclerosis pain	1 (2)	IV	50	
Other and trauma	2 (4; 1)	IV	75; 100	

Pain assessment used at least one of VAS (visual analogue scale); MPQ (McGill pain questionnaire); N1T (N-of-1 trial); HRQoL, health-related quality of life; NRS, numerical rating scale. Only VAS-related outcomes using a threshold of >50% improvement are shown here.

Table 2.5 Summary of efficacy and safety of deep brain stimulation by indication from other, older studies. (after Bittar *et al.* 2005) [37]

Indication	Volume of evidence (no. patients)	Success on initial stimulation	Success on chronic stimulation	Long-term percentage success
Amputation pain (phantom and stump)	9	7	4	44
Post-stroke pain	45	24	14	31
FBSS	59	54	46	78
Peripheral nerve injury	44	36	31	70
Post-herpetic neuralgia	11	6	4	36
Intercostal neuralgia	4	3	1	25
Brachial plexus damage/avulsion	12	9	6	50
Malignancy pain	23	19	15	65
Facial pain (trigeminopathic)	32	21	12	38
Central pain of spinal cord origin	47	28	20	43
Other	35	28	22	63

Table 2.6 Summary of efficacy and anatomical targets from other, older studies. (after Bittar *et al.* 2005 [5])

Anatomical site of DBS	Volume of evidence no. patients	Number successful long term	Percentage success
PVG	148	117	79
PVG and ST or IC	55	48	87
ST	100	58	58
ST or IC	16	6	38

PVG, periventricular grey matter; ST, sensory thalamus; IC, internal capsule.

the risk for epidural haematoma and renders easier the use of electrophysiological techniques to localize the central sulcus, usually with SEPs concomitant to MRI-guided neuronavigation. Intraoperative cortical stimulation with clinical assessment or EMG recordings can help to determine the position of the electrodes. One or two quadripolar electrodes are implanted over the motor representation of the painful area, either parallel or orthogonal to the central sulcus. The electrode is connected to a subcutaneous IPG. The stimulation parameters are optimized postoperatively, keeping the intensity below motor threshold, and the stimulation is usually set on cyclic mode (alternating on/off periods).

The mechanism of action of MCS remains hypothetical. Tsubokawa et al. [40] showed that MCS attenuated abnormal thalamic hyperactivity after spinothalamic transection in cats, and considered that the effect involved retrograde activation of somatosensory cortex by cortico-cortical axons [41]. However, positron-emission tomography and SEPs failed to show any significant activation of the sensory-motor cortex during MCS, while a strong focal activation was observed in the thalamus, insula, cingulate-orbitofrontal junction and brain stem [42, 43], suggesting that MCS-induced pain relief may relate to top-down activation of descending pain control systems going from motor cortex to thalamus, and perhaps to motor brain stem nuclei, and also blunting of affective reactions to pain via activation of orbitofrontal-perigenual cingulate cortex [43]. Both hypotheses have received recent support from studies in animals and in humans [44, 45, 46]. The fact that many of the regions activated by MCS contain high levels of opioid receptors suggests that long-lasting MCS effects may also involve secretion of endogenous opioids.

Eligible patients should be resistant or intolerant to the main drugs used for neuropathic pain [1, 2]. Some studies include pre-operative sessions of transcranial magnetic stimulation, which is thought to be predictive of the MCS outcome (see Repetitive transcranial magnetic stimulation, below). Candidates for MCS have sometimes experienced failure of other neurosurgical procedures, such as radicellectomy (DREZ lesion), antero-lateral cordotomy, trigeminal nerve surgery or SCS.

Evidence

Our search disclosed no systematic review or meta-analysis, but found a relatively large number of studies (mostly case-series) on CPSP and facial neuropathic pain. In CPSP, we extracted 143 non-overlapping patients from 20 case-series: the average success rate was ~50%. Slightly better results (60% of responders, based on 60 patients from 8 series) were obtained in facial neuropathic pain, both central and peripheral. Most of these case series were Class IV. Two studies can be classified as Class III, because they had a comparator (results of other treatments, surgical or pharmacological), and outcome assessment and treatment were dissociated: Katayama et al. [39] had a 48% success rate in patients with CPSP and Nuti et al. [4] a 52% success rate in 31 patients with various neuropathic pain conditions, mostly CPSP. One of these papers provided follow-up results up to 4 years [4].

In phantom pain, brachial plexus or nerve trunk lesion, spinal cord lesions or CRPS, we only found case reports. Most common undesired events were related to some malfunction of the stimulating apparatus (e.g., unexpected battery depletion). Seizures, wound infection, sepsis, extradural haematoma and pain induced by MCS have also been reported. Overall, 20% of patients experience one or more complications, in general of benign nature. Details of the search with summary of benefits/harms can be found in Table 2.7 and 2.8.

Recommendations

There is Level C evidence (two convincing Class III studies, 15–20 convergent Class IV series) that MCS is useful in 50–60% of patients with CPSP and central or peripheral facial neuropathic pain, with only a small risk of medical complications. The evidence about any other condition remains insufficient.

Repetitive transcranial magnetic stimulation

The use of rTMS in patients with chronic pain aims at producing analgesic effects by means of non-invasive cortical stimulation [47]. Stimulation is performed by applying on the scalp, above a targeted cortical region, the coil of a magnetic stimulator. A focal stimulation using a figure-of-eight coil is mandatory. The intensity of stimulation is expressed as a percentage of the motor threshold of a muscle at rest in the painful territory. The

Table 2.7 Summary of efficacy and safety of MCS in CPSP.

Indication	Volume of evidence [no. trials (no. patients)]	EFNS class	Summary of efficacy	Summary of harms	Comments
CPSP	Systematic review and meta-analysis	All class IV (unless indicated otherwise)	Case series (8–45 cases) Satisfactory pain relief (≥50%) reported in 0–100% of cases (all series)	Most common complications: 26% (battery failure, seizures, wound infection and sepsis)	Many patient duplications or reinterventions making total nb of cases difficult to calculate. Reports with duplicated data were pooled
	None		In series with $n > 20$ cases satisfactory pain relief in 48–52% of patients	Pain induced by MCS	Efficacy related to pre-operative response to drugs? (Yamamoto 1997, $n = 28$)
	Primary studies (1991–2006)			Phantom pain	
	No RCT			Extradural haematoma	
	[20 cases series, with much overlap (143 non-overlapping patients)]			Seizures	
	Rasche et al. 2006, Nuti et al. 2005 [4] (+Mertens et al. 1999 +G-Larrea et al. 1999) [43]	III		Hardware malfunction	Efficacy related to sensory symptoms? (Druot 2002, $n = 11$)
	Saitoh et al. 2003 (+Saitoh et al. 2001)			Overall 20% of patients experience one or more complications and in general of benign nature	Efficacy related to motor symptoms? (Katayama 1998, $n = 31$)
	Fukaya et al. 2003 +Katayama et al. 2001 [39] +Katayama et al. 1998 +Yamamoto et al. 1997	III			
	Nguyen et al. 2000 +Nguyen et al. 2000 +Nguyen et al. 1999 +Nguyen et al. 1997				
	Nandi et al. 2002				
	Carroll et al. 2000				
	Fujii et al. 1997				
	Katayama et al. 1994				
	Tsubokawa et al. 1993 +Tsubokaw et al. 1991				
	Drouot et al. 2002				

CPSP, central post-stroke pain; MCS, motor cortex stimulation.

Table 2.8 Summary of efficacy and safety of motor cortex stimulation in facial pain.

Indication	Volume of evidence [no. trials (no. patients)]	EFNS class	Summary of efficacy	Summary of harms	Comments
Facial pain	Systematic review and meta-analysis: None Primary studies (1991–2006) No RCT *Case series (60 patients)* Rasche *et al.* 2006 (3/50) Brown Ptiliss 2005 (10/60) Nuti *et al.* 2005 [4] (5/60) Drouot *et al.* 2002 (15) Nguyen *et al.* 2000a (12/83) +Nguyen *et al.* 2000b same +Nguyen *et al.* 1999 same +Nguyen *et al.* 1997 (7/100) Ebel *et al.* 1996 (7/43) Katayama *et al.* 1994 (3/66) Meyersonl 1993 (5/100)	All class IV	Case series Satisfactory pain relief (≥50%) reported in 43–100% of cases (all series) No series with $n > 20$ cases Mean percent of patients with satisfactory pain relief: 66%	Most common complications: 26% (battery failure, seizures, wound infection and sepsis) Pain induced by MCS Extradural haematoma Seizures Hardware malfunction Overall 20% of patients experience one or more complications, in general of benign nature	Many patient duplications or reinterventions making total nb of cases difficult to calculate. Reports with duplicated data were pooled. Small series but sometimes long follow-up: 72 m

MCS, motor cortex stimulation.

stimulation is performed just below motor threshold. The frequency and the total number of delivered pulses depend on the study. A single session should last at least 20 min and should include at least 1,000 pulses. Daily sessions can be repeated for one or several weeks. There is no induced pain and no need for anaesthesia or for hospital stay during the treatment.

The rationale is the same as for implanted MCS. The stimulation is thought to activate fibres that run through the motor cortex and project to remote structures involved in some aspects of neuropathic pain processing (emotional or sensori-discriminative components). The method is non-invasive and can be applied to any patient with drug-resistant, chronic neuropathic pain, who could be a candidate for the implantation of a cortical stimulator. As the clinical effects are rather modest and short-lasting beyond the time of a single session of stimulation, this method cannot be considered a therapy, except if the sessions of stimulation are repeated for several days or weeks.

Evidence

We identified some reviews (none systematic) and 14 controlled studies that used sham stimulations in crosso-

ver or parallel groups, comprising 280 patients with definite neuropathic pain (CPSP, spinal cord lesions, trigeminal nerve, brachial plexus or limb nerve lesions, phantom pain and CRPS II). Efficacy, rather than varying between pain conditions, mostly depends on stimulation parameters. There is consensus from two RCTs in patients with CPSP or various peripheral nerve lesions that rTMS of the primary motor cortex, when applied at low frequency (1 Hz or less), is ineffective (Class II) [48, 49]. Focal-coil stimulations at high rate (5–20 Hz), of long duration (at least 1,000 pulses) and possibly repeated sessions, induces pain relief (>30%) in ~50% of patients (Class II/III) [50, 51, 52]. The effect begins after a few days and its duration is short (<1 week after a single session). Another important aspect is that a positive response to high-frequency rTMS is probably predictive of a positive outcome of subsequent chronic epidural MCS (Class II) [49].

There is insufficient evidence for other indications or techniques, including magnetic stimulation of the dorso-lateral prefrontal cortex or the parietal cortex, as well as transcranial direct current stimulation. The efficacy and safety outcomes of transcranial magnetic stimulation are detailed in Tables 2.9 and 2.10.

Table 2.9 Summary of efficacy and safety of rTMS, primary motor cortex stimulation, 1 Hz or less.

Indication	Volume of evidence [no. trials (no. patients)]	EFNS class	Summary of efficacy	Summary of harms	EFNS grade	Comments
Stroke (n = 32), Spinal cord lesion (n = 4), Trigeminal nerve lesion (n = 1), Brachial plexus or limb nerve lesion (n = 8), Phantom limb pain (n = 14)	New primary studies Three sham-controlled trials All negative (59 p.) Lefaucheur et al. 2001a André-Obadia et al. 2006 Irlbacher et al. 2006	II II III	No efficacy *Pain relief ≥30%*: 5% (mean pain relief: 4%)	No reported complications	B	No significant effect compared with sham stimulation

Table 2.10 Summary of efficacy and safety of rTMS, primary motor cortex stimulation, 5 Hz or more.

Indication	Volume of evidence [no. trials (no. patients)	EFNS class	Summary of efficacy	Summary of harms	EFNS grade	Comments
Stroke (n = 98), Spinal cord lesion (n = 24), Trigeminal nerve lesion (n = 60), Brachial plexus or limb nerve lesion (n = 36) CRPS (n = 10)	New primary studies [11 sham-controlled trial (281 p.)] Positive studies (228 p.) Lefaucheur et al. 2001a Lefaucheur et al. 2001b Lefaucheur et al. 2004a Pleger et al. 2004 Khedr et al. 2005 Hirayama et al. 2006 Lefaucheur et al. 2006a Lefaucheur et al. 2006b	II II II III II II II	*Pain relief ≥30%*: 46% (mean pain relief: 26%) 104 responders/206 patients. Efficacy regarding indication: idem for stroke vs. trigeminal nerve lesion (Lefaucheur et al. 2004; Khedr et al. 2005) or brachial plexus lesion (Lefaucheur et al. 2004); better for thalamic vs. brainstem stroke (Lefaucheur et al. 2004) poorer results for spinal cord lesion (Lefaucheur et al. 2004) CRPS: no significant difference with the other causes (Pleger et al. 2004)	No reported complications	B	No significant effect compared to sham stimulation in case of circular coil (Rollnik et al. 2002) or 5 Hz-rTMS (Irlbacher et al. 2006) and <1000 pulses per session (Rollnik et al. 2002; Irlbacher et al. 2006) Better pain relief in case of repeated sessions (Khedr et al. 2005) or stimulation of adjacent cortical area (Lefaucheur et al. 2006b) Pain relief duration: less than one week after a single session; about two weeks after one week of stimulation
Stroke (n = 20), Spinal cord lesion (n = 6), Trigeminal nerve lesion (n = 1), Brachial plexus or limb nerve lesion (n = 8) Phantom limb pain (n = 15), CRPS (n = 2), non-neuropathic (n = 1)	Negative studies (53 p.): Rollnik et al. 2002 André-Obadia et al. 2006 Irlbacher et al. 2006	III II III				

rTMS, repetitive transcranial magnetic stimulation; CRPS, complex regional pain syndrome.

Recommendations

There is moderate evidence that rTMS of the motor cortex, using a figure-of-eight coil and high frequency (5–20 Hz), induces significant pain relief in CPSP and several other neuropathic pain conditions (Level B). However, because the effect is modest and short-lasting, rTMS should not be used as the sole treatment in chronic neuropathic pain. It may be proposed for short-lasting pains or to identify suitable candidates for an epidural implant (MCS). In contrast, in the same pain conditions, low-frequency rTMS is probably ineffective (Level B).

General comments

Most trials on neurostimulation for pain relief did not comply with the requirements of evidence-based medicine (EBM), often because of the difficulty in using an adequate comparator for these stimulations. Level B recommendations could, however, be drawn for some procedures in some pain conditions. Some neurostimulation procedures are relatively new, and consequently the evidence is still sparse and it would be premature to draw negative conclusions (Figure 2.1). Peripheral stimulations have been used very little in neuropathic pain. Acupuncture-like stimulations are probably more efficacious than high-frequency TENS, but we do not have strong evidence for this. Unlike some other neurostimulation procedures, TENS is extremely easy to apply and without risk, which explains why TENS is so widely used in acute and chronic pain patients, with little concern for whether the improvements are due to a placebo effect or not. This may also hold true for neuropathic pain patients. SCS has Class II RCT evidence. Its efficacy has been demonstrated in two conditions, which are not definitely neuropathic: FBSS and CRPS type I. Pain in FBSS is usually mixed and it is difficult to extract the neuropathic component, whereas CRPS I is still a 'putative neuropathic' pain.

Spinal cord stimulation, DBS and MCS are typically used when all other treatments have failed. This context should be taken into account when making recommendations. We analysed only published evidence. Thousands of stimulators are implanted every year and only a tiny minority appears in published studies. Absence of evidence is not evidence of absence of effect, and low-level evidence (i.e., case-series) should be given some credence.

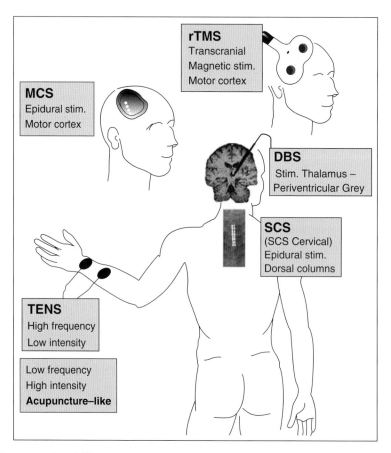

Figure 2.1 Schematic representation of different neurostimulation procedures, e.g. for a patient with pain in the left hand because of peripheral nerve injury.

For some indications, there was a considerable body of positive case-series findings, sometimes over long periods. Furthermore, the whole field has been largely characterized by a heavy dependence on the outcome measure (50% pain relief) as a threshold indicator of success, after both trial and definitive stimulation, which may distort the true picture. Others have found 30% pain relief to correspond to clinically meaningful success [5], and factors beyond changes in pain intensity are also relevant.

Although not a new therapy, DBS has changed considerably over the last decade, in line with advances in both stimulator technology and neuroimaging techniques, leading to improved efficacy and fewer complications. DBS should be performed in experienced, specialist centres, willing to publish their results, and using established outcome measures. Whereas its efficacy in CPSP is controversial, DBS appears more promising for phantom limb and trigeminal neuropathic pains.

Motor cortex stimulation is useful in CPSP and in central or peripheral facial pain. Interestingly, the proportion of good and excellent results increases consistently in patients with facial pain relative to all other classes. The reason is not yet established. Candidates for MCS have neuropathic pain that is resistant to drugs and often to other interventions. In view of the potential development of this method, it is of the utmost importance that placebo-controlled, double-blind studies are produced to increase the level of evidence, particularly because MCS, not being perceived by the patient, allows a perfect placebo.

As with TENS, the efficacy of rTMS seems to increase with dose: higher frequency, longer duration of the session and more sessions tend to yield better results. Because the clinical effects are rather modest and short-lasting, rTMS cannot be considered as a therapeutic method for the long term, except if the sessions are repeated for several days or weeks. Currently, rTMS can be proposed as a non-invasive pre-operative therapeutic test for patients with drug-resistant chronic pain who are candidates for surgically implanted chronic MCS.

Concerning harms (detailed in the tables), TENS and rTMS are virtually risk-free. SCS, DBS and MCS do entail adverse events in a large proportion of patients (up to 20% with MCS and 40% with SCS experience). However, most of these are simple lead migration or battery depletion that do not produce physical harm and can usually be solved. Real harms are few, usually wound infection

(3.4% with SCS, 7.3% with DBS, 2.2% with MCS) and very rare – often single – cases of aseptic meningitis, transient paraparesis, epidural haematoma, epileptic seizures and skin reactions, none being life-threatening. Our search disclosed one case only of death 20 years ago [53]. Indeed, one of the reasons for the use of neurostimulation therapy is that the application of low-intensity electrical currents is not associated with any of the side-effects entailed by drugs.

Finally, we feel that neurostimulation therapy will prove to be useful for a broader indication than is suggested by our search. We hope that future trials are designed bearing in mind the EBM requirements. Although it is difficult to find a credible placebo for neurostimulation therapy, the investigators may compare their procedure to other treatments. Furthermore, we recommend that investigators pay attention to definition of diagnosis, inclusion criteria, blind assessment of the outcomes and impact on patient- related variables such as quality of life and daily living activities.

Conflicts of interest

RST has a consultant contract with Medtronic, as an expert in Health Care Policy and Clinical Trial Design.

PH, LGL, JPL and BS received an honorarium from Medtronic for lectures or advisory boards. The other authors have nothing to declare.

Supplementary material

The following supplementary material is available for this article: Appendix 1. SCS search strategies. Appendix 2. Full list of studies. This material is available as part of the online article from www.blackwell-synergy.com/doi/abs/10.1111/j.1468-1331.2007.01916.x (this link will take you to the article abstract).

Blackwell Publishing are not responsible for the content or functionality of any supplementary materials supplied by the authors. Any queries (other than missing material) should be directed to the corresponding author for the article.

References

1. Finnerup, NB, Otto, M, McQuay, HJ, *et al*. Algorithm for neuropathic pain treatment: an evidence-based proposal. *Pain* 2005; **118**:289–305.

2. Attal, N, Cruccu, G, Haanpaa, M, *et al.* EFNS guidelines on pharmacological treatment of neuropathic pain. *Eur J Neurol* 2006; **13**:1153–69.

3. Cruccu, G, Anand, P, Attal, N, *et al.* EFNS guidelines on neuropathic pain assessment. *Eur J Neurol* 2004; **11**:153–62.

4. Nuti, C, Peyron, R, Garcia-Larrea, L, *et al.* Motor cortex stimulation for refractory neuropathic pain: four year outcome andpredictors of efficacy. *Pain* 2005; **118**:43–52.

5. Farrar, JT, Young, JP, Jr., LaMoreaux, L, *et al.* Clinical importance of change in chronic pain intensity measured on an 11-point numerical pain rating scale. *Pain* 2001; **94**:149–58.

6. Brainin, M, Barnes, M, Baron, JC, *et al.* Guideline Standards Subcommittee of the EFNS Scientific Committee. Guidance for the preparation of neurological management guidelines by EFNS scientific task forces – revised recommendations. *Eur J Neurol* 2004; **11**:577–81.

7. Melzack, R, Wall, PD. Pain mechanisms: a new theory. *Sciences (New York)* 1965; **150**:971–9.

8. Fukazawa, Y, Maeda, T, Hamabe, W, *et al.* Activation of spinal anti-analgesic system following electroacupuncture stimulation in rats. *J Pharmacol Sci* 2005; **99**:408–14.

9. Zhang, GG, Yu, C, Lee, W, *et al.* Involvement of peripheral opioid mechanisms in electro-acupuncture analgesia. *Explore (NY)* 2005; **1**:365–71.

10. McQuay, HJ, Moore, RA, Eccleston, C, *et al.* Systematic review of outpatient services for chronic pain control. *Health Technol Assess* 1997; **1**:1–135.

11. Reichstein, L, Labrenz, S, Ziegler, D, *et al.* Effective treatment of symptomatic diabetic polyneuropathy by highfrequency external muscle stimulation. *Diabetologia* 2005; **48**:824–8.

12. Kumar, D, Marshall, HJ. Diabetic peripheral neuropathy: amelioration of pain with transcutaneous electrostimulation. *Diabetes Care* 1997; **20**:1702–5.

13. Hamza, MA, White, PF, Craig, WF, *et al.* Percutaneous electrical nerve stimulation: a novel analgesic therapy for diabetic neuropathic pain. *Diabetes Care* 2000; **23**:365–70.

14. Forst, T, Nguyen, M, Forst, S, *et al.* Impact of low frequency transcutaneous electrical nerve stimulation on symptomatic diabetic neuropathy using the new salutaris device. *Diabetes Nutr Metab* 2004; **17**:163–8.

15. Cheing, GL, Luk, ML. Transcutaneous electrical nerve stimulation for neuropathic pain. *J Hand Surg* 2005; **30**:50–5.

16. Thorsteinsson, G, Stonnington, HH, Stillwell, GK, *et al.* Transcutaneous electrical stimulation: a double-blind trial of its efficacy for pain. *Arch Phys Med Rehabil* 1977; **58**:8–13.

17. Rutgers, MJ, Van Romunde, LKJ, Osman, PO. A small randomized comparative trial of acupuncture versus transcutaneous electrical neurostimulation in postherpetic neuralgia. *Pain Clinic* 1988; **2**:87–9.

18. Bloodworth, DM, Nguyen, BN, Garver, W, *et al.* Comparison of stochastic vs. conventional transcutaneous electrical stimulation for pain modulation in patients with electromyographically documented radiculopathy. *Am J Phys Med Rehabil* 2004; **83**:584–91.

19. Sindou, MP, Mertens, P, Bendavid, U, *et al.* Predictive value of somatosensory evoked potentials for long-lasting pain relief after spinal cord stimulation: practical use for patient selection. *Neurosurgery* 2003; **52**:1374–83.

20. Cameron, T. Safety and efficacy of spinal cord stimulation for the treatment of chronic pain: a 20-year literature review. *J Neurosurg* 2004; **100**(3 Suppl. Spine):254–67.

21. Taylor, RS, Van Buyten, JP, Buchser, E. Systematic review and meta-analysis of the effectiveness of spinal cord stimulation in the management of failed back surgery syndrome. *Spine* 2005; **30**:152–60.

22. Taylor, RS, Van Buyten, JP, Buchser, E. Spinal cord stimulation for complex regional pain syndrome: a systematic review of the clinical and cost-effectiveness literature and assessment of prognostic factors. *Eur J Pain* 2006; **10**:91–101.

23. Simpson, BA. Spinal cord stimulation. *Pain Rev* 1994; **1**:199–230.

24. Simpson, BA. Spinal cord and brain stimulation, in *Textbook of Pain* (eds PD Wall, R Melzack), 4th edn, 1999; Churchill Livingstone, London, pp. 1253–381.

25. Simpson, BA, Meyerson, BA, Linderoth, B. Spinal cord and brain stimulation, in *Wall and Melzack's Textbook of Pain* (eds SB McMahon, M Koltzenburg), 5th edn, 2006; Elsevier Churchill Livingstone, London, pp. 563–82.

26. North, RB, Kidd, DH, Farrokhi, F, *et al.* Spinal cord stimulation versus repeated lumbosacral spine surgery for chronic pain: a randomized, controlled trial. *Neurosurgery* 2005; **56**:98–106.

27. Kumar, K, North, R, Taylor, R, *et al.* Spinal cord stimulation versus conventional medical management: a prospective, randomised, controlled, multicentre study of patients with failed back surgery syndrome (PROCESS study). *Neuromodulation* 2005; **8**:213–18.

28. Kumar, K, Taylor, RS, Jacques, L, *et al.* Spinal cord stimulation versus conventional medical management for neuropathic pain: a multicentre randomised controlled trial in patients with failed back surgery syndrome. *Pain* 2007; **132**:179–88.

29. Kemler, MA, Barendse, GAM, Van Kleef, M, *et al.* Spinal cord stimulation in patients with chronic reflex sympathetic dystrophy. *N Engl J Med* 2000; **343**:618–24.

30. Kemler, MA, de Vet, HC, Barendse, GA, *et al.* Spinal cord stimulation for chronic reflex sympathetic dystrophy – five-year follow-up. *N Engl J Med* 2006; **354**: 2394–6.

31. Heath, RG, Mickle, WA. (1960) Evaluation of seven years' experience with depth electrode studies in human patients, in *Electrical Studies on the Unanesthetized Brain* (eds ER Ramey, DS O'Doherty), 1960; Paul B. Hoeber, New York, pp. 214–47.

32. Hosobuchi, Y, Adams, JE, Rutkin, B. Chronic thalamic stimulation for the control of facial anesthesia dolorosa. *Arch Neurol* 1973; **29**:158–61.

33. Richardson, DE, Akil, H. Long term results of periventricular gray self-stimulation. *Neurosurgery* 1977; **1**:199–202.

34. Green, AL, Wang, S, Owen, SL, *et al.* Stimulating the human midbrain to reveal the link between pain and blood pressure. *Pain* 2006; **124**, 349–59.

35. Owen, SL, Green, AL, Nandi, D, *et al.* Deep brain stimulation for neuropathic pain. *Neuromodulation* 2006; **9**:100–6.

36. Owen, SL, Green, AL, Stein, JF, *et al.* Deep brain stimulation for the alleviation of post-stroke neuropathic pain. *Pain* 2006; **120**:202–6.

37. Bittar, RG, Kar-Purkayastha, I, Owen, SL, *et al.* Deep brain stimulation for pain relief: a meta-analysis. *J Clin Neurosci* 2005; **12**:515–19.

38. Hamani, C, Schwalb, JM, Rezai, AR. Deep brain stimulation for chronic neuropathic pain: long-term outcome and the incidence of insertional effect. *Pain* 2006; **125**:188–96.

39. Katayama, Y, Yamamoto, T, Kobayashi, K, *et al.* Motor cortex stimulation for post-stroke pain: comparison of spinal cord and thalamic stimulation. *Stereotact Funct Neurosurg* 2001; **77**:183–6.

40. Tsubokawa, T, Katayama, Y, Yamamoto, T, *et al.* Treatment of thalamic pain by chronic motor cortex stimulation. *Pacing Clin Electrophysiol* 1991; **14**:131–4.

41. Tsubokawa, T, Katayama, Y, Yamamoto, T, *et al.* Chronic motor cortex stimulation in patients with thalamic pain. *J Neurosurg* 1993; **78**:393–401.

42. Peyron, R, Garcia-Larrea, L, Deiber, MP, *et al.* Electrical stimulation of precentral cortical area in the treatment of central pain: electrophysiological and PET study. *Pain* 1995; **62**:275–86.

43. Garcia-Larrea, L, Peyron, R, Mertens, P, *et al.* Electrical stimulation of motor cortex for pain control: a combined PET-scan and electrophysiological study. *Pain* 1999; **83**:259–73.

44. Rusina, R, Vaculin, S, Yamamotova, A, *et al.* The effect of motor cortex stimulation in deafferentated rats. *Neuro Endocrinol Lett* 2005; **26**:283–8.

45. Senapati, AK, Huntington, PJ, Peng, YB. Spinal dorsal horn neuron response to mechanical stimuli is decreased by electrical stimulation of the primary motor cortex. *Brain Res* 2005; **1036**:173–9.

46. Peyron, R, Faillenot, I, Mertens, P, *et al.* Motor cortex stimulation in neuropathic pain. Correlations between analgesic-effect and hemodynamic changes in the brain. A PET study. *Neuroimage* 2007; **34**:310–21.

47. Lefaucheur, JP. The use of repetitive transcranial magnetic stimulation (rTMS) in chronic neuropathic pain. *Neurophysiol Clin* 2006; **36**:117–24.

48. Lefaucheur, JP, Drouot, X, Keravel, Y, *et al.* Pain relief induced by repetitive transcranial magnetic stimulation of precentral cortex. *Neuroreport* 2001; **12**:2963–5.

49. Andre-Obadia, N, Peyron, R, Mertens, P, *et al.* Transcranial magnetic stimulation for pain control. Doubleblind study of different frequencies against placebo, and correlation with motor cortex stimulation efficacy. *Clin Neurophysiol* 2006; **117**:1536–44.

50. Khedr, EM, Kotb, H, Kamel, NF, *et al.* Longlasting antalgic effects of daily sessions of repetitive transcranial magnetic stimulation in central and peripheral neuropathic pain. *J Neurol Neurosurg Psychiatry* 2005; **76**:833–8.

51. Lefaucheur, JP, Drouot, X, Nguyen, JP. Interventional neurophysiology for pain control: duration of pain relief following repetitive transcranial magnetic stimulation of the motor cortex. *Neurophysiol Clin* 2001; **31**:247–52.

52. Lefaucheur, JP, Drouot, X, Menard-Lefaucheur, I, *et al.* Neurogenic pain relief by repetitive transcranial magnetic cortical stimulation depends on the origin and the site of pain. *J Neurol Neurosurg Psychiatry* 2004; **75**:612–16.

53. Levy, RM, Lamb, S, Adams, JE. Treatment of chronic pain by deep brain stimulation: long term follow-up and review of the literature. *Neurosurgery* 1987; **21**:885–93.

CHAPTER 3

Trigeminal neuralgia management

G. Cruccu,[1] G. Gronseth,[2] J. Alksne,[3] C. Argoff,[4] M. Brainin,[5] K. Burchiel,[6] T. Nurmikko[7] and J. M. Zakrzewska[8]

[1]La Sapienza University, Rome, Italy; [2]University of Kansas, Kansas City, USA; [3]University of California, San Diego, USA; [4]New York University School of Medicine and North Shore University Hospital, MA, USA; [5]Donau-Universität Krems, Krems, Austria; [6]Oregon Health & Science University, Portland, USA; [7]University of Liverpool, Liverpool, UK; [8]University College London Hospitals Eastman Dental Hospital, London, UK

Introduction

The American Academy of Neurology (AAN) and the European Federation of Neurological Societies (EFNS) decided to develop scientifically sound, clinically relevant guidelines to aid specialists and non-specialists in the management of trigeminal neuralgia (TN) by addressing its diagnosis, pharmacological treatment and surgical treatment.

The International Association for the Study of Pain (IASP) defines TN as sudden, usually unilateral, severe, brief, stabbing, recurrent episodes of pain in the distribution of one or more branches of the trigeminal nerve [1]. The annual incidence of TN is 4–5/100,000 [2]. It is the most common neuralgia. In the latest classification of the International Headache Society [3], a distinction is made between *classical* and *symptomatic* TN: classical TN (CTN) includes all cases without an established aetiology (i.e., idiopathic), as well as those with potential vascular compression of the fifth cranial nerve, whereas the diagnosis of symptomatic TN (STN) is made in cases secondary to tumour, MS, structural abnormalities of the skull base, and the like. It should be noted that categorization of TN into *typical* and *atypical* forms is based on symptom constellation,

not aetiology, and will not be discussed further in this review.

The first issue facing the clinician caring for a patient with TN is accurately distinguishing symptomatic from classical TN. The diagnostic portion of this parameter addresses the following questions:

1. How often does routine neuroimaging (CT, MRI) identify a cause (excluding vascular contact) of TN?

2. Which clinical or laboratory features accurately identify patients with STN?

3. For patients with classical TN, does high-resolution MRI accurately identify patients with neurovascular compression?

The first-line therapy of trigeminal neuralgia is pharmacological, if for no other reason than in most cases it is immediately available and usually effective. Introduction of phenytoin in the 1940s and carbamazepine in the 1960s changed the management of TN considerably, which previously had been almost exclusively surgical. The pharmacological portion of this parameter addresses the following questions:

4. Which drugs have shown efficacy in the treatment of CTN?

5. Which drugs have shown efficacy in the treatment of STN?

European Handbook of Neurological Management: Volume 2, Second Edition. Edited by Nils Erik Gilhus, Michael P. Barnes, Michael Brainin.
© 2012 Blackwell Publishing Ltd. Published 2012 by Blackwell Publishing Ltd.

6. Is there evidence of efficacy of intravenous drugs in acute exacerbations of TN?

When medical treatment fails due to poor pain control or because of intolerable side-effects, surgery is often considered the next option. The timing and choice of surgery is the next issue to face the patient. Surgical interventions are varied and are best classified according to the principal target: peripheral techniques targeting portions of the trigeminal nerve distal to the Gasserian ganglion; percutaneous Gasserian ganglion techniques targeting the ganglion itself; gamma knife radiosurgery targeting the trigeminal root and posterior fossa vascular decompression techniques.

7. When should surgery be offered?

8. Which surgical technique gives the longest pain free period with fewest complications and good quality of life?

9. Which surgical techniques should be used in patients with multiple sclerosis?

Search methods

The AAN and EFNS identified an expert panel of TN experts and general neurologists with methodological

expertise. Conflicts of interest were disclosed. Panel members were not compensated.

We searched Medline, EMBASE and the Cochrane Library. Searches extended from the time of database inception to 2006. All searches used the following synonyms for TN: trigeminal neuralgia, tic douloureux, facial pain and trigeminal neuropathy. Search terms were used as text words or MESH headings as appropriate. The primary search was supplemented by a secondary search using the bibliography of retrieved articles and knowledge from the expert panel. Only full original communications were accepted. Panel members reviewed abstracts and titles for relevance. Then, at least two panel members reviewed papers meeting inclusion criteria. An additional panel member arbitrated disagreements.

The methods of classifying evidence adopted by AAN and EFNS are very similar; those of grading the recommendations, though largely compatible, differ in a few points. A detailed comparison of the two methods of classification and grading can be found in the online Supplementary Material, Appendix 1. The classification of the identified studies was agreed by American and European authors (see Tables 3.1–9). This was not possible for the grading of recommendations. The present

Table 3.1 Diagnosis: frequency at which neuroimaging identified patients with symptomatic TN.

First Author Year	Class	Sampling	Population	Data collection	TN criteria	Modality	Total TN Patients	STN Patients (CI)
Cruccu 2006 [5]	III	Consecutive patients with TN	Referral centre	Prospective	IHS	MRI	120	16 MS 6 tumours
Sato 2004 [8]	III	Consecutive patients with TN	University	Retrospective	IASP	MRI or CT	61	7 tumours
Goh 2001 [6]	III	Consecutive patients with TN and MRI	National dental centre	Retrospective	Not stated	MRI	40[a]	4 masses
Majoie 1998 [7]	III	Consecutive patients with TN and MRI	University	Retrospective	Not stated	MRI	22	3 tumours 1 aneurysm
Nomura 1994 [10]	IV	Consecutive patients with TN	University	Retrospective	Not stated (non-TN neurological signs)	MRI or CT	164	22 masses
Pooled Class III							37/243 Yield	15% (11 to 20)

[a]Patients with non-trigeminal symptoms or signs eliminated. CI: 95% confidence interval.

article, meant for the *European Journal of Neurology*, used the EFNS grading of recommendations [4].

Results

Diagnosis

Question 1. For patients with trigeminal neuralgia without non-trigeminal neurological symptoms or signs, how often does neuroimaging (CT, MRI) identify a cause (excluding vascular contact)?

Evidence: Five articles (one graded Class IV) reported the results of head imaging on consecutive patients diagnosed with TN (Table 3.1). Four studies included cohorts of TN patients assembled at university and tertiary centres with a presumed interest in TN. Because more complicated and potentially less representative TN patients are treated at such centres, these studies were judged to be at risk for referral bias and thus graded Class III [5, 6, 7, 8]. Yields of brain imaging ranged from 10% to 18%. Combining Class III studies results in a pooled estimate of 15% (95% CI, 11–20).

Conclusions: For patients with trigeminal neuralgia without non-trigeminal neurological symptoms, routine neuroimaging possibly identifies a cause in up to 15% of patients (four Class III studies).

Question 2. For patients with trigeminal neuralgia, which clinical or laboratory features accurately identify patients with STN?

Evidence: We found seven papers (one graded Class IV) studying the diagnostic accuracy of clinical characteristics for distinguishing STN from CTN (Table 3.2). Potential clinical characteristics studies included the presence of sensory deficits, age of onset, first division of trigeminal nerve affected, bilateral trigeminal involvement and unresponsiveness to treatment.

One study was graded Class III because of a case-control design with a narrow spectrum of patients [9]. Four studies were judged to have a moderately low risk of bias because of a cohort design with a broad spectrum of patients. However, these studies collected data retrospectively and were thus graded Class II [6, 8, 10, 11]. We found one prospective Class I study [5]. In these studies involvement of the first trigeminal division and unresponsiveness to treatment were not associated with a significant increase in the risk of STN. Younger age was significantly associated with increased risk of STN.

However, in these studies there was considerable overlap in the age ranges of patients with CTN and STN. Thus, although younger age increases the risk of finding STN, the diagnostic accuracy of age as a predictor of STN was too low to be clinically useful. The presence of trigeminal sensory deficits and bilateral involvement was significantly more common in patients with STN. However, many patients with STN had normal sensation and unilateral involvement of the trigeminal nerve (Figure 3.1).

Nine studies looked at the diagnostic accuracy of electrophysiological testing in distinguishing STN from CTN patients. Five studies addressed the accuracy of trigeminal reflex testing (Table 3.3); one study used a prospective design and was graded Class I [5]; the remaining studies, using a case-control design with a narrow spectrum of patients or retrospective data collection, were graded Class II or III [12, 13, 14, 15]. The diagnostic accuracy of trigeminal reflexes for identifying STN patients in most studies was relatively high (sensitivity 59–100%, specificity 93–100%). Pooled sensitivity 94% (95% CI, 91–97); pooled specificity 87% (95% CI, 77–93). Four studies addressed the accuracy of evoked potential (Table 3.4), two attaining Class II and two Class III [12, 16, 17, 18]. The diagnostic accuracy of evoked potentials for identifying STN patients was moderate (sensitivity 60–100%, specificity 49–76%). Pooled sensitivity 84% (95% CI, 73–92); pooled specificity 64% (95% CI, 56–71).

Conclusions: For patients with TN, involvement of the first division of the trigeminal nerve and unresponsiveness to treatment are probably not associated with an increased risk of STN (one Class I, two Class II). Younger age (one Class I, three Class II) and abnormal trigeminal nerve evoked potentials (two Class II and two Class III) are probably associated with an increased risk of STN. However, there is too much overlap in patients with CTN and STN for these predictors to be considered clinically useful. The presence of trigeminal sensory deficits or bilateral involvement of the trigeminal nerves probably increases the risk of STN. However, the absence of these features does not rule out STN (one Class I, two Class II). Because of a high specificity (94%) and sensitivity (87%) abnormal trigeminal reflexes are probably useful in distinguishing STN from CTN (one Class I and two Class II).

Question 3. For patients with classical TN, does high-resolution MRI accurately identify patients with neurovascular compression?

Table 3.2 Diagnostic accuracy of clinical features for distinguishing symptomatic TN from classic TN.

First Author Year	Class	Design	Spectrum	CTN/STN	Number	Age mean ± SD	Sensory deficits	First division	Bilateral	Poor rx response
Cruccu 2006 [5]	I	CO P	Broad	CTN	96	62 ± 12	0/96	28/136	0/96	–
				STN	24 (mixed)	51 ± 10	2/24	9/33	0/24	
De Simone 2005 [9]	III	CC P	Narrow	CTN	13	60 ± 12	4/13	8/25	0/13	–
				STN	15 (MS)	43 ± 11	10/15	3/23	0/15	
Sato 2004 [8]	II	CO R	Broad	CTN	43					3/43
				STN	7 (tumours)					2/7
Ogutcen-Toller 2004 [11]	II	CO R	Broad	CTN	31				0/31	
				STN	7 (masses)				1/7	
Goh 2001 [6]	II	CO R	Broad	CTN	36	60 ± 13	0/36		0/36	10/35
				STN	6 (masses)	54 ± 11	2/6		0/6	3/6
Hooge 1995 [83]	IV	CS R	Narrow	CTN	0	–	–		–	–
				STN	35 (MS)	51	3/35		5/35	2/20
Nomura 1994 [10]	II	CO R	Broad	CTN	142	47 ± 13 (n = 58)	1/142	11/58	0/58	
				STN	22 (masses)	48 ± 16	11/22	6/22	0/22	
Pooled classes I-III					P assoc	<0.0001	<0.001	NS	<0.001	NS
					Sen% (CI)		37 (27–49)	23 (15 to 34)	1.4 (0–7)	39 (18 to 65)
					Spe% (CI)		98 (96–99)	79 (73 to 84)	100 (98–100)	83 (74 to 9)
					Pos LR		18.5	1.1	Large	2.3

CO: cohort survey. CC: case control. CS: Case series. P: Prospective data collection. R: Retrospective or not described data collection. CI: 95% confidence intervals. P assoc: probability of statistically significant association between the presence of the characteristic and the presence of symptomatic STN. Sen: sensitivity. Spe: specificity. Sensitivities calculated for presence of characteristic in symptomatic TN. Specificities calculated for absence of characteristic in classical TN. Pos LR: positive likelihood ratio.

Evidence: Sixteen papers studied TN patients with high-resolution MRI, usually prior to microvascular decompression. Nine studies were graded Class IV because they relied on the unmasked findings of the

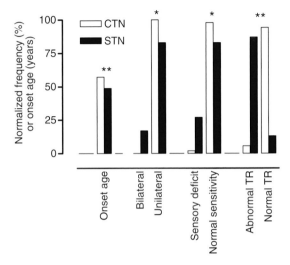

Figure 3.1 Differential diagnosis between classical (CTN) and symptomatic trigeminal neuralgia (STN). Response to treatment and involvement of first trigeminal division are similar in the two populations. Onset age is lower in CTN than STN (**$P < 0.0001$). Bilateral neuralgia and sensory deficits only occur in STN (*$P < 0.001$). Trigeminal reflexes (TR) are abnormal in STN (87%) and normal in CTN (94%) (**$P < 0.0001$). Data from 10 trials (Class I–III) in 628 patients, detailed in Tables 3.2 and 3.3.

operating surgeon to determine the presence of vascular contact; in these studies, the surgeon always found a blood vessel contacting the trigeminal nerve. Table 3.5 lists the seven higher-quality studies and their methodological characteristics. One study employed a case-control design with a narrow spectrum of patients and another was retrospective (Class III) [7, 19]. Five studies were masked cohort surveys with prospective data collection (Class I) [20, 21, 22, 23, 24]. The most common reference standard in these Class I studies was the masked comparison of the MRI of the symptomatic side to the asymptomatic side.

Pooled data showed a highly significant association between the presence of a MRI-identified vascular contact and the presence of TN ($P < 0.0001$). But sensitivities and specificities in the Class I–III studies varied widely (sensitivity 52–100%; specificity 29–93%) and in three Class I studies the association was not significant. The heterogeneity in results may come from differences in the various MRI techniques employed. Currently, it is not possible to establish which MRI technique is most reliable.

Conclusions: Because of inconsistency of results, there is insufficient evidence to support or refute the usefulness of MRI to identify vascular contact in CTN or to indicate the most reliable technique. Given the significance of pooled data, however, we suggest patients considered suitable for MVD undergo high-resolution MRI.

Table 3.3 Diagnostic accuracy of trigeminal reflex testing for distinguishing symptomatic TN from classic TN.

First Author Year	class	Design	Spectrum	Ref. Standard	STN A/T	CTN A/T	P assoc	Spe (CI)	Sen (CI)
Kimura 1970 [14]	III	CC P	narrow	Clinical	1/1	1/14	NS	93%	100%
Ongerboer de Visser 1974 [15]	III	CC R	narrow	Clinical	16/16	0/11	<0.0001	100%	100%
Kimura 1983 [13]	II	CC P	broad	Clinical	10/17	4/93	<0.0001	96%	59%
Cruccu 1990 [12]	II	CC P	broad	Clinical imaging	4/4	2/30	<0.0003	93%	100%
Cruccu 2006 [5]	I	CO P	broad	Clinical MRI	23/24	7/96	<0.0001	93%	96%
Pooled classes I–III					54/62	14/244	<0.0001	94% (91 to 97)	87% (77 to 93)

Trigeminal reflex testing: R1 early blink reflex after supraorbital stimulation (for ophthalmic division), SP1 early masseter inhibitory reflex after infraorbital stimulation (for maxillary division), and SP1 early masseter inhibitory reflex after mental stimulation or mandibular tendon reflex (for mandibular division). A/T: abnormal/total. CO: cohort survey. CC: case control. P: Prospective data collection. R: Retrospective or not described data collection. CI: 95% confidence intervals. P assoc: probability of statistically significant association between the presence of the characteristic and the presence of symptomatic STN. Sen: sensitivity. Spe: specificity. Sensitivities calculated for presence of abnormal trigeminal reflexes in symptomatic TN. Specificities calculated for absence of abnormal trigeminal reflexes in classical TN.

Table 3.4 Diagnostic accuracy of evoked potentials for distinguishing symptomatic TN from classic TN.

Author year	class	Method	Design	Spectrum	Ref. Standard	STN A/T	CTN A/T	P assoc	Sen (CI)	Spe (CI)
Leandri 1988 [43]	III	electrical-TEPs	CC P	narrow	imaging	18/23	9/38	<0.0001	78%	76%
Cruccu 1990 [12]	III	electrical-TEPs	CC P	broad	imaging	4/4	9/30	<0.05	100%	70%
Cruccu 2001 [16]	II	laser-EPs	CC P	broad	MRI	20/20	24/47	<0.0001	100%	49%
Mursch 2002 [84]	II	electrical-TEPs	CO R	broad	Not stated	6/10	13/37	NS	60%	65%
Pooled II-III						48/57	55/152	<0.0001	84% (73 to 92)	64% (56 to 71)

TEPs, trigeminal evoked potentials; A/T, abnormal/total; CO, cohort survey; CC, case control; P, prospective data collection; R, retrospective or not described data collection; CI, 95% confidence intervals; P assoc, probability of statistically significant association between the presence of the characteristic and the presence of symptomatic STN; Sen, sensitivity; Spe, specificity. Sensitivities calculated for presence of abnormal evoked potentials in symptomatic TN. Specificities calculated for absence of abnormal evoked potentials in classical TN.

Recommendations on diagnosis

For patients with TN without non-trigeminal neurological symptoms, routine imaging may be considered to identify STN (Level C). Younger age at onset, involvement of the first division of the trigeminal nerve, unresponsiveness to treatment and abnormal trigeminal-evoked potentials should be disregarded as useful for disclosing STN (Level B). Determining the presence of trigeminal sensory deficits or bilateral involvement of the trigeminal nerves should be considered useful to distinguish STN from CTN. However, the absence of these features should be disregarded as useful for distinguishing STN from CTN (Level B). Measuring trigeminal reflexes in a qualified electrophysiological laboratory should be considered useful for distinguishing STN from CTN (Level B). There is insufficient evidence to support or refute the usefulness of MRI to identify CTN patients who are more likely to respond to MVD.

Pharmacological treatment

Question 4. Which drugs have shown efficacy in the treatment of classical trigeminal neuralgia (CTN) in general?

Evidence: Our search strategy identified 15 randomized controlled trials studying the effectiveness of various medications for TN. In three of these the number of patients was too small (*n* = 3–6). Of the remaining 12,

eight were placebo-controlled trials and four used carbamazepine as the comparator (Tables 3.6 and 3.7).

Phenytoin was the first drug to be used for CTN with positive effects, but no randomized controlled trials have ever been published (four Class III open studies; cf. Sindrup and Jensen [25]).

Four placebo-controlled studies (Class I or II) totalling 147 patients demonstrated efficacy of carbamazepine (CBZ) [18, 26, 27, 28]. The treatment response in these trials was robust, with the number needed to treat (NNT) to attain important pain relief being 1.7– 1.8 [25, 29, 30]. CBZ reduced both the frequency and intensity of painful paroxysms and was equally efficacious on spontaneous and trigger-evoked attacks [26]. The efficacy of CBZ is compromised by poor tolerability with numbers-needed-to-harm (NNHs) of 3.4 for minor and of 24 for severe adverse events [29, 30, 31]. The use of older antiepileptic drugs such as CBZ is often complicated by pharmacokinetic factors and frequent adverse events [29, 30]. The issue of balance between effect and adverse reactions is particularly important in elderly patients with TN.

Oxcarbazepine (OXC) is often used as initial treatment for TN [32]. Its preference over CBZ is mainly related to its documented efficacy in epilepsy and accepted greater tolerability and decreased potential for drug interactions (Class I) [17]. Three RCTs using a double-blind design

Table 3.5 Diagnostic accuracy of MRI for identifying abnormal vascular contact in classic TN.

Author year	class	Method	Design	Spectrum	Masked	Ref. Standard	Symptomatic NVC/T	Asymptomatic NVC/T	P assoc	Sen (CI)	Spe (CI)
Korogi 1995 [22]	I	3D-TOF	COP	broad	Yes	Symptomatic side	12/16	4/16	<0.012	75%	75%
Masur 1995 [23]	I	3D-FLASH	COP	broad	Yes	Symptomatic side	12/18	10/18	NS	67%	44%
Majoie 1997 [85]	III	3D-FISP MP-RAGE	CCP	narrow	Yes	clinical	10/13	8/113	<0.0001	77%	93%
Yamakami 2000 [24]	I	CISS-3D-TOF	COP	broad	Yes	Symptomatic side	14/14	7/30	<0.0001	100%	77%
Benes 2005 [21]	I	3D-Fiesta 3D-FSPGR	COP	broad	Yes	Symptomatic side	11/21	10/21	NS	52%	52%
Anderson 2006 [20]	I	3D-TOF 3D-Gad	COP	broad	Yes	Symptomatic side	42/48	34/48	NS	88%	29%
Erbay 2006 [19]	III	CISS-MPR	COR	broad	Yes	Symptomatic side	30/40	10/40	<0.0001	75%	75%
Pooled	I-III						131/170	83/286	<0.0001	77% (70–83)	71% (65–76)

NVC/T: neurovascular contact/total. CO: cohort survey. CC: case control. P: Prospective data collection. R: Retrospective or not described data collection. CI: 95% confidence intervals. P assoc: probability of statistically significant association between the presence of the characteristic and the presence of TN. Sen: sensitivity. Spe: specificity. Sensitivities calculated for presence of neurovascular contact on the symptomatic side. Specificities calculated for absence of neurovascular contact on the asymptomatic side.

Table 3.6 Medical treatment. Placebo-controlled trials.

Author/ year	class	No patients	Intervention	Design	Allocation conceal	No. drop-outs	Outcomes	Improved on active	Improved on placebo	Duration of treatment arm & long-term Follow up
Campbell et al. 1966 [26]	I	70 (77 patients recruited); age range 20–84	CBZ 300–800 mg/d	R, D-B, double C-O	Not stated	Not stated, possibly none	Severity of pain, No paroxysms, Trigger inactive	58% 68% 68%	26% 26% 40%	4 weeks No F/U
Killian & Fromm 1968 [27]	II	24 (30 patients recruited); age range 36–83	CBZ 400–1000 mg/d	R, D-B, initially C-O, followed by closed label extension	Not stated	3 on active, placebo not stated	Global pain response	24/24 (complete or v.good)	0/24 ('response in all minimal or absent')	C-O, 5 days Extension, 2 weeks to 36 months
Nicol 1969 [18]	II	44 (of 54 entered)	CBZ 100–2400 mg/d	R, D-B, modified C-O, followed by closed label extension	Not stated	10 insufficient follow up	Global pain response	15/20 (good or excellent)	6/7 (good or excellent)	C-O, 2 weeks F/U up to 46 months
Rockcliff & Davis, 1966 [28]	II	9; age range 37–81	CBZ 600 mg/d	R, D-B, C-O, sequential design	Independent pharmacist	No drop outs	Patient preference	8/9	0/9	3 days F/U 7–10 months, median 9 months
Fromm et al. 1984 [36]	II	10; age range 59–78	Baclofen 40–80 mg/d	Randomization unclear, D-B, C-O	Not stated	No drop outs	No. paroxysms	7/10 reduction	1/10 reduction	1 week No F/U
Zakrzewska et al. 1997 [37]	II	14; age range 44–75	Lamotrigine 400 mg/d	R, D-B, C-O, add on	Not stated	1 on placebo	Composite index, global response	7/13	1/14	2 weeks No F/U
Fromm 1993 [40]	III	11; age range 41–83; most pts had undergone surgery or were on concurrent medications	Tizanidine 12 mg/d	Randomization unclear, D-B, C-O	Not stated	1 on placebo	Frequency of paroxysms	8/10 reduction	4/10 reduction	1 week F/U 6 patients (effect lost 1–3 months)
Kondziolka et al. 1994 [41]	I	47; age range 26–82	Proparacaine 0.5% eyedrops	R, D-B, C-O	Not stated	No drop outs	Pain score, frequency	6/25	5/25	30 days No F/U

R, randomized; D-B, double-blind; C-O, cross-over; PG, parallel group; CBZ, carbamazepine; NK, not known.

Table 3.7 Medical treatment (comparator studies against carbamazepine).

Author/year	class	No patients	Intervention	Design	Allocation concealment	No. drop outs	Outcomes	Improved on study drug	Improved on comparator	Duration of treatment arm & long-term Follow up
Lindstrom & Lindblom 1987 [39]	III	12; age range 41–78	Tocainide 20 mg/ kg/d	R, D-B, C-O	Not stated	TOC 0 CBZ 0	Global pain	9/12	10/12	2 weeks No F/U
Lechin et al. 1989 [38]	II	48; age range 48–68	Pimozide 4–12 mg/d vs. CBZ 0.3–1.2 g/d	R, D-B, C-O	Not stated	PMZ 0 CBZ not stated	Composite 'TN score'	48/48	27/48	8 weeks Duration of F/U not stated
Liebel 2001 [35]	II	48, age range 38–83	OXC 600 mg/d increased to 'optimal' vs. CBZ 400 mg/d to 'optimal'	R, D-B, PG	Not stated	OXC 0 CBZ 2	50% reduction in TN attacks	24/24	19/20	6–32 weeks
Beydoun et al. 2000, 2002 [33, 34]	II	130 (meta-analysis of 3 studies)	OXC 700– 900 mg/d vs. CBZ 500– 1200 mg/d	R, D-B, PG	Not stated		No. weekly attacks, (evoked pain global efficacy)	63/69	54/61	6–8 weeks

R, randomized; D-B, double-blind; C-O, cross-over; PG, parallel group, CBZ, carbamazepine; OXC, oxcarbazepine; PMZ, pimozide; TOC, tocainide; NK, not known.

including a total of 130 patients compared oxcarbazepine (OXC) 600–1,800 mg/day to CBZ in CTN patients (Class II and meta-analysis) [33, 34, 35]. The reduction in number of attacks and global pain assessments were equally good for both CBZ and OXC (88% of patients achieving a reduction of attacks by >50%). These studies used as comparator CBZ rather than placebo, disallowing calculations for NNT values for OXC.

Other drugs have each been studied in single trials: baclofen was superior to placebo in reducing the number of painful paroxysms (Class II) [36]; lamotrigine (400 mg/day) was effective as add-on therapy on a composite index of efficacy (Class II) [37]; pimozide was more effective than CBZ (Class II) [38]; and tocainide was as effective as CBZ (Class III) [39]. In a small group of patients (most having already undergone trigeminal surgery or taking concurrent medications) tizanidine was better than placebo, but its effect decayed within 1–3 months (Class III) [40].

Small, open-label studies (Class IV) have suggested therapeutic benefit from other antiepileptic drugs (clonazepam, gabapentin, valproate), but in general the proportion of patients improving was lower than that yielded by CBZ.

Topical ophthalmic anaesthesia was ineffective in a Class I placebo-controlled RCT [41].

Conclusions: Carbamazepine is established as effective for controlling pain in patients with TN (multiple Class I and II). Oxcarbazepine (one meta-analysis and one Class II) is probably effective, and baclofen, lamotrigine and pimozide are possibly effective for controlling pain in patients with TN (one Class II). Topical ophthalmic anaesthesia is probably ineffective for controlling pain in patients with TN (one Class I). There is insufficient evidence to support or refute the efficacy of clonazepam, gabapentin, phenytoin, tizanidine, topical capsaicin and valproate for controlling pain in patients with TN.

Considering the relatively narrow mechanism of action of the available drugs, combination treatments might be useful. However, there are no published studies directly comparing polytherapy with monotherapy [42].

Question 5. Which drugs have shown efficacy in the treatment of STN?

Evidence: There are no placebo-controlled studies in patients with STN. The existing studies all deal with TN associated with multiple sclerosis and are small, open-

label trials (Class IV). Lamotrigine has been reported to be more effective than CBZ in 18 patients [86]. Three trials (comprising a total of 19 patients) have reported an effect of gabapentin alone or associated with CBZ [44, 45, 46]. One study reported efficacy of topiramate in six patients [47]. Finally, two Class IV studies reported efficacy of misoprostol (a prostaglandin-E1 analogue) in a total of 25 patients [48, 49].

Conclusion: There is insufficient evidence to support or refute the effectiveness of gabapentin, lamotrigine, misoprostol and topiramate in treating pain in symptomatic TN (Class IV studies).

Question 6. Is there evidence of efficacy of intravenous administration of drugs in acute exacerbations of TN?

Evidence: We were unable to find published RCTs on the use of intravenous opioids, TCAs, benzodiazepines, antiepileptic drugs or non-opioid analgesics. Textbooks make a passing reference to the use of i.v. antiepileptic drugs in the emergency management of TN, and Cheshire [50] has reported three patients who responded quickly to i.v. fosphenytoin (Class IV).

Conclusion: There is insufficient evidence to support or refute the efficacy of i.v. fosphenytoin or other i.v. medications for the acute treatment of pain from TN (Class IV).

Recommendations on pharmacological treatment

Carbamazepine is established as effective (Level A) and oxcarbazepine is probably effective (Level B) for controlling pain in CTN. Baclofen, lamotrigine and pimozide may be considered to control pain in patients with CTN (Level C). Topical ophthalmic anaesthesia is probably ineffective in controlling pain in patients with CTN (Level B). There is insufficient evidence to support or refute the efficacy of other medications in CTN, of any medication in STN and of any intravenous medication for the acute treatment of pain from TN.

Evidence translated in a clinical context: In line with the recent EFNS Guidelines [51], the two drugs to consider as first-line therapy in CTN are CBZ (200–1,200 mg/day) and OXC (600–1,800 mg/day). Although the evidence for CBZ is stronger than for OXC, the latter may pose fewer safety concerns. If any of these sodium-channel blockers is ineffective, referral for a surgical consultation would be a reasonable next step. In cases where surgical intervention is unlikely (e.g., because of the frailty of the patient) there are insufficient data to recommend the next step. Limited evidence supports add-on therapy with lamotrigine or a switch to baclofen (pimozide being no longer in use). The effect of other drugs commonly used in neuropathic pain, such as gabapentin, pregabalin, serotonin-noradrenaline reuptake inhibitors or tricyclic antidepressants, is unknown.

Because spontaneous recovery in typical CTN is rare and the condition is cyclical, with periods of partial or complete remission and recurrence, it is reasonable to encourage patients to adjust the dosage to the frequency of attacks.

Surgical treatment

Our literature search on surgical procedures revealed three Class I prospective RCTs, one Class II prospective cohort study and a handful of Class III studies where the outcome was independently assessed (explicitly stated). The vast majority of the evidence was Class IV.

Question 7. When should surgery be offered?

Evidence: There are no studies dealing specifically with this issue. Some guidance can be found in two studies (Class III) that asked patients after surgery whether they preferred the surgical option [52, 53]. Zakrzewska and Patsalos [53] followed up a cohort of 15 patients for over 15 years who were initially treated medically and then where offered surgery when medical management failed to control their pain. Twelve patients underwent a variety of surgical procedures of whom eight stated that they should have had surgery earlier. In a large study of patients who underwent posterior fossa surgery, >70% of 245 patients treated with microvascular decompression would have preferred to have treatment earlier. [52]

Conclusion: Patients with TN refractory to medical therapy possibly prefer a surgical option early (two Class III).

Question 8. Which surgical technique gives the longest pain-free period with fewest complications and a good quality of life?

Evidence: The evidence from direct comparisons between different surgical procedures is insufficient [54, 55, 56]. Demographics of the patients included in our analysis can be found in Table 3.8 and complications in Table 3.9 and Figure 3.2.

Peripheral techniques: These techniques involve block or destruction of portions of the trigeminal nerve distal to the Gasserian ganglia. Two small RCTs (Class I) on the

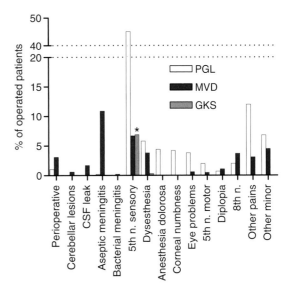

Figure 3.2 Complications of surgery. Frequency (%) of complications with surgical procedures for trigeminal neuralgia. PGL: percutaneous gasserian lesions (includes radiofrequency thermocoagulation, glycerol rhizotomy, balloon compression). MVD: Microvascular Decompression. GKS: Gamma Knife Surgery. Data from 14 trials (Class III) in 2,785 operated patients, detailed in Table 3.9. *: many Class IV studies on GKS report trigeminal sensory disturbances in 9–37% of patients.

use of streptomycin and lidocaine compared with lidocaine alone showed no effect on pain [57, 58]. Other peripheral lesions, including cryotherapy, neurectomies, alcohol injection, phenol injection, peripheral acupuncture, radiofrequency thermocoagulation, have been reported as case-series but with no independent outcome assessment (Class IV). These studies showed that 50% of patients had a recurrence of pain after one year. The morbidity associated with the peripheral procedures was low. There are no data on quality of life.

Percutaneous procedures on the Gasserian ganglion

These techniques [59] (also called percutaneous rhizotomies) involve penetration of the foramen ovale with a cannula and then controlled lesion of the trigeminal ganglion or root by various means: thermal (radiofrequency thermocoagulation, RFT) [60], chemical (injection of glycerol) [61] or mechanical (compression by a balloon inflated into Meckel's cave) [62]. Notwithstanding the thousands of patients who underwent and currently undergo these procedures, we only found uncontrolled

Table 3.8 Surgical treatment: demographics of patients in the Class III studies.

	Mittal et al. 1986 [64]	Zakrzewska et al. 1999 [66]	North et al. 1990 [65]	de Siqueira 2006 [63]	Barker et al. 1996 [75]	Broggi et al. 2000 [76]	Piatt et al. 1984 [77]	Zakrzewska et al. 1993 [78]	Zakrzewska et al. 2005 [52]	Maesawa et al. 2001 [69]	Petit et al. 2003 [70]	Regis et al. 2006 [71]
Technique	RFT	RFT	GR	BC	MVD	MVD	MVD	MVD	MVD	GKS	GKS	GKS
No. of patients	229	48	85	105	1185	250	104	65	245	220	112	110
No. of interventions	280	48	109	105	1204		105	66	245			
Male %	42.9	40		42	40	48.6	42	37.0	34	42.0	37.5	57
Female %	57.1	60		57	60	51.4	63	63.0	66	66.0	62.5	43
Right side %	57	58	59	69	61	54.7	60	65.0		60.9	48	53
Left side %	43	38	41	29	37	45.3	43	33.0		39.1	49	47
Bilateral %	2.8	4	0	1	2	1.4	1	2.0			3	0
mean duration (yrs)	7.5		9.2	9.5	8	8.5	4		6.7	8.0		6
duration 1–5yrs %	50	65										
duration >6yrs %	50	35										
range duration (yrs)	0.4–32		1–50	0.05–30	1–44		1–44			0.4–47	0.2–40	0.7–44
Mean/median age op	60.5		62	61	57	56.0	56.7	54	59	70	64	68
age range at op	18–91		30–89	35–85	5–87	20–74	25–78	21–75	ns	26–92	24–95	29–90
Atypical %	0	35.4	12.9		0	4	0	0	0	7.3	30	7
MS %	5.6	0	4.7		0			0	0			
symptomatic %	5	0			0			6		0		
previous surgery %	ns	ns	39		28	45	32	ns	20	61.4	31	44
pre-op sensory changes %	ns	ns			37			ns	ns	37.8		64
mean/median follow up (months)	44	30	36	7	74		48.3	45	5.3	22	30	
range of follow up months	4–96	7–55	0.5–4.5	0–7	26–246	12–94		37–53	6–240	6–78	8–66	12–?
lost to follow up %	7	10	ns	10	10	4.8	8	5	10	0	14	8
data collection	question.	question.	interview	question. interview	question.	telephone	question.	question.	question.	telephone	telephone	question. exam

case-series. Only two reports on RFT, one on glycerol injection and one on balloon compression employed independent outcome assessors (Class III) [63–66]. Ninety per cent of patients attain pain relief from the procedures. Failure is often due to technical difficulties. At one year 68–85% of patients will be pain-free, but by 3 years this has dropped to 54–64%. At 5 years, around 50% of patients undergoing RFT are still pain-free. Sensory loss after these percutaneous procedures is present in almost half of patients (Figure 3.2). Less than 6% develop troublesome dysesthesiae. The incidence of anaesthesia dolorosa is around 4%. Postoperatively, 12% of patients report discomfort described as burning, heavy, aching or tiring. Corneal numbness, with the risk of keratitis, occurs in 4% of patients. Problems with other cranial nerves are low, and the major perioperative complication is meningitis, mainly aseptic (0.2%). Up to 50% of patients undergoing balloon compression suffer temporary and rarely chronic masticatory problems [63]. Mortality is extremely low [67].

Gamma knife surgery: This is the only non-invasive technique; it aims a focused beam of radiation at the trigeminal root in the posterior fossa. There is one Class I RCT comparing two different regimes [68]. This study showed no major differences between the gamma knife techniques used. Additionally, we found three case-series (Class III) which used independent outcome assessment and provided long-term follow-up [69, 70, 71]. At one year after gamma knife therapy complete pain relief with no medication occurs in up to 69% of patients, falling to 52% at 3 years. Pain relief can be delayed for a mean of one month [72]. In the Class III studies sensory complications averaged 6%. But in large Class IV series facial numbness is reported in 9–37% of patients (though it tends to improve with time) and troublesome sensory loss and/or paraesthesiae are reported in 6–13% (by contrast, anaesthesia dolorosa is practically absent) [56, 72, 73, 74]. No complications outside the trigeminal nerve have been reported. Quality of life improves and 88% are satisfied with the outcome [71].

Microvascular decompression: This is a major neurosurgical procedure and entails craniotomy to reach the trigeminal nerve in the posterior fossa. Vessels compressing the nerve are identified and moved out of contact. The procedure aims to preserve trigeminal nerve function. Five reports were identified which used independent outcome assessment (Class III) [52, 75, 76, 77, 78]. Ninety per cent of patients obtain pain relief and >80% will still be pain-free at 1 year, 75% at 3 years and 73% at 5 years. The average mortality associated with the operation is 0.2%, though it may rise to 0.5% in some reports [67, 79]. Postoperative morbidity is lowest in high-volume units [79]. Up to 4% of patients incur major problems, such as CSF leaks, infarcts or hematomas. Aseptic meningitis is the commonest complication (11%). Diplopia due to 4th or 6th nerve damage is often transient and 7th nerve palsy is rare. Sensory loss occurs in 7% of patients [80]. The major long-term complication is ipsilateral hearing loss, which can be as high as 10% depending on how it is evaluated (i.e., audiometry or subjective reports) (Figure 3.2).

Recurrence of pain after surgery: Recurrence of pain after surgical intervention, particularly ablative procedures, is common, occurring in up to 50% of patients after 5 years. A few studies were identified that dealt with recurrences but their quality was poor and there were no studies that used independent observers [67].

Conclusions: Percutaneous procedures on the Gasserian ganglion, gamma knife and microvascular decompression are possibly effective in the treatment of TN (multiple Class III studies). Microvascular decompression possibly provides the longest pain-free duration compared to other surgical techniques. (multiple Class III studies). The evidence about peripheral techniques is negative (two Class I about streptomycin/lidocaine) or insufficient (Class IV studies for all the other peripheral techniques).

Question 9. Which surgical techniques should be used in patients with multiple sclerosis?

Evidence: There are only small case-series reporting treatment outcomes in patients with multiple sclerosis (MS), with a general tendency towards lesser efficacy in this population. Most authors recommend the use of Gasserian ganglion procedures unless a definitive vascular compression of the trigeminal nerve is identified on MRI. Case reports of the benefit of microvascular decompression in patients with MS suggest poorer efficacy than in non-MS patients [81, 82].

Conclusion: There is insufficient evidence to support or refute the effectiveness of the surgical management of TN in patients with MS. Due to uncertainty of surgical outcome, we believe that in this patients population pharmacotherapy should be carefully assessed and only

Table 3.9 Surgical treatment: complications.

Reference	Procedure	no.	mortality	perioperative	cerebellar oedema or haematoma	sinus thrombosis	CSF leak	reoperation for CSF leak	aseptic meningitis
Mittal Thomas 1985 [64]	RFT	265	1	1					
Zakrzewska et al. 1999 [66]	RFT	31	0						
Zakrzewska et al. 1999 [66]	RFT	17	0						
North et al. 1990 [65]	GR	85	0	4					
de Siqueira et al. 2006 [63]	BC	105	0	1	0	0	0	0	1
total	PGL	503	1	5	0	0	0	0	1
percent			0.2	1	0	0	0	0	0.2
Barker 1996 [75]	MVD	1185	2	31	8	0	17		198
Barker 1997 [80]	MVD								
Broggi et al. 1999 [76]	MVD	250	0	14	1	1	12	5	
Piatt & Wilkins 1984 [77]	MVD	104	1	13	2	2	2		3
Zakrzewska 1993 [78]	MVD	66	0						
Zakrzewska 2005 [52]	MVD	245	0						
total	MVD	1850	3	58	11	3	31	5	201
percent			0.2	3.1	0.6	0.2	1.7	0.3	10.9
Maesawa et al. 2001 [69]	GKS	220	0						
Petit 2003 [70]	GKS	112							
Regis 2006 [71]	GKS	100	0	0					
total	GKS	432	0	0					
percent			0	0					

BC: balloon compression; GKS: gamma knife surgery; GR: glycerol rhizolysis; MVD: microvascular decompression; PGL: percutaneous Gasserian lesions; RFT: radiofrequency thermocoagulation; ad: anaesthesia dolorosa; perioperative complications include: pneumonia, deep vein thrombosis, GI bleed, those expected after any surgery not specific to this surgery; box with number 0 indicates that the text specifically reports absence of that kind of complication; empty box indicates that the complication is not mentioned; we assumed that the Authors would have reported all complications, i.e. in calculating percentages we considered empty boxes equal 0; box with question mark indicates that we did not consider it in calculating percentages because the text left some doubt.

patients with compelling evidence of drug-resistant TN be considered for surgical procedures.

Recommendations on surgical treatment

For patients with TN refractory to medical therapy early surgical therapy may be considered (Level C). Percutaneous procedures on the Gasserian ganglion, gamma knife and microvascular decompression may be considered (Level C). Microvascular decompression may be considered over other surgical techniques to provide the longest duration of freedom from pain (Level C). Although the evidence regarding the surgical management of TN in patients with MS is insufficient, we recommend that before surgical intervention pharmacological avenues be thoroughly explored (good practice point).

bacterial meningitis	4th nerve	6th nerve	diplopia	7th nerve	other	8th perm.	sensory	dysesthesia	ad	5th motor	corneal bumbness	eye	other facial pain	other minor complication
		2		1		1	135	15	22	2	16	10		28
						2	24	2	0	2	0	2	3	
						1	14	4	0	4	0	4	12	
			1				3	3	0		5		33	
0	0	0	0	0	3	7	?	5	0	2		3	?	6
0	0	2	1	1	3	11	178	29	22	10	21	19	48	34
0	0	0.5	0.2	0.2	0.6	2	45	5.8	4.4	2	4.2	3.8	12	6.8
4	13	2		6	1	15		7	0					
							78	48					39	
		6		3	1	8	16	0	2				?	
0	0	0		2	4	15	9	2	0	0	0	0	?	1
						6	12	3	0	4	0	2	7	25
						24	9	10	0	5	0	10		57
4	13	2	6	11	6	68	124	70	2	9	0	12	46	83
0.2	0.7	0.1	0.3	0.6	0.3	3.7	6.7	3.8	0.1	0.5	0	0.6	3.1	4.5
							17	1	0	0				
							7							
							6	4	0	0				
							30	5	0	0				
							6.9	0.3	0	0				

Conclusion and recommendations for future research

The presence of trigeminal sensory deficits, bilateral involvement or abnormal trigeminal reflexes are useful indicators of symptomatic TN, whereas younger age of onset, involvement of the first division, unresponsiveness to treatment and abnormal trigeminal-evoked potentials are not. We recommend the use of carbamazepine or oxcarbazepine as first-choice pharmacological treatment in classical TN, and baclofen or lamotrigine as second choice. Although all the surgical procedures are inherently supported by low-level evidence, the results in thousands of patients indicate that the surgical treatments for trigeminal neuralgia are efficacious and acceptably safe. An evidence-based direct comparison between the different surgical procedures is so far impossible. To briefly differentiate them, however, we may summarize that the percutaneous Gasserian lesions can be safely performed in the elderly but often result in facial numbness, microvascular decompression provides the longest-lasting pain relief but involves some risk of major neurological complications, while gamma knife is the least invasive and safest procedure but pain relief may take one month to develop.

To improve the management of TN, a number of studies would be useful: population-based studies of TN patients to determine true prevalence of STN in TN patients without non-trigeminal symptoms; more prospective cohort surveys of TN patients to determine which clinical characteristics and electrophysiological studies identify STN patients; cohort surveys of CTN patients planning MVD, all having high resolution pre-op MRI with characterization of vascular contact, if any; RCTs of newer drugs compared to carbamazepine with adequate assay sensitivity and focus on all relevant outcomes including tolerability, safety and quality of life; studies directly addressing the definition of pharmacoresistance and the appropriateness of referral to surgery; RCTs in symptomatic TN patients; RCTs comparing different surgical techniques; long-term cohort studies to determine how quickly medical management fails.

Finally, we regard this first attempt to produce joint AAN–EFNS guidelines largely successful. All the specific problems of trigeminal neuralgia and the search results reported here were agreed by American and European authors. Difficulties only arose with the grading of recommendations, which eventually led to two slightly different documents. We feel that AAN and EFNS should make further efforts to overcome the remaining problems. This chapter reports the published results of a joint AAN-EFNS task force [87].

Conflicts of interest

The following authors gave lectures or participated in advisory boards for the following pharmaceutical companies:
GC: Lundbeck, Novartis, Pfizer
GG: Böhringer, GlaxoSmithKline, Pfizer
TN: Allergan, Astra-Zeneca, GlaxoSmithKline
GW: Pharma, Napp, Novartis, Pfizer, Renovis, SchwarzPharma, Wyeth
JMZ: UCB Pharma.

Supplementary material

The following supplementary material is available online: Appendix S1. Comparison of the AAN and EFNS methods of classifying evidence and grading recommendations. Appendix S2. Extended list of references. The material is available as part of the online article from: http://www.blackwell-synergy.com/doi/abs/10.1111/j.1468-1331.2008.02185.x (this link will take you to the article abstract).

Blackwell Publishing are not responsible for the content or functionality of any supplementary materials supplied by the authors. Any queries (other than missing material) should be directed to the corresponding author for the article.

References

1. Merskey, H, Bogduk, N. *Classification of Chronic Pain. Descriptions of Chronic Pain Syndromes and Definitions of Pain Terms*, 1994; IASP Press, Seattle, pp. 59–71.
2. Katusic, S, Williams, DB, Beard, CM *et al.* Epidemiology and clinical features of idiopathic trigeminal neuralgia and glossopharyngeal neuralgia: similarities and differences, Rochester, Minnesota, 1945–1984. *Neuroepidemiology* 1991; **10**:276–81.
3. Headache Classification Subcommittee of the International Headache Society The International classification of Headache Disorders, 2nd edition. *Cephalalgia* 2004; **24**(Suppl 1):9–160.
4. Brainin, M, Barnes, M, Baron, JC, *et al.* Guideline Standards Subcommittee of the EFNS Scientific Committee. Guidance for the preparation of neurological management guidelines by EFNS Scientific Task Forces – revised recommendations 2004. *Eur J Neurol* 2004; **11**:577–81.
5. Cruccu, G, Biasiotta, A, Galeotti, F. *et al.* Diagnostic accuracy of trigeminal reflex testing in trigeminal neuralgia. *Neurology* 2006; **60**:139–41.
6. Goh, BT, Poon, CY, Peck, RH. The importance of routine magnetic resonance imaging in trigeminal neuralgia diagnosis. *Oral Surg Oral Med Oral Pathol Oral Radiol Endod* 2001; **92**:424–9.
7. Majoie, CB, Hulsmans, FJ, Castelijns, JA, *et al.* Symptoms and signs related to the trigeminal nerve: diagnostic yield of MR imaging. *Radiology* 1998; **209**:557–62.
8. Sato, J, Saitoh, T, Notani, K, *et al.* Diagnostic significance of carbamazepine and trigger zones in trigeminal neuralgia. *Oral Surg Oral Med Oral Pathol* 2004; **97**:18–22.
9. De Simone, R, Marano, E, Brescia Morra, V, *et al.* A clinical comparison of trigeminal neuralgic pain in patients with

and without underlying multiple sclerosis. *Neurol Sci* 2005; **26**(Suppl 2):s150–s151.

10. Nomura, T, Ikezaki, K, Matsushima, T, *et al.* Trigeminal neuralgia: differentiation between intracranial mass lesions and ordinary vascular compression as causative lesions. *Neurosurg Rev* 1994; **17**:51–7.

11. Ogutcen-Toller, M, Uzun, E, Incesu, L. Clinical and magnetic resonance imaging evaluation of facial pain. *Oral Surg Oral Med Oral Pathol Oral Radiol Endod* 2004; **97**:652–8.

12. Cruccu, G, Leandri, M, Feliciani, M, *et al.* Idiopathic and symptomatic trigeminal pain. *J Neurol Neurosurg Psychiatry* 1990; **53**:1034–42.

13. Kimura, J. Clinical uses of the electrically elicited blink reflex. *Adv Neurol* 1983; **39**:773–86.

14. Kimura, J, Rodnitzky, RL, Van Allen, MW. Electrodiagnostic study of trigeminal nerve. Orbicularis oculi reflex and masseter reflex in trigeminal neuralgia, paratrigeminal syndrome, and other lesions of the trigeminal nerve. *Neurology* 1970; **20**:574–83.

15. Ongerboer de Visser, BW, Goor, C. Electromyographic and reflex study in idiopathic and symptomatic trigeminal neuralgias: latency of the jaw and blink reflexes. *J Neurol Neurosurg Psychiatry* 1974; **37**:1225–30.

16. Cruccu, G, Leandri, M, Iannetti, GD, *et al.* Small-fiber dysfunction in trigeminal neuralgia: carbamazepine effect on laser-evoked potentials. *Neurology* 2001; **56**:1722–6.

17. Kutluay, E, McCague, K, D_Souza, J, *et al.* Safety and tolerability of oxcarbazepine in elderly patients with epilepsy. *Epilepsy Behav* 2003; **4**:175–80.

18. Nicol, CF. A four year double blind study of tegretol in facial pain. *Headache* 1969; **9**:54–7.

19. Erbay, SH, Bhadelia, RA, Riesenburger, R, *et al.* Association between neurovascular contact on MRI and response to gamma knife radiosurgery in trigeminal neuralgia. *Neuroradiology* 2006; **48**:26–30.

20. Anderson, VC, Berryhill, PC, Sandquist, MA, *et al.* Highresolution three-dimensional magnetic resonance angiography and three-dimensional spoiled gradient-recalled imaging in the evaluation of neurovascular compression in patients with trigeminal neuralgia: a double-blind pilot study. *Neurosurgery* 2006; **58**:666–673.

21. Benes, L, Shiratori, K, Gurschi, M, *et al.* Is preoperative highresolution magnetic resonance imaging accurate in predicting neurovascular compression in patients with trigeminal neuralgia? A single-blind study. *Neurosurg Rev* 2005; **28**:131–6.

22. Korogi, Y, Nagahiro, S, Du, C, *et al.* Evaluation of vascular compression in trigeminal neuralgia by 3D time-of-flight MRA. *J Comput Assist Tomogr* 1995; **19**:879–84.

23. Masur, H, Papke, K, Bongartz, G, *et al.* The significance of three-dimensional MR-defined neurovascular compression

for the pathogenesis of trigeminal neuralgia. *J Neurol* 1995; **242**:93–8.

24. Yamakami, I, Kobayashi, E, Hirai, S, *et al.* Preoperative assessment of trigeminal neuralgia and hemifacial spasm using constructive interference in steady state-threedimensional Fourier transformation magnetic resonance imaging. *Neurol Med Chir (Tokyo)* 2000; **40**:545–56.

25. Sindrup, SH, Jensen, TS. Pharmacotherapy of trigeminal neuralgia. *Clin J Pain* 2002; **18**:22–7.

26. Campbell, FG, Graham, JG, Zilkha, KJ. Clinical trial of carbamazepine (tegretol) in trigeminal neuralgia. *J Neurol Neurosurg Psychiatry* 1966; **29**:265–7.

27. Killian, JM, Fromm, GH. Carbamazepine in the treatment of neuralgia. *Arch Neurol* 1968; **19**:129–36.

28. Rockcliff, BW, Davis, EH. Controlled sequential trials od carbamazepine in trigeminal neuralgia. *Arch Neurol* 1996; **15**:129–36.

29. Wiffen, P, Collins, S, Carroll, D, *et al.* Anticonvulsant drugs for acute and chronic pain. *Cochrane Database Syst Rev* 2005; **3**. Art. No.:CD001133.- pub2. DOI: 10.1002/14651858. CD001133.

30. Wiffen, P, McQuay, H, Moore, R. Carbamazepine for acute and chronic pain. *Cochrane Database Syst Rev* 2005; **3**. Art. No.: CD005451. DOI: 10.1002/14651858.CD005451.

31. McQuay, H, Carroll, D, Jadad, AR, *et al.* Anticonvulsant drugs for management of pain: a systematic review. *BMJ* 1995; **311**:1047–52.

32. Jensen, TS. Anticonvulsants in neuropathic pain: rationale and clinical evidence. *Eur J Pain* 2002; **6**(Suppl A):61–8.

33. Beydoun, A. Clinical use of tricyclic anticonvulsants in painful neuropathies and bipolar disorders. *Epilepsy Behav* 2002; **3**:S18–S22.

34. Beydoun, A. Safety and efficacy of oxcarbazepine: results of randomized, double-blind trials. *Pharmacotherapy* 2000; **20**:152S–158S.

35. Liebel, JT, Menger, N, Langohr, H. Oxcarbazepine in der Behandlung der Trigeminusneuralgie. *Nervenheilkunde* 2001; **20**:461–5.

36. Fromm, GH, Terrence, CF, Chattha, AS. Baclofen in the treatment of trigeminal neuralgia: double-blind study and long-term follow-up. *Ann Neurol* 1984; **15**:240–4.

37. Zakrzewska, JM, Chaudhry, Z, Nurmikko, TJ, *et al.* Lamotrigine (Lamictal) in refractory trigeminal neuralgia: results from a double-blind placebo controlled crossover trial. *Pain* 1997; **73**:223–30.

38. Lechin, F, van der Dijs, B, Lechin, ME, *et al.* Pimozide therapy for trigeminal neuralgia. *Arch Neurol* 1989; **46**:960–3.

39. Lindstrom, P, Lindblom, U. The analgesic effect of tocainide in trigeminal neuralgia. *Pain* 1987; **28**:45–50.

40. Fromm, GH, Aumentado, D, Terrence, CF. A clinical and experimental investigation of the effects of tizanidine in trigeminal neuralgia. *Pain* 1993; **53**:265–71.

41. Kondziolka, D, Lemley, T, Kestle, JR, *et al.* The effect of single-application topical ophthalmic anesthesia in patients with trigeminal neuralgia. A randomized double-blind placebo-controlled trial. *J Neurosurg* 1994; **80**: 993–7.

42. Nurmikko, TJ, Eldridge, PR. Trigeminal neuralgia– pathophysiology, diagnosis and current treatment. *Br J Anaesth* 2001; **87**:117–32.

43. Leandri, M, Parodi, CI, Favale, E. Early trigeminal evoked potentials in tumours of the base of the skull and trigeminal neuralgia. *Electroencephalogr Clin Neurophysiol* 1988; **71**:114–24.

44. Khan, OA. Gabapentin relieves trigeminal neuralgia in multiple sclerosis patients. *Neurology* 1998; **51**:611–14.

45. Solaro, C, Lunardi, GL, Capello, E. An open-label trial of gabapentin treatment of paroxysmal symptoms in multiple sclerosis patients. *Neurology* 1998; **51**:609–11.

46. Solaro, C, Messmer Uccelli, M, *et al.* Low-dose gabapentin combined with either lamotrigine or carbamazepine can be useful therapies for trigeminal neuralgia in multiple sclerosis. *Eur Neurol* 2000; **44**:45–8.

47. Zvartau-Hind, M, Din, MU, Gilani, A, *et al.* Topiramate relieves refractory trigeminal neuralgia in MS patients. *Neurology* 2000; **55**:1587–8.

48. DMKG study group. Misoprostol in the treatment of trigeminal neuralgia associated with multiple sclerosis. *J Neurol*, 2003; **250**:542–45.

49. Reder, AT, Arnason, BG. Trigeminal neuralgia in multiple sclerosis relieved by a prostaglandin E analogue. *Neurology* 1995; **45**:1097–100.

50. Cheshire, WP, Jr Fosphenytoin: an intravenous option for the management of acute trigeminal neuralgia crisis. *J Pain Sympt Manage* 2001; **21**:506–10.

51. Attal, N, Cruccu, G, Haanpaa, M, *et al.* EFNS guidelines on pharmacological treatment of neuropathic pain. *Eur J Neurol* 2006; **13**:1153–69.

52. Zakrzewska, JM, Lopez, BC, Kim, SE, *et al.* Patient reports of satisfaction after microvascular decompression and partial sensory rhizotomy for trigeminal neuralgia. *Neurosurgery* 2005; **56**:1304–11.

53. Zakrzewska, JM, Patsalos, PN. Long-term cohort study comparing medical (oxcarbazepine) and surgical management of intractable trigeminal neuralgia. *Pain* 2002; **95**: 259–66.

54. Aryan, HE, Nakaji, P, Lu, DC, Alksne, JF. Multimodality treatment of trigeminal neuralgia: impact of radiosurgery and high resolution magnetic resonance imaging. *J Clin Neurosci* 2006; **13**:239–44.

55. Burchiel, KJ, Steege, TD, Howe, JF, *et al.* Comparison of percutaneous radiofrequency gangliolysis and microvascular decompression for the surgical management of tic douloureux. *Neurosurgery* 1981; **9**:111–19.

56. Henson, CF, Goldman, HW, Rosenwasser, RH, *et al.* Glycerol rhizotomy versus gamma knife radiosurgery for the treatment of trigeminal neuralgia: an analysis of patients treated at one institution. *Int J Radiat Oncol Biol Phys* 2005; **63**:82–90.

57. Bittar, GT, Graff-Radford, SB. The effects of streptomycin/ lidocaine block on trigeminal neuralgia: a double blind crossover placebo controlled study. *Headache* 1993; **33**:155–60.

58. Stajcic, Z, Juniper, RP, Todorovic, L. Peripheral streptomycin/ lidocaine injections versus lidocaine alone in the treatment of idiopathic trigeminal neuralgia. A double-blind controlled trial. *J Craniomaxillofac Surg* 1990; **18**:243–6.

59. Lopez, BC, Hamlyn, PJ, Zakrzewska, JM. Systematic review of ablative neurosurgical techniques for the treatment of trigeminal neuralgia. *Neurosurgery* 2004; **54**:973–82.

60. Sweet, WH, Wepsic, JG. Controlled thermocoagulation of trigeminal ganglion and rootlets for differential destruction of pain fibers. 1. Trigeminal neuralgia. *J Neurosurg* 1974; **40**:143–56.

61. Hakanson, S. Trigeminal neuralgia treated by the injection of glycerol into the trigeminal cistern. *Neurosurgery* 1981; **9**:638–46.

62. Mullan, S, Lichtor, T. Percutaneous microcompression of the trigeminal ganglion for trigeminal neuralgia. *J Neurosurg* 1983; **59**:1007–12.

63. de Siqueira, SR, da Nobrega, JC, de Siqueira, JT, *et al.* Frequency of postoperative complications after balloon compression for idiopathic trigeminal neuralgia: prospective study. *Oral Surg Oral Med Oral Pathol Oral Radiol Endod* 2006; **102**:e39–e45.

64. Mittal, B, Thomas, DG. Controlled thermocoagulation in trigeminal neuralgia. *J Neurol Neurosurg Psychiatry* 1986; **49**:932–6.

65. North, RB, Kidd, DH, Piantadosi, S, *et al.* Percutaneous retrogasserian glycerol rhizotomy. Predictors of success and failure in treatment of trigeminal neuralgia. *J Neurosurg* 1990; **72**:851–6.

66. Zakrzewska, JM, Sawsan, J, Bulman, JS. A prospective, longitudinal study on patients with trigeminal neuralgia who underwent radiofrequency thermocoagulation of the Gasserian ganglion. *Pain* 1999; **79**:51–8.

67. Zakrzewska, JM. Trigeminal neuralgia, in *Assessment and Management of Orofacial Pain* (eds JM Zakrzewska, SD Harrison), 2002; Elsevier, Amsterdam, pp. 267–76.

68. Flickinger, JC, Pollock, BE, Kondziolka, D, *et al.* Does increased nerve length within the treatment volume improve

trigeminal neuralgia radiosurgery? A prospective double-blind, randomized study. *Int J Radiat Oncol Biol Phys* 2001; **51**:449–54.

69. Maesawa, S, Salame, C, Flickinger, JC, *et al.* Clinical outcomes after stereotactic radiosurgery for idiopathic trigeminal neuralgia. *J Neurosurg* 2001; **94**:14–20.

70. Petit, JH, Herman, JM, Nagda, S, *et al.* Radiosurgical treatment of trigeminal neuralgia: evaluating quality of life and treatment outcomes. *Int J Radiat Oncol Biol Phys* 2003; **56**:1147–53.

71. Regis, J, Metellus, P, Hayashi, M, *et al.* Prospective controlled trial of gamma knife surgery for essential trigeminal neuralgia. *J Neurosurg* 2006; **104**:913–24.

72. Lopez, BC, Hamlyn, PJ, Zakrzewska, JM. Stereotactic radiosurgery for primary trigeminal neuralgia: state of the evidence and recommendations for future reports. *J Neurol Neurosurg Psychiatry* 2004; **75**:1019–24.

73. Shehan, J, Pan, HC, Stroila, M, *et al.* Gamma knife surgery for trigeminal nerulagia: outcomes and prognostic factors. *J Neurosurg* 2005; **102**:434–41.

74. Tawk, RG., Duffy-Fronckowiak, M, Scott, BE, *et al.* Stereotactic gamma knife surgery for trigeminal neuralgia: detailed analysis and treatment response. *J Neurosurg* 2005; **102**:442–9.

75. Barker, FG, Jannetta, PJ, Bissonette, DJ, *et al.* The longterm outcome of microvascular decompression for trigeminal neuralgia. *N Engl J Med* 1996; **334**:1077–83.

76. Broggi, G, Ferroli, P, Franzini, A, *et al.* Microvascular decompression for trigeminal neuralgia: comments on a series of 250 cases, including 10 patients with multiple sclerosis. *J Neurol Neurosurg Psychiatry* 2000; **68**:59–64.

77. Piatt, JH, Jr, Wilkins, RH. Microvascular decompression for tic douloureux. *Neurosurgery* 1984; **15**:456.

78. Zakrzewska, JM, Thomas, DG. Patient's assessment of outcome after three surgical procedures for the management of trigeminal neuralgia. *Acta Neurochir (Wien)* 1993; **122**:225–30.

79. Kalkanis, SN, Eskandar, EN, Carter, BS, *et al.* Microvascular decompression surgery in the United States, 1996 to 2000: mortality rates, morbidity rates, and the effects of hospital and surgeon volumes. *Neurosurgery* 2003; **52**: 1251–61.

80. Barker, FG, Jannetta, PJ, Bissonette, DJ, *et al.* Trigeminal numbness and tic relief after microvascular decompression for typical trigeminal neuralgia. *Neurosurgery* 1997; **40**: 39–45.

81. Broggi, G, Ferroli, P, Franzini, A, *et al.* Operative findings and outcomes of microvascular decompression for trigeminal neuralgia in 35 patients affected by multiple sclerosis. *Neurosurgery* 2004; **55**:830–9.

82. Eldridge, PR, Sinha, AK, Javadpour, M, *et al.* Microvascular decompression for trigeminal neuralgia in patients with multiple sclerosis. *Stereotact Funct Neurosurg* 2003; **81**: 57–64.

83. Hooge, JP, Redekop, WK. Trigeminal neuralgia in multiple sclerosis. *Neurology* 1995; **45**:1294–6.

84. Mursch, K, Schafer, M, Steinhoff, BJ, *et al.* Trigeminal evoked potentials and sensory deficits in atypical facial pain – a comparison with results in trigeminal neuralgia. *Funct Neurol* 2002; **17**:133–6.

85. Majoie, CB, Hulsmans, FJ, Verbeeten, B, *et al.* Trigeminal neuralgia: comparison of two MR imaging techniques in the demonstration of neurovascular contact. *Radiology* 1997; **204**:455–60.

86. Leandri, M, Lundardi, G, Inglese, M. *et al.* Lamotrigine in trigeminal neuralgia secondary to multiple sclerosis. *J Neurol* 2000; **247**:556–8.

87. Cruccu, G, Gronseth, G, Alksne J. *et al.* AAN-EFNS guidelines on trigeminal neuralgia management. *Eur J Neurol* 2008; **15**:1013–28.

CHAPTER 4

Molecular diagnosis of neurogenetic disorders: general issues, Huntington's disease, Parkinson's disease and dystonias

H. F. Harbo,[1] J. Finsterer,[2] J. Baets,[3,4] C. Van Broeckhoven,[4] S. Di Donato,[5] B. Fontaine,[6] P. De Jonghe,[3,4] A. Lossos,[7] T. Lynch,[8] C. Mariotti,[5] L. Schöls,[9] A. Spinazzola,[5] Z. Szolnoki,[10] S. J. Tabrizi,[11] C. Tallaksen,[1] M. Zeviani,[5] J-M. Burgunder[12] and T. Gasser[9]

[1]Oslo University Hospital, and University of Oslo, Oslo, Norway; [2]Rudolfstiftung and Danube University, Krems, Vienna, Austria; [3]University Hospital of Antwerp, Antwerp, Belgium; [4]Institute Born-Bunge and University of Antwerp, Antwerp, Belgium; [5]IRCCS Foundation Neurological Institute Carlo Besta, Milan, Italy; [6]Assistance Publique-Hôpitaux de Paris, Centre de référence des canalopathies musculaires, Groupe Hospitalier Pitié-Salpêtrière, Paris, France; [7]Hadassah University Hospital, Jerusalem, Israel; [8]Mater Misericordiae University, Beaumont & Mater Private Hospitals, Dublin, Ireland; [9]University of Tübingen, Tübingen, Germany; [10]Pandy County Hospital, Gyula, Hungary; [11]Institute of Neurology and National Hospital for Neurology and Neurosurgery, Queen Square, London, UK; [12]University of Bern, Bern, Switzerland

Introduction

In 2001, the first two European Federation of Neurological Societies (EFNS) guideline papers on the molecular diagnosis of inherited neurological diseases were published [1, 2]. Since then, the progress of the field has been nothing less than astounding, so an updated series of guidelines is needed. The aim of this chapter is to provide a summary of the current possibilities and limitations of molecular genetic diagnosis of Huntington's disease, Parkinson's disease and dystonias, and recommendations for genetic testing.

Search strategy

To collect data about the molecular diagnosis of different neurogenetic disorders, literature searches were performed in various electronic databases, such as MEDLINE,

OMIM and GENETEST. Original papers and meta-analyses, review papers and guideline recommendations were reviewed.

Method for reaching consensus

Consensus about the recommendations was reached using a stepwise approach. First, members of the task force met at the EFNS congresses in 2007 and 2008 to discuss the preparations of the guidelines. Second, experts in the specific topics wrote proposals for chapters for each group of disorders. Third, these chapters were distributed and discussed in detail among all task force members until a final consensus had been reached.

Results and recommendations

Recommendations are based on the criteria established by the EFNS [3], with some modifications to account for

European Handbook of Neurological Management: Volume 2, Second Edition. Edited by Nils Erik Gilhus, Michael P. Barnes, Michael Brainin.
© 2012 Blackwell Publishing Ltd. Published 2012 by Blackwell Publishing Ltd.

the specific nature of genetic tests. As genetic testing is, by definition, the gold standard for diagnosing a genetically defined disease (barring the rare event of a lab error), its diagnostic accuracy cannot be tested against another diagnostic method. Therefore, the level of recommendations will be based on the quality of available studies (for a definition see supplementary material [3]) that investigate the proportion of cases of a clinically defined group of patients, which are explained by a specific molecular diagnostic test. As practically all of these studies have been retrospective (i.e. looking for a specific mutation in a previously ascertained and clinically diagnosed cohort of patients) the highest level of recommendation will be at level B [3]. References for the studies forming the basis of our recommendations are given both in tables and in the separate chapters. If only small case series studying genotype–phenotype correlations are available, the level of recommendation will be at level C. If only case reports could be found, but experts still felt that they could give a recommendation, the level of recommendation will be 'good practice point'.

General guidelines for molecular diagnosis of neurogenetic disorders

For the neurologist, the availability of molecular testing for an increasing number of diseases is the most challenging consequence of the recent progress in the molecular genetic sciences. In clinical practice, the benefits and limitations of molecular diagnosis depend on the degree of genetic complexity of the disorder under investigation. Some diseases, such as Huntington's disease, are caused by a specific mutation in a single gene [4], and routine molecular diagnosis can be provided by a simple and cheap polymerase chain reaction (PCR)-based assay. In other cases, such as in the spastic paraplegias, many different mutations in different genes may be causative ('allelic' and 'locus of non-allelic' heterogeneity, respectively). Depending on the size and number of the gene(s) involved, this may render molecular diagnosis costly and time-consuming. The treating physician therefore has to be able to weigh the probability that a test that is ordered will actually detect a mutation against its costs.

Despite these caveats, and despite the fact that today only a small percentage of neurogenetic disorders can be treated effectively, molecular diagnosis is increasingly important because it may provide valuable information for the affected individuals and their families on prognosis and recurrence risks, and may help to make informed decisions on life and family planning.

Today, molecular testing will usually be helpful only if a 'monogenic' disease or a rare monogenic variant of an otherwise common disease is suspected, although considerable progress has also been made in recent years in defining relevant genetic risk factors for the development of the more common 'genetically complex' diseases. Those variants are not discussed here, despite their potential relevance for developing future therapies.

Genetic counselling

The primary goal of molecular diagnosis is always to provide help for the individual patient, client (usually an affected or at-risk individual) and/or the families. Reducing the prevalence of inherited disorders in a population or in subsequent generations may be a secondary effect, but must never be allowed to guide the process of genetic counselling.

A genetic diagnosis affects not only the patient, but also the entire family, so genetic counselling is essential. Sensitive and informed counselling provides patients and families with a foundation for decisions about testing. Patients should be counselled about the clinical features and course of the suspected disease, as well as the potential consequences for the family, taking into consideration the most important genetic parameters such as mode of inheritance, penetrance or variability of clinical expression. Thorough experience in both the human genetics and the specific neurological aspects of a disorder is necessary for qualified counselling.

Informed consent

As is true for all diagnostic procedures, the essential prerequisite for molecular diagnosis is the informed and voluntary consent of the patient. Therefore, the neurologist should establish that a patient or lawful surrogate is capable of comprehending relevant information and of exercising informed choices. Genetic tests should not be performed at the request of members of the patients' families or other third parties (e.g. insurers, employers) without the expressed written consent of the patient.

Confidentiality

Test results suggesting that patients or family members carry mutations that indicate or predict a major neurological disorder or a susceptibility to a neurological disease are highly sensitive. Therefore, rigorous measures to ensure confidentiality should be taken. Test results should never be disclosed to a third party without explicit written consent from the patient or his or her lawful surrogates.

Presymptomatic diagnosis

The identification of disease genes allows for presymptomatic (predictive) diagnosis in many cases. Guidelines for presymptomatic diagnosis have been issued by the International Huntington's Disease Society and the World Federation of Neurology for Huntington's disease [5]. These guidelines, which include extensive pre- and post-test counselling, should be followed in all cases of presymptomatic diagnosis. Involvement of an experienced genetic counsellor is essential. If no clear therapeutic consequences can be envisioned, presymptomatic testing should not be performed in minors.

Other sources of information on genetic testing

Genetic classifications in these guidelines follow, if applicable, the most comprehensive catalogue of human hereditary diseases, the 'Online Mendelian Inheritance in Man (MIM)' (http://omim.nih.org), which is maintained by the National Center of Biotechnology Information (NCBI). 'MIM numbers' are given for easy reference.

Further information can be obtained on several useful websites:
- www.geneclinics.org: 'GeneClinics', a clinical information resource relating genetic testing to diagnosis, management and genetic counselling.
- www.eurogentest.org: 'EuroGentest', an EU-funded network of excellence that intends to harmonize genetic testing across Europe. The website provides information about availability and quality assurance of genetic test.
- www.orpha.net: 'OrphaNet' a searchable database of over 5000 rare diseases, which includes information about genetic testing.
- http://omim.nih.org: 'Online Mendelian Inheritance in Man, OMIM'. Online catalogue of mendelian disorders and traits in humans.

- www.mitomap.org: MITOMAP: a human mitochondrial genome database, Center for Molecular Medicine.

Technical aspects of molecular testing

If the gene causing a neurological disorder is known, molecular diagnosis can be performed by mutational analysis. Only DNA from the affected or at-risk individual is required. Usually, exons that are known to harbour mutations (point mutations or small deletions or insertions) will be amplified from genomic DNA, which has been extracted from peripheral blood leukocytes by PCR. Depending on its type, the mutation will then be detected either by gel electrophoresis (e.g. in the case of trinucleotide repeat expansions) or by DNA sequencing. Heterozygous deletions or multiplications of entire exons, or even entire genes, are increasingly recognized as a rather common type of pathogenic mutation. These mutations cannot be detected by routine sequencing, and must be sought by exon or gene dosage assays. If a gene is very large (genes with more than 30 exons are not uncommon) and mutations are scattered throughout the entire gene, mutational analysis can be very costly and time-consuming with current routinely used methods. In these cases, routine sequence analysis is sometimes offered only for those portions of a gene where mutations are known to be clustered.

The patient confirms his or her informed consent to the procedure in writing. Usually, 10–20 ml of whole blood (usually using EDTA) is drawn. The blood can be sent to a laboratory without freezing or refrigeration. A delay of 3–5 days before DNA extraction is acceptable. It is crucial that the tubes are clearly labelled and that the clinical information, including family history and informed consent, are included in the shipment.

Molecular diagnosis of Huntington's disease

Huntington's disease (HD, MIM 143 100) is the 'prototypic' neurogenetic disorder (Table 4.1). It is usually characterized by the triad of choreic movements, cognitive decline and personality changes. Clinical manifestations may be highly variable, however, and, particularly in juvenile patients, akinesia, rigidity or epileptic seizures may occur. The disease is caused by the expansion of a

Table 4.1 Molecular diagnosis of Huntington's disease (HD) and HD-like disorders.

Disease	Inheritance	Position	Mutation	Gene product	Reference	Remarks	MIM number
Huntington's disease (HD)	AD	4p16.3	Trinuc	Huntingtin	[4]	In HD cases with early onset, large expansions should be searched for by suitable techniques	143 100
Huntington disease-like (HDL) disorder 1 (HDL1)	AD	20pter-p12	Octapeptide expansion	Prion protein	[15]	Only one family, but octapeptide insertions in the PrP gene have been described in other HD-phenocopy series	603 218
Huntington's disease like (HDL) disorder 2 (HDL2)	AD	16q24.3	Trinuc	Junctophilin 3	[12]	Described to date only in patients of African ancestry	606 438
Spinocerebellar (SCA) 17 (HDL4)	AD	6q27	Trinuc	TATA box-binding protein	[13]	Cerebellar atrophy	607 136
Dentatorubro-pallidoluysian atrophy (DRPLA)	AD	12p13.31	Trinuc	Atrophin 1	[14]	Cerebellar atrophy	125 370

AD, autosomal dominant; Trinuc, trinucleotide-repeat expansion.

CAG triplet in the first exon of the *HTT* gene (formerly *HD* or *IT15*), which encodes huntingtin, leading to the formation of an elongated polyglutamine (polyQ) sequence within the protein [4]. This highly polymorphic CAG repeat ranges between 10 and 28 copies on normal chromosomes, but is expanded to a range of 36–121 on HD chromosomes. Adult-onset patients usually have 40–55 repeats, with juvenile-onset patients having more than 60. CAG repeats >40 are fully penetrant, although there is a borderline repeat range between 36 and 39 repeats with reduced penetrance. CAG-repeat lengths vary from generation to generation, with both expansion and contraction, but there is a tendency for repeat lengths to increase, particularly when transmitted through the paternal lineage.

The instability of the CAG expansion with the tendency to expand during transmission underlies the phenomenon of anticipation, i.e. increasing severity and earlier onset of an inherited disease in subsequent generations. CAG-repeat instability during paternal trans-mission is important in the development of large expansions associated with juvenile HD, and approximately 80% of juvenile HD patients inherit the HD gene from their father. There is a negative correlation between the CAG repeat size and age at onset. However, CAG-repeat length does not completely explain variations in age of onset, clinical phenotype or rate of clinical progression, suggesting that other modifying genes may play an important role [6].

Diagnostic testing for HD is usually requested by neurologists when patients present with neurological signs and symptoms of the disease. Adequate genetic counselling and informed consent in these situations are important. In some instances there may be no previously known family history of HD, so the diagnosis comes as a shock to the person and the family. In these situations partners and other family members should be involved early in the diagnostic counselling process, because a confirmatory result of HD has profound implications for siblings and offspring.

Indications and consequences of diagnostic and pre-symptomatic molecular diagnosis have been studied widely in HD (reviewed in Hayden and Bombard [7]). There are numerous issues relating to insurance, employment and genetic discrimination of people at risk for HD [8]. In suspected HD patients with early onset, it must be remembered that parents may carry smaller repeat expansions and thus may manifest the disease after their offspring. Molecular diagnosis in a young individual may therefore result in inadvertent presymptomatic testing in a parent [9].

The wide availability of genetic testing has allowed detailed genotype/phenotype studies in HD. It has also increased our understanding of disorders that present with a similar clinical picture to HD (HD phenocopies) with similar cognitive, psychiatric and motor features, but HD gene negative (reviewed in Wild and Tabrizi [10]). HD phenocopies occur in approximately 1% of large genetic screens of individuals with clinical signs of HD [11].

Expansions of CTG/CAG triplets in a variably spliced exon of the *JPH3* gene (junctophilin 3) are responsible for Huntington disease-like-2 (HDL2, MIM 606 438), but have been found only in rare patients of African ancestry [12]. Spinocerebellar ataxia (SCA) 17 (MIM 607 136) is caused by a CAG-repeat expansion in the TATA-binding protein (TBP) gene, which may resemble HD, and in fact has also been termed HDL-4 [13]. Other autosomal dominant diseases that may mimic HD are dentatorubro-pallidoluysian atrophy (DRPLA, MIM 125 370), which is caused by a CAG-repeat expansion in the atrophin-1 gene [14].

Other disorders that may more rarely resemble HD are SCA1 and SCA3. Inherited prion disorders may also cause HD phenocopies. Specifically, a 192-nucleotide insertion in the prion protein gene encoding 8 octapeptide repeats was described to cause an HD-like disease, and was called HDL-1. It is essentially an early onset prion disease with prominent psychiatric features [15]

Other causes of HD phenocopies include neuroacanthocytosis (MIM 200 150), where autosomal recessive cases have been associated with mutations in the chorein gene on chromosome 9 [16]. Lastly, a recently described disorder in the north of England, neuroferritinopathy (MIM 606 159), caused by mutations in the ferritin light chain polypeptide [17], has clinical features that overlap with HD. Despite the increasing number of recognized

genetic disorders that resemble HD, achieving a genetic diagnosis in HD phenocopy cases is still difficult, with currently less than 3% of cases having a confirmatory genetic result [18].

Summary of recommendations concerning molecular diagnosis of Huntington's disease

Diagnostic testing for HD is recommended (level B) when a patient presents with an otherwise unexplained clinical syndrome of a progressive choreic movement disorder and neuropsychiatric disturbances with or without a positive family history of the disease [11]. Previously established guidelines for presymptomatic molecular diagnosis should be followed [5]. In mutation-negative cases, no general recommendation can be given to test for any of the rare genes causing HD phenocopies.

Molecular diagnosis of inherited parkinsonian syndromes

Until recently, the role of genetic factors in the aetiology of Parkinson's disease (PD) has not been widely recognized. Today it is well established that mutations in several genes are able to cause monogenic forms of PD [19] (Table 4.2).

Point mutations [20], but also duplications and triplications [21], of the gene for α-synuclein (SNCA) can cause an autosomal-dominant form of PD clinically indistinguishable from the sporadic disease (MIM 168 601). Point mutations and triplications are rare and have mostly been found in cases with a strong dominant family history and a high prevalence of dementia, but SNCA duplications can cause late-onset typical PD. Nevertheless, SNCA mutations are very rare [22, 23], so molecular diagnosis should be considered only for clearly familial cases.

Mutations in the gene for leucine-rich repeat kinase 2 (LRRK2; *PARK8*, MIM 607060) are much more common, accounting for approximately 5–15% of familial and (due to reduced penetrance and late onset) 1–2% of apparently sporadic patients with PD [24–26]. In some genetically isolated populations, such as the Ashkenazi Jews or North African Arabs, the proportion of carriers of the most common mutation, *G2019S*, can be as high as 30–40% [27]. The clinical and pathological picture is most

Table 4.2 Molecular diagnosis of Parkinson's disease (PD) and dystonias.

Disease	Locus	Inheritance[1]	Position	Gene product	Reference	Remarks	MIM number
Familial Parkinson's disease, dominant	PARK1/4	AD	4q21	α-Synuclein	[20]	Point mutations as well as gene duplications and triplications found	601 508
	PARK8	AD	12p12	LRRK2, dardarin	[24]	Most common form of dominant PD	607 060
Familial Parkinson's disease, recessive	PARK2	AR	6q25-27	Parkin	[45]	Early onset	602 544
	PARK6	AR	1p33	PINK1	[46]	Early onset	605 909
	PARK7	AD	1p34	DJ-1	[47]	Early onset	606 324
Familial parkinsonism, other	PARK9	AR	1p36	ATP13A2	[48]	Multisystem degeneration, Kufor–Rakeb syndrome	606 693
	GBA	AD	1q21	Glucocerebrosidase	[30, 31]	Heterozygous carriers of pathogenic mutations in Gaucher's associated gene GBA	
Primary torsion dystonia	DYT1	AD	9q34	Torsin A	[32]	A single GAG deletion responsible for all cases	128 100
X-chromosomal dystonia–Parkinson's syndrome	DYT3	XL	Xq11.2	TAF1	[49]	Very rare, only in Filipinos	314 250
Dopa-responsive dystonia	DYT5, DRD	AD	14q22	GTP cyclohydrolase I	[36]	Pharmacological testing should precede genetic testing	600 225
Dopa-responsive dystonia	DYT5, DRD	AR	11p15.5	Tyrosine hydroxylase	[37]	Rare, often more complex phenotype	191 290
Myoclonus dystonia	DYT11, MD	AD	7q21	SGCE	[39]	Maternal imprinting causes reduced penetrance upon maternal transmission	159 900
Rapid-onset dystonia–parkinsonism	DYT12, RDP	AD	19q13	ATP1A3	[42]	Often new mutations	128 235
Paroxysmal dystonia, non-kinesiogenic	DYT8, PNKD	AD	2q35	MR-1	[43]	Attacks precipitated by coffee, alcohol, exertion	118 800
Paroxysmal exercise-induced dystonia	DYT17, PED	AD	1p35	Glut1	[43]	Treatable by ketogenic diet	612 126

AD, autosomal dominant; AR, autosomal recessive; XL, X linked.

commonly indistinguishable from idiopathic PD, as is the age of onset of around 60 years. As the gene is very large and the frequency of mutations varies between populations, the decision to seek molecular diagnosis will depend on the specific circumstances. In Europeans, molecular diagnosis will be feasible only in familial cases suggestive of dominant inheritance, whereas in some populations testing for specific high-prevalence mutations (e.g. the *G2019S* mutation among Ashkenazim) is an already established clinical routine [28].

The most common cause of early onset recessive parkinsonism are mutations in the parkin gene on chromosome 6 (MIM 600116). The vast majority of patients with parkin mutations have disease onset before age 35, so genetic testing should be limited to early onset cases [29]. As a substantial proportion of the mutations are whole exon or even whole gene rearrangements, genetic testing should include appropriate methods for the detection of these copy number variations. Mutations in the other recessive PD genes (*PINK1*, MIM 605909, and *DJ1*, MIM 606324) cause a clinically similar phenotype of early onset parkinsonism; their prevalence is less well studied, but appears to be lower than that of parkin. Only homozygous or compound heterozygous mutations can be confidently considered to be pathogenic, because the role of heterozygous parkin mutations as risk factors for sporadic PD is still controversial.

In addition, mutations in the gene for glucocerebrosidase (GBA), which causes Gaucher's disease in homozygous or compound heterozygous individuals, clearly increase the risk for PD [30, 31]. Again there is a markedly higher prevalence of these variants in Ashkenazi Jews. Penetrance of these variants is not, however, clear, making counselling difficult.

Summary of recommendations concerning molecular diagnosis of Parkinson's disease

In Europeans, molecular testing for LRRK2 is recommended (level B) in familial cases with dominant inheritance of parkinsonian syndromes [25, 26]. Testing for the LRRK2 *G2019S* mutation is recommended in familial and sporadic patients in specific populations, e.g. in the Ashkenazim or North African Arabs (level B) [27].

Testing for mutations in recessive PD genes (parkin, *PINK1*, *DJ-1*) is recommended (level B) in families suggestive of recessive inheritance (affected sib pairs)

or in sporadic patients with very early onset (<35 years) [29].

Molecular diagnosis of the dystonias

A growing number of genes are being found to cause familial forms of dystonias (see Table 4.2). Consequently, molecular diagnosis of these disorders is becoming increasingly important, although in clinical practice it is still restricted to a relatively small proportion of patients with a clearly defined familial disease, while the contribution of genetic factors in the more common focal dystonias remains poorly defined.

The primary dystonias

Primary dystonias are characterized by involuntary muscle contractions, leading to twisting and repetitive movements with no discernible structural or metabolic cause.

A specific mutation, a deletion of the trinucleotide GAG (encoding glutamic acid) in the gene for torsin A on chromosome 9q34, is the major cause of early onset generalized dystonia (DYT1) [32]. Patients usually have disease onset in an extremity before age 24, with relatively rapid progression to a generalized form. Molecular testing will identify the mutation in more than 90% of Ashkenazi Jewish patients with this phenotype, due to a common founder mutation [33], and in about 30–50% of non-Jewish white patients [34], although no specific mutations are found in those with the much more common adult-onset cervical or cranial dystonias [35]. Due to the reduced penetrance of about 30% of the GAG deletion, *DYT1* mutation carriers often have a negative family history, and a positive family history is NOT a prerequisite for genetic testing in a patient with a typical phenotype. This also must be taken into account during the counselling process.

Dystonia-plus syndromes

The genetic basis of several relatively rare forms of hereditary dystonia with specific additional clinical or biochemical features has been elucidated, providing the basis for molecular diagnosis. In clinically typical patients, mutations can be detected in about 40–80% of cases, whereas genetic testing is rarely helpful in clinically unclassifiable patients.

Dopa-responsive dystonia (DRD) (MIM 128 230) is most commonly caused by point mutations or exon deletions in the gene for GTP cyclohydrolase I (dominant with reduced penetrance) [36], but can rarely also be due to recessive mutations in the genes for tyrosine hydroxylase [37]. Given these genetic parameters, family history is not a good predictor for a positive test result, so a convincing response to levodopa treatment should be documented before molecular testing is initiated. Other than by their dopa response, these patients cannot reliably be distinguished from DYT1 patients. Conspicuous diurnal fluctuations of symptom severity (getting worse during the day) may be a clue. The clinical picture may also mimic cerebral palsy (CP), which is why any patient with CP should be given a trial with levodopa. In a patient with typical DRD, mutations can be found in up to 80% of cases [38].

If the phenotype is characterized by very rapid ('lightning-like') myoclonic jerks affecting predominantly the muscles of the trunk, neck and proximal extremities, a diagnosis of *myoclonus–dystonia* (M-D) (MIM 159 900) should be considered [39]. If the family history is positive, mutations are identified in the gene for ε-sarcoglycan (*SGCE*) in a significant proportion of cases [40, 41]. The genetic basis of some other dystonia-plus syndromes, such as 'rapid-onset dystonia-parkinsonism' (MIM 128 235) [42], or some of the paroxysmal dystonias [43], has also been elucidated, but these disorders are exceedingly rare and mutational analysis is usually offered only in a research setting.

Summary of recommendations concerning molecular diagnosis of dystonia

Molecular testing for the GAG deletion in the *TOR1A* gene is recommended (level B) in patients with early (<26 years) and limb-onset generalized dystonia regardless of family history. Testing for *GCH1* mutations including gene dosage studies is recommended (level B) in patients with early onset generalized dystonia with a clear response to levodopa, regardless of the family history. Sequencing and gene dosage studies of the *SGCE* gene is recommended (level B) only in patients with a typical clinical picture of M-D syndrome *and* a suggestive family history. No genetic tests can be recommended in more common focal dystonias (good practice point).

Other movement disorders

Sequence analysis of the ATP7B gene causing *Wilson's disease* (MIM 277 900) can confirm the diagnosis in a patient with a diagnosis of WD for family counselling purposes [44]. Blood and urine chemistry, particularly copper excretion in urine, is still the diagnostic method of choice in most cases. Approximately 55% of patients in a white population harbour mutations in exons 7, 8, 14, 15 or 18. Identification of a mutation in an index patient allows presymptomatic testing in other at-risk family members, which may be particularly important in this disease, because preventive and therapeutic measures are of help.

Although *essential tremor* (MIM 190 300) and the *restless legs syndrome* (MIM 102 300) are the most common movement disorders, no disease-causing mutations that would allow genetic testing have been identified so far. Identified risk alleles cannot be used for individual diagnosis.

Conclusion

The presented guidelines on the molecular diagnosis of Huntington's disease, Parkinson's disease and dystonias have been created in response to the increasing amount of data on the genetic background of these disorders, the increasing need of the clinical neurologist to learn about the genetic perspective and the increasing availability of commercial molecular diagnosis for the daily routine.

Conflicts of interest

Member of this Task Force have no conflicts of interest related to the recommendations given in this paper.

References

1. Gasser, T, Dichgans, M, Finsterer, J, *et al.* EFNS Task Force on Molecular Diagnosis of Neurologic Disorders: guidelines for the molecular diagnosis of inherited neurologic diseases. Second of two parts. *Eur J Neurol* 2001; **8**:407–24.
2. Gasser, T, Dichgans, M, Finsterer, J, *et al.* EFNS Task Force on Molecular Diagnosis of Neurologic Disorders: guidelines

for the molecular diagnosis of inherited neurologic diseases. First of two parts. *Eur J Neurol* 2001; **8**:299–314.

3. Brainin, M, Barnes, M, Baron, JC, *et al.* Guidance for the preparation of neurological management guidelines by EFNS scientific task forces–revised recommendations 2004. *Eur J Neurol* 2004; **11**:577–81.

4. The Huntington's Disease Collaborative Research Group. A novel gene containing a trinucleotide repeat that is expanded and unstable on Huntington's disease chromosomes. *Cell* 1993; **72**:971–83.

5. International Huntington Association (IHA) and the World Federation of Neurology (WFN) Research Group on Huntington's Chorea. Guidelines for the molecular genetics predictive test in Huntington's disease. *Neurology* 1994; **44**:1533–6.

6. Wexler, NS, Lorimer, J, Porter, J, *et al.* Venezuelan kindreds reveal that genetic and environmental factors modulate Huntington's disease age of onset. *Proc Natl Acad Sci U S A* 2004; **101**:3498–503.

7. Hayden, MR, Bombard, Y. Psychosocial effects of predictive testing for Huntington's disease. *Adv Neurol* 2005; **96**: 226–39.

8. Harper, PS, Gevers, S, de Wert, G, Creighton, S, Bombard, Y, Hayden, MR. Genetic testing and Huntington's disease: issues of employment. *Lancet Neurol* 2004; **3**:249–52.

9. Scheidtmann, K, Schwarz, J, Holinski, E, Gasser, T, Trenkwalder, C. Paroxysmal choreoathetosis–a disorder related to Huntington's disease? *J Neurol* 1997; **244**:395–8.

10. Wild, EJ, Tabrizi, SJ. Huntington's disease phenocopy syndromes. *Curr Opin Neurol* 2007; **20**:681–7.

11. Kremer, B, Goldberg, P, Andrew, SE, *et al.* A worldwide study of the Huntington's disease mutation. The sensitivity and specificity of measuring CAG repeats. *N Engl J Med* 1994; **330**:1401–6.

12. Holmes, SE, O'Hearn, E, Rosenblatt, A, *et al.* A repeat expansion in the gene encoding junctophilin-3 is associated with Huntington disease-like 2. *Nat Genet* 2001; **29**:377–8.

13. Stevanin, G, Fujigasaki, H, Lebre, AS, *et al.* Huntington's disease-like phenotype due to trinucleotide repeat expansions in the TBP and JPH3 genes. *Brain* 2003; **126**(Pt 7):1599–603.

14. Koide, R, Ikeuchi, T, Onodera, O, *et al.* Unstable expansion of CAG repeat in hereditary dentatorubral-pallidoluysian atrophy (DRPLA). *Nat Genet* 1994; **6**:9–13.

15. Moore, RC, Xiang, F, Monaghan, J, *et al.* Huntington disease phenocopy is a familial prion disease. *Am J Hum Genet* 2001; **69**:1385–8.

16. Ueno, S, Maruki, Y, Nakamura, M, *et al.* The gene encoding a newly discovered protein, chorein, is mutated in chorea-acanthocytosis. *Nat Genet* 2001; **28**:121–2.

17. Curtis, AR, Fey, C, Morris, CM, *et al.* Mutation in the gene encoding ferritin light polypeptide causes dominant adult-onset basal ganglia disease. *Nat Genet* 2001; **28**:350–4.

18. Wild, EJ, Mudanohwo, EE, Sweeney, MG, *et al.* Huntington's disease phenocopies are clinically and genetically heterogeneous. *Mov Disord* 2008; **23**:716–20.

19. Gasser, T. Update on the genetics of Parkinson's disease. *Mov Disord* 2007; **22**(suppl 17):S343–50.

20. Polymeropoulos, MH, Lavedan, C, Leroy, E, *et al.* Mutation in the alpha-synuclein gene identified in families with Parkinson's disease. *Science* 1997; **276**:2045–7.

21. Singleton, AB, Farrer, M, Johnson, J, *et al.* alpha}-Synuclein locus triplication causes Parkinson's disease. *Science* 2003; **302**:841.

22. Berg, D, Niwar, M, Maass, S, *et al.* Alpha-synuclein and Parkinson's disease: implications from the screening of more than 1,900 patients. *Mov Disord* 2005; **20**:1191–4.

23. Ibanez, P, Lesage, S, Janin, S, *et al.* Alpha-synuclein gene rearrangements in dominantly inherited parkinsonism: frequency, phenotype, and mechanisms. *Arch Neurol* 2009; **66**:102–8.

24. Zimprich, A, Biskup, S, Leitner, P, *et al.* Mutations in LRRK2 cause autosomal-dominant parkinsonism with pleomorphic pathology. *Neuron* 2004; **44**:601–7.

25. Berg, D, Schweitzer, K, Leitner, P, *et al.* Type and frequency of mutations in the LRRK2 gene in familial and sporadic Parkinson's disease*. *Brain* 2005; **128**(Pt 12):3000–11.

26. Gilks, WP, Abou-Sleiman, PM, Gandhi, S, *et al.* A common LRRK2 mutation in idiopathic Parkinson's disease. *Lancet* 2005; **365**:415–16.

27. Ozelius, LJ, Senthil, G, Saunders-Pullman, R, *et al.* LRRK2 G2019S as a cause of Parkinson's disease in Ashkenazi Jews. *N Engl J Med* 2006; **354**:424–5.

28. Orr-Urtreger, A, Shifrin, C, Rozovski, U, *et al.* The LRRK2 G2019S mutation in Ashkenazi Jews with Parkinson disease: is there a gender effect? *Neurology* 2007; **69**:1595–602.

29. Lucking, CB, Durr, A, Bonifati, V, *et al.* Association between early-onset Parkinson's disease and mutations in the parkin gene. *N Engl J Med* 2000; **342**:1560–7.

30. Aharon-Peretz, J, Rosenbaum, H, Gershoni-Baruch, R. Mutations in the glucocerebrosidase gene and Parkinson's disease in Ashkenazi Jews. *N Engl J Med* 2004; **351**:1972–7.

31. Mata, IF, Samii, A, Schneer, SH, *et al.* Glucocerebrosidase gene mutations: a risk factor for Lewy body disorders. *Arch Neurol* 2008; **65**:379–82.

32. Ozelius, LJ, Hewett, JW, Page, CE, *et al.* The early-onset torsion dystonia gene (DYT1) encodes an ATP-binding protein. *Nat Genet* 1997; **17**:40–8.

33. Bressman, SB, Sabatti, C, Raymond, D, *et al.* The DYT1 phenotype and guidelines for diagnostic testing. *Neurology* 2000; **54**:1746–52.

34. Valente, EM, Warner, TT, Jarman, PR. *et al.* The role of DYT1 in primary torsion dystonia in Europe. *Brain* 1998; **121**: 2335–9.

35. Grundmann, K, Laubis-Herrmann, U, Bauer, I. *et al.* Frequency and phenotypic variability of the GAG deletion of the DYT1 gene in an unselected group of patients with dystonia. *Arch Neurol* 2003; **60**:1266–70.

36. Ichinose, H, Ohye, T, Matsuda, Y, *et al.* Characterization of mouse and human GTP cyclohydrolase I genes. Mutations in patients with GTP cyclohydrolase I deficiency. *J Biol Chem* 1995; **270**:10062–71.

37. Knappskog, PM, Flatmark, T, Mallet, J, Ludecke, B, Bartholome, K. Recessively inherited L-DOPA-responsive dystonia caused by a point mutation (Q381K) in the tyrosine hydroxylase gene. *Hum Mol Genet* 1995; **4**:1209–12.

38. Hagenah, J, Saunders-Pullman, R, Hedrich, K, *et al.* High mutation rate in dopa-responsive dystonia: detection with comprehensive GCHI screening. *Neurology* 2005; **64**: 908–11.

39. Zimprich, A, Grabowski, M, Asmus, F, *et al.* Mutations in the gene encoding epsilon-sarcoglycan cause myoclonus-dystonia syndrome. *Nat Genet* 2001; **29**:66–9.

40. Asmus, F, Zimprich, A, Tezenas Du, MS, *et al.* Myoclonus-dystonia syndrome: epsilon-sarcoglycan mutations and phenotype. *Ann Neurol* 2002; **52**:489–92.

41. Grunewald, A, Djarmati, A, Lohmann-Hedrich, K, *et al.* Myoclonus-dystonia: significance of large SGCE deletions. *Hum Mutat* 2008; **29**:331–2.

42. de Carvalho, AP, Sweadner, KJ, Penniston, JT, *et al.* Mutations in the Na⁺/K⁺-ATPase alpha3 gene ATP1A3 are associated with rapid-onset dystonia parkinsonism. *Neuron* 2004; **43**:169–75.

43. Suls, A, Dedeken, P, Goffin, K, *et al.* Paroxysmal exercise-induced dyskinesia and epilepsy is due to mutations in SLC2A1, encoding the glucose transporter GLUT1. *Brain* 2008; **131**(Pt 7):1831–44.

44. Tanzi, RE, Petrukhin, K, Chernov, I, *et al.* The Wilson disease gene is a copper transporting ATPase with homology to the Menkes disease gene. *Nat Genet* 1993; **5**:344–50.

45. Kitada, T, Asakawa, S, Hattori, N, *et al.* Mutations in the parkin gene cause autosomal recessive juvenile parkinsonism. *Nature* 1998; **392**:605–8.

46. Valente, EM, bou-Sleiman, PM, Caputo, V, *et al.* Hereditary early-onset Parkinson's disease caused by mutations in PINK1. *Science* 2004; **304**:1158–60.

47. Bonifati, V, Rizzu, P, van Baren, MJ, *et al.* Mutations in the DJ-1 gene associated with autosomal recessive early-onset parkinsonism. *Science* 2003; **299**:256–9.

48. Ramirez, A, Heimbach, A, Grundemann, J, *et al.* Hereditary parkinsonism with dementia is caused by mutations in ATP13A2, encoding a lysosomal type 5 P-type ATPase. *Nat Genet* 2006; **38**:1184–91.

49. Makino, S, Kaji, R, Ando, S, *et al.* Reduced neuron-specific expression of the TAF1 gene is associated with X-linked dystonia-parkinsonism. *Am J Hum Genet* 2007; **80**:393–406.

CHAPTER 5

Molecular diagnosis of mitochondrial disorders

J. Finsterer,[1] H. F. Harbo,[2] J. Baets,[3,4] C. Van Broeckhoven,[4] S. Di Donato,[5] B. Fontaine,[6] P. De Jonghe,[3,4] A. Lossos,[7] T. Lynch,[8] C. Mariotti,[5] L. Schöls,[9] A. Spinazzola,[5] Z. Szolnoki,[10] S. J. Tabrizi,[11] C. Tallaksen,[1] M. Zeviani,[5] J-M. Burgunder[12] and T. Gasser[9]

[1]Rudolfstiftung and Danube University, Krems, Vienna, Austria; [2]Oslo University Hospital, and University of Oslo, Oslo, Norway; [3]University Hospital of Antwerp, Antwerp, Belgium; [4]Institute Born-Bunge and University of Antwerp, Antwerp, Belgium; [5]IRCCS Foundation Neurological Institute Carlo Besta, Milan, Italy; [6]Assistance Publique-Hôpitaux de Paris, Centre de référence des canalopathies musculaires, Groupe Hospitalier Pitié-Salpêtrière, Paris, France; [7]Hadassah University Hospital, Jerusalem, Israel; [8]Mater Misericordiae University, Beaumont & Mater Private Hospitals, Dublin, Ireland; [9]University of Tübingen, Tübingen, Germany; [10]Pandy County Hospital, Gyula, Hungary; [11]Institute of Neurology and National Hospital for Neurology and Neurosurgery, Queen Square, London, UK; [12]University of Bern, Bern, Switzerland

Objectives

These European Federation of Neurological Sciences (EFNS) guidelines on the molecular diagnosis of mitochondrial disorders (MIDs) are designed to summarize the possibilities and limitations of molecular genetic techniques and to provide diagnostic criteria for deciding in which cases a molecular diagnostic work-up is indicated.

Background

Since the publication of the first EFNS guidelines about the molecular diagnosis of inherited neurological diseases in 2001, [1, 2] rapid progress has been made in this field, necessitating the creation of an updated version of these guidelines, which follows the EFNS Scientific Committee recommendations for guideline papers [3].

Search strategy

To collect data about planning, conditions and performance of molecular diagnosis of MIDs a literature search in various electronic databases, such as Cochrane library, MEDLINE, OMIM, GENETEST and EMBASE, was carried out and original papers, meta-analyses, review papers and guideline recommendations were reviewed.

Method for reaching consensus

Consensus about the recommendations was reached using a stepwise approach. First, task force members met at the EFNS congresses in 2007 and 2008 to discuss the preparations of the guidelines. Second experts in the field of genetics of MIDs wrote a guideline proposal. Third these recommendations were discussed in detail among all task force members until a final consensus had been reached.

European Handbook of Neurological Management: Volume 2, Second Edition. Edited by Nils Erik Gilhus, Michael P. Barnes, Michael Brainin.
© 2012 Blackwell Publishing Ltd. Published 2012 by Blackwell Publishing Ltd.

Results and recommendations

Recommendations follow the criteria established by the EFNS [3], with some modifications to account for the specific nature of genetic tests. As genetic testing is by definition the gold standard for diagnosing a genetic disease, its diagnostic accuracy cannot be tested against another diagnostic method. Therefore, the level of recommendations will be based on the quality of available studies [3], which investigate the proportion of cases of a clinically defined group of patients that are explained by a specific molecular diagnostic test. As almost all of these studies have a retrospective design and look for a specific mutation in a previously ascertained and clinically diagnosed cohort of patients, the highest achievable recommendation level will be B [3]. If only small case series studying genotype–phenotype correlations are available, the level of recommendation will be C. If only case reports are available but experts still provided recommendations, the recommendation level is assessed as 'good practice point'.

Genetic background of mitochondrial disorders

Primary MIDs comprise a wide range of phenotypes due to mutations in mitochondrial DNA (mtDNA)- or nuclear DNA (nDNA)-located genes, resulting in respiratory chain (RC) or oxidative phosphorylation (OXPHOS) defects. MIDs are regarded as one of the most common groups of inherited metabolic disease. The prevalence of mtDNA point mutations that cause disease is estimated as 1/5000–10 000 and the frequency of mtDNA mutations among healthy individuals as 1/200 [4]. The high prevalence of MIDs urges the clinician to accurately diagnose these disorders, which is difficult in the light of highly variable and overlapping phenotypes, transmission patterns and molecular backgrounds. In the following, the authors describe the genetic background of human MIDs and provide recommendations for a diagnostic algorithm for a suspected MID.

Classification

The RC/OXPHOS pathway is conducted by two separated and partially autonomous genetic systems, the nuclear and mitochondrial genomes. Identification of mutations in mtDNA- or nDNA-located genes provides the basis for the current classification of MIDs (Figure 5.1). The first group of MIDs is due to sporadic or maternally transmitted mtDNA mutations and the second to sporadic or Mendelian nDNA mutations.

The mtDNA mutations

Mutations may be present in either all mtDNA copies (homoplasmy) or only part of the mtDNA copies (heteroplasmy, coexistence of wild-type and mutated mtDNA within a mitochondrion, cell or tissue). Only if mutated mtDNA copies accumulate above a critical threshold (threshold level), which depends on age and tissue, is a mutation phenotypically expressed. This is why heteroplasmic mtDNA mutations behave as 'recessive-like' traits. However, phenotypic expression may vary according to the intrinsic pathogenicity of a mutation, its tissue distribution, the variable aerobic energy demand of different tissues or organs, and the individual genetic background. Homoplasmic mtDNA mutations usually manifest as single-organ- or even single-cell-type failure, similar to retinal ganglion cells in Leber's hereditary optic neuropathy (LHON), which may be due to primary or secondary LHON mutations. The mtDNA mutations may be either classified as large-scale rearrangements or as point mutations.

The mtDNA rearrangements

Large-scale mtDNA rearrangements comprise single, partial, mtDNA deletions and, more rarely, partial duplications, which are both heteroplasmic. Three main phenotypes are associated with single mtDNA deletions: *Kearns–Sayre syndrome* (KSS), *sporadic progressive external ophthalmoplegia* (PEO) and *Pearson's syndrome* (Table 5.1).

KSS is a sporadic, severe MID characterized by the invariant triad of PEO, pigmentary retinopathy and onset at age over 20 years. Frequent additional features include progressive cerebellar syndrome, dysphagia, myopathy, endocrine dysfunction (diabetes, short stature), atrioventricular block, increased cerebrospinal fluid (CSF) protein or lactacidosis. Muscle biopsy shows ragged-red fibres (RRFs).

Sporadic PEO is characterized by bilateral ptosis and ophthalmoplegia, and is frequently associated with muscle weakness and exercise intolerance. Occasio-

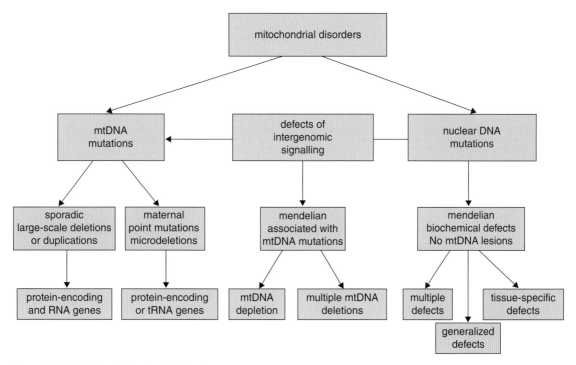

Figure 5.1 Classification of mitochondrial disorders.

nally, patients present with additional signs, such as ataxia, cataract, retinitis pigmentosa, hearing loss or cardiomyopathy.

Pearson's syndrome is a rare sporadic disorder of early infancy, characterized by sideroblastic anaemia, or pancytopenia and exocrine pancreatic insufficiency. Infants surviving into childhood develop features of KSS.

MIDs caused by mtDNA rearrangements occur in most cases sporadically, most likely during oogenesis in the patient's mother, during repair of damaged mtDNA rather than during replication [5]. However, mother-to-child transmission of mtDNA duplications or deletions has been occasionally reported and may be responsible for a 5% recurrence risk of these conditions. The mtDNA rearrangements in KSS or PEO can be exclusively detected in muscle and in Pearson's syndrome exclusively in blood cells.

The mtDNA point mutations
Point mutations are usually maternally inherited, and either affect protein synthesis genes (tRNA, rRNA) or

protein-encoding genes. Mutated protein synthesis genes impair translation of all mtDNA-encoded polypeptides, thereby determining defects of multiple respiratory chain complexes (RCCs). Mutated protein-encoding genes affect only the activity of the RCC that houses the mutant protein. Despite the large number of pathogenic mtDNA mutations in humans (see www.mitomap.org), only four of them occur frequently in various human populations: 3243A>G (MELAS), 8344A>G (MERRF), 8993T>G (NARP) and 11778A>G (LHON) (see Table 5.1).

Mitochondrial encephalomyopathy, lactic acidosis and *stroke-like episodes* (MELAS) is characterized by the presence of stroke-like episodes (SLEs), lactacidosis or RRFs. Additional manifestations include confusional state, dementia, psychosis, seizures, basal ganglia calcification, migraine-like headache, ataxia, optic atrophy, retinopathy, deafness, myopathy, diabetes, intestinal pseudo-obstruction or cardiomyopathy. In approximately 80% of the cases MELAS syndrome is caused by the heteroplasmic transition 3243A>G in the $tRNA^{Leu(UUR)}$ gene. The second most frequent mtDNA mutation is the transition 3271T>C. Other mtDNA genes mutated in MELAS

Table 5.1 Mitochondrial disorders (MIDs).

MID syndrome	MIM	Trait	Type of mutation	Mutated gene	Characteristics	Reference
Mitochondrial DNA (mtDNA)						
Chronic progressive external ophthalmoplegia (mtPEO)	252110, 220110, 252011	Spor	deletion, duplication	*mtDNA*	Molecular genetic analysis should be performed in muscle	[16]
Kearns–Sayre syndrome (KSS)	530000	Spor	deletion, duplication	*mtDNA*	Molecular genetic analysis should be performed in muscle	[17]
Pearson's bone marrow–pancreas syndrome (PS)	557000	Spor	deletion, duplication	*mtDNA*	Surviving infants may later develop KSS	[18]
Mitochondrial encephalomyopathy with lactacidosis and 'stroke-like episodes' (MELAS)	540000	Mat	np 3243, np 3271	*tRNA^Leu*	Other point mutations have been described in rare cases	[19]
Myoclonus epilepsy with ragged red fibres (MERRF)	545000	Mat	np 8344	*tRNA^lys*	Other point mutations have been described in rare cases	[20]
Leber's hereditary optic neuropathy (LHON)	535000	Mat	np 117 78, np 3460, np 14 484	RCCI subunits	Other point mutations have been described in rare cases	[21]
Neurogenic weakness, ataxia and retinitis pigmentosa (NARP)	551500	Mat	np 8993	*ATPase6*	High percentage of this mutation may lead to MILS	[22]
Maternally inherited Leigh's syndrome (MILS)	590050	Mat	np 8993	*ND1-6, COXIII, ATPase6, tRNAs*		[23]
Nuclear DNA (nDNA)						
Autosomal dominant PEO (AD PEO)	157640, 609283, 609286, 610131	AD	4q34-35, 10q23-24, 15q25	*ANT1, PEO1, POLG1*	Multiple deletions of mtDNA	[24–27]
Autosomal recessive PEO (AR PEO)		AR	15q25	*POLG1*	Multiple deletions of mtDNA	[28]
Myoneurogastrointestinal encephalomyopathy (MNGIE)	603041	AR	22q13-qter	*TYMP*	Multiple deletions or depletion of mtDNA	[29]
Mitochondrial depletion syndrome (DPS)	609560	AR	15q25, 2p23-p21, 4q34-35, 8q23.1, 13q12.2-q13 2p11.2, 2p13, 16q22	*POLG1, MPV17, PEO1, RRM2B, SUCLA2, SUCLG1, DGUOK, TK2*	Reduction of the mtDNA copy number	[30, 31]
Leigh's syndrome (LS)	256000	AR	22q13, 17p13-p12 17p12-p11.2, 10q24, 5p15, 9q34 and others	*SCO2, SCO1, COX10, COX15 NDUFS, NDUFV, SDH, SURF1, CoQ*	Genetically extremely heterogeneous	[32]
Dominant optic atrophy (ADOA)	165500	AD	3q28	*OPA1*	Mitochondrial biogenesis	[33]

Note that this compilation of MIDs is not complete. The selection of MIDs was chosen at random to provide the reader with an orientation. The speed at which progress is achieved in molecular genetics allows such tables to become outdated quickly. In cases of doubt, it is recommended that current publications or specialized centres be consulted. For many if not most of the diseases listed here, mutations in other currently unknown genes may also be responsible.

AD, autosomal dominant; AR, autosomal recessive; X, X-chromosomal; mat, maternal transmission; np, nucleotide position; spor, sporadic; Pm, point mutation; Del, deletion; Ins, insertion; np, nucleotide position.

syndrome include the *tRNA^Phe^*, *tRNA^Val^*, *tRNA^Lys^*, *COXII*, *COXIII*, *ND1*, *ND5*, *ND6* and *rRNA* genes. The genotype–phenotype correlation of the 3243A>G mutation is weak, because it also causes maternally inherited PEO, KSS, maternally inherited diabetes and deafness (MIDD), Leigh's syndrome (LS), cluster headache, isolated myopathy, cardiomyopathy, renal failure or pancreatitis. In single cases polymerase-gamma (POLG1) mutations may cause MELAS.

Myoclonus epilepsy with ragged-red fibres (MERRF) is a maternally inherited encephalomyopathy characterized by myoclonus, epilepsy, myopathy, cerebellar ataxia, deafness and dementia. Additional features include SLEs, basal ganglia atrophy, optic atrophy, pyramidal signs, polyneuropathy, cardiomyopathy, heart block, pancytopenia and lipomatosis. The most common mtDNA mutation causing MERRF syndrome is the *tRNA^Lys^* transition 8344A>G. Other mutations include the transitions 8356T>C and 8363G>A. Although the genotype–phenotype correlation of the 8344A>G mutation is tighter than that of other mtDNA mutations, it also causes phenotypes as different as LS, isolated myoclonus, familial lipomatosis or myopathy.

Neurogenic weakness, ataxia and retinitis pigmentosa (NARP) is a maternally inherited MID arising from the heteroplasmic m8993T>G transversion in the *ATPase6* gene. If the heteroplasmy rate is >95%, the mutation manifests as *maternally inherited Leigh's syndrome (MILS)*. MILS patients present with dysmorphism, developmental delay, epilepsy, SLEs, dystonia, ophthalmoparesis, myopathy and polyneuropathy. NARP and MILS may coexist within the same family. RRFs are absent on muscle biopsy (see Table 5.1).

LHON is characterized by bilateral, acute or subacute loss of vision due to retinal ganglia degeneration or demyelination, or optic nerve atrophy. Occasionally, the heart is affected. The penetrance of LHON is approximately 40% in males and approximately 10% in females, and onset is usually in the second or third decade. Although about 20 mtDNA mutations potentially cause LHON, 3 are most commonly found in all human populations – np11778 (*ND4*, RCCI), np3460 (*ND1*, RCCI) and np14484 (*ND6*, RCCI) – and considered as high risk (primary LHON mutations).

Several other mtDNA point mutations have been detected in single patients or pedigrees affected with a number of other syndromic and non-syndromic MIDs.

Disorders due to nDNA mutations

MIDs due to nDNA mutations include disorders due to:
- mutated RC subunits
- mutated ancillary proteins
- faulty intergenomic communication affecting mtDNA maintenance or expression
- mutated biosynthetic enzymes for lipids or cofactors
- coenzyme Q deficiency
- defective mitochondrial trafficking or transport machinery
- mutant proteins involved in mitochondrial biogenesis
- defective apoptosis.

Mutations in RC subunits

Although 72 of 85 subunits of the RC/OXPHOS system are nDNA encoded, nDNA mutations have been identified only in a minority of MID patients so far. Isolated RCCI deficiency is the most common biochemical finding in RC/OXPHOS disease, being present in about a third of the cases. RCCI is composed of 45 proteins, 7 of which are encoded by mtDNA and the remaining 38 by nDNA genes. Only 20% of children with RCCI deficiency harbour mtDNA mutations in ND genes, suggesting that the vast majority of patients carry mutations in nDNA genes encoding for structural RCCI subunits (*NDUFS1*, *NDUFS2*, *NDUFS3*, *NDUFS4*, *NDUFS6*, *NDUFS8*, *NDUFV1*, *NDUFV2*) or assembly factors. Most patients present with variable non-syndromic MIDs with early onset hypotonia, cardiomyopathy, ataxia, psychomotor delay or LS. Lactacidosis is only a rare finding. RCCI deficiency may be also due to splice-site mutations in the *NDUFA11* or *NDUFA1* gene respectively, phenotypically presenting as encephalocardiomyopathy with severe lactacidosis [6]. RCCII is composed of four nuclear encoded subunits. Mutations in *SDHA*, encoding for the 75-kDa flavoprotein subunit of RCCII, have been occasionally found in children with LS or late-onset neurodegenerative disease. An autosomal recessive (AR), non-lethal phenotype of severe psychomotor retardation, extrapyramidal signs, dystonia, athetosis and ataxia, mild axial hypotonia and dementia has been associated with a missense mutation in *UQCRQ*, one of ten nDNA genes encoding RCCIII subunits. Mutations in nDNA-encoded COX (cytochrome *c* oxidase) subunits are assumed to be incompatible with extrauterine survival. Recently, however, a mutation in one such subunit, COX6B1, manifested clinically as severe infantile encephalomyopathy [7].

Mutations in ancillary proteins

Mitochondrial ancillary proteins are not part of RCCs, but involved in RCC formation, turnover and function. The most important gene of this group is *SURF1*, which encodes a COX assembly factor. Mutations in *SURF1* manifest as LS and are associated with severe COX deficiency. The SURF-1 protein is absent in all tissues of these individuals [8].

Leigh's syndrome, also known as subacute necrotizing encephalomyopathy, is an early onset, infantile, progressive neurodegenerative disorder manifesting as severe psychomotor delay, cerebellar and pyramidal signs, seizures, dystonia, respiratory abnormalities, ophthalmoparesis, floppy infant, polyneuropathy, cardiomyopathy, dysphagia or recurrent vomiting. Magnetic resonance imaging (MRI) shows focal symmetrical lesions in the basal ganglia, thalamus, brain stem, cerebellum and posterior columns of the spinal cord. RRFs are consistently absent, except for cases with MILS [9]. LS is a genetically heterogeneous entity. In some cases it is attributable to mtDNA mutations (8993T>G 'NARP/MILS'), in others it arises from an AR defect. In still other cases LS is X-linked or sporadic in case of the mutated E1α subunit of the pyruvate dehydrogenase complex.

All defects described to date in patients with LS affect the terminal oxidative metabolism and are likely to impair ATP production. Other COX assembly factors include SCO1, SCO2, COX10 and COX15. These factors are associated with COX-deficient LS or other multisystem fatal infantile disorders, in which encephalopathy is accompanied by cardiomyopathy (SCO2, COX15), nephropathy (COX10) or hepatopathy (SCO1). Mutations in a RCCIII assembly protein, known as BCS1L, have also been associated with Leigh-like syndromes as well as with lethal infantile growth retardation, aminoaciduria, cholestasis, iron overload, lactacidosis and early death (GRACILE) syndrome. Only in two RCCV assembly genes have pathogenic mutations been identified so far. A mutation in the *ATP12* gene was associated with congenital lactacidosis and fatal infantile multisystem disease, involving brain, liver, heart and muscle. *TMEM70* mutations cause isolated ATP synthase deficiency and neonatal encephalocardiomyopathy. LS may be also due to mutations in the RCCI assembly factors *NDUFA12L*, *NDUFAF1* and *C6ORF66*. *NDUFA12L* mutations manifest phenotypically as leucencephalopathy.

NDUFAF1 and *C6ORF66* mutations manifest as severe cardioencephalomyopathy. Mutated *C20ORF7* was made responsible for lethal congenital encephalopathy due to a RCCI defect.

Defects of intergenomic signalling

Maintenance of mtDNA requires the concerted activity of several nuclear-encoded factors that participate in its replication as part of the mitochondrial replisome or by supplying dNTPs (deoxynucleotide triphosphates) to mitochondria. Autosomal disorders classified as defects of nuclear–mitochondrial intergenomic communication may be associated with either accumulation of multiple, large-scale mtDNA deletions in muscle or brain (mtDNA breakage syndromes) or severe reduction of the mtDNA copy number (mtDNA depletion syndromes). A third group is due to mutations in genes encoding for proteins involved in the protein synthesis machinery.

Some mtDNA breakage syndromes
Autosomal dominant and autosomal recessive PEO

Most autosomal PEO families carry heterozygous mutations in *ANT1*, *POLG1* or *twinkle* genes. *ANT1* encodes the muscle-heart-specific mitochondrial adenine nucleotide translocator, *twinkle* a mtDNA helicase and *POLG1* the catalytic subunit of the mtDNA-specific POLGI. *POLG1* is particularly relevant because *POLG1* mutations are the most common cause of Mendelian PEO (see http://dirapps.niehs.nih.gov/polg/index.cfm) and specific mutations or a combination of mutations can be associated with a wide phenotypic spectrum, including autosomal dominant or recessive PEO, sensory ataxic neuropathy, dysarthria, ophthalmoplegia (SANDO), spinocerebellar ataxia and epilepsy with or without ophthalmoplegia (SCAE), or recessive, infantile Alpers–Huttenlocher syndrome (AHS), characterized by myopathy, hepatopathy, epilepsy, migraine, intractable seizures and learning disability (hepatic poliodystrophy). Although *POLG1*-associated PEO is characterized by accumulation of multiple mtDNA deletions, the latter syndromes are associated with tissue-specific mtDNA depletion. The phenotypic heterogeneity is explained by the complexity of the enzyme, which is composed of an exonuclease domain with predominantly proofreading functions and a polymerase domain that primarily mediates mtDNA replication. Only a single heterozygous dominant mutation has been identified in *POLG2*, which encodes the accessory subunit of POLG.

MNGIE

MNGIE is an AR multisystem disorder of young adults characterized by PEO, peripheral neuropathy, leucencephalopathy and severe gastrointestinal dysmotility, leading to cachexia and early death. The gene responsible for MNGIE encodes the thymidine phosphorylase (*TYMP*), which promotes the phosphorylation of thymidine into thymine and deoxyribose phosphate. *TYMP* defects result in systemic accumulation of thymidine and deoxyuridine, which leads to a deoxynucleotide pool imbalance and mtDNA instability, manifesting as point mutations, multiple mtDNA deletions or partial mtDNA depletion in the skeletal muscle. In addition, an MNGIE-like phenotype has been associated with *POLG1* mutations [10].

The mtDNA depletion syndromes

The mtDNA depletion syndromes (DPSs) are early onset, age-specific syndromes and are phenotypically quite heterogeneous. Southern blot analysis or quantitative polymerase chain reaction (PCR) is diagnostic, demonstrating severe reduction of mtDNA in affected tissues (up to 98% in most severe forms). So far, DPSs have been linked to mutations in nine genes (*POLG1*, *PEO1* (*twinkle*), thymidine kinase (*TK2*), *DGUOK*, *SUCLA2*, *SUCLG1*, *MPV17*, *RRM2B*). Three main clinical presentations are differentiated: a myopathic, an encephalomyopathic and a hepatocerebral form. Consistent with the different phenotypes, mtDNA depletion affects either a specific tissue (most commonly muscle, liver or brain) or multiple organs including the heart, brain or kidneys.

Myopathic DPS

Myopathic DPS is due to mutations in the *TK2* or *RRM2B* genes. *TK2* mutations are responsible for approximately 20% of the myopathic DPS cases. Recently, mutations in p53-dependent ribonucleotide reductase (*RRM2B*) have been reported in children with mtDNA depletion in muscle, manifesting as developmental delay, microcephaly or proximal tubulopathy.

Encephalomyopathic DPS

Encephalomyopathic DPS is due to mutations in the *SUCLA2* or *SUCLG1* genes. *SUCLA2* encodes the β subunit of the ADP-forming succinyl-CoA ligase and manifests phenotypically as Leigh-like syndrome with muscle hypotonia, lactacidosis, dystonia and moderate methylmalonic aciduria. Mutations in the *SUCLG1* gene, encoding for the α subunit of GDP-forming succinyl-CoA ligase, manifest as fatal infantile lactacidosis, dysmorphism and methylmalonic aciduria with muscle and liver mtDNA depletion.

Hepatocerebral DPS

Hepatocerebral DPS is due to mutations in the *PEO1*, *POLG1*, *DGUOK* or *MPV17* genes [11]. Phenotypes of *POLG1* mutations were described above. Mutations in PEO1 may cause an AR Alpers-like phenotype. *MPV17* encodes a protein of unknown function located at the inner mitochondrial membrane. *MPV17* mutations manifest as hepatic failure, hypoglycemia, muscle hypotonia, ataxia, dystonia or polyneuropathy. Hepatocerebral DPS from *MPV17* mutations is allelic to Navajo neurohepatopathy, characterized by hepatopathy, polyneuropathy, corneal anaesthesia and scarring, acral mutilation, leucencephalopathy, failure to thrive, recurrent metabolic acidosis and intercurrent infections. Mutations in the *TYMP* gene may cause not only multiple mtDNA deletions but also mtDNA depletion, manifesting clinically as MNGIE.

Defective mitochondrial protein synthesis machinery

Autochthonous translation of mtDNA proteins is carried out by an apparatus composed of tRNAs and rRNAs, synthesized *in situ* from mtDNA genes and numerous proteins encoded by nDNA genes, including 77 mitoribosomal proteins, several tRNA maturation enzymes (e.g. pseudouridylate synthases), the aminoacyl-tRNA synthetases, and translation initiation, elongation and termination factors. Mutations in the *PUS1* gene, encoding the catalytic domain of the pseudouridylate synthase-1, cause AR mitochondrial myopathy and sideroblastic anaemia (MLASA). Mutations in *DARS2*, the gene encoding mitochondrial aspartyl-tRNA synthetase, manifest as leucencephalopathy with brain-stem and spinal cord involvement and lactacidosis (LBSL) syndrome. Lactacidosis in LBSL is due to RC defects in tissues other than muscle or skin. Missplicing mutations in the *RARS2* gene, encoding the mitochondrial arginine-tRNA synthetase, cause AR pontocerebellar hypoplasia

(PCH) with prenatal onset, cerebellar/pontine atrophy/hypoplasia, microcephaly, neocortical atrophy and severe psychomotor impairment. Impaired RNA processing is speculated to preferentially affect the brain because of a tissue-specific vulnerability of the splicing machinery.

Defects of the mitochondrial lipid milieu

Barth's syndrome is an X-linked recessive disorder characterized by mitochondrial myopathy, hypertrophic or dilated cardiomyopathy, left ventricular hypertrabeculation/non-compaction, growth retardation, leukopenia and methylglutaconic aciduria. Barth's syndrome is caused by mutations in the *G4.5* gene, encoding one of the tafazzins. Tafazzins are homologous to phospholipids acyltransferases, which are involved in the biosynthesis of cardiolipin, a phospholipid species present on the inner mitochondrial membrane. Cardiolipin is required for structural stabilization and functional modulation of RCCV.

CoQ defects

Coenzyme Q_{10} (CoQ), a lipid-soluble component of virtually all cell membranes, transports electrons from RCCI and RCCII to RCCIII, and is essential for stabilizing RCCIII. Primary CoQ deficiency causes AR MIDs, such as: encephalomyopathy with recurrent myoglobinuria, brain involvement and RRF; a severe infantile multisystem MID; cerebellar ataxia; and LS. So far, mutations in *COQ2*, *COQ8* (*ADCK3*, *CABC1*, *PDSS1*, *PDSS2* genes encoding enzymes of CoQ biosynthesis) have been reported in primary CoQ deficiency [12]. Secondary CoQ deficiency is due to mutations in genes not directly related to ubiquinone biosynthesis, such as *APTX* (cerebellar ataxia), *ETFDH* (pure myopathy) and *BRAF* (cardiofaciocutaneous syndrome). In most CoQ deficiencies, however, the causative molecular genetic defect remains elusive. Most cases with primary or secondary CoQ deficiency respond favourably to CoQ supplementation.

Mitochondrial transport machinery defects

An example of such a defect is the X-linked deafness–dystonia syndrome (DDS), also known as Mohr–Tranebjaerg syndrome, which is due to loss-of-function mutations in the *DDP1/TIMM8A* gene. The gene product is involved in the transport and sorting of proteins to the inner mitochondrial membrane [13]. RC functions and ATP synthesis are intact. Patients present with childhood-onset progressive deafness, dystonia, spasticity, mental deterioration and blindness. Another example is X-linked sideroblastic anaemia with ataxia (XLSA/A), which is caused by partial inactivating mutations in the *ABCB7* gene, encoding the ATP-binding cassette transporter, responsible for iron transport from the mitochondrion to the cytoplasm [14]. Mutations in the mitochondrial phosphate carrier SLC25A3, which transports inorganic phosphate into the mitochondrial matrix, causes congenital lactacidosis, hypertrophic cardiomyopathy and muscle hypotonia. Biochemically, muscular ATP synthesis is impaired.

Defects in mitochondrial biogenesis

Mitochondria are dynamic organelles, which constantly fuse and divide. The equilibrium between fusion and fission controls the morphology of mitochondria, which appear as either corpuscles or elongated tubules depending on the prevailing process. Mitochondrial fusion requires the concerted action of three GTPases: mitofusin-1, mitofusin-2 and OPA1. For mitochondrial fission, another GTPase called dynamin-like protein-1 (DLP1) is required. Mutations in 'fusion' genes result in fragmentation of mitochondria due to ongoing fission but absent fusion. Disruption of 'fission' proteins results in tubulized, 'spaghetti-like' mitochondria, excessively long and interconnected. Heterozygous mutations in *MFN2* cause Charcot–Marie–Tooth neuropathy 2A, whereas *OPA1* mutations cause an optic atrophy, the most common inherited optic atrophy. In some cases, optic atrophy may be associated with myopathy, PEO, hearing loss, ataxia and accumulation of multiple mtDNA deletions in skeletal muscle. *DLP1* mutations may cause severe infantile encephalopathy and, as *DLP1* is also expressed in peroxisomes, elongated mitochondria and elongated peroxisomes.

Defects in apoptosis

Mutated proteins involved in mitochondrial apoptosis have been recently shown to cause MIDs. In a patient with developmental delay, asymmetrical cerebral atrophy, epilepsy, hemiplegia and myopathy with COX deficiency, a mutation in the *FASTKD2* gene, encoding a protein localized in the mitochondrial inner compartment, was the cause. Preliminary data indicate that this protein plays a role in mitochondrial apoptosis. In staurosporine-induced apoptosis experiments, decreased nuclear fragmentation was detected in treated mutant fibroblasts.

Summary of recommendations for the genetic diagnosis of MIDs

Diagnostic work-up for suspected MID is a stepwise procedure. The first step comprises a comprehensive individual and family history and clinical investigations by specialists in neurology, ophthalmology, otology, endocrinology, cardiology, gastroenterology, nephrology, haematology or dermatology. Important instrumental procedures include chemical investigations of the serum, CSF and urine, electrophysiological investigations, functional and imaging studies of the cerebrum, and muscle biopsy [15]. Based on their results the probability for

the presence of an MID can be assessed according to the Nijmegen, Bernier or Walker diagnostic criteria.

In a second step clinicians need to decide whether an individual phenotype conforms to any of the syndromic MIDs or represents a non-syndromic MID; they also need to determine if the phenotype occurred sporadically or followed a Mendelian or maternal trait of inheritance.

Genetic testing is the third step and depends on steps 1 and 2. If the phenotype suggests syndromic MID due to mtDNA point mutations (MELAS, MERRF, NARP, LHON), DNA microarrays using allele-specific oligonucleotide hybridization, real-time PCR or single-gene sequencing are indicated. If the phenotype suggests syndromic MID due to mtDNA deletion (mtPEO, KSS, Pearson's syndrome), mtDNA analysis starts with restriction fragment length polymorphism (RFLP) or Southern blot analysis from appropriate tissues (Figure 5.2). The

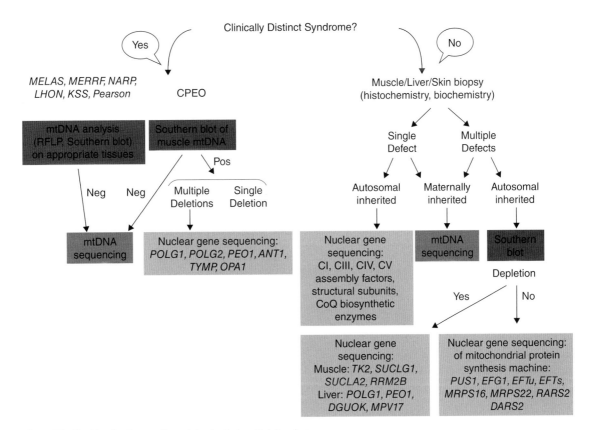

Figure 5.2 Algorithm for the genetic analysis of mitochondrial disorders.

mtDNA deletions with low heteroplasmy rate may be detected only by long-range PCR. If neither a single deletion nor multiple deletions are found, mtDNA sequencing is recommended (level B).

If RFLP or Southern blot analysis of muscle mtDNA detects multiple mtDNA deletions (breakage syndromes), sequencing of POLG I (autosomal dominant and recessive PEO, SANDO, SCAE, AHS), POLG2, PEO1 (autosomal dominant PEO), ANT1 (autosomal dominant PEO), TYMP (MNGIE) or OPA1 (ADOAD) genes should follow (level B). Sequencing should start with the POLG1 gene, because it is the most likely to carry a mutation. Sequencing of TYMP should be done only if serum thymidine is elevated. If the phenotype suggests LS, appropriate nDNA genes encoding RCC subunits or assembly factors (SURF1, ATP12, SCO1, SCO2, COX10, COX15 NDUFS, NDUFV, SDH) need to be sequenced. Sequencing of appropriate nDNA genes is also required if the phenotype suggests GRACILE (TMEM70), IOSCA (PEO1), MLASA (PUS1), Barth's syndrome (TAZ/G4.5), DDS/Mohr–Tranebjaerg syndrome (DDP1), MIRAS (POLG1) or CMT2A (mitofusin-2) (level B).

If an individual presents with a non-syndromic phenotype, biochemical investigations of the most affected tissues (muscle, liver, brain, skin) should clarify whether a single or multiple RCCs are defective (level B). If a single autosomally inherited defect is present, sequencing of appropriate structural subunits or assembly factors of RCCI, -III, -IV or -V is necessary (level B). If biochemical investigations in muscle tissue suggest CoQ deficiency, sequencing of genes involved in CoQ biosynthesis (most frequently ETFDH) should be carried out (level B).

If the single RRC defect is maternally inherited, one should proceed with mtDNA sequencing of appropriate mtDNA genes (level B). If multiple, autosomally inherited, biochemical defects are found, a Southern blot analysis or quantitative PCR should clarify whether or not there is mtDNA depletion. If these investigations detect mtDNA depletion, sequencing of the TK2 or RRM2B genes is indicated if the skeletal muscle is the primary affected organ and if creatine kinase is elevated. If muscle and cerebrum are the most affected organs, sequencing of the SUCLG1, SUCLA2 genes is indicated. If the liver is the primary affected organ, sequencing of the POLG1, PEO1, DGUOK and MPV17 genes is recommended (level B – see Figure 5.2).

If Southern blot analysis fails to detect mtDNA depletion, sequencing of genes involved in the mitochondrial protein synthesis machinery (PUS1, EFT, EFG1, EFTs, MRPS16, MRPS22, RARS2, DARS2) is recommended (level B – see Figure 5.2). Corresponding proteins of the MRPS22, EFT and EFTs genes are involved in the initiation and elongation of peptides during protein synthesis and are responsible for the group of elongation factor disorders. In the case of PCH and severe psychomotor impairment, the RARS2 gene should be sequenced for splice-site mutations. Sequencing of the FASTKD2 gene is required in cases with developmental delay, asymmetrical cerebral atrophy, epilepsy, hemiplegia and myopathy with COX deficiency after exclusion of other causes of COX deficiency. Tissues most frequently chosen are blood (MELAS, MERRF, NARP, LHON, Pearson's syndrome) or muscle (KSS). Availability of muscle tissue for mtDNA analysis is mandatory in patients with phenotypes associated with large-scale mtDNA rearrangements, which can be easily missed in leukocytes except for Pearson's syndrome. Alternative tissues for DNA analysis are cells from the urine sediment, buccal mucosa or hair follicles. Although mtDNA point mutations can also be detected in blood samples, the percentage of mutant mtDNA in maternally inherited phenotypes associated with heteroplasmic point mutations is often significantly higher in muscle than in other tissues.

Conclusions

This second part of the EFNS guidelines should not only familiarize clinicians with mitochondrial genetics but also enable them to implement this knowledge into daily practice, when investigating the genotype of a suspected MID. The guidelines should allow them to collect essential and useful information for geneticists and confront neurologists with the limitations of the methods and incompleteness of currently available insight despite the rapid developments in the understanding of mitochondrial genetics. As a result of the rapid developments in this field, there will be a need to regularly update these guidelines, provide information about laboratories offering genetic testing and provide algorithms for cost-effective diagnostic work-up. To stimulate and support ongoing or future basic or therapeutic trials for human MIDs, Europe-wide networks and databases are required.

References

1. Gasser, T, Dichgans, M, Finsterer, J, et al. EFNS task force on molecular diagnosis of neurologic disorders. Guidelines for the molecular diagnosis of inherited neurologic diseases. First of two parts. *Eur J Neurol* 2001; **8**:407–24.

2. Gasser, T, Dichgans, M, Finsterer, J, et al. EFNS Task Force on Molecular Diagnosis of Neurologic Disorders: guidelines for the molecular diagnosis of inherited neurologic diseases. First of two parts. *Eur J Neurol* 2001; **8**:299–314.

3. Brainin, M, Barnes, M, Baron, JC, et al. Guidance for the preparation of neurological management guidelines by EFNS scientific task forces–revised recommendations 2004. *Eur J Neurol* 2004; **11**:577–81.

4. Elliott, HR, Samuels, DC, Eden, JA, Relton, CL, Chinnery, PF. Pathogenic mitochondrial DNA mutations are common in the general population. *Am J Hum Genet* 2008; **83**: 254–60.

5. Krishnan, KJ, Reeve, AK, Samuels, DC, et al. What causes mitochondrial DNA deletions in human cells? *Nat Genet* 2008; **40**:275–9.

6. Berger, I, Hershkovitz, E, Shaag, A, Edvardson, S, Saada, A, Elpeleg, O. Mitochondrial complex I deficiency caused by a deleterious NDUFA11 mutation. *Ann Neurol* 2008; **63**:405–8.

7. Massa, V, Fernandez-Vizarra, E, Alshahwan, S, et al. Severe infantile encephalomyopathy caused by a mutation in COX6B1, a nucleus-encoded subunit of cytochrome c oxidase. *Am J Hum Genet* 2008; **82**:1281–9.

8. Tiranti, V, Jaksch, M, Hofmann, S, et al. Loss-of-function mutations of SURF-1 are specifically associated with Leigh syndrome with cytochrome c oxidase deficiency. *Ann Neurol* 1999; **46**:161–6.

9. Tsao, CY, Herman, G, Boué, DR, et al. Leigh disease with mitochondrial DNA A8344G mutation: case report and brief review. *J Child Neurol* 2003; **18**:62–4.

10. Van Goethem, G, Dermaut, B, Löfgren, A, Martin, JJ, Van Broeckhoven, C. Mutation of POLG is associated with progressive external ophthalmoplegia characterized by mtDNA deletions. *Nat Genet* 2001; **28**:211–12.

11. Spinazzola, A, Zeviani, M. Disorders of nuclear-mitochondrial intergenomic communication. *Biosci Rep* 2007; **27**:39–51.

12. Mollet, J, Delahodde, A, Serre, V, et al. CABC1 gene mutations cause ubiquinone deficiency with cerebellar ataxia and seizures. *Am J Hum Genet* 2008; **82**:623–30.

13. Blesa, JR, Solano, A, Briones, P, Prieto-Ruiz, JA, Hernández-Yago, J, Coria, F. Molecular genetics of a patient with Mohr-Tranebjaerg Syndrome due to a new mutation in the DDP1 gene. *Neuromol Med* 2007; **9**:285–91.

14. Boultwood, J, Pellagatti, A, Nikpour, M, et al. The role of the iron transporter ABCB7 in refractory anemia with ring sideroblasts. *PLoS ONE* 2008; **3**:e1970.

15. Finsterer, J, Jarius, C, Eichberger, H. Phenotypic variability in 130 adult patients with respiratory chain disorders. *J Inherit Metab Dis* 2001; **24**:560–76.

16. Holt, IJ, Harding, AE, Morgan-Hughes, JA. Deletions of muscle mitochondrial DNA in patients with mitochondrial myopathies. *Nature* 1988; **331**:717–19.

17. Zeviani, M, Moraes, CT, DiMauro, S, et al. Deletions of mitochondrial DNA in Kearns-Sayre syndrome. *Neurology* 1988; **38**:1339–46.

18. Rotig, A, Colonna, M, Bonnefont, JP, et al. Mitochondrial DNA deletion in Pearson's marrow/pancreas syndrome. *Lancet* 1989; **i**:902–3.

19. Goto, Y, Nonaka, I, Horai, S. A mutation in the tRNA(Leu)(UUR) gene associated with the MELAS subgroup of mitochondrial encephalomyopathies. *Nature* 1990; **348**:651–3.

20. Shoffner, JM, Lott, MT, Lezza, AM, Seibel, P, Ballinger, SW, Wallace, DC. Myoclonic epilepsy and ragged-red fiber disease (MERRF) is associated with a mitochondrial DNA tRNA(Lys) mutation. *Cell* 1990; **61**:931–7.

21. Wallace, DC, Singh, G, Lott, MT, et al. Mitochondrial DNA mutation associated with Leber's hereditary optic neuropathy. *Science* 1988; **242**:1427–30.

22. Holt, IJ, Harding, AE, Petty, RK, Morgan-Hughes, JA. A new mitochondrial disease associated with mitochondrial DNA heteroplasmy. *Am J Hum Genet* 1990; **46**:428–33.

23. Tatuch, Y, Christodoulou, J, Feigenbaum, A, et al. Heteroplasmic mtDNA mutation (T>G) at 8993 can cause Leigh disease when the percentage of abnormal mtDNA is high. *Am J Hum Genet* 1992; **50**:852–8.

24. Suomalainen, A, Kaukonen, J, Amati, P, et al. An autosomal locus predisposing to deletions of mitochondrial DNA. *Nat Genet* 1995; **9**:146–51.

25. Kaukonen, J, Zeviani, M, Comi, GP, Piscaglia, MG, Peltonen, L, Suomalainen, A. A third locus predisposing to multiple deletions of mtDNA in autosomal dominant progressive external ophthalmoplegia. *Am J Hum Genet* 1999; **65**:256–61.

26. Zeviani, M, Servidei, S, Gellera, C, Bertini, E, DiMauro, S, DiDonato, S. An autosomal dominant disorder with multiple deletions of mitochondrial DNA starting at the D-loop region. *Nature* 1989; **339**:309–11.

27. Servidei, S, Zeviani, M, Manfredi, G, et al. Dominantly inherited mitochondrial myopathy with multiple deletions of mitochondrial DNA: clinical, morphologic, and biochemical studies. *Neurology* 1991; **41**:1053–9.

28. Van Goethem, G, Schwartz, M, Löfgren, A, Dermaut, B, Van Broeckhoven, C, Vissing, J. Novel POLG mutations in progressive external ophthalmoplegia mimicking

mitochondrial neurogastrointestinal encephalomyopathy. *Eur J Hum Genet* 2003; **11**:547–9.

29. Nishino, I, Spinazzola, A, Hirano, M. Thymidine phosphorylase gene mutations in MNGIE, a human mitochondrial disorder. *Science* 1999; **283**:689–92.

30. Copeland, WC. Inherited mitochondrial diseases of DNA replication. *Annu Rev Med* 2008; **59**:131–46.

31. Zeviani, M, Di Donato, S. Mitochondrial disorders. *Brain* 2004; **127**:2153–72.

32. Oldfors, A, Tulinius, M. Mitochondrial encephalomyopathies. *Handbook Clin Neurol* 2007; **86**:125–65.

33. Alexander, C, Votruba, M, Pesch, UE, *et al.* OPA1, encoding a dynamin-related GTPase, is mutated in autosomal dominant optic atrophy linked to chromosome 3q28. *Nat Genet* 2000; **26**:211–15.

CHAPTER 6

Molecular diagnosis of ataxias and spastic paraplegias

T. Gasser,[1] J. Finsterer,[2] J. Baets,[3,4,4'] C. Van Broeckhoven,[4,4'] S. Di Donato,[5] B. Fontaine,[6]
P. De Jonghe,[3,4] A. Lossos,[7] T. Lynch,[8] C. Mariotti,[9] L. Schöls,[1] A. Spinazzola,[10]
Z. Szolnoki,[11] S. J. Tabrizi,[12] C.M.E. Tallaksen,[13] M. Zeviani,[10] J-M. Burgunder[14]
and H. F. Harbo[13]

[1]University of Tübingen, and German Center for Neurodegenerative Diseases (DZNE), Tübingen, Germany; [2]Rudolfstiftung and Danube University, Krems, Vienna, Austria; [3]University Hospital of Antwerp, Antwerpen, Belgium; [4]VIB, Antwerpen, Belgium; [4']Institute Born-Bunge, University of Antwerp, Antwerp, Belgium; [5]Fondazione-IRCCS, Istituto Neurologico Carlo Besta, Milan, Italy; [6]Assistance Publique-Hôpitaux de Paris, Centre de référence des canalopathies musculaires, Groupe Hospitalier Pitié-Salpêtrière, Paris, France; [7]Hadassah University Hospital, Jerusalem, Israel; [8]Mater Misericordiae University, Beaumont & Mater Private Hospitals, Dublin, Ireland; [9]IRCCS Foundation, Neurological Institute Carlo Besta, Milan, Italy; [10]IRCCS Foundation Neurological Institute Carlo Besta, Milan, Italy; [11]Pandy County Hospital, Gyula, Hungary; [12]Institute of Neurology and National Hospital for Neurology and Neurosurgery, Queen Square, London, UK; [13]Oslo University Hospital, and Faculty of Medicine, University of Oslo, Oslo, Norway; [14]University of Bern, Bern, Switzerland

Introduction

Since the publication of the first two EFNS guideline papers on the molecular diagnosis of neurological diseases in 2001 [1, 2], rapid progress has been made, necessitating an updated series of guidelines. This chapter provides updated guidelines for molecular testing of ataxias and hereditary spastic paraplegias. Criteria will be presented which help to make the decision when a molecular diagnostic work-up should be initiated, and tables summarize information on the genetic basis of the disorders discussed below.

For a more general introduction to molecular genetic testing, including questions of genetic counselling, the reader is referred to 'EFNS guidelines on the molecular diagnosis of neurogenetic disorders: General issues, Huntington's disease, Parkinson's disease and dystonias' (Harbo et al., in press).

Search strategy

To collect data about the molecular diagnosis of different neurogenetic disorders literature searches were performed in various electronic databases, including Medline, OMIM and GENETEST. Original papers, meta-analyses, review paper and guideline recommendations were reviewed.

Method for reaching consensus

Consensus on recommendations was reached using a step-wise approach. First, members of the Task Force met at the EFNS congresses in 2007 and 2008 to discuss the preparation for the guidelines. Second, experts in the specific topics wrote proposals for chapters for each group of disorders. Then, the chapters were distributed and discussed in detail by all Task Force members until a consensus was reached.

Results and recommendations

Recommendations are based on the criteria established by the EFNS [3], with modifications to account for the specific nature of genetic tests. As genetic testing is by definition the gold standard in the diagnosis of a genetically defined disease (barring the rare event of a laboratory error), its diagnostic accuracy cannot be tested against another method. Therefore, the level of recommendations is based on the quality of the studies [3] investigating the proportion of cases of a clinically defined group of patients who can be diagnosed by a specific test. As practically all studies are retrospective (i.e., look for a specific mutation in a previously ascertained diagnosed cohort) the highest level of recommendation is Level B [3]. If only small case-series studying genotype–phenotype correlations are available, the level of recommendation is Level C. Where only case reports could be found, but experts still felt that they could give a recommendation, the level of recommendation is good practice point.

Molecular diagnosis of hereditary ataxias

The hereditary ataxias are a heterogeneous group of neurological disorders (Table 6.1), characterized by imbalance, progressive gait and limb lack of coordination, dysarthria and disturbances of eye movements. The phenotype is often complicated by the presence of additional neurological and systemic signs, which depend on both the specific genetic subtype and individual characteristics. Approximately 10 loci for autosomal recessive phe-notypes and more than 25 loci for the autosomal dominant forms [4, 5] have been found. The estimated prevalence varies greatly between countries, from 1/50,000 for Friedreich ataxia (FRDA1) in Europe to 1/100,000 for ataxia telangiectasia (AT) and the dominant spinocerebellar ataxias (SCAs) worldwide. X-linked ataxias are rare. In exceptional instances cerebellar ataxia may represent the main clinical finding of mitochondrial diseases (Finsterer *et al.*, in press). Detailed family and medical history, physical examination, neuroimaging and laboratory tests may guide molecular screening.

Autosomal dominant cerebellar ataxias

In the current genetic classification, the autosomal dominant cerebellar ataxias are designated as spinocerebellar ataxias (SCAs) and episodic ataxias (EAs).

Spinocerebellar ataxias

So far 27 genetic loci for SCAs have been identified: SCA1-8, SCA10-23, SCA25-30 [5, 6]. In addition, dentato-rubro-pallidoluysian atrophy (DRPLA) is commonly included in this group [7] (Table 6.1). Three major classes of SCAs have been recognized. The first includes DRPLA and SCA1, 2, 3, 6, 7, 17 caused by a CAG repeat expansion in the coding region. This type of mutation represents the most common cause of dominantly inherited ataxias. Longer expansions are associated with earlier onset and more severe disease. A second category of repeat expansions is localized outside the protein-coding region. This group includes SCA8, 10 and 12. A third category is represented by the dominant ataxias SCA5, 11, 13, 14, 15/16 and 27, caused by conventional deletion, missense, nonsense and splice-site mutations in their respective genes. The clinico-genetic heterogeneity of the SCAs has led to some uncertainty concerning the assigned loci/genes: SCA15 and 16 are due to mutations in the same gene; and SCA19 and SCA22 have been suggested to be the same disease, while two different non-allelic diseases have been mapped to the 16q22.1 locus [8, 9] (Table 6.1).

Molecular testing should be guided by taking into account the main associated symptoms (Table 6.1): SCA6 patients have relatively pure cerebellar ataxia, SCA1, 2 and 3 patients show variable involvement of the extrapyramidal, pyramidal and peripheral nervous system, while those with SCA7 are typically distinguished by retinal

Table 6.1 Molecular diagnosis of cerebellar ataxias.

Disease	Inheri-tance[1]	Gene	Position	Mutation[2]	Main associated symptoms	Age at onset	Paraclinical test	MIM number
SCA1	AD	ATXN1	6p23	Trinuc	Dementia, nystagmus, slow saccades pyramidal signs, neuropathy	4–74		164400
SCA2	AD	ATXN2	12q24.1	Trinuc	Dementia, slow saccades, hyporeflexia, amyotrophy, neuropathy, myoclonus, rare Parkinsonism	6–67		183090
SCA3	AD	ATXN3	14q24.3–q31	Trinuc	Nystagmus, diplopia, ophthalmoplegia, eyelid retraction, Parkinsonism, spasticity neuropathy	5–65		607047
SCA4[3]	AD	Unknown	16q22.1	Unknown	Cerebellar syndrome associated with axonal sensitive neuropathy	19–72		600223
16q-linked ADCA[3]	AD	Puratrophin–1 PLEKHG4[1]	16q22.1	Pm, C > T in the 5'UTR	Late-onset cerebellar syndrome, often associated with sensorineural hearing impairment	>50		117210
SCA5	AD	β–III Spectrin (SPTBN2)	11q13	Pm; Del	Pure cerebellar syndrome, downbeat nystagmus, bulbar symptoms in juvenile cases. Slow progression	15–50		600224
SCA6	AD	CACNA1A	19p13	Trinuc	Pure cerebellar syndrome, downbeat positioning nystagmus, sometimes episodic ataxia at onset, double vision, pyramidal signs, deep sensory loss, migraine. (Disease is allelic to episodic EA2 and familial hemiplegic migraine)	19–77		601011
SCA7	AD	ATXN7	3p14–p21.1	Trinuc	Retinal degeneration, ophthalmoplegia, pyramidal signs	0.1–76		164500
SCA8	AD	ATXN8 (Kelch-like)	13q21	Trinuc	Sensory neuropathy, slow progression	0–73		608768
SCA10	AD	ATXN10	22q13	ATTCT expansion	Seizures, pyramidal and extrapyramidal signs	10–40		603516
SCA11	AD	TTBK2	15q14–21.3	Pm; Del; Ins	Pure cerebellar syndrome, hyperreflexia, very slow progression	17–33		604432
SCA12	AD	PPP2R2B	5q31–q33	Trinuc	Dementia, tremor of head and upper extremities, parkinsonism, hyperreflexia, neuropathy	8–55		604326
SCA13	AD	KCNC3	19q13.3–q13.4	Pm	Delayed motor development, mental retardation in some, seizures	4–60		605259
SCA14	AD	PRKCG	19q13.4–qter	Pm	Cognitive deficits, depression, facial myokymia, rare myoclonus and focal dystonia	10–59		605361
SCA15/ SCA16	AD	ITPR1	3p26–p25	Del; Pm	Pure cerebellar syndrome or associated with head tremor. Slow progression	10–66		606658

continued

Table 6.1 continued

Disease	Gene	Inheritance[1]	Position	Mutation[2]	Main associated symptoms	Age at onset	Paraclinical test	MIM number
SCA17	TBP	AD	6q27	Trinuc	Dementia, psychosis, chorea, seizures, Huntington disease-like symptoms	10–70		607136
SCA18	Unknown	AD	7q22–q32	Unknown	Limb weakness, axonal sensory neuropathy (EMG shows denervation)	13–27		607458
SCA19[4]	Unknown	AD	1p21–q21	Unknown	Dementia	20–45		607346
SCA20	Unknown	AD	11p13–q11	Unknown	Dysphonia, palatal tremor, spasmodic cough, bradikynesia, dentate calcification	19–64		608687
SCA21	Unknown	AD	7p21.3–p15.1	Unknown	Cognitive impairment, parkinsonism	6–30		607454
SCA22[4]	Unknown	AD	1p21–q23	Unknown	Pure cerebellar syndrome	10–46		607346
SCA23	Unknown	AD	20p13–12.3	Unknown	Pure cerebellar syndrome or associated with pyramidal signs, sensory loss	43–56		610245
SCA25	Unknown	AD	2p15–p21	Unknown	Sensory neuropathy	1.5–39		608703
SCA26	Unknown	AD	19p13.3	Unknown	Pure cerebellar syndrome, slow progression	26–60		609306
SCA27	FGF14	AD	13q34	Pm	Tremor, dyskinetic movements, psychiatric signs	12–40		609307
SCA28	AFG3L2[5]	AD	18p11.22–q11.2	Pm	Ophthalmoplegia, hyperreflexia, slow progression	12–36		610246
SCA29	Unknown	AD	3p26	Unknown	Non progressive, highly variable phenotype	congenital		117360
SCA30[6]	Unknown	AD	4q34–q35	Unknown	Minor pyramidal signs	45–76		
DRPLA	DRPLA	AD	12p13.31	Trinuc	Dementia, chorea, myoclonus, seizures	10–59		125370
EA1	KCNA 1	AD	12p13	Pm; Del	Muscle spasms, interictal myokymia and jerking movements, chorea at onset. Attack duration: seconds to minutes	2–15		160120
EA2	CACNA1A	AD	19p13	Pm; Trinuc	Downbeat nystagmus, dysarthria, vertigo, muscle weakness, migraine. Interictal ataxia and nystagmus Attack duration: hours to days	2–20		108500
EA3	Unknown	AD	1q42	Unknown	Myokymia, migraine, tinnitus, vertigo, dysarthria. Attack duration: 1min–6h	1–42		606554
EA4/ PATX	Unknown	AD	Unknown	Unknown	Vertigo, diplopia. Interictal nystagmus and saccadic smooth pursuit. Attack duration: brief	23–60		606552
EA5	CACNB4β4	AD	2q22–23	Pm	Vertigo. Interictal nystagmus, ataxia, epilepsy. Attack duration: hours	3–19		601949
EA6	SLC1A3 (EAAT1)	AD	5p13	Pm	Cognitive impairment. Interictal epilepsy, migraine, ataxia, motor delayed milestones. Attack duration: hours/day	<20		600111
EA7	Unknown	AD	19q13	Unknown	Vertigo, dysarthria, muscle weakness. Attack duration: hours/days	13–19		611907

Disease	Gene	Inheritance	Locus	Mutation	Clinical features	Repeat	Biomarker	OMIM
FRDA	FRDA1 (Frataxin)	AR	9q13–q21.1	Trinuc; Pm	Saccadic smooth pursuit, fixation instability, saccadic dysmetria, dysarthria, Babinski sign, deep sensory loss, neuropathy cardiomyopathy, diabetes	2–55		229300
AVED	αTTP	AR	8q13.1–q13.3	Del; Ins; Pm	Head titubation, nystagmus, saccadic smooth pursuit, retinopathy	2–52	Low plasma levels of vit.E	277460
ABL	MTP	AR	4q22–24	Pm	Steatorrhea, areflexia, sensory ataxia, retinal degeneration, dissociated nystagmus on lateral gaze, slow saccades, neuropathy	0–20	Acanthocytes, reduced serum LDL and VLDL	200100
AOA1	APTX	AR	9p13	Ins; Del; Pm	Oculomotor apraxia, fixation instability, saccadic pursuit, gaze-evoked nystagmus, hypometric saccades, neuropathy, choreoathetosis, mild mental retardation	1–29	Hypercholesterolemia, hypoalbuminemia	606350
AOA2	SETX	AR	9q34	Pm; Del	Oculomotor apraxia (rare), saccadic pursuit, slow saccades, fixation instability, choreoathetosis, motor neuropathy with amyotrophy	3–30	Increased AFP	608465
AT	ATM– gene	AR	11q22–q23	Del; Ins; Pm	Telangiectasia, immune deficiency, predisposition to cancer, oculomotor apraxia, increased latency of saccades.	1–4	Chromosomal instability, increased AFP	208900
ATLD	MRE11	AR	11q21	Pm	Similar to AT, milder course	1–7	Possible chromosomal instability, normal AFP	600814
FXTAS	FMR1	X-linked	Xq27.3	Trinuc	Intention tremor, nystagmus, mild parkinsonism, neuropathy	>50		300623

[1]AD: autosomal dominant; AR: autosomal recessive

[2]Pm: point mutations; Del: deletions; Ins: insertions; Trinuc: trinucleotide–repeat expansions

[3]See [8]

[4]SCA19 and SCA22 may be the same disease. See [9]

[5]Di Bella D, et al. AFG3L2 mutations cause autosomal dominant SCA28 and reveal an essential role of the m–AAA AFG3L2 homocomplex in the cerebellum. (Abstract N.216, presented at the annual meeting of The American Society of Human Genetics, 11–15 November, 2008, Philadelphia, Pennsylvania). Available at: www.ashg.org/2008meeting/abstracts/fulltext

[6]Not yet catalogued in OMIM. See [6]

Abbreviations AFP: alpha-fetoprotein ATLD: ataxia–telangiectasia-like disorder ATTP: α-tocopherol transfer protein ATXN 1/2/3/7/8/10: Ataxin1/2/3/7/8/10 CACNA1A: calcium channel, alpha-1a subunit CACNB4β4: calcium channel, beta-4 subunit EAAT1: excitatory amino acid transporter 1 FGF14: fibroblast growth factor 14 FMR1: fragile X mental retardation ITPR1: inositol 1,4,5–triphosphate receptor, type 1 KCNA 1: potassium voltage-gated channel KCNC3: potassium channel, 3 MRE11: meiotic recombination 11 MTP: microsomal transfer protein PLEKHG4: pleckstrin domain-containing protein PPP2R2B: protein phosphatase 2, subunit B PRKCG: protein kinase Cγ SETX SLC1A3: glial high-affinity glutamate transporter 3 SPTBN2: spectrin, beta, nonerythrocytic 2 TBP: TATA box-binding protein TTBK2: tau tubulin kinase 2 degeneration [5,10, 11, 12]. An additional criterion guiding molecular tests is to consider the geographic origin of the family, since some SCA genotypes are more frequent in particular populations [5]. Genetic testing for SCA1, 2, 3, 6, 7 and 17 is technically reliable and available in many laboratories as a routine procedure. Large clinico-genetic series have been reported to support this selection of genes [10, 11, 12]. For the other SCAs, insufficient data do not allow general recommendations.

Recommendations for genetic testing in spinocerebellar ataxias

Where there is a family history compatible with autosomal dominant inheritance, genetic testing should include SCA1, 2, 3, 6, 7 and 17, which represent the majority of the presently identified SCA genotypes in Europe (Level B) [10, 11, 12]. Among those, priorities should be chosen according to associated clinical features.

Episodic ataxias

The episodic ataxias (EA) are characterized by recurrent attacks of ataxia, giddiness and vertigo. Attacks may last minutes (EA1) to several hours (EA2) and can be provoked by rapid movements in EA1 and by exercise, emotional stress, alcohol and caffeine in EA2. In the interval, myokymia is present in hand muscles when analysed by EMG in EA1, whereas EA2 patients present with interictal gaze-evoked nystagmus. The current classification recognizes seven distinct subtypes (Table 6.1) [13]. Four genes have been identified, including the potassium channel gene KCNA1 (EA1), the calcium channel genes CACNA1A (EA2) and CACNB4 (EA5) and the glutamate transporter gene SLC1A3 (EA6) [13, 14]. EA2 is allelic to SCA6 and familial hemiplegic migraine (FHM1). In these disorders clinical phenotypes are highly overlapping: both ataxia and hemiplegic migraine may occur in the same patient, and EA2 phenotype or SCA6 features have been described in the same family [14].

Severity and frequency of attacks may be reduced by acetazolamide.

Recommendations for genetic test in episodic ataxias

Genetic testing for EA1 and EA2 available in specialized or research laboratories is recommended in patients with a family history suggesting dominant inheritance and recurrent attacks of ataxia and vertigo (Level C) [14].

Autosomal recessive cerebellar ataxias

Autosomal recessive ataxias are a heterogeneous group of rare neurodegenerative diseases, mostly characterized by early-onset cerebellar ataxia associated with various neurological, ophthalmological or systemic signs (Table 6.1). Neurological features include optic atrophy, extrapyramidal and pyramidal signs, peripheral neuropathy, cognitive impairment or epilepsy. These diseases are usually caused by a 'loss of function' of specific cellular proteins involved in metabolic homeostasis, cell-cycle and DNA repair or protection [4, 15]. The more common recessive forms in Europe are Friedreich ataxia (FRDA), ataxia telangiectasia (AT) and ataxia with oculomotor apraxia (AOA).

Friedreich's ataxia (FRDA)

FRDA (MIM 229300) is the most common hereditary ataxia in Caucasian populations. The classical clinical features are onset before age 25, progressive gait and limb ataxia, dysarthria, absent deep tendon reflexes, sensory loss and pyramidal weakness. Ataxia is of the afferent, rather than the cerebellar type. Cardiomyopathy is present in the majority of patients. Axonal sensory neuropathy, distal wasting, scoliosis, sensorineural deafness, optic atrophy and diabetes are common. In most cases the disease is caused by a GAA-trinucleotide-repeat expansion in the first intron of the FRDA gene on chromosome 9q13-21 [15]. FRDA patients carry expanded alleles with 90–1,300 repeats. Over 90% of FRDA patients carry the expansion on both alleles. Only a few patients are compound heterozygous, harbouring point mutations or microdeletions on one allele and the GAA expansion on the other. The expansion size has been shown to be inversely correlated with age of onset and age of confinement to wheelchair, and directly correlated with the incidence of cardiomyopathy.

Ataxia with oculomotor apraxia type 1 and type 2 (AOA1–AOA2)

The disease is characterized by ataxia, oculomotor apraxia and choreoathetosis. AOA has been recently associated with two distinct genetic forms: AOA1 and AOA2 [16]. AOA1 (MIM 208920) has an early age at onset and is characterized by cerebellar ataxia, sensorimotor neuropathy, nystagmus, variable oculomotor apraxia, extrapyramidal signs and mild cognitive impairment. Patients may present with hypoalbuminaemia, hypercholesterolaemia and normal alpha-fetoprotein. The disease is caused by mutations in the aprataxin gene, *APTX*, on chromosome 9p13. The protein is believed to play a role in DNA repair.

Ataxia with oculomotor apraxia type 2 (MIM 606002) presents with a similar phenotype as type 1, but age at onset is in the early teens and laboratory studies show normal albumin and high serum alpha-fetoprotein. The disease is caused by mutations in the gene encoding senataxin, *SETX,* on chromosome 9q34. Although the functional role of human senataxin is unknown, its yeast orthologue, *Sen1p,* is implicated in DNA transcription, repair and processing.

Ataxia telangiectasia (AT)

Ataxia telangiectasia (MIM 208900) has an estimated prevalence of 1/40,000–1/100,000. The disease is characterized by cerebellar ataxia, ocular apraxia, telangiectasias, immune defects and a predisposition to malignancy. Patients present in early childhood with progressive cerebellar ataxia and later develop telangiectasias and progressive neurological degeneration. Choreoathetosis or dystonia or both occur in 90% of patients. High serum alpha-fetoprotein is typical. The disease results from mutations in the AT-mutated gene (ATM) on chromosome 11q22–23. The protein is involved in the DNA damage-response pathway. The phenotype can vary in severity depending on the amount of the ATM protein expressed [17]. A significant feature is susceptibility to cancer, with a risk of approximately 40%. Most frequent malignancies are leukaemia or lymphoma. Patients and heterozygote relatives should be advised to avoid any kind of radiation, including unnecessary x-ray.

Ataxia with vitamin E deficiency

Ataxia with vitamin E deficiency (AVED, MIM 277460) presents with a phenotype similar to Friedreich's ataxia with age at onset before 20, yet the concentration of vitamin E in serum is typically reduced. Most patients are from the Mediterranean area. Decreased visual acuity or retinitis pigmentosa may occur. The disease is caused by mutations of the alpha-tocopherol transfer protein gene on chromosome 8q13. Supplementation with vitamin E slows the progression of the disease [18].

Abeta-lipoproteinaemia

Abeta-lipoproteinaemia (ABL, MIM 200100) is caused by mutations in the gene for the large subunit of the microsomal triglyceride transfer protein, on chromosome 4q22–24, which functions in the assembly of apolipoprotein-B containing very low-density lipoproteins and chylomicrons. The neurological phenotype is similar to that observed in vitamin E deficiency, but is associated with lipid malabsorption, hypocholesterolaemia and acanthocytosis. Treatment involves dietary modification and vitamin E replacement, which may prevent neurological complications [4].

Recommendations for genetic test in autosomal recessive ataxias

In cases presenting with early onset ataxia, peripheral sensory neuropathy and absence of marked cerebellar atrophy at MRI, genetic test for FRDA mutation is recommended (Class B) [4, 15].

Molecular testing for ATM, AOA1 and AOA2 is recommended when guided by positive biochemical findings, such as reduced levels of albumin and increased levels of cholesterol or alpha-fetoprotein (Level C) [16, 17]. AVED can usually be diagnosed reliably by measuring vitamin E levels in serum. Molecular diagnosis can be helpful for early detection in siblings of patients with an established diagnosis (Level C) [18].

X-linked ataxias

Fragile X tremor/ataxia syndrome (FXTAS, MIM 300623) is caused by an expanded CGG-trinucleotide-repeat in the FMR1 gene, ranging in size from 55 to 200 repeats ('premutations'). Full-repeat expansions (>200 repeats) result in fragile X mental retardation syndrome. Men with a fragile X premutation present in the sixth decade with progressive intention tremor, ataxia and parkinsonism, cognitive decline and peripheral neuropathy [19]. Symmetric regions of increased T2 signal intensity in the middle cerebellar peduncles and adjacent cerebellar white matter are considered typical of this neurological condition.

Recommendations for FXTAS genetic testing

Genetic testing for the X-linked FXTAS is recommended when there is a clinical suspicion and is readily available in many laboratories (Class B) [19].

Molecular diagnosis of hereditary spastic paraplegias

The hereditary spastic paraplegias (HSP) are a heterogeneous group of neurodegenerative disorders (Table 6.2), characterized by a slowly progressive pyramidal tract dysfunction, occurring either in 'pure' or 'complicated' form, the latter being associated with a variety of other neurological signs and symptoms [19]. Classifications based on phenotypes have been gradually replaced by a genetic classification [20]. To date, about 40 genetically distinct forms have been recognized, and 17 of the genes have been identified. There are about as many autosomal dominant (AD) as recessive (AR) forms, in addition to at least three X-linked HSPs (Table 6.2). Most of the AD-HSPs present clinically as pure HSP, while most of the AR-HSPs are complicated forms. If the family history is negative, a thorough work-up of the differential diagnosis is mandatory. Adrenomyeloneuropathy (AMN), mitochondrial disorders, multiple sclerosis, vitamin B_{12} deficiency and myelopathy due to cervical pathology are the most important.

X-linked forms of HSP

Symptoms caused by mutations in the spastic paraplegia gene 1 (SPG1) (MIM 303350) start in infancy. SPG1 is allelic to MASA (mental retardation, aphasia, shuffling gait, adducted thumbs) and X-linked hydrocephalus, caused by different mutations in the *L1-CAM* gene, encoding a neural cell adhesion molecule. Mutations in the *proteolipid protein (PLP)* gene (MIM 312920) cause SPG2. PLP mutations disturb myelination and are associated with a wide variety of phenotypes, ranging from severe infantile forms of Pelizaeus-Merzbacher disease (PMD, MIM 312080) with complex oculomotor disturbance, spastic weakness, ataxia, choreoathetosis, optic atrophy and psychomotor retardation to relatively mild pure spastic paraplegia of adult onset.

For both SPG1 and SPG2, clinical diagnosis depends on the typical neurological findings, X-linked inheritance pattern and abnormal myelination on MRI [21].

AD forms of HSP

The most frequent form of HSP reported worldwide is SPG4, where either point mutations or deletions in the *SPAST* gene are found (MIM 182601). It accounts for approximately 50% of AD-HSP [22]. Most patients carry point mutations or small deletions or insertions, but in about 20% of SPG4 families the disease is caused by deletions of one or more entire exons in the *SPAST* gene [23]. Interestingly, a large number of *SPAST* variants have been reported in HSP patients without a family history of gait disorders, although there appear to be very few de novo mutations. This may be due to the presence of 20% asymptomatic mutation carriers and to the remarkable heterogeneity in the clinical presentation with regard to age at onset and severity of disease. Onset has been reported from 1 to 76 years of age, but occurs mostly in early adulthood (20–40 years). As a rule there are no additional neurological symptoms except for urinary urgency and leg cramps, which are considered to be part of pure HSP. A few SPG4 families with complicated HSP (neuropathy, mild ataxia, dementia) have been described. Progression tends to be more rapid with later onset.

The second most frequent AD-HSP is SPG3, caused by mutations in the *SPG3A* gene, encoding the protein atlastin (MIM 182600). SPG3 is a pure form, sometimes associated with neuropathy with onset in childhood or adolescence (<20 years). The course of the disease is often mild, but can be severe. SPG3 represents about 40% of young-onset AD-HSP when SPG4 has been excluded [24].

SPG31 with mutations in the *REEP1* gene is the next frequent form of HSP and accounts for 8% of all AD-HSP [25].

SPG10 with mutations in *KIF5A* coding for the kinesin heavy chain is less frequent, and association with an axonal neuropathy is reported [26]. The other forms of AD-HSP (Table 6.2) have been reported in only one or a few families, and for many forms the gene is not yet identified. A variant in the gene *ZFYVE27*, which was hypothesized to cause SPG33 [27], is probably a rare polymorphism [33].

AR forms of HSP

About 15 forms of AR-HSP are described (see Table 6.2), and for most of them no gene has been identified. As a rule, most recessive forms are complicated.

SPG7 (MIM 607259) is caused by mutations in the gene encoding paraplegin. SPG7 has a wide range of onset (8–42 years) and mainly presents as pure HSP, but may include cerebellar and cerebral atrophy, optic atrophy and bulbar symptoms. Interestingly, the encoded protein is highly homologous to the yeast mitochondrial

Table 6.2 Hereditary spastic paraplegia. (Autosomal dominant AD, recessive AR, X-linked).

Name	Locus/Gene/Protein	Heredity	Onset (years)	Phenotype	MIM number
SPG1	Xq28/L1-CAM[1]	X	1–5	MASA[2], MR[3]	303350
SPG2	Xq21/PLP1[4]	X	1–18	Hydrocephalus, allelic with Pelizaeus–Merzbacher	312920
SPG3A	14q11.2/atlastin	AD	2–50	Pure HSP, neuropathy	182600
SPG4	2p22– p21/SPAST/spastin	AD	1–74	Pure HSP, Rarely cognitive impairment, neuropathy, thin corpus callosum	182601
SPG5A	8p12–q13/CYPB1	AR	1–30	Pure HSP	270800
SPG6	15q11.1/NIPA1	AD	12–35	Pure HSP	600363
SPG7	16q24.3/SPG7/ paraplegin	AR	8–42	Complex or pure HSP: Optic atrophy, ophthalmoplegia, bulbar symptoms, scoliosis, cortical and cerebellar atrophy	607259
SPG8	8q23-q24/ KIAA0196/ strumpellin	AD	20–40	Pure HSP	603563
SPG9	10q23.3-q24.1	AD	1–40	Cataract, distal amyotrophy, neuropathy, short stature, gastroesophageal reflux	601162
SPG10	12q13/KIF5A/kinesin heavy chain	AD	2–51	Neuropathy	604187
SPG11	15q13-q15/KIAA1840/ spatacsin	AR	4–21	Thin corpus callosum, white matter lesions, cognitive impairment, dysarthria	604360
SPG12	19q13	AD	1–22	Pure HSP	604805
SPG13	2q24-q34/ HSPD1/HSP60	AD	17–68	Pure HSP	605280
SPG14	3q27-q28	AR	30	Mild MR[3], distal neuropathy, pes cavus	605229
SPG15	14q22-q24/ZFYVE26/spastizin	AR	8–35	Kjellins syndrome, cognitive impairment, macula pigmentation, cerebellar ataxia, neuropathy and distal amyotrophy, cerebral atrophy, thin corpus callosum	270700
SPG16	Xq11.2	X	1–5	Complex HSP: Severe	300266
SPG17	11q12-q14/ BSCL2/seipin	AR–AD	8–40	Silver's syndrome, distal amyotrophy. Allelic with DSMAV	270685
SPG19	9q33-q34	AD	36–55	Pure HSP	607152
SPG20	13q12.3/SPG20/spartin	AR	1–10	Troyer's syndrome, distal amyotrophy	275900
SPG21	15q22.31/SPG21/ maspardin	AR	1–30	Progressive dementia, cerebellar and extrapyramidal symptoms, thin corpus callosum	248900
SPG23	1q24-q32	AR	1	Mild MR[3], postural tremor, pigmentary skin abnormalities,	270750
SPG24	13q14	AR	1	Pure HSP	607584

continued

Table 6.2 continued

Name	Locus/Gene/Protein	Heredity	Onset (years)	Phenotype	MIM number
SPG25	6q23–q24.1	AR	30–46	Pain, discs prolapses, spondylosis	608220
SPG26	12p11.1–12q14	AR	6–11	Mild cognitive impairment, dysarthria, atrophy of hand muscles	609195
SPG27	10q22.1–10q24.1	AD	25–45	Dysarthria	609041
SPG28	14q21.3–q22.3	AR	6–15	Pure HSP	609340
SPG29	1p31.1–21.1	AD	11–30	Hypacusis, paraesophagal hernia and vomiting	609727
SPG30	2q37.3	AR	12–21	Mild cerebellar ataxia and neuropathy	610357
SPG31	2p12/REEP1	AD	1–60	Pure HSP	610250
SPG32	14q12–q21	AR	6–7	Mild MR[3], pseudobulbar symptoms, slow progression, cerebral atrophy, thin corpus callosum, hypoplastic pons	611252
SPG33?	See text				610244
SPG35	16q21–q23	AR	6–11	Cognitive impairment, epilepsy	612319
SPG37	8p21.1–q13.3	AD	8–60	Pure HSP	611945
SPG38	4p16–p15	AD	7–23	Hand muscle atrophy	612335
SPG39	19p13.3/PNPLA6	AR	childhood	Distal amyotrophy	612020
SPG42	3q24–q26/SLC33A1	AD	4–42	Pure HSP	612539
SPAX1	12p13	AD	10–20	Spastic ataxia	108600
ARSACS[5]	13q12/SACS/sacsin	AR	1–70	Spastic ataxia, retinopathy, neuropathy	270550
IAHSP[6]	2q33/ALS2/alsin	AR	1–2	Tetraplegia, dysphagia, anarthria	607225
AHDS	Xq13.2	X	Infancy	Allan–Herndon syndrome	300523

[1]Neural cell adhesion molecule L1 gene
[2]Mental retardation, Aphasia, 'Shuffling gait', Adducted thumbs
[3]Mental retardation
[4]Proteolipid protein gene
[5]Spastic ataxia of Charlevoix-Saguenay
[6]Infantile ascending hereditary spastic paraplegia

ATPases, which have both proteolytic and chaperon-like activities at the inner mitochondrial membrane. Analysis of muscle biopsies from two patients carrying paraplegin mutations showed typical signs of mitochondrial OXPHOS defects, suggesting a mitochondrial mechanism for neurodegeneration in HSP-type disorders. SPG7 was found with a frequency of 7% in sporadic Dutch cases of HSP with adult onset [28].

SPG11 (MIM 182601) appears to be the most frequent form of AR-HSP in the European population (21%) [29]. The gene *KIAA1840* codes for the protein spatacsin, but its function is unknown. It is a complicated form of HSP, with early onset (generally <25 years) and moderate to severe disability. Typical associated findings are thin corpus callosum (TCC), cognitive impairment, dysarthria and atrophy of hand muscles.

SPG15 (MIM 270700) may be the second most frequent form of complicated HSP with TCC [30]. It is similar to SPG11, with cognitive impairment in most patients, neuropathy and distal amyotrophy, mild cerebellar signs, pigmentary retinal degeneration and TCC and/or white matter hyperintensities. This clinical presentation was previously described in the literature as Kjellin syndrome. The gene *ZFYVE26* coding for the protein spastizin has recently been identified [30].

Autosomal-recessive spastic ataxia of Charlevoix-Saguenay (ARSACS, MIM 270550) was described as a common type of ataxia in north-eastern Quebec. It has also been reported in other countries, including Africa and Japan, and showed a high frequency in Dutch patients with early-onset spastic ataxia [31]. The *SACS* gene codes for the protein sacsin. Clinical features suggesting ARSACS are spasticity, cerebellar atrophy, neuropathy and retinopathy.

Summary of recommendations concerning molecular diagnosis of HSP

Dominant forms

Patients with pure HSP and a family history of spastic paraparesis should be tested for SPG4 (Level B). If direct sequencing of the *SPAST* gene is negative, a multiplex ligation-dependent probe amplification assay (MLPA) should be applied to assess genomic deletions (Level B). As a third step, sequencing of *Atlastin* (SPG3) in subjects with a pure form and onset before 20 years of age is recommended (Level B). Sequencing of REEP1 and KIF5A can be considered in remaining mutation-negative dominant families, the latter particularly when a neuropathy is present (Level C).

X-linked and recessive forms

Testing for mutations in *L1-CAM* and *PLP* (SPG 1 and SPG2) should be proposed in early-onset complex forms of HSP with typical radiological findings (Level B). Molecular testing first for SPG11 and then SPG15 is recommended in recessive HSP and thin corpus callosum (Level B). SPG7 may be tested especially when cerebellar features are present (Level C). For other recessive and X-linked HSP forms no general recommendation can be given.

Apparently sporadic spastic paraplegia

Sporadic subjects with progressive spastic paraparesis where other causes of spasticity have been carefully excluded should be tested for SPG4 mutations including MLPA (Level B) [32]. In negative cases, sequencing of SPG7 may be proposed (Level C).

Conflicts of interest

Member of this Task Force have no conflicts of interest related to the recommendations given in this chapter.

Web links

• www.geneclinics.org: GeneClinics, a clinical information resource relating genetic testing to diagnosis, management, and genetic counselling. University of Washington, Seattle.
• www.eurogentest.org: EuroGentest, an EU-funded network of excellence with the aim of harmonizing genetic testing across Europe. The website provides information about the availability and quality assurance of genetic tests.
• www.orpha.net: OrphaNet is a searchable database of over 5,000 rare diseases and includes information about genetic testing (methods, laboratories) on most neurogenetic diseases.
• omim.nih.org: Online Mendelian Inheritance in Man (OMIM) is an online catalogue of Mendelian disorders and traits.

Acknowledgements

This article was written with support of the EUROSCA network.

References

1. Gasser T, Dichgans M, Finsterer J, *et al.* EFNS Task Force on Molecular Diagnosis of Neurologic Disorders: guidelines for the molecular diagnosis of inherited neurologic diseases. Second of two parts. *Eur J Neurol* 2001; **8**:407–24.

2. Gasser T, Dichgans M, Finsterer J, *et al.* EFNS Task Force on Molecular Diagnosis of Neurologic Disorders: guidelines for the molecular diagnosis of inherited neurologic diseases. First of two parts. *Eur J Neurol* 2001; **8**:299–314.

3. Brainin M, Barnes M, Baron JC, *et al.* Guidance for the preparation of neurological management guidelines by EFNS scientific task forces – revised recommendations 2004. *Eur J Neurol* 2004; **11**:577–81.

4. Fogel BL, Perlman S. Clinical features and molecular genetics of autosomal recessive cerebellar ataxias. *Lancet Neurol* 2007; **6**:245–57.

5. Soong BW, Paulson HL. Spinocerebellar ataxias: an update. *Curr Opin Neurol* 2007; **20**:438–46.

6. Storey E, Bahlo M, Fahey M, *et al.* A new dominantly inherited pure cerebellar ataxia, SCA30. *J Neurol Neurosurg Psychiatry* 2009; **80**:408–11.

7. Koide R, Ikeuchi T, Onodera O, *et al.* Unstable expansion of CAG repeat in hereditary dentatorubral–pallidoluysian atrophy (DRPLA). *Nat Genet* 1994; **6**:9–13.

8. Hellenbroich Y, Bernard V, Zühlke C. Spinocerebellar ataxia type 4 and 16q–linked Japanese ataxia are not allelic. *J Neurol* 2008; **255**:612–13.

9. Schelhaas HJ, Verbeek DS, Van de Warrenburg BPC, Sinke RJ. SCA19 and SCA22: evidence for one locus with a worldwide distribution. *Brain* 2004; **127**:e6.

10. Moseley ML, Benzow KA, Schut LJ, *et al.* Incidence of dominant spinocerebellar and Friedreich triplet repeats among 361 ataxia families. *Neurology* 1998; **51**:1666–71.

11. Silveira I, Miranda C, Guimarães L, *et al.* Trinucleotide repeats in 202 families with ataxia: a small expanded (CAG) n allele at the SCA17 locus. *Arch Neurol* 2002; **59**:623–9.

12. Brusco A, Gellera C, Cagnoli C *et al.* Molecular genetics of hereditary spinocerebellar ataxia: mutation analysis of SCA genes and CAG/CTG repeat expansion detection (RED) in 225 Italian families. *Arch Neurol* 2004; **61**:727–73.

13. Jen JC. Recent advances in the genetics of recurrent vertigo and vestibulopathy. *Curr Opin Neurol* 2008; **21**:3–7.

14. Jen JC, Graves TD, Hess EJ, *et al.* Primary episodic ataxias: diagnosis, pathogenesis and treatment. *Brain* 2007; **130**:2484–93.

15. Pandolfo M. Friedreich ataxia. *Semin Pediatr Neurol* 2003; **10**:163–72.

16. Le Ber, I, Brice A, Durr A. New autosomal recessive cerebellar ataxias with oculomotor apraxia. *Curr Neurol Neurosci Rep* 2005; **5**:411–17.

17. Taylor AM, Byrd PJ. Molecular pathology of ataxia telangiectasia. *J Clin Pathol* 2005; **58**:1009–15.

18. Cavalier L, Ouahchi K, Kayden HJ, *et al.* Ataxia with isolated vitamin E deficiency: heterogeneity of mutations and phenotypic variability in a large number of families. *Am J Hum Genet* 1998; **62**:301–10.

19. Berry-Kravis E, Abrams L, Coffey SM, *et al.* Fragile X–associated tremor/ataxia syndrome: clinical features, genetics, and testing guidelines. *Mov Disord* 2007; **22**:2018–30.

20. Fink JK. Hereditary spastic paraplegia. *Curr Neurol Neurosci Rep* 2006; **6**:65–76.

21. Stevanin G, Ruberg M, Brice A. Recent advances in the genetics of spastic paraplegias. *Curr Neurol Neurosci Rep* 2008; **8**:198–210.

22. Woodward KJ. The molecular and cellular defects underlying Pelizaeus–Merzbacher disease. *Expert Reviews in Molecular Medicine* 2008; **10**:e14.

23. Patrono C, Scarano V, Cricchi F, *et al.* Autosomal dominant hereditary spastic paraplegia: DHPLC–based mutation analysis of SPG4 reveals eleven novel mutations. *Hum Mutat* 2005; **25**:506.

24. Beetz C, Nygren AO, Schickel J, *et al.* High frequency of partial SPAST deletions in autosomal dominant hereditary spastic paraplegia. *Neurology* 2006; **67**:1926–30.

25. Durr A, Camuzat A, Colin E, *et al.* Atlastin1 mutations are frequent in young–onset autosomal dominant spastic paraplegia. *Arch Neurol* 2004; **61**:1867–72.

26. Beetz C, Schule R, Deconinck T, *et al.* REEP1 mutation spectrum and genotype/phenotype correlation in hereditary spastic paraplegia type 31. *Brain* 2008; **131**:1078–86.

27. Schule R, Kremer BP, Kassubek J, *et al.* SPG10 is a rare cause of spastic paraplegia in European families. *J Neurol Neurosurg Psychiatry* 2008; **79**:584–7.

28. Mannan AU, Krawen P, Sauter SM, *et al.* ZFYVE27 (SPG33), a novel spastin-binding protein, is mutated in hereditary spastic paraplegia. *Am J Hum Genet* 2006; **79**:351–7.

29. Brugman F, Scheffer H, Wokke JH, *et al.* Paraplegin mutations in sporadic adult-onset upper motor neuron syndromes. *Neurology* 2008; **71**:1500–5.

30. Stevanin G, Azzedine H, Denora P, *et al.* Mutations in SPG11 are frequent in autosomal recessive spastic paraplegia with thin corpus callosum, cognitive decline and lower motor neuron degeneration. *Brain* 2008; **131**:772–84.

31. Hanein S, Martin E, Boukhris A, *et al.* Identification of the SPG15 gene, encoding spastizin, as a frequent cause of complicated autosomal–recessive spastic paraplegia, including Kjellin syndrome. *Am J Hum Genet* 2008; **82**:992–1002.

32. Vermeer S, Meijer RP, Pijl BJ, *et al.* ARSACS in the Dutch population: a frequent cause of early-onset cerebellar ataxia. *Neurogenetics* 2008; **9**:207–14.

33. Depienne C, Tallaksen C, Lephay JY, *et al.* Spastin mutations are frequent in sporadic spastic paraparesis and their spectrum is different from that observed in familial cases. *J Med Genet* 2006; **43**:259–65.

34. Martignoni M, Riano E, Rugarli EI. The role of ZFYVE27/protrudin in hereditary spastic paraplegia. *Am J Hum Genet* 2008; **83**:127–8.

CHAPTER 7

Molecular diagnosis of channelopathies, epilepsies, migraine, stroke and dementias

J-M. Burgunder,[1] J. Finsterer,[2] Z. Szolnoki,[3] B. Fontaine,[4] J. Baets,[5,6,7] C. Van Broeckhoven,[6,7] S. Di Donato,[8] P. De Jonghe,[5,6,7] T. Lynch,[9] C. Mariotti,[10] L. Schöls,[11] A. Spinazzola,[12] S. J. Tabrizi,[13] C. Tallaksen,[14,15] M. Zeviani,[12] H. F. Harbo[15] and T. Gasser[16]

[1]University of Bern, Bern, Switzerland; [2]KA Rudolfstiftung, Vienna, and Danube University Krems, Austria; [3]Pandy County Hospital, Gyula, Hungary; [4]Assistance Publique-Hôpitaux de Paris, Centre de référence des canalopathies musculaires, Groupe Hospitalier Pitié-Salpêtrière, Paris, France; [5]University Hospital of Antwerp, Antwerp, Belgium; [6]VIB, Antwerp, Belgium; [7]Laboratory of Neurogenetics, Institute Born-Bunge, and University of Antwerp, Antwerp, Belgium; [8]Fondazione-IRCCS, Istituto Neurologico Carlo Besta, Milan, Italy; [9]The Dublin Neurological Institute, Mater Misericordiae University, Beaumont and Mater Private Hospitals, Dublin, Ireland; [10]Unit of Genetic of Neurodegenerative and Metabolic Diseases, IRCCS Foundation, Neurological Institute Carlo Besta, Milan, Italy; [11]Centre of Neurology and Hertie-Institute for Clinical Brain Research, University of Tübingen, Tübingen, Germany; [12]Division of Molecular Neurogenetics, IRCCS Foundation Neurological Institute Carlo Besta, Milan, Italy; [13]Institute of Neurology and National Hospital for Neurology and Neurosurgery, London, UK; [14]Ullevål University Hospital, Oslo, Norway; [15]Oslo University Hospital, Ullevål, Oslo, Norway; [16]Hertie-Institute for Clinical Brain Research, University of Tübingen, Tübingen, Germany

Introduction

Since the publication of the first EFNS guidelines on the molecular diagnosis of inherited neurological diseases in 2001 [1, 2] rapid progress has been made, necessitating the creation of an updated version of these guidelines, which follows the EFNS Scientific Committee recommendations for guideline papers [3].

Objectives

These EFNS guidelines on the molecular diagnosis of channelopathies, including epilepsy and migraine, as well as stroke and dementia, are designed to summarize the possibilities and limitations of molecular genetic techniques and to provide diagnostic criteria for making the decision when a molecular diagnostic work-up is indicated in adults.

Search strategy

To collect data about planning, conditions and performance of molecular diagnosis of these disorders, a literature search of various electronic databases, including the Cochrane Library, Medline, OMIM, GENETEST and EMBASE, was carried out and original papers,

European Handbook of Neurological Management: Volume 2, Second Edition. Edited by Nils Erik Gilhus, Michael P. Barnes, Michael Brainin.
© 2012 Blackwell Publishing Ltd. Published 2012 by Blackwell Publishing Ltd.

meta-analyses, review papers and guideline recommen-dations were reviewed.

Method for reaching consensus

Consensus on the recommendations was reached by a step-wise approach. First, Task Force members met at the EFNS congresses in 2007 and 2008 to discuss the prepara-tions for the guidelines. Second, experts in the genetics of the disorders mentioned above wrote a guideline pro-posal. Then their recommendations were distributed and discussed in detail among all Task Force members until a consensus was reached.

Results and recommendations

Recommendations follow the criteria established by the EFNS [3], with some modifications to account for the specific nature of genetic tests. Since genetic testing is by definition the gold standard to diagnose a genetically defined disease, its diagnostic accuracy cannot be tested against another diagnostic method. Therefore, the level of recommendations was based on the quality of availa-ble studies [3] and the proportion of cases of a clinically defined group of patients explained by a specific molecu-lar diagnostic test was estimated. As nearly all of these studies have a retrospective design and look for a specific mutation in a previously ascertained and clinically diag-nosed cohort of patients, the highest achievable recom-mendation level was Level B [3]. If only small case-series studying genotype–phenotype correlations were availa-ble, the level of recommendation was Level C. If only case reports could be found, but experts still felt that they could give a recommendation, the level of recommenda-tion was assessed as good practice point.

Channelopathies

Ion channels are transmembrane proteins, which allow fluxes between the intra- and extracellular spaces with specific conductance for different ions, including sodium, calcium, chloride and others. Voltage-gated activation modulates membrane excitability, allowing intercellular communication and impulse propagation. Ion channel gene mutations have been found in neurological disor-ders, which have in common episodic or paroxysmal clinical manifestations. Muscle channelopathies include periodic paralysis, non-dystrophic myotonia, Andersen-Tawil syndrome and congenital myasthenia. Disorders affecting the central nervous system comprise episodic ataxia, migraine and epilepsy. Molecular diagnosis is now available for many neurological channelopathies (Table 7.1).

Muscular channelopathies

Hypokalaemic periodic paralysis is an autosomal domi-nantly hereditary disease [4] characterized by episodic muscle paralysis concomitant with a decrease in blood potassium levels and facilitated by muscle exercise or sugar ingestion. Between attacks, muscle examination is normal. The disease may be caused by specific mutations either in the calcium channel α1S-subunit (*CACNA1S*) gene, localized on chromosome 1, or in the sodium channel α1-subunit (*SCN4A*) on chromosome 17. Mutations in *CACNA1S*, found in 70–90% of patients from different ethnic backgrounds, are the most frequent. Patients with *SCN4A* mutations tend to have muscle aches and drug-induced symptom aggravation [5]. *In vitro* expression of mutated channels suggests a loss of function mechanism and an increased 'leakiness' of the channels [6]. Mechanisms underlying blood potassium level changes are not well understood. Electromyography following sensitization by a long exercise test allows diag-nosis of periodic paralysis even between attacks and may predict channel-type mutation [7]. Treatment relies on the avoidance of provocative factors and the use of chlo-ride potassium salts and acetazolamide.

Hyperkalaemic periodic paralysis, paramyotonia con-genita and sodium channel myotonia are caused by dis-tinct mutations of the sodium channel gene *SCN4A* on chromosome 17 [8–10]. Overlapping syndromes with different degrees of paralysis and myotonia occur depending on the mutation. Hyperkalaemic periodic paralysis is characterized by episodic attacks of muscle weakness concomitant with increased blood potassium levels. Provocation factors include muscle exercise, cold, alcohol, potassium-rich food, stress or steroids. Paramyotonia congenita is characterized by prolonged muscle contraction aggravated by exercise (paradoxical

Table 7.1 Neurological channelopathies.

Disease	Gene	Mode of inheritance	Gene locus	Mutated protein	OMIM
Hypokalaemic periodic paralysis (HOKPP)	CACNA1S	AD	1q32	Calcium channel α1S subunit type 1	170400
	SCN4A	AD	17q23	Sodium channel α-subunit type 4	170400
Hyperkalaemic periodic paralysis (HYPP)	SCN4A	AD	17q23	Sodium channel α-subunit type 4	170500
					168300
Paramyotonia Congenita (PMC)					608390
Sodium channel myotonia or potassium-aggravated myotonia					
Myotonia congenita	CLCN1	AD (Thomsen)	7q35	Chloride channel type 1	160800
		AR (Becker)	7q35		255700
Andersen-Tawil syndrome (ATS)	KCNJ2	AD	17q23	Potassium channel subfamily J member 2	170390
Congenital myasthenic syndrome (CMS)	SCN4A	AD	17q23	Sodium channel α-subunit type 4	603967
Benign neonatal epilepsy (BNE1, 2)	KCNQ2	AD	20q13	Potassium channel subfamily Q member 2	121200
	KCNQ3	AD	8q24		121201
				Potassium channel subfamily Q member 3	
Benign familial neonatal-infantile seizures	SCN2A	AD	2q24	Sodium channel α-subunit type 2	607745
Generalized epilepsy with febrile seizure-plus (GEFS+)	SCN1B	AD	19q13	Sodium channel α-subunit type 1	604233
	SCN1A	AD	2q24	Sodium channel α-subunit type 1	
Severe myoclonic epilepsy of infancy	SCN1A	AD	2q24	Sodium channel α-subunit type 1	607208
Juvenile myoclonic epilepsy	CLCN2	AR	3q26	Chloride channel type 2	606904
Childhood absence epilepsy	CLCN2	AR	3q26	Chloride channel type 2	607682

myotonia) and cold. Distinct patterns of spontaneous activity, possibly related to the mutation type, may be recorded on needle electromyography [11]. All these disorders are transmitted with an autosomal dominant mode of inheritance and are caused by mutations in *SCN4A* distinct from the ones implicated in hypokalaemic periodic paralysis. Although there may be variations between and within families, there is a good genotype–phenotype correlation. *In vitro* expression of mutated channels has revealed that they may activate early or inactivate late or incompletely, resulting in increased excitability of the cell membrane. A slight increase in excitability will result in an increased number of action potentials and thus myotonia. Treatment is based on the avoidance of provoking factors, mild exercise at onset of an attack or intake of carbohydrates. Acetazolamide may prevent the attacks of muscle weakness. Blockers of the open states of the sodium channel (mexiletine, carbamazepine and diphenylhydantoin) can alleviate myotonia [12].

Neuronal channelopathies

Neuronal channelopathies comprise a variety of disorders, including episodic ataxias, migraine and some forms of epilepsy [13]. Ataxias are discussed in another paper in this series and migraine is discussed below. Rare inherited forms of epilepsy are increasingly recognized as channelopathies. Benign infantile neonatal epilepsy

(*EBN1*, *EBN2*) is an autosomal dominant condition, in which newborns develop tonic-clonic seizures within the first days of life. Neurological development is normal and the seizures are easily controlled by antiepileptic medication. The disease is caused by loss-of-function mutations in either the potassium channel gene *KCNQ2* or *KCNQ3* (Table 7.1). In autosomal dominant benign familial neonatal–infantile seizures, mutations have been found in the gene encoding the neuronal sodium channel α1-subunit (*SCN2A*) on chromosome 2. Generalized epilepsy with febrile seizures-plus (GEFS+) is an autosomal dominant condition with different types of seizures (febrile seizures, generalized seizures or partial seizures). Mutations were found in the genes encoding the α1-subunit of the sodium channel (*SCN1B*), the α1-subunit of the neuronal sodium channel (*SCN1A*), and in the *GABRG2* gene. In severe myoclonic epilepsy of infancy (SMEI), seizures are refractory to medication and patients develop neurological deterioration due to de novo mutations in the gene encoding the α1-subunit of the neuronal sodium channel *SCN1A* on chromosome 2. Juvenile myoclonic epilepsy has an onset in adolescence with a combination of myoclonic, generalized and absence seizures. Mutations were found in the gene encoding the chloride channel *CLCN2* on chromosome 3. Mutations in *CLCN2* have also been linked to childhood absence epilepsy, a condition of good prognosis characterized by multiple absences beginning in mid-childhood with generalized 3Hz spike-and-wave complexes.

Recommendations

There is good evidence to suggest that a thorough clinical and electrophysiological investigation may lead to the choice of the gene to be tested in patients with periodic paralysis (Level B). In myotonic disorders it is recommended that myotonic dystrophy is searched for, as well as clinical and electrophysiological phenotype characterization to guide molecular genetic testing (Level B).

Molecular investigations are possible and in some cases may help to diagnose the condition, but with regard to the large number of different mutations in different genes should not be considered as a routine procedure. Furthermore, diagnosis can be made more easily by clinical and physiological investigations (good practice point). One exception of note is the diagnosis of SMEI, in which mutations are found in *SCN1A* in 80% of patients (Level B).

Cerebrovascular diseases

Cerebral autosomal dominant arteriopathy with subcortical infarcts and leukencephalopathy

The main clinical features of cerebral autosomal dominant arteriopathy with subcortical infarcts and leukencephalopathy (CADASIL) include migraine with aura in the third decade of life, recurrent ischaemic stroke or transitoric ischaemic attacks 10 years later, followed by dementia 20 years after onset. The disorder results from mutations in the gene coding for Notch3 located on chromosome 19q12 (Table 7.2). Mutations are localized in coding regions for epidermal growth factor (EGF)-like repeat domains. Most (70%) of the mutations are clustered within exons 3 and 4. Direct sequencing of these two exons is suggested as a first step if clinical suspicion is high. Multiple small subcortical infarcts with leukoaraiosis are typically found in the frontal poles [14]. The diagnosis may also be supported by skin biopsy showing typical osmiophilic granula.

Amyloid angiopathies

Cerebral amyloid angiopathy (CAA), Dutch type, is caused by a point mutation within the amyloid precursor protein (*APP*) gene (guanine-to-cytosine at nucleotide 1852), resulting in a substitution of glutamine for glutamic acid at position 693 (Table 7.2). Several other *APP* mutations in Alzheimer's disease (AD) are associated with a strong microvascular amyloid involvement [15]. Icelandic-type CAA results from a point mutation within the *Cystatin C* gene with a change of leucine in position 68 to glutamine. CAA should be considered in patients with early-onset recurrent cerebral haemorrhages in association with prominent white matter changes.

Cerebral cavernous malformations

Cerebral cavernous malformations (CCM) are vascular malformations causing haemorrhagic or ischaemic strokes. Approximately half of the cases are inherited as an autosomal dominant trait with incomplete penetrance. Most of the CCM cases result from mutations in the *KRIT1* gene (Table 7.2), localized on chromosome 7q21-22 (CCM1) [16]. Mutations seem to be distributed over the entire coding sequence. Mutational analysis can

Table 7.2 Main genetic causes of stroke and migraine.

Disease	Gene product	Mutation	Position	Mode of transmission	OMIM
Cerebral autosomal dominant arteriopathy with subcortical infarcts and leukoencephalopathy (CADASIL)	Notch3	PM	19q12	AD	125 310
Cerebral amyloid angiopathy (CCA, Dutch type)	Amyloid precursor protein	np 1852	21q21	AD	104 760
Cerebral amyloid angiopathy (CCA, Icelandic type)	Cystatin C	As 68	20p11.2	AD	105 150
Cerebral cavernous malformations	CCM1	Point mutations deletions	7q21-22	AD (incomplete penetrance)	116 860
Cerebral cavernous malformations	CCM2	Point mutations deletions	7p13-15	AD (incomplete penetrance)	603 284
Cerebral cavernous malformations	CCM3	Point mutations deletions	3q25.2 ± 27	AD (incomplete penetrance)	603 285
Familial hemiplegic migraine (FMH)	CACNA1A	Point mutations,	19p13	AD	141 500
Elevated level of serum homocysteine	methylenetetrahydrofolate reductase enzyme (MTHFR)	Point mutations	1p36.3	AR	607093
Elevated level of serum homocysteine	cystatione β-synthetase enzyme (CBS)	Missense, nonsense, splicing, deletion, insertion mutations	21q22.3	AR	236200

be considered in patients with multiple cavernomas or a family history of cerebral haemorrhages. However, at-risk individuals may also be identified by MRI. Two additional loci, CCM2 (OMIM 603 284) and CCM3 (OMIM 603 285), have been localized to chromosomes 7p13-15 and 3q25.2-27, respectively.

Fabry's disease

Fabry's disease is an X-linked systematic disorder resulting from deficiency of the lysosomal enzyme alpha-galactosidase A. Early clinical features, such as angiokeratoma and hypohidrosis, typically occur in childhood. Kidney, heart, and brain involvement may develop in mid-adulthood. Cerebrovascular involvement includes both large- and small-vessel disease, resulting in ischaemic lesions or vascular demyelization of the white matter. Diagnosis can be confirmed by measuring alpha galactosidase A activity or by screening for mutations.

Due to X-linked inheritance, in females mutation screening may be required.

Homocystinuria

Homocystinuria mostly results from a reduced activity of the cystatione β-synthetase and methylenetetrahydrofolate reductase enzymes, which are associated with a highly or mildly elevated level of serum homocysteine (>15 micromol/L). The cystatione β-synthetase enzyme deficiency has been associated with several missense, nonsense, splicing, deletions or insertions mutations. A permanent or temporary (thermo-sensitive) decrease in the activity of the methylenetetrahydrofolate reductase enzyme can also result from C677T or A1298C mutations. These relatively frequent mutations are associated with mostly autosomal recessive enzyme deficiencies. The majority of the patients with a highly elevated serum homocystein level have a thromboembolic stroke or stroke-like episodes if not treated. Screening for mutations in the cystatone β-synthetase and methylenetetrahydrofolate reductase gene is available. Correlation between mutations, homocystein serum level and clinical phenotype is influenced by several biochemical conditions such as folic acid and vitamin B daily uptake.

Ehlers-Danlos syndrome

Ehlers-Danlos syndrome type IV is an autosomal dominant disorder caused by mutations in the *COL3A1* gene. The main clinical features are easy bruising, hyperextensibility of joints, thin skin with visible veins and rupture of arteries, uterus or intestine. Arterial dissection in large- and medium-sized arteries can account for ischaemic stroke.

Recommendations

Direct sequencing of exons 3 and 4 in the Notch3 gene is suggested as a first step if clinical suspicion for CADASIL is high (Level B). CCA should be considered in patients with early onset, recurrent cerebral haemorrhages in association with prominent white matter lesions without classic clinical risk factors. In such cases the *KRIT1* gene should be screened for causative mutations (Level B). Genetic tests for Fabry's disease are suggested in the case of neuropathic pain, hypohydrosis, acroparaesthesia, corneal opacities, cataract, renal failure, cardiac failure, ischaemic stroke or TIAs (Level B). Mutation screening in Ehlers-Danlos syndrome can be performed in the presence of clinical implications (easy bruising, hyperestensibility of joints, thin skin with visible veins, rupture of arteries, uterus or the intestine, and arterial dissection) (good practice point). In the event of a stroke attack with elevated level of serum homocysteine (>15 micromol/L), screening for mutations in cystatone beta-synthetase and methylenetetrahydrofolate reductase is suggested (Level B).

Migraine

Familial hemiplegic migraine

FHM is inherited in an autosomal dominant way. Most of the cases are linked to a locus on chromosome 19p13, and in some instances point mutations have been described in the alpha1 subunit of the calcium channel gene (*CACNA1A*). Point mutations in the same gene cause episodic ataxia type 2 (EA2), and the expansion of a CAG-repeat is responsible for spinocerebellar ataxia

type 6 (SCA6). Clinical presentation and genetic findings overlap between all three conditions. A minority of affected families are linked to a second locus on chromosome 1q23 (*ATP1A2*), and a mutation in the neuronal voltage-gated sodium channel gene (*SCN1A*) has recently been described (Table 7.2).

Recommendations

The diagnosis of familial hemiplegic migraine can be confirmed with sequencing the hot spots of the most often affected gene (*CACNA1A*) (good practice point).

Inherited dementias

The majority of degenerative dementias occur with an autosomal dominant inheritance pattern and similar phenotypes to sporadic disease. The proportion of familial occurrence varies between 2% and 50%, depending on the dementia subtype. In dementing disorders, it is particularly important to ensure adequate genetic counselling and obtain consent from the patient or family caregiver prior to any attempt of molecular genetic diagnosis [17]. It also needs to be pointed out that a postmortem diagnosis of the cause of a familial degenerative dementia can provide critically important information for future counselling of the family and should be discussed. In most instances, molecular genetic diagnosis will only be feasible in patients with a clear family history indicative of a monogenic form of the disease or in sporadic occurrences with an unusually early age of onset. Due to reduced penetrance, however, some known dominant mutations can also cause seemingly sporadic late-onset disease in some populations, even in a surprisingly high proportion of cases.

Alzheimer's disease

Alzheimer's disease is the most common type of primary degenerative dementia. Clinical features include a slow, progressive amnesic syndrome and variable combinations of other cortical cognitive deficits but also include behavioural changes and affective symptoms. Mutations in three genes have been found to cause an autosomal dominant form of the disease (sometimes referred to as AD type 1, 3 and 4) [18], and together these account for <5% of all cases (Table 7.3) (www.molgen.ua.ac.be/

Table 7.3 Genetics of hereditary dementias.

Disorder	Abbreviation	Mode of inheritance	Gene locus	Mutated protein	Type of mutation	OMIM
Familial Alzheimer's disease	AD1	AD	21q21	Amyloid precursor protein	Pm, Dupl	104760
	AD2	AD	19q13.2	ApoE	CV	104310
	AD3	AD	14q24.3	Presenilin 1	Pm, exonic deletions	104311
	AD4	AD	1q31-q42	Presenilin 2	Pm	600759
Frontotemporal dementia with parkinsonism	FTPD-17	AD	17q21	MAPTau	Pm, Del, Ins	601630
Frontotemporal dementia with ubiquitinated lesions	FTD-U	AD	17q21	Progranulin	Pm, genomic Del	607485
Fam. Creutzfeld-Jakob disease	PRNP	AD	20pter-p12	Prion-Protein	Pm, Ins	123400

AD: autosomal dominant; Pm: point mutation; Del: deletion; Ins: insertion, CV: common variant.

ADMutations). Among them, AD3, which is caused by mutations in the presenilin 1 gene (*PSEN1*) on chromosome 14, is the most common. In contrast, AD1, due to mutations in the gene for the amyloid precursor protein (*APP*, OMIM 104760, chromosome 21) and AD4 mutations in the presenilin 2 gene (*PSEN2*, OMIM 600759, chromosome 1) are rare [19]. *APP* encodes a transmembrane protein that gives rise, after proteolytic cleavage, to Aß-fragments that pathologically aggregate in amyloid plaques thought to be at the centre of the pathogenic cascade in AD [20]. Point mutations in coding regions, as well as whole-gene duplications and promoter mutations increasing transcriptional activity, have been shown to lead to AD [15, 21]. The presenilins are part of the proteolytic complex known as the γ-secretase that cleaves APP and releases the Aß-fragment. *PSEN1* mutations are probably pathogenic due to the fact that they increase the relative ratio of the more amyloidogenic $Aß_{1-42}$ fragment to $Aß_{1-40}$. An earlier onset age between 30 and 60 years is common in monogenic forms, although *PSEN1* mutations have also been detected in patients with onset at ages over 60–70 years. When accompanied by a positive family history, molecular genetic testing should be considered. Several specialized laboratories across Europe provide such testing. Here, the probability of identifying a mutation in one of the three AD genes is approximately 10%; where the patient has a clear autosomal dominant

heritance, the incidence increases to 20%. Mutation screening can also be offered to apparently sporadic patients with a diagnosis age of <70 years, with a chance of approximately 5% to find a mutation. In addition to the mutations mentioned above that can cause AD with high penetrance, a common variant of the apolipoprotein E gene (*APOE*) known as the ε4-allele has been clearly established as a risk factor for early- and late-onset AD (AD2). As the *APOE* ε4-allele is neither necessary nor sufficient to cause AD, however, there is a wide consensus that at present there is no clear benefit in *APOE* genotyping to assist with diagnosis [22] or presymptomatic risk assessment. One exception involves *APOE* genotyping in individuals carrying a causal mutation in *PSEN1*, *APP* or *PSEN2*, because the *APOE* ε4-allele can lower the age of onset by 5 years in mutation carriers. A growing number of other loci (AD5–15 in the 'OMIM' catalogue) and genes have been suggested. Most of these were identified through association studies, but none is currently relevant for genetic testing in clinical practice (AlzGene Database www.alzforum.org/res/com/gen/alzgene/default.asp).

Fronto-temporal lobar degeneration

The heterogeneous group of frontotemporal lobar degeneration (FTLD) disorders are characterized by predominantly frontotemporal distribution of cortical cerebral atrophy and a clinical picture of prominent behavioural changes, frontal deficits and/or speech disturbances. Consensus criteria have been published and are widely accepted to distinguish three clinical variants. The behavioural variant (bv FTLD or FTD) is also called frontal variant with prominent behavioural disturbances. The two variants with prominent language disorders include semantic dementia (SD), characterized mainly by a fluent dysphasic syndrome, and primary non-fluent aphasia (PNFA). In all these variants, however, other signs and symptoms of an atypical parkinsonian syndrome, often in the form of a corticobasal syndrome (CBS), or of a syndrome resembling progressive supranuclear palsy (PSP) or motor neuron degeneration (MND) may occur and even dominate the clinical picture. The most common presentation is an early change in personality and social behaviour, and language dysfunction, but with relative preservation of memory functions. Historically, at least a subset of these patients had been subsumed under the heading of Pick's disease. Today, the term frontotemporal lobar degeneration (FTLD) is suggested as an umbrella term.

Pathologically, the majority of patients with FTLD show ubiquitinated deposits of the protein TDP-43 (designated FTLD-TPD). In a substantial proportion of patients, however, deposition of the microtubule-associated protein tau (MAPT) is found; in these patients, the disease is termed FTLD-tau. Further, in a small subset of patients with FTLD-U pathology, the ubiquitinated inclusions are negative for TDP-43 and tau, and consist of an as yet elusive protein composition. A wide spectrum of loss-of-function mutations (haploinsufficiency), often small deletions or insertions leading to a premature stop codon in the progranuline gene (PGRN) [23, 24], have been found in FTLD-TDP. In contrast, missense or splice-site mutations MAPT have been recognized as a cause of FTLD-tau (Table 7.3).

The relationship between genotype, pathology and clinical phenotype in FTLD is complex. Clinical features associated with a particular genetic cause or pathology vary widely, even within families. As a general rule, prominent extrapyramidal symptoms are somewhat more likely to predict a tauopathy, whereas behavioural problems and semantic dementia are more likely to predict a TDP-43 proteinopathy [25]. On the other hand, parkinsonism was found in 30% of patients with PRGN mutations in a large series [26]. The fact that approximately 30–50% of patients with FTLD, depending on the clinical subtype, have a positive family history suggests autosomal-dominant inheritance. The proportion is highest in those with FTD-ALS and lowest in semantic dementia [27]. Mutations in the MAPT gene can be found in 10–43% of patients with a positive family history of FTLD, but in only about 3% of all FTLD patients. PGRN mutations account for 13–26% of familial and 1–11% of all FTLD cases (3.2% in apparently sporadic cases) [28]. Therefore, genetic screening of the PRGN and MAPT genes is clearly indicated and useful for genetic counselling in patients with autosomal-dominant FTLD. It can also be considered in sporadic cases, although mutations are found in <10%. Other genes associated with familial forms of FTLD include the CHMP2B gene on chromosome 3 and the gene for the valosin-containing protein on chromosome 9. In the latter, FTLD is often found in conjunction with an inclusion body myopathy and early-onset Paget's disease. Both of these forms of familial FTLD are very rare.

Prion diseases

Prion diseases (spongiform encephalopathies, in humans usually known as Creutzfeld-Jakob disease, CJD) are a group of usually rapidly progressive dementias manifesting as idiopathic, acquired or inherited disorders. A clearly positive family history of a dominant inheritance is found in 10–20% of cases. Different mutations in the prion protein gene on chromosome 20 have been identified in these families (Table 7.3). Complete sequencing of the prion protein gene is provided by several centres and can be offered, given the appropriate counselling, in cases with a strong clinical suspicion of familial CJD.

Clinical heterogeneity

Occasionally, mutations in genes typically implicated in one neurodegenerative disorder can be identified in patients clinically presenting with another neurodegenerative disorder. Examples include the MAPT Arg406Trp mutation associated with Alzheimer's disease phenotype and PSEN1 Gly183Val in a patient with pathologically confirmed Pick's disease. Patients with PGRN loss of function mutations also display a broad phenotypic spectrum. Thus, if a mutation screening of known genes is negative but there is a strong indication of familial inheritance, it is recommended to extend the mutation screening to genes implicated in other neurodegenerative diseases.

Recommendations

In the setting of a clinical diagnosis of AD, mutational screening first in *PSEN1*, then in *APP*, and finally (if negative) in *PSEN2* can be useful for genetic counselling in cases of early-onset autosomal-dominant AD (Level B). Genetic screening in sporadic cases with early onset can be considered (good practice point). If the clinical diagnosis is frontotemporal dementia, genetic testing for mutations in *PRGN* and *MAPT* is clearly indicated and useful for genetic counselling in patients with autosomal-dominant FTLD (Level B), regardless of the presence of severity of extrapyramidal features. Testing can also be considered in familial and sporadic cases, although mutations are found only in <5% (good practice point).

References

1. Gasser, T, Dichgans, M, Finsterer, J, *et al.* EFNS task force on molecular diagnosis of neurologic disorders: guidelines for the molecular diagnosis of inherited neurologic diseases. First of two parts. *Eur J Neurol* 2001; **8**:299–314.

2. Gasser, T, Dichgans, M, Finsterer, J, *et al.* EFNS task force on molecular diagnosis of neurologic disorders: guidelines for the molecular diagnosis of inherited neurologic diseases. Second of two parts. *Eur J Neurol* 2001; **8**:407–24.

3. Brainin, M, Barnes, M, Baron, JC, *et al.* Guidance for the preparation of neurological management guidelines by EFNS Scientific Task Forces – revised recommendations 2004. *Eur J Neurol* 2004; **11**:577–81.

4. Fontaine, B, Fournier, E, Sternberg, D, *et al.* Hypokalemic periodic paralysis: a model for a clinical and research approach to a rare disorder. *Neurotherapeutics* 2007; **4**:225–32.

5. Sternberg, D, Maisonobe, T, Jurkat-Rott, K, *et al.* Hypokalaemic periodic paralysis type 2 caused by mutations at codon 672 in the muscle sodium channel gene SCN4A. *Brain* 2001; **124**:1091–9.

6. Sokolov, S, Scheuer, T, Catterall, WA. Gating pore current in an inherited ion channelopathy. *Nature* 2007; **446**:76–8.

7. Fournier, E, Arzel, M, Sternberg, D, *et al.* Electromyography guides toward subgroups of mutations in muscle channelopathies. *Ann Neurol* 2004; **56**:650–61.

8. Fontaine, B, Khurana, TS, Hoffman, EP, *et al.* Hyperkalemic periodic paralysis and the adult muscle sodium channel alpha-subunit gene. *Science* 1990; **250**:1000–2.

9. Ricker, K, Moxley, RT, III, Heine, R, Lehmann-Horn, F. Myotonia fluctuans. A third type of muscle sodium channel disease. *Arch Neurol* 1994; **51**:1095–102.

10. Rudel, R, Lehmann-Horn, F. Paramyotonia, potassium-aggravated myotonias and periodic paralyses. 37th ENMC International Workshop, Naarden, The Netherlands, 8–10 December 1995. *Neuromuscul Disord* 1997; **7**:127–32.

11. Fournier, E, Viala, K, Gervais, H, *et al.* Cold extends electromyography distinction between ion channel mutations causing myotonia. *Ann Neurol* 2006; **60**:356–65.

12. De Luca, A, Pierno, S, Liantonio, A, *et al.* New potent mexiletine and tocainide analogues evaluated in vivo and *in vitro* as antimyotonic agents on the myotonic ADR mouse. *Neuromuscul Disord* 2004; **14**:405–16.

13. Bernard, G, Shevell, MI. Channelopathies: a review. *Pediatr Neurol* 2008; **38**:73–85.

14. Dichgans, M. Cerebral autosomal dominant arteriopathy with subcortical infarcts and leukoencephalopathy: phenotypic and mutational spectrum. *J Neurol Sci* 2002; **203–4**: 77–80.

15. Theuns, J, Marjaux, E, Vandenbulcke, M, *et al.* Alzheimer dementia caused by a novel mutation located in the APP C-terminal intracytosolic fragment. *Hum Mutat* 2006; **27**: 888–96.

16. Labauge, P, Krivosic, V, Denier, C, *et al.* Frequency of retinal cavernomas in 60 patients with familial cerebral cavernomas: a clinical and genetic study. *Arch Ophthalmol* 2006; **124**:885–6.

17. AGS Genetic testing for late-onset Alzheimer's disease. AGS eEhics Committee. *J Am Geriatr Soc* 2001; **49**:225–6.

18. Brouwers, N, Sleegers, K, Van Broeckhoven, C. Molecular genetics of Alzheimer's disease: an update. *Ann Med* 2008; **40**:562–83.

19. Hardy, J, Gwinn-Hardy, K. Genetic classification of primary neurodegenerative disease. *Science* 1998; **282**:1075–9.

20. Hardy, J, Selkoe, DJ. The amyloid hypothesis of Alzheimer's disease: progress and problems on the road to therapeutics. *Science* 2002; **297**:353–6.

21. Rovelet-Lecrux, A, Hannequin, D, Raux, G, *et al.* APP locus duplication causes autosomal dominant early-onset Alzheimer disease with cerebral amyloid angiopathy. *Nat Genet* 2006; **38**:24–6.

22. Campion, D, Dumanchin, C, Hannequin, D, *et al.* Early-onset autosomal dominant Alzheimer disease: prevalence, genetic heterogeneity, and mutation spectrum. *Am J Hum Genet* 1999; **65**:664–70.

23. Cruts, M, Van Broeckhoven, C. Loss of progranulin function in frontotemporal lobar degeneration. *Trends Genet* 2008; **24**:186–94.

24. Gijselinck, I, van der Zee, J, Engelborghs, S, *et al.* Progranulin locus deletion in frontotemporal dementia. *Hum Mutat* 2008; **29**:53–8.

25. McKeith, IG, Morris, CM. Apolipoprotein E genotyping in Alzheimer's disease. *Lancet* 1996; **347**:1775.

26. Josephs, KA. Frontotemporal dementia and related disorders: deciphering the enigma. *Ann Neurol* 2008; **64**:4–14.

27. Le Ber, I, van der Zee, J, Hannequin, D, *et al.* Progranulin null mutations in both sporadic and familial frontotemporal dementia. *Hum Mutat* 2007; **28**:846–55.

28. Goldman, JS, Farmer, JM, Wood, EM, *et al.* Comparison of family histories in FTLD subtypes and related tauopathies. *Neurology* 2005; **65**:1817–19.

CHAPTER 8

Molecular diagnosis of neurogenetic disorders: motoneuron, peripheral nerve and muscle disorders

J-M. Burgunder,[1] L. Schöls,[2] J. Baets,[3,4,5] P. Andersen,[6] T. Gasser,[7] Z. Szolnoki,[8] B. Fontaine,[9] C. Van Broeckhoven,[4,5] S. Di Donato,[10] P. De Jonghe,[3,4,5] T. Lynch,[11] C. Mariotti,[12] A. Spinazzola,[12] S. J. Tabrizi,[13] C. Tallaksen,[14] M. Zeviani,[15] H. F. Harbo,[13] and J. Finsterer[15]

[1]University of Bern, Switzerland; [2]University of Tübingen, Tübingen, Germany; [3]University Hospital of Antwerp, Antwerp, Belgium; [4]VIB; Antwerp, Belgium; [5]Institute Born-Bunge, and University of Antwerp, Antwerp, Belgium; [6]Umeå University, Umeå, Sweden; [7]University of Tübingen, Tübingen, Germany; [8]Pandy County Hospital, Gyula, Hungary; [9]Assistance Publique-Hôpitaux de Paris, Centre de référence des canalopathies musculaires, Groupe Hospitalier Pitié-Salpêtrière, Paris, France; [10]Fondazione-IRCCS, Istituto Neurologico Carlo Besta, Milan, Italy; [11]Mater Misericordiae University, Beaumont & Mater Private Hospitals, Dublin, Ireland; [12]IRCCS Foundation, Neurological Institute Carlo Besta, Milan, Italy; [13]Institute of Neurology and National Hospital for Neurology and Neurosurgery, London, UK; [14]University Hospital, Ullevål, Oslo, Norway Faculty Division Ullevål University Hospital, University of Oslo, Oslo, Norway; [15]KA Rudolfstiftung, Vienna and Danube University Krems, Austria

Introduction

Since the publication of the first EFNS guidelines on the molecular diagnosis of inherited neurological diseases in 2001 [1, 2] rapid progress has been made in this field, necessitating the creation of an updated version of these guidelines, which follows the EFNS Scientific Committee recommendations for guideline papers [3].

Objectives

These EFNS guidelines on the molecular diagnosis of motoneuron disorders, polyneuropathies and myopa-thies are designed to summarize the possibilities and limitations of molecular genetic techniques and to provide diagnostic criteria for deciding when a molecular diagnostic work-up is indicated.

Search strategy

To collect data about planning, conditions and perform-ance of molecular diagnosis of motoneuron disorders, polyneuropathies and myopathies a literature search in various electronic databases, including the Cochrane Library, Medline, OMIM, GENETEST and EMBASE, was carried out and original papers, meta-analyses, review papers and guideline recommendations reviewed.

European Handbook of Neurological Management: Volume 2, Second Edition. Edited by Nils Erik Gilhus, Michael P. Barnes, Michael Brainin.
© 2012 Blackwell Publishing Ltd. Published 2012 by Blackwell Publishing Ltd.

Method for reaching consensus

Consensus about the recommendations was reached by a step-wise approach. First, Task Force members met at the EFNS congresses in 2007 and 2008 to discuss the preparations of the guidelines. Second, experts in the field of genetics of neuromuscular disorders and myopathies wrote a guideline proposal. Then these recommendations were distributed and discussed in detail among all Task Force members until a consensus was reached.

Results and recommendations

Recommendations follow the criteria established by the EFNS [3], with some modifications to account for the specific nature of genetic tests. Since genetic testing is by definition the gold standard in the diagnosis of a genetically defined disease, its diagnostic accuracy cannot be tested against another diagnostic method. Therefore, the level of recommendations will be based on the quality of available studies [3], which investigate the proportion of cases of a clinically defined group of patients explained by a specific molecular diagnostic test. As nearly all of these studies have a retrospective design and look for a specific mutation in a previously ascertained and clinically diagnosed cohort of patients, the highest achievable recommendation level is Level B [3]. If only small case-series studying genotype–phenotype correlations are available, the level of recommendation is Level C. If only case reports could be found, but experts still felt that they could give a recommendation, the level of recommendation was assessed as a good practice point. The more frequent genes have been included in the paper (Tables 8.1–8.4), while a more comprehensive list of known genes is included in Supplementary Material online, Tables S1–S4.

Molecular diagnosis of motoneuron diseases

Amyotrophic lateral sclerosis

Familial forms are presented by 5–10% of cases with amyotrophic lateral sclerosis (ALS). ALS-1 is the most common, represents about 12–23% of familial ALS and is caused by mutations in the gene for superoxide dis-

mutase 1 (*SOD1*) on chromosome 21q21-22 (Table 8.1). Additionally, about 1–4% of sporadic ALS cases carry *SOD1* mutations. So far, some 158 mutations have been identified in the *SOD1* gene, of which 142 are believed to be pathogenic. All other forms of monogenetic ALS are rare (Table S1) [4]. Juvenile forms of ALS have been characterized as ALS-2, ALS-4, ALS-5 and ALS-X. *SOD1* mutations may be inherited as an autosomal dominant trait with complete or incomplete penetrance, as an autosomal recessive disease or as a *de novo* mutation, with some degree of genotype–phenotype correlation [5]. Hereditary forms of ALS show equal gender distribution, tend to start earlier than sporadic ALS (mean age 46 vs. 60 years) and initially present with bulbar signs in 20–30% of cases, but are otherwise clinically indistinguishable from sporadic ALS. ALS may be coincident with frontotemporal dementia (FTD) in 5–15% of cases. Different loci for ALS-FTD including genes involving the tau metabolism have been identified to provide susceptibility to ALS (Table 8.1 and Table S1) [6]. At present there is no specific therapy for patients with *SOD1* gene mutations. A number of specific phase 1 clinical trials in patients with *SOD1* gene mutations are in progress to modulate *SOD1* gene expression.

Proximal spinal muscular atrophy

Proximal spinal muscular atrophy (SMA) is one of the most common and severe autosomal-recessive diseases of children. The frequency is between 1/8,000 and 1/10,000. The pathology involves dysfunction and loss of anterior horn cells, leading to muscle atrophy and weakness. Four forms of SMA are recognized (Table 8.2): SMA I (infantile, Werdnig-Hofmann type), II (intermediate type), III (juvenile, Kugelberg-Welander type) and IV (adult type). Early-onset forms (SMA I–III) are frequently caused by a homozygous deletion of exon 7 of the telomeric copy of the survival motorneuron gene (*SMN1*). In the remaining 2–5% of cases the disease is caused by point mutations or small deletions or insertions in this gene. Most of these cases are compound heterozygotes with the common *SMN1* deletion on one chromosome and another mutation on its homologue. Spinal muscular atrophy with respiratory distress (SMARD1) [7], with mutations in the immunoglobulin mu binding protein 2 gene (*IGHMBP2*) gene and other forms of SMA, significantly overlap with distal hereditary motor neuropathy (see below).

Table 8.1 Genetic subtypes amyotrophic lateral sclerosis (ALS) (except rare forms: see Supplementary Table 1 online).

Disease	Inheritance	Chromosomal position	Gene product	Frequency and ethnicity	Molecular diagnosis	Age at onset [years]	Remarks	OMIM
ALS 1	AD AR	21q	SOD1	Most common autosomal dominant form, 6% of all ALS cases	B	Mean: 46–48 Range: 6–94	Incomplete penetrance with some mutations	105400
ALS 5	AR	15q15	Unknown	Most common autosomal recessive from	D	10–20	Predominant lower motor neuron, late bulbar involvement	602099
ALS 9	AD	14q11	Angiogenin	Most identified in Irish, Italian and Scottish families	C	27–76		611895
ALS-FTD	AD	17q21	MAPT		C		Frontotemporal dementia and Parkinsonism more common than ALS	600274
FTLDU	AD	17q21	Progranulin	>150 families	C	35–87	Prominent frontotemporal dementia, mild parkinsonism, ALS rare	607485

Abbreviations: AD = autosomal dominant; AR = autosomal recessive; *MAPT* = microtubule-associated protein tau; *SOD1* = superoxide dismutase 1

Availability of molecular diagnosis:

A: Routine procedure, commercially available, results usually within 4 weeks

B: Routine procedure, but may be time-consuming and expensive, usually due to occurrence of multiple mutations; results may take several months

C: Usually available only within research setting

D: Not yet available

Table 8.2 Genetics of Spinal muscular atrophy (SMA).

Disease	Inheritance	Chromosomal position	Gene product	Frequency and ethnicity	Molecular diagnosis	Age at onset [years]	Remarks	OMIM number
Spinal muscular atrophy SMA I (Werdnig-Hoffmann): SMA II (intermediate form): SMA III (Kugelberg-Welander)	AR	5q11.2-13	Survival motoneuron (SMN1)	Common	A	SMA I: infantile SMA II: 0–3 SMA III: 3–30	Deletion of the SMN1 gene	253300 253400
SMA IV (adult form)	?	Unknown	Unknown		D	SMA: >30	Rarely deletions of SMN1	271150
Spinal and bulbar muscular atrophy (SBMA), Kennedy disease	X-linked	Xq11-q12	Androgen receptor		A	20–50	CAG repeat expansion	313200
Spinal muscular atrophy with respiratory distress (SMARD1)	AR	11q13	IGHMBP2	>50 families	B	Congenital – 2 months	Allelic with dHMN6	604320

Abbreviations: AD = autosomal dominant; AR = autosomal recessive;
Availability of molecular diagnosis:
A: Routine procedure, commercially available, results usually within 4 weeks
B: Routine procedure, but may be time-consuming and expensive, usually due to occurrence of multiple mutations; results may take several months
C: Usually available only within research setting
D: Not yet available

Spinal and bulbar muscular atrophy (SBMA), Kennedy disease

SBMA is an X-linked recessive disorder, affecting males with progressive limb and bulbar weakness, fasciculations (in particular on the chin and periorally, where fasciculations are rarely seen in ALS and SMA type IV) and muscle wasting. Patients have variable involvement of the lower motor and sensory neurons and endocrine systems, including diabetes mellitus, gynaecomastia and reduced fertility. Motor deficits mimic those of ALS and dominate the clinical presentation. The main difference is the absence of upper motoneuron involvement, a rather benign course of the disease and the X-linked inheritance in SBMA [8]. SBMA is caused by the expansion of a CAG trinucleotide repeat in the first exon of the androgen receptor (AR) gene (abnormal range ≥ 35 repeats; normal alleles 9–34 repeats).

Recommendations

Currently, molecular diagnosis mainly has implications for genetic counselling rather than for therapy. However, when more directed aetiological therapies become available, establishing a correct genetic diagnosis in a given patient will be essential. Despite the rather low prevalence, sequencing of the small *SOD1* gene should be considered in ALS patients with dominant inheritance in order to offer presymptomatic or prenatal diagnosis, if this is requested by the family (Level B). Screening for *SMN1* deletions is indicated in SMA I–III to confirm the diagnosis and provide genetic counselling (Level B). In patients with spinal muscular atrophies with respiratory distress starting in the first months of life sequencing of *IGHMBP2* is likely to provide a molecular diagnosis (Level C). In adult-onset SMA genetic testing for SBMA should be considered in males with bulbar manifestations, gynaecomastia and X-linked inheritance (Level B).

Molecular diagnosis of inherited neuropathies

Introduction

Inherited peripheral neuropathies form a clinically and genetically heterogeneous group of disorders, which is the most common group of inherited neuromuscular diseases and has an estimated prevalence of 1/2,500 [9]. Based on clinical observations, they can be classified into four main categories: hereditary motor and sensory neuropathy (HMSN, or CMT after the first describers Charcot, Marie and Tooth), characterized by progressive distal weakness and atrophy, with gait disorder, areflexia and sensory loss with a distal to proximal gradient; distal hereditary motor neuropathy (HMN), hereditary sensory and autonomic neuropathy (HSAN) and the hereditary episodic neuropathies. In total, up to 40 genes have been identified causing the different variants of hereditary neuropathy (Table 8.3 with the most common forms and Table S3; see also www.molgen.ua.ac.be/CMTMutations). In general, AR mutations lead to loss of function. In AD forms, however, many of the mutated proteins result in a toxic gain of function that cannot be deduced directly from the normal function of the gene product. Several genes encode ubiquitously expressed proteins, raising the question of how mutations cause such selective damage to the peripheral nervous system. Nonetheless, some common pathways are emerging: structural myelin proteins, protein synthesis, protein sorting and degradation, transport and cytoskeleton, mitochondrial dynamics, RNA/DNA metabolism and nerve growth regulation [10].

Charcot-Marie-Tooth disease

Disease onset in CMT is usually in the first two decades of life and progression is slow, resulting in mild to moderate impairment. The motor nerve conduction velocity (NCV) in the median nerve is markedly reduced (<38 m/s) in demyelinating CMT (CMT1) and normal or only slightly decreased in axonal CMT (CMT2) in which decreased amplitudes of the compound muscle action potentials (CMAPs) are found. In addition, intermediate forms have been described, displaying overlap between CMT1 and CMT2. Inheritance can be autosomal (mostly dominant in non-consanguineous families and outbred populations) and X-linked. *De novo* mutations seem to be frequent, affecting up to one third of patients depending on the series [11]. In general, recessive inheritance is rarer than dominant and is related to a more severe course of the disease with onset in early infancy, delayed motor milestones, loss of ambulation and variable associated signs [12]. Disease onset and severity show considerable variability. The earliest and most severe form is the rare congenital hypomyelinating neuropathy (CHN) in which disease starts shortly after birth with hypotonia and muscle wasting, resulting in

Table 8.3 Genetics of the most frequent hereditary neuropathies (rare forms: see Supplementary Table 3 online).

Gene	Gene product	Locus	Phenotype	Additional features	Alternative	OMIM
Charcot-Marie Tooth (CMT)						
Demyelinating forms (CMT1) – autosomal dominant (AD)						
PMP22 duplication/ point mutation*	Peripheral myelin protein 22	17p11.2	CMT1A		HNPP (deletion)	601097
*MPZ**	Myelin Protein Zero	1q22	CMT1B, CMT1E	Late onset (axonal forms), pupillary abnormalities (CMT2J)	Axonal (CMT2I, CMT2J) and intermediate (CMTDI3)	159440
Axonal forms (CMT2) – autosomal dominant (AD)						
*MFN2**	Mitofusin 2	1p36.2	CMT2A2	Optic atrophy, pyramidal tract signs		608507
X-linked forms (CMTX)						
*GJB1**	Gap Junction associated protein B1	Xq13.1	CMTX1	more severe phenotype in males (demyelinating)		304040
Inherited focal episodic neuropathies						
*PMP22 deletion**	Peripheral myelin protein 22	17p11.2	HNPP		CMT1A (duplication)	162500
SEPT9	Septin-9	17q25	HNA			604061

*genes offered as routine genetic diagnostics.

feeding and breathing difficulties and sometimes premature death. Another severe phenotype, known as Déjerine-Sottas neuropathy, has early infantile onset. Several additional features can be present in certain sub-forms of CMT which can sometimes help to guide molecular diagnosis (e.g., vocal cord paralysis, cranial nerve involvement, upper limb predominance, pyramidal tract signs, optic atrophy, etc.) [13].

Information on gene and mutation distribution in the different forms of hereditary neuropathy to be used for guideline formulation is based on a limited number of studies. The most common form, CMT1A, is caused by a duplication of the *PMP22* gene on chromosome 17 (Table 8.3) and accounts for 43% of all CMT cases and up to 70% of AD CMT1 [11]. The high frequency of *de novo* duplication or deletions on chromosome 17 stresses the importance of suspicion of genetic disease in isolated patients with compatible phenotype. The second most common genotype corresponds to mutations in *GJB1* (Table 8.3) causing X-linked CMT found in approximately 10% of all CMT patients [14]. Point mutations in *MPZ* and *PMP22* correspond to 5% and 2.5% of CMT1

patients respectively. CMT2 accounts for at least a third of hereditary neuropathies with CMT2A2 caused by mutations in *MFN2* (Table 8.3), representing 20–30% in the CMT2 subgroup [15]. In a smaller proportion of patients mutations in *GJB1* and *MPZ* can be found [11]. In the intermediate forms of CMT *GJB1* and *MPZ* are the most likely genes to be involved. Mutations in other genes are reported in only a small minority of patients and reliable population data are lacking (Table S3), overall a molecular diagnosis can be made in as much as 65% of adults with a CMT phenotype by performing *PMP22* duplication and *GJB1* mutation analysis. This number rises to 80% in patients with demyelinating CMT [11].

Given the rarity of AR CMT in the European population, routine diagnostic screening of the many known genes is currently not feasible (see Table S3 for a comprehensive listing). Most patients are isolated due to the small size of kinships, making the distinction with *de novo* mutations or reduced penetrance in AD CMT very difficult. Molecular diagnosis can be guided by the presence of particular clinical, neuropathological and electrophysiological features [12]. In more selected consanguineous populations the relative proportion of AR CMT is substantially higher, thus potentially increasing the yield of mutation screening in recessive genes, even if data on the relative frequency of each sub-form are still lacking [12].

Hereditary motor neuropathy

HMN is a mostly AD, rare pure peripheral motor disorder with a distal predominance, accounting for 10% of all hereditary neuropathies. It is sometimes accompanied by pyramidal tract signs, vocal cord paralysis or hand predilection. Nerve conduction studies are indicative of an axonal neuropathy more or less selectively affecting the motor nerves [16]. Two mutations in exon 3 of *BSCL2* (Seipin) have been found in HMN, and this is with 7% the most frequently mutated gene in this disorder (Table S3). Mutations are found in 15% of the patients presenting with accompanying pyramidal tract involvement [17].

Hereditary sensory-autonomic neuropathy

HSAN is characterized by variable sensory and autonomic symptoms due to selective degeneration of peripheral sensory and autonomic neurons. Hallmark features are progressive sensory loss with marked insensitivity to pain, skin changes with chronic ulceration and sometimes more severe complications, such as osteomyelitis, necessitating amputations [18].

Limited information is available on gene and mutations distribution in HSAN (Table S3). In a recently performed study the cumulative mutation frequency in all known genes for a large cohort of HSAN patients was 19% [19]. Mutations in *NTRK1* (neurotrophic tyrosine kinase receptor type 1) correspond to a very specific and homogeneous phenotype, congenital insensitivity to pain with anhidrosis (CIPA). Mutations in *RAB7* can be found in CMT2B, a motor and sensory neuropathy that is often considered to be part of the spectrum of HSAN due to the pronounced sensory abnormalities and associated ulceromutilations (Table S3). *RAB7* (Ras-Associated protein Rab7) and *NTRK1* mutations account each for 7% of patients in the selected cohort [19].

Recurrent focal neuropathies

A final subgroup consists of hereditary recurrent focal neuropathies [20], including hereditary neuropathy with susceptibility to pressure palsies (HNPP), related to CMT1 and due to a deletion in the same region of chromosome 17, and hereditary neuralgic amyotrophy (HNA) with recurrent attacks of pain, weakness and sensory disturbances following the distribution of the brachial plexus. Both present with an AD inheritance.

HNPP is a genetically homogeneous disorder. The overwhelming majority of patients with a clinically established diagnosis of HNPP carry the *PMP22* deletion on chromosome 17 (Table 8.3). Rare patients with loss-of-function point mutations in *PMP22* can also be found [20]. Mutations in *SEPT9* (Septin 9) are known to cause HNA (Table S3). However, this disorder is genetically heterogeneous since several families have been reported that do not map to the locus harbouring this gene [20]. No population data are available for HNA.

Recommendations

Diagnosis in hereditary neuropathies is based on patient and family history (including ethnicity) and clinical examination revealing the various hallmarks of neuropathy. Gait disturbance, foot deformities (e.g., pes cavus and hammer toes), distal atrophy, weakness and sensory loss in lower and upper limbs and areflexia. Special attention for additional or unusual features is warranted. Nerve conduction studies differentiating the predominant phenotypes (i.e., motor or sensory, axonal or demyelinating) are essential to orient molecular genetic analyses. Concentric needle EMG recordings are usually indicative of chronic neurogenic changes and may help to distinguish between HMN and distal myopathies. Although the distinction between different disease entities is not always straightforward,

most patients can be assigned to one of the categories described above.

Currently, molecular genetic testing can be offered for several of the more prevalent CMT genes. There are numerous rare genes (especially for AR forms) for which analysis is unlikely to be offered routinely. Screening of these genes is usually restricted to a handful of research laboratories.

In patients presenting with CMT1, *PMP22* duplication should be examined first, followed by sequencing of *GJB1* (if no male-to-male transmission is present), *MPZ* and *PMP22* (Level B). In the case of CMT2, *MFN2* is the first gene to be screened, followed by *MPZ*, since a limited number of specific mutations in this gene are known to cause axonal CMT (Level B). Mutations in GJB1, especially in women, also often present as CMT2. In patients with intermediate CMT, *GJB1* and *MPZ* should be screened (Level B).

HNPP caused by a *PMP22* deletion on chromosome 17 is investigated simultaneously with the screening for *PMP22* duplication (CMT1A) and is thus offered as a routine diagnostic procedure (Level B).

For both HMN and HSAN overall mutation frequencies are too low to make routine diagnostic screening feasible. If screenings are conducted, *BSCL2* is the first candidate to screen in HMN [17]; for HSAN, *NTRK1* can be screened in CIPA patients and *RAB7* in CMT2B patients [19] (Level B). The *SEPT9* gene is not part of routine diagnostics but could be screened in the context of HNA (Level C).

Molecular diagnosis of myopathies

Introduction

During the last couple of years, a tremendous increase in data on numerous hereditary myopathies has been produced. Other than in the most common hereditary myopathies, prevalence data on the involvement of different genes in different populations are not yet known. In general, the clinical diagnosis can be complemented by quite precise morphological and protein expression data during muscle biopsy, suggesting a particular gene being involved. (Regularly actualized tables can be found online: www.musclegenetable.org.)

Muscle dystrophies
Duchenne/Becker muscular dystrophy (DMD/BMD)

Duchenne/Becker muscular dystrophy is an X-linked recessive condition (Table 8.4). The frequency of DMD is 1/3,000 and BMD 1/20,000. The age of onset of DMD in most of the cases is <5 years. Characteristic of the clinical features are progressive muscular weakness, mainly proximal, calf pseudohypertrophy, as well as markedly elevated serum creatine kinase. In BMD the onset is later and the course of the disease is generally milder, but there is a remarkable variability of clinical expression. Muscle biopsy demonstrates the typical dystrophic changes, with absence of dystrophin in DMD and variably decreased dystrophin in BMD. The dystrophin gene, which spans 2.4 Mb of DNA, is very large, with 85 exons and maps to chromosome Xp21, shows deletions of variable size in approximately 60% of cases, duplications are found in 5–10% and point mutations are responsible in the remainder.

In a typical case of a young patient with a clinical presentation suggestive of DMD or BMD including an X-chromosomal inheritance, a molecular diagnosis can be made from blood DNA without the need for a biopsy.

If a PCR-based assay for deletions is negative, it is worthwhile performing dystrophin analysis based on immunohistochemistry and on immunoblot from a muscle biopsy. In the case of abnormal dystrophin expression more complex analysis, including multiplex ligation-dependent probe amplification, may lead to the diagnosis [21]. As there is a high probability of gonadal mosaicism, prenatal diagnosis is offered, not only to the confirmed carriers but also to women who previously gave birth to affected boys (isolated cases) and DNA analysis has shown that they are not the carriers.

Facioscapulohumeral muscular dystrophy (FSHD)

FSHD is an autosomal dominant condition. The frequency is 1/20,000 in the Netherlands. Distribution of muscle weakness and wasting reveals descending progression involving the face, shoulder girdle, hip girdle and peroneal muscles [22].

The gene for FSHD is located on chromosome 4q35 (Table 8.4), but is still not known. In affected persons, Southern blots of DNA digested with EcoRI and probed with p13E-11 reveal a decreased fragment between 10 and 38 kb. This is probably due to a deletion of variable size in a 3.3 kb repetitive sequence (D_4Z_4). Interpretation of molecular studies in FSHD is not straightforward because 30% of the subjects with the deletion are asymptomatic. Furthermore, there is a highly homologous polymorphic repeat on chromosome 10, with observations of exchange between the two chromosomes, and a bi-allelic variation on chromosome 4q35, which stresses the need of the use of more complex molecular methods to diagnose FSH. On the other hand, a deletion has been detected only in 95% of the patients affected with FSHD.

Myotonic dystrophy

Myotonic dystrophy is one of the most frequent muscular dystrophies affecting adults and children. Besides wasting

Table 8.4 Genetics of the myopathies (except rare forms: see Supplementary Table 4 online).

Gene	Gene product	Locus	Phenotype	Additional features and/or Alternative phentoypes	OMIM
Muscular dystrophies					
X chromosomal					
DYS	Dystrophin	Xp21.2	Duchenne muscle dystrophy	Cardiomyopathy dilated Becker	310200
EMD	Emerin	Xq28	Emery Dreifuss muscle dystrophy		310300
Autosomal dominant (AD)					
DMPK	Myotonic dystrophy protein kinase	19q13.3	Myotonic dystrophy		160900
FSHD	FSHD	4q35	Facio scapulohumeral muscle dystrophy		158900
MYOT	myotilin	5q31	LGMD1A	Myofibrillar myopathy Hyperckemia, idiopathic	159000
CAV3	caveolin-3	3p25	LGMD1C	Muscular dystrophy Rippling muscle disease	601253
Autosomal recessive (AR)					
CAPN3	calpain3	15q15	LGMD2A		253600
DYSG	dysferlin	2p13	LGMD2B	Miyoshi myopathy. Distal myopathy, with anterior tibial onset	603009
SGCG	γ-sarcoglycan	13q12	LGMD2C		253700
SGCA	α-sarcoglycan	17q12-q21.33	LGMD2D		600119
SGCB	β-sarcoglycan	4q12	LGMD2E		604286
SGCD	δ-sarcoglycan	5q33-q34	LGMD2F		601287
Congenital muscular dystrophies					
Autosomal dominant					
DNM2	Dynamin 2	19p13.2	Congenital muscular dystrophy with dynamin 2 defect	Charcot-Marie-Tooth disease, dominant intermediate B Myopathy, centronuclear, autosomal dominant	NA
Autosomal recessive					
TGA7	Integrin a7	12q	Integrin a7 deficiency		613204
LAMA2	Laminin a2 chain of merosin	6q22-q23	Merosin deficient CMD		607855
FKRP	Fukutin related protein	19q1	CMD + secondary merosin deficiency	Walker-Warburg Syndrome	606612
FCMD	Fukutin	9q31-q33	Fukuyama congenital muscular dystrophy	Muscular dystrophy, limbgirdle, type 2L Walker-Warburg syndrome	253800
COL6A1	alpha 1 type VI collagen	21q22.3	Ullrich Syndrome	Bethlem myopathy (also AD)	254090
					continued

Table 8.4 continued

Gene	Gene product	Locus	Phenotype	Additional features and/or Alternative phentoypes	OMIM
Congenital myopathies					
Autosomal recessive					
TPM3	tropomyosin 3	1q21-q23	Nemaline myopathy 1		609284
ACTA1	alpha actin, skeletal muscle	1q42.13-q42.2	Nemaline myopathy 1	congenital myopathy with excess of thin myofilaments congenital myopathy with fiber-type disproportion	161800
RYR1	ryanodine receptor 1	19q13.1	Central core disease	Malignant hyperthermia susceptibility 1	117000
MYH7	myosin, heavy polypeptide 7, cardiac muscle, beta	14q12	Hyaline body myopathy	Cardiomyopathy, dilated Myopathy, distal 1 Myosin storage myopathy	608358
Autosomal recessive					
NEB	nebulin	2q22	Nemaline myopathy 2		256030
X chromosomal					
MTM1	myotubularin	Xq28	Myotubular myopathy		310400
Distal myopathies					
Autosomal dominant					
TTN	titin	2q31	Tibial muscular dystrophy	Cardiomyopathy, dilated, Udd Myopathy LGMD2J	600334
MYOT	myotilin	5q31	Distal myopathy with myotilin defect	LGMD1A LGMD1	609200
DNM2	dynamin	2 19p13.2	Dynamin2 related distal myopathy	Charcot-Marie-Tooth disease, dominant intermediate B Myopathy, centronuclear, autosomal dominant	160150
Autosomal recessive					
DYSF	dysferlin	2p12-14	Distal recessive myopathy	Miyoshi myopathy LGMD2B	254130
Myofibrillar myopathies					
Autosomal dominant					
DES	desmin	2q35	Myofibrillar myopathy, desmin-related myopathy		601419
PABP2	Poly(A) binding protein 2	14q11.2-q13	Oculopharyngeal muscle dystrophy		164300

Other abbreviations: LGMD: limb-girdle muscle dystrophy.

and myotonia in skeletal muscles in a characteristic distribution (facial muscles, mostly temporal, masseter and sternocleidomastoid, as well as distal limb muscles) the disease also affects several other organ systems. Additional features are male baldness, often cataract, cognitive changes, hormonal disturbances, cardiomyopathy and visceral symptoms.

The genetic basis for DM1 is a CTG repeats expansion in the DMPK gene on 19q13 (Table 8.4). Normal alleles vary from 5 to 37 CTGs; 38–49 is considered as subclinical permutation, expansion over 50 is usually associated with clinical manifestations.

DM2, another autosomal dominant disorder, closely resembles DM1, except that muscle weakness is predominantly proximal and less pronounced, while hypertrophy of calves is frequent, has been described as proximal myotonic myopathy (DM2). It is caused by an expansion of CCTG repeat in the zinc finger protein-9, which can be directly examined in typical cases, or in DM cases without CTG expansion in the DMPK gene (Table 8.4).

Emery-Dreifuss-type muscular dystrophy

The clinical features are: joint contractures, mostly in elbows, knees, ankles, neck; and moderate weakness and wasting of muscles, mostly of a proximal distribution in the upper extremities and a distal pattern in the legs. Cardiac symptoms also occur. The first symptoms start usually in childhood as contractures. Cardiac symptoms may occur also in otherwise asymptomatic heterozygous female carriers.

The disease is genetically heterogeneous – the main mode of transmission is X-linked (Table 8.4 and Table S4). In these cases, deletions are found in a small gene on Xq28 (Emerin). Most mutations are private (i.e., different in each affected family) and complete sequencing is usually necessary.

Limb-girdle muscular dystrophies

The limb-girdle muscular dystrophies (LGMDs) form a group of genetically determined disorders with the common feature of a progressive proximal muscle weakness. The prevalence is about 1/15,000 and varies among populations. There is a high variety of clinical phenotypes, with a large number of mutations in different genes described so far (Table 8.4 and Table S4). Four of the autosomal recessive inherited forms result from mutations in the genes coding for dystrophin-associated

proteins, sarcoglycans (SG) α, β, γ, δ, and cardiac involvement is known. The subset of autosomal recessive LGMD without SG involvement is represented by several variants (Table 8.4 and Table S4). One of them is caused by mutations in the calpain 3 (*CANP3*) gene, another variant results from mutations in the dysferlin (*DYSF*) gene; and 5–10% of LGMDs are inherited in an autosomal dominant fashion. The prevalence of mutations in Caveolin-3 (*CAV3*), the first gene to be known in this group, and the others is not known. Furthermore, overlap with other phenotypes and cardiac involvement has been well established. The first step in the molecular diagnosis of LGMD is to use a comprehensive panel of immunological tests in the muscle biopsy. The absence or severe reduction of immunoreactivity using immunohistochemistry or immunoblot of one of the sarcoglycans will point to the most likely mutated gene, while a more subtle change may be secondary to the destabilization of the complex. If *SGs* appear normal, the use of antibodies recognizing *CANP3* and *DYSF* in muscles is recommended. Once the candidate has been recognized at the protein level, mutation search can be performed selectively.

Congenital muscular dystrophies

Several forms of variable muscle dystrophies with an autosomal recessive inheritance, manifesting early in life with a progressive variable phenotype including hypotonia, weakness, contractures, elevated creatine kinase and dystrophic features at muscle biopsy, are usually grouped as congenital muscular dystrophies. So far 13 forms of congenital muscular dystrophies (CMD) with overlapping phenotypes have been genetically characterized (Table 8.4 and Table S4). In a typical mixed cohort of patients, fewer than half could be diagnosed at the molecular level using immunological studies of muscle protein and molecular genetic testing [23].

Congenital myopathies

This is a large group of rare diseases having as a common clinical denominator congenital floppiness, muscle weakness, slimness and frequent skeletal dysmorphism. The usually slowly progressive clinical phenotype is variable and overlapping among the different forms, including central-core disease, multi-minicore disease, congenital fibre type disproportion and newly described entities such as actin aggregate myopathy or desmin myopathy

(Table 8.4 and Table S4). The diagnosis is based on specific morphological abnormalities found in the muscle biopsy.

Central core disease (CCD, Table 8.4) is transmitted as an autosomal dominant trait. The characteristic feature of muscle histopathology is an amorphous area in the centre of the fibre. CCD is caused by mutations in the ryanodine receptor on chromosome 19q13 and is allelic (different mutations in a single gene) to one form of malignant hyperthermia susceptibility (MHS). Patients with CCD are at risk for malignant hyperthermia and both conditions may appear in the same family. MHS is genetically heterogeneous. It has been estimated that approximately 50% of cases are due to mutations in the ryanodine receptor. Identification of a particular mutation in a family with an individual known to be susceptible to malignant hyperthermia may be helpful to counsel family members and obviate a muscle biopsy.

The characteristic histopathological feature of nemaline myopathy (Table 8.4) is the presence of small rods, originating from the Z-band of the muscle fibre, staining red by the Gomori technique. The disease is transmitted as an autosomal recessive (maps to 2q21.2–2q22) or autosomal dominant trait (maps to 1q 21–23). The gene product is ⟨-tropomyosine). The course is quite variable, with very severe, usually lethal neonatal, childhood and adult forms.

In myotubular or centronuclear myopathy (Table 8.4) the nuclei are situated centrally, surrounded by a pale halo. The muscle fibres show signs of immaturity. There are several different forms of myotubular myopathy, including X-linked (mapped to Xq28), recessive and autosomal dominant forms. Actin or desmin aggregates are demonstrated in the muscle biopsy.

Other myopathies

Distal myopathies form a group of mainly muscular dystrophies with dorsal or ventral involvement of distal upper and lower extremities. The incidence is regionally variable and the age of onset is typically in adulthood. The phenotype may overlap with other myopathies and vacuoles are commonly found at muscle biopsy. Myofibrillar myopathies are characterized by specific cytoplasmatic inclusions. Similar to other hereditary myopathies, morphological features complement clinical phenotype description to guide molecular diagnostics (Table 8.4 and Table S4).

Recommendations

In the presence of a typical phenotype, which includes data from both the patient and the family, a molecular diagnosis can be made without further investigations. This includes a male patient with muscular dystrophy, whose uncle had a similar phenotype, a patient with the typical presentation of a myotonic dystrophy or of a facio-scapulohumeral dystrophy. In such cases an analysis of the respective gene should be performed without a muscle biopsy (Level B). In limb-girdle dystrophies, in congenital dystrophies and in congenital myopathies, a biopsy is needed in order to collect data on the morphological and molecular phenotype through microscopic and protein expression analysis. These data will then guide the choice of the appropriate gene testing (Level B).

Conflicts of interest

Member of this Task Force have no conflicts of interest related to the recommendations given in this chapter.

References

1. Gasser, T, Dichgans, M, Finsterer, J, et al. EFNS task force on molecular diagnosis of neurologic disorders: guidelines for the molecular diagnosis of inherited neurologic diseases. First of two parts. Eur J Neurol 2001; 8:299–314.
2. Gasser, T, Dichgans, M, Finsterer, J, et al. EFNS task force on molecular diagnosis of neurologic disorders: guidelines for the molecular diagnosis of inherited neurologic diseases. Second of two parts. Eur J Neurol 2001; 8:407–24.
3. Brainin, M, Barnes, M, Baron, JC, et al. Guidance for the preparation of neurological management guidelines by EFNS scientific task forces – revised recommendations 2004. Eur J Neurol 2004; 11:577–81.
4. Schymick, JC, Talbot, K, Traynor, BJ. Genetics of sporadic amyotrophic lateral sclerosis. Hum Mol Genet 2007; 16(2):R233–R242.
5. Andersen, PM, Borasio, GD, Dengler, R, et al. Good practice in the management of amyotrophic lateral sclerosis: clinical guidelines. An evidence-based review with good practice points. EALSC Working Group. Amyotroph Lateral Scler 2007; 8:195–213.
6. Valdmanis, PN, Rouleau, GA. Genetics of familial amyotrophic lateral sclerosis. Neurology 2008; 70:144–52.
7. Kaindl, AM, Guenther, UP, Rudnik-Schoneborn, S, et al. Spinal muscular atrophy with respiratory distress type 1 (SMARD1). J Child Neurol 2008; 23:199–204.
8. Chahin, N, Klein, C, Mandrekar, J, Sorenson, E. Natural history of spinal-bulbar muscular atrophy. Neurology 2008; 70:1967–71.

9. Martyn, CN, Hughes, RA. Epidemiology of peripheral neuropathy. *J Neurol Neurosurg Psychiatr* 1997; **62**:310–18.

10. Niemann, A, Berger, P, Suter, U. Pathomechanisms of mutant proteins in Charcot-Marie-Tooth disease. *Neuromolecular Med* 2006; **8**:217–42.

11. Szigeti, K, Nelis, E, Lupski, JR. Molecular diagnostics of Charcot-Marie-Tooth disease and related peripheral neuropathies. *Neuromolecular Med* 2006; **8**:243–54.

12. Dubourg, O, Azzedine, H, Verny, C, *et al.* Autosomal-recessive forms of demyelinating Charcot-Marie-Tooth disease. *Neuromolecular Med* 2006; **8**:75–86.

13. Pareyson, D, Scaioli, V, Laura, M. Clinical and electrophysiological aspects of Charcot-Marie-Tooth disease. *Neuromolecular Med* 2006; **8**:3–22.

14. Kleopa, KA, Scherer, SS. Molecular genetics of X-linked Charcot-Marie-Tooth disease. *Neuromolecular Med* 2006; **8**: 107–22.

15. Verhoeven, K, Claeys, KG, Zuchner, S, *et al.* MFN2 mutation distribution and genotype/phenotype correlation in Charcot-Marie-Tooth type 2. *Brain* 2006; **129**:2093–102.

16. Irobi, J, Dierick, I, Jordanova, A, *et al.* Unraveling the genetics of distal hereditary motor neuronopathies. *Neuromolecular Med* 2006; **8**:131–46.

17. Dierick, I, Baets, J, Irobi, J, *et al.* Relative contribution of mutations in genes for autosomal dominant distal hereditary motor neuropathies: a genotype–phenotype correlation study. *Brain* 2008; **131**:1217–27.

18. Auer-Grumbach, M, Mauko, B, Auer-Grumbach, P, Pieber, TR. Molecular genetics of hereditary sensory neuropathies. *Neuromolecular Med* 2006; **8**:147–58.

19. Rotthier, A, Baets, J, De Vriendt, E, *et al.* Genes for hereditary sensory and autonomic neuropathies: a genotype-phenotype correlation. *Brain* 2009; **132**:2699–711.

20. Chance, PF. Inherited focal, episodic neuropathies: hereditary neuropathy with liability to pressure palsies and hereditary neuralgic amyotrophy. *Neuromolecular Med* 2006; **8**:159–74.

21. Okizuka, Y, Takeshima, Y, Awano, H, *et al.* Small mutations detected by multiplex ligation-dependent probe amplification of the dystrophin gene. *Genet Test Mol Biomarkers* 2009; **13**:427–31.

22. Kissel, JT. Facioscapulohumeral dystrophy. *Semin Neurol* 1999; **19**:35–43.

23. Peat, RA, Smith, JM, Compton, AG, *et al.* Diagnosis and etiology of congenital muscular dystrophy. *Neurology* 2008; **71**:312–21.

CHAPTER 9

Intravenous immunoglobulin in the treatment of neurological diseases

I. Elovaara,[1] S. Apostolski,[2] P. van Doorn,[3] N. E. Gilhus,[4] A. Hietaharju,[5] J. Honkaniemi,[6] I. N. van Schaik,[7] N. Scolding,[8] P. Soelberg Sørensen,[9] and B. Udd[1]

[1]Tampere University Hospital and School of Medicine, University of Tampere, Tampere, Finland; [2]School of Medicine, University of Belgrade, Belgrade, Serbia; [3]Erasmus Medical Centre, Rotterdam, The Netherlands; [4]Haukeland University Hospital, Bergen, Norway; [5]Tampere University Hospital, Tampere, Finland; [6]Vaasa Central Hospital, Vaasa, Finland; [7]Academic Medical Center, University of Amsterdam, Amsterdam, The Netherlands; [8]University of Bristol Institute of Clinical Neuroscience, Frenchary Hospital UK, Bristol, UK; [9]National University Hospital, Rigshospitalet, Copenhagen, Denmark

Background

Intravenous immunoglobulin (IVIG) has been successfully used to treat a number of immune-mediated diseases of the central and peripheral nervous system. Although the underlying mechanisms of the action of IVIG have not been fully explained, it is known that it can interfere with the immune system at several levels. The effect of IVIG in any particular disease may not be attributed to only one of its action mechanism, because the pathophysiology of these diseases is complex. IVIG has been used as a first-line therapy in Guillain-Barré syndrome (GBS), chronic inflammatory demyelinating polyradiculoneuropathy (CIDP), multifocal motor neuropathy (MMN) and dermatomyositis (DM). It may be used also in diseases of neurotransmission, multiple sclerosis (MS) and in some rare neurological disorders of adults and children, including Rasmussen's encephalitis (RE), stiff-person syndrome (SPS) and post-polio syndrome (PPS). In this chapter we review the available literature on the use of IVIG in treatment of neurological diseases and offer evidence-based recommendations for its use in these disorders.

Search strategy

The Task Force systematically searched Ovid Medline and several other sources to a set of predefined key questions. The final search was performed in December 2007. Recent papers of high relevance were reviewed. Consensus was reached by discussions during a Task Force meeting. Evidence was classified as Class I–IV and recommendations as Level A–C according to the current EFNS guidelines [1]. When only Class IV evidence was available the Task Force has offered advice as good practice points.

Mechanisms of action of IVIG in neurological diseases

Despite over 25 years' usage in autoimmunity, how concentrated non-host immunoglobulins, delivered intravenously, produce their clinical effect remains unknown. Of many potential mechanisms of action [2], whether one (unlikely), all (also unlikely) or several in combination are important remains obscure. It is likely that different effects are relevant in different disorders. We here

European Handbook of Neurological Management: Volume 2, Second Edition. Edited by Nils Erik Gilhus, Michael P. Barnes, Michael Brainin.
© 2012 Blackwell Publishing Ltd. Published 2012 by Blackwell Publishing Ltd.

consider the range of possible actions of IVIG, highlighting effects that appear especially pertinent in specific neurological disorders.

The possibility that IVIG works through non-immune mechanisms [3] (e.g., binding and removal of microbial toxins or targeting their surface antigens) is perhaps less relevant in neurology. However, direct actions on oligodendrocyte progenitors have been postulated to explain an effect in promoting experimental remyelination [4, 5], although alternative mechanisms are possible [6–9].

More direct, immune-modulating effects are generally considered more neurologically relevant. T-cell proliferation is reduced by IVIG [10], various pro-inflammatory cytokines are suppressed, including interleukin-1, tumour necrosis factor-α and γ-interferon, and lymphocyte and monocyte apoptosis is induced [11]. Endogenous immunoglobulin production and B-cell differentiation are suppressed, and IgG catabolism is accelerated by IVIG [3]. Therapeutic immunoglobulins exert Fc region-mediated inhibition of antibody production; they also modulate anti-idiotypic networks vital to immune tolerance.

In addition, IVIG contains anti-idiotypic antibodies that bind to F(ab) to neutralize autoantibodies – a mechanism involved in GM1-related neuropathy and perhaps GBS [12, 13]. Finally considering cytopathic immune effectors, IVIG interferes with the complement system: the beneficial effects of IVIG are associated with the disappearance of complement in the muscles [14], involved suppression of macrophage function through induction of increased $\Phi Fc\gamma RII$-B expression, reducing phagocytic activity.

Guillain-Barré syndrome

The proposed autoimmune aetiology led to the introduction of immunotherapy. Before its introduction, 10% of patients died and 20% were left seriously disabled [15]. Plasma exchange (PE) was introduced as a possible treatment in 1978 and was shown to offer significant benefit by a randomized trial published in 1985 [16, 17]. It became the gold standard against which other treatments were measured [18].

Intravenous immunoglobulin was introduced for GBS in 1988 [19]. In 1992, the first randomized trial comparing IVIG and PE showed similar effects for each treatment [20]. In five trials (total 582 participants), the improvement on the disability grade scale with IVIG was very similar to that with PE, (95% CI 20.25–0.20) [20–24]. The effectiveness of IVIG has been shown in GBS patients unable to walk unaided (GBS disability score ≥3) who were started on IVIG within the first 2 weeks after onset of weakness. Results from PE studies indicate that PE is also effective when applied in patients less severely affected [25] and in patients who are treated within the first 4 weeks from onset [17]. This has not been investigated in studies of IVIG treatment. Although PE was more frequently discontinued, there was also no significant difference between IVIG and PE for other outcome measures [23]. One trial compared PE alone with PE followed by IVIG: the 128 patients who received both treatments did not had significant extra benefit after 4 weeks of treatment compared with the 121 patients who received PE alone [22].

In children, who may have a better prognosis than adults, limited evidence from three open trials suggests that IVIG hastens recovery compared with supportive care alone [26–28], a finding supported by a good quality observational study [29].

A recent trial reported possible minor short-term benefit when high-dose intravenous methylprednisolone was combined with IVIG [30]. The significance of this benefit has been debated [31].

The comparisons of IVIG and PE showed no difference in the long-term outcome. Neither IVIG, PE nor any other treatment significantly reduces mortality, which ranged from 5% to 15% in hospital and population-based studies [32].

Only limited information is available concerning the dosage of IVIG. The usual IVIG regimen is 0.4 g/kg/day for 5 days. In a French trial, 3 days of 0.4 g/kg daily was slightly, but not significantly, less effective than 6 days of 0.4 g/kg daily [25].

In retrospective studies, patients with antibodies to ganglioside GM1 or GM1b treated with IVIG recovered faster than those treated with PE [33–35]. There is no evidence that it is better to administrate IVIG (2 g/kg) in 2 or in 5 days. There is some indication that administration in 2 days may lead to a greater proportion of patients with a relapse [28].

Information is also lacking about how to treat patients who deteriorate or fail to improve after being treated with

IVIG or PE. It is common practice to re-treat patients who improve or stabilize and then relapse with IVIG (2 g/kg in 2–5 days) or PE. There is some indication that relapses occurring after 9 weeks may indicate that the patient had acute-onset CIDP [36]. Some centres treat patients again if they fail to improve after about 2–3 weeks, but evidence for this is lacking [37]. Whether mildly affected GBS patients (able to walk unaided) or patients with Miller Fisher syndrome should be treated with IVIG has not been studied. There is also no study available indicating that a second IVIG course is justified in patients who seem to be unresponsive to IVIG.

Recommendations

IVIG 0.4 g/kg/day for 5 days or PE can be used as first-line treatment and are considered to be equally effective (Level A). IVIG has milder side-effects than PE and this would favour IVIG over PE treatment (Level B). IVIG treatment after PE, as standard combination, does not produce significant extra benefit and cannot be recommended (Level B). Combining high-dose intravenous methylprednisolone with IVIG may have a minor short-term benefit (Level C). Children, who generally have a better prognosis, should be treated with IVIG as first-line treatment (Level C). Patients who improve after IVIG and then relapse should preferentially be treated with a second course of IVIG (good practice point). In patients who seem to be unresponsive to the first course of IVIG a second course may be tried, but evidence supporting this is lacking (good practice point). No recommendations can be given for whether mildly affected GBS patients or patients with Miller Fisher syndrome should be treated with IVIG.

Chronic inflammatory demyelinating polyradiculoneuropathy

Seven randomized controlled trials (RCT) with IVIG have been performed, including 284 patients with CIDP, and have been summarized in a Cochrane systematic review [38, 39, 40, 41, 42, 43, 44]. Four RCTs compared 2 g/kg bodyweight of IVIG [40, 42, 43, 44, 45], administered over 2 or 5 days with placebo, one compared IVIG with a 6-week course of oral prednisolone tapering from 60 to 10 mg daily [41], and one compared 1.8 g/kg bodyweight of IVIG in a course of 6 weeks with PE twice weekly for 3 weeks then once weekly for another 3 weeks [38]. Each study used different outcome measures impeding assessment.

Meta-analysis of the five placebo-controlled trials (232 patients) showed that IVIG produces significant improvement in disability lasting 2–6 weeks with a relative benefit of 2.0, 95% CI 1.48–2.71 (Class I) [39]. The benefit difference is 27%, which gives the number needed to treat (NNT) of 3.7, 95% CI 2.36–6.4. The two crossover trials comparing PE with IVIG and prednisolone with IVIG did not show a significant short-term difference, but the samples were too small to establish equivalence (both Class II) [39]. Both trials had other methodological issues. However, there are many observational studies reporting a beneficial effect from corticosteroids except in pure motor CIDP in which they have sometimes appeared to be harmful (Classes III and IV) [46, 47]. Apart from the treatment of pure motor forms of CIDP, there is no evidence to justify a different approach for other variants of CIDP [46].

Controlled long-term data on disability are available from the largest trial only ($n = 117$) [45]. The initial loading dose of 2 g/kg was followed by a maintenance dose of 1 g/kg every 3 weeks. After 24 weeks of treatment, mean change from baseline disability was −1.1 (SD 1.8) in the IVIG treatment group and −0.3 (SD 1.3) in the placebo treatment group (weighted mean difference −0.8 [95% CI −1.37 to −0.23]). In the second part of the study, after patients were again randomized for IVIG or placebo, a similar effect was found. A long-term, open follow-up in 84 CIDP patients responding to IVIG treatment reported remission in most patients. Seventy-three patients (87%) needed at least two courses; median time to remission was 2.1 years; and 10% of patients needed IVIG for more than 8.7 years [48].

Recommendations

Patients with very mild symptoms which do not or only slightly interfere with activities of daily living may be monitored without treatment (good practice point). Treatment should be considered for patients with moderate or severe disability. IVIG (2 g/kg in 2–5 days) (Level A) or corticosteroids (1 mg/kg or 60 mg daily) (Level B) can be used as first-line treatment in sensorimotor CIDP. The presence of relative contraindications to either treatment should influence the choice (good practice point). For pure motor CIDP, IVIG treatment should be first choice and if corticosteroids are used, patients should be monitored closely for deterioration (good practice point). If a patient responds to IVIG, attempts should be made at intervals to reduce the dose to discover whether the patient still needs

IVIG and what dose is needed (good practice point). It is important to avoid deterioration sometimes seen just before the next IVIG course. The treatment intervals should be such that this does not occur. If a patient becomes stable on intermittent IVIG, the dose should be reduced before the frequency of administration is lowered (good practice point). These recommendations are in line with the EFNS guideline on the management of CIDP previously published [46].

Multifocal motor neuropathy

There are few treatment options for people with MMN. MMN does usually not respond to steroids or PE, and patients may deteriorate when they receive these treatments [49, 50, 51, 52]. The efficacy of IVIG has been suggested by many open, uncontrolled studies; in 94 case reports (487 MMN pts), published between 1990 and 2004, an improvement of muscle weakness was seen in 81% of patients and an improvement of disability was seen in 74% (Class IV) [53]. Four RCTs of IVIG for treating MMN have been performed [54, 55, 56, 57]. These four trials encompass 45 patients, of whom 34 were randomly assigned to IVIG or placebo and have been summarized in a Cochrane systematic review [53]. Different disability scales were used, making the primary end-point of change in disability difficult to assess. Disability showed a trend for improvement with IVIG, however this was not significant ($P = 0.08$). IVIG treatment was significantly superior to placebo in achieving an improvement in muscle strength ($P = 0.0005$; NNT 1.4, 95% CI 1.1–1.8) (Class I). As weakness is the only determinant of disability in patients with MMN, it is to be expected that in patients whose muscle strength improves after IVIG treatment, disability will improve as well.

Elevated anti-ganglioside GM1 antibodies and definite conduction block have been shown to be correlated with a favourable response to IVIG (Class IV) [58]. Approximately a third of patients have a sustained remission (>12 months) with IVIG alone; approximately half of patients need repeated IVIG infusions and, of them, half need additional immunosuppressive treatment [59]. The effect of IVIG declines during prolonged treatment even when dosage is increased, probably due to ongoing axonal degeneration [60, 61]. However, in one retrospective study, treatment with higher than normal mainte-

nance doses of IVIG (1.6–2.0 g/kg over 4–5 days) promoted re-innervation, decreased the number of conduction blocks and prevented axonal degeneration in 10 MMN patients for up to 12 years [62].

Recommendations

As there is no other treatment of proven benefit, the recommendation is to use IVIG (2 g/kg in 2–5 days) as a first-line treatment (Level A). If the initial IVIG treatment is effective, repeated infusions should be considered (Level C). A considerable number of patients need prolonged treatment, but attempts should be made to decrease the dose to discover whether a patient still needs IVIG (good practice point). Furthermore, the frequency of maintenance therapy should be guided by the individual response, whereby typical treatment regimens are 1 g/kg every 2–4 weeks or 2 g/kg every 4–8 weeks (good practice point). A recent European guideline on the management of MMN summarizes the other treatment options [63].

Paraproteinaemic demyelinating neuropathy

Paraproteinaemia, also known as monoclonal gammopathy, is characterized by the presence of abnormal immunoglobulin (M protein) produced by bone marrow cells in blood. The different types of immunoglobulin are classified according to the heavy chain class as IgG, IgA or IgM. The non-malignant paraproteinaemias are generally referred to as monoclonal gammopathy of undetermined significance (MGUS).

Paraproteins are found in up to 10% of patients with peripheral neuropathy not secondary to another primary illness [64]. In about 60% of patients with MGUS-related neuropathy the paraprotein belongs to the IgM subclass [65]. In almost half of patients who have IgM MGUS and a peripheral neuropathy, the M protein reacts against myelin-associated glycoprotein [66]. The most common type of IgM MGUS-related peripheral nerve involvement is a distal, symmetrical demyelinating neuropathy. Patients with IgG or IgA paraproteinaemic neuropathy usually have both proximal and distal weakness and sensory impairment that is indistinguishable from CIDP.

Two randomized placebo-controlled crossover trials with IVIG have been performed, encompassing 33 patients with IgM paraproteinaemic demyelinating neuropathy [67, 68] (Class II). A third randomized study was an open parallel group trial with 20 patients, which compared IVIG and recombinant interferon-α [69] (Class II). The results of these three trials have been summarized in a Cochrane review [70], which concluded that IVIG is relatively safe and may produce some short-term benefit. There are six Class IV studies [71, 72, ,73, 74, 75, 76] with 56 patients treated with IVIG. Of these, 26 showed improvement ranging from transient relief of paraesthesiae to a clear-cut response with a marked gain in daily activities. In an EFNS guideline article the use of IVIG in IgM paraproteinaemic demyelinating neuropathy was recommended only in patients with significant disability or rapid worsening [77].

No controlled trials were available on the effects of IVIG in IgG or IgA paraproteinaemic neuropathy. There is one retrospective review of 20 patients with IgG MGUS neuropathy treated with IVIG; beneficial response was found in 8 [78] (Class IV). An open prospective trial of IVIG reported clinical improvement in 2 of 4 patients with IgG MGUS [72] (Class IV). In a review which included 124 patients with IgG MGUS neuropathy, 81% of the 67 patients with a predominantly demyelinating neuropathy responded to the same immunotherapies used for CIDP (including IVIG) as compared with 20% of those with axonal neuropathy [79] (Class IV). A Cochrane review states that observational or open trial data provide limited support for the use of immunotherapy, including IVIG, in patients with IgG and IgA paraproteinaemic neuropathy [80]. The EFNS guideline concludes that the detection of IgG or IgA MGUS does not justify a different approach from CIDP without a paraprotein [77].

Paraneoplastic syndromes

Due to the low incidence of immunologically mediated paraneoplastic diseases, there are very few prospective, randomized, double-blind and placebo-controlled studies. Paraneoplastic syndromes involving peripheral nervous system, such as Lambert-Eaton myasthenic syndrome (LEMS) and neuromyotonia, are considered to respond best to immunosupressive treatment. However, there is only one report showing the beneficial but short-term effect of IVIG on the muscle strength in LEMS (Class II) [81]. Nevertheless, a recent Cochrane review has concluded that limited data from one placebo-controlled study show improvement in muscle strength after IVIG [82]. The IVIG response regarding improvement of muscle strength probably does not differ in paraneoplastic and non-paraneoplastic LEMS. Only one case report describes the beneficial effect of IVIG in patient with neuromyotonia [83], while another demonstrated worsening after IVIG therapy [84]. Symptoms in paraneoplastic opsoclonusataxia syndrome in paediatric neuroblastoma patients are stated to improve, although data on the long-term benefits of the treatment are lacking (Class IV) [85]. In adults the response is less immunosuppressive, although IVIG is suggested to accelerate recovery (Class IV) [86]. Evidence for the effect of IVIG in paraneoplastic cerebellar degeneration, limbic encephalitis and sensory neuropathy is scarce. In previously published reports, patients were treated with a combination of immunosupressive or immunomodulatory drugs, including IVIG, with a poor response (Class IV) [87].

Recommendations

Intravenous immunoglobulin therapy may be tried in paraneoplastic LEMS and opsoclonus-ataxia, especially in paediatric neuroblastoma patients (good practice point). No clear recommendations of the effect of IVIG in paraneoplastic neuromyotonia, cerebellar degeneration, limbic encephalitis or sensory neuropathy can be made due to lack of data.

Inflammatory myopathies

Three categories of inflammatory myopathy are reviewed based on published IVIG trials: DM, polymyositis and sporadic inclusion body myositis (IBM). Common

Recommendations

IVIG should be considered as the initial treatment of demyelinating IgM MGUS-related neuropathy (Level B). While the long-term effects and cost-benefit aspects are unknown, routine use of IVIG cannot be recommended in patients without significant disability (good practice point). However, in patients with significant disability or rapid worsening, IVIG may be tried, although its efficacy is not proven (good practice point). In patients with CIDP-like neuropathy, the detection of paraproteinaemia does not justify a different therapeutic approach from CIDP without a paraprotein.

diagnostic criteria based on neuropathological muscle biopsy findings are widely accepted in DM and in s-IBM, whereas there are diverging opinions regarding nosology of polymyositis.

Dermatomyositis

Published data are available on one RCT, one non-RCT, one retrospective chart review and four case-series. One 3-month, randomized crossover trial compared IVIG and prednisone to placebo and prednisone in 15 therapy-resistant patients [88]. Patients on IVIG significantly improved by symptom scale ($P = 0.035$) and a modified MRC scale ($P = 0.018$) (Class II). One retrospective chart review [89] and two case-series [90, 91] tried IVIG as an add-on therapy (Class III). Together, 82% improved clinically in these studies. One non-randomized trial and one case-series included patients with DM or polymyositis [92, 93]. The outcome in both was positive but as these were pooled data results on patients with DM could not be separated (Class IV).

Recommendations

IVIG is recommended as a second-line treatment in combination with prednisone for patients with DM who have not adequately responded to corticosteroids (Level B). IVIG is recommended, in combination with immunosuppressive medication, as a measure to reduce the dose of steroids in patients with DM (Level C). IVIG is not recommended as a monotherapy for DM (good practice point). In severe, life-threatening DM, IVIG can be considered as the first-line treatment together with other immunosuppressive therapy (good practice point).

Inclusion body myositis

Three RCTs with small-to-moderate numbers of patients were published. Two were crossover trials comparing IVIG to placebo in 19 patients [94] and 22 patients [95] (Class II). The outcome was negative even if some symptomatic positive effects were recorded. In one RCT, IVIG plus prednisone was compared with placebo plus prednisone in 35 patients [96] (Class II). Here too the outcome was negative.

The available data provide results of three fairly small randomized trials. The overall outcome was negative even though a small number of patients reported benefits regarding swallowing difficulties.

Recommendation

IVIG cannot be recommended for the treatment of sporadic IBM (Level A).

Polymyositis

Only one non-RCT [97] (Class III) and two case-series (Class IV) (see above, DM) on IVIG therapy for polymyositis have been published. Only the first used IVIG exclusively in patients with polymyositis. This study reported clinical improvement in 71% of patients, with significant improvement in muscle strength, muscle disability scores and creatinine kinase levels ($P < 0.01$). Steroid doses could be reduced after IVIG ($P < 0.05$).

Intravenous immunoglobulin can apparently be considered as an alternative in patients who do not respond to conventional immunosuppressive treatment. Dose and duration of the treatment are as recommended for DM.

Recommendation

IVIG may be considered among the treatment options for patients with polymyositis not responding to first-line immunosuppressive treatment (Level C).

Myasthenia gravis

Myasthenia gravis (MG) is caused by autoantibodies against antigen in the post-synaptic neuromuscular membrane; in most patients against the acetylcholine receptor (AChR), in 5% against muscle-specific tyrosin kinase (MuSK) and in 5% against undefined antigen(s). A direct induction of muscle weakness by the autoantibodies has been shown. PE with removal of autoantibodies has a well-documented effect [98].

An improvement of muscle weakness in MG by IVIG treatment has been documented by five controlled, prospective studies, comprising 338 patients. The three largest studies represent Class I evidence [99, 100, 101], the other two smaller studies Class II evidence [102, 103]. The only placebo-controlled study examined short-term treatment of 51 MG patients with increasing weakness. A significant improvement of a quantitative MG score for disease severity was found due to an effect in the patients with more severe disease. The effect was present after 2 weeks and was maintained after 4 weeks. The other four studies showed that IVIG had roughly the same efficacy as PE as acute treatment for MG exacerbations (Class I). It has a tendency for a slightly slower effect of IVIG, and also fewer side effects. No MG-specific side-effects were reported. There was no significant superiority of IVIG 2 g/kg over 2 days compared with 1 g/kg on a single day, but a trend for the slight superiority for the higher dose [100]. The changes of anti-AChR antibody titre were not significant [99, 102].

There are several additional reports on prospective or retrospective MG patient materials treated with IVIG for acute exacerbations, some of them comparing with other treatments (Class III and IV). The dose used was mostly 2 g/kg. These studies show a significant improvement after IVIG in all muscle groups, the improvement starting after 3–6 days [104, 105, 106, 107, 108, 109].

For MG patients with anti-MuSK antibodies there are case reports of a positive effect of IVIG [110, 111]. In the only placebo-controlled prospective study, 14 patients with anti-MuSK antibodies and 13 patients without detectable antibodies were included [101]. Results were not reported for antibody subgroups, but overall results indicate an improvement also in the non-AChR antibody positive MG patients (Class IV).

A recent EFNS guideline document and two recent Cochrane reviews concluded that IVIG is a well-documented, short-term treatment for acute exacerbations of MG and for severe MG [98, 112]. It has been discussed whether PE has a more rapid effect than IVIG for MG crisis, but this has not been convincingly established in controlled studies.

Intravenous immunoglobulin is often used to prepare MG patients for thymectomy or other types of surgery. This is especially recommended for those with severe weakness, bulbar symptoms, poor pulmonary function or a thymoma. There are no controlled studies for this practice. However, the well-documented, short-term effect of IVIG in acute exacerbations is useful in the postoperative situation (good practice point). IVIG is widely recommended for severe MG or MG exacerbations during pregnancy and also before giving birth. This is partly due to its effect on muscle strength, partly to its safety profile. Similarly, IVIG has been recommended for neonatal MG [113] (good practice point).

Intravenous immunoglobulin has been proposed as long-term maintenance therapy for MG. Such treatment

has only been examined in open-label studies, including a small number of patients with severe MG. These studies report significant improvement starting after a few days and continuing for up to 2 years [114, 115, 116] (Class IV). Maintenance IVIG treatment was given every 1–4 months. However, no control groups were included, the number of patients was low and the patients received other immunoactive and symptomatic therapy as well. Recent EFNS Task Force guidelines, a Cochrane review and other guideline documents conclude that there is insufficient evidence to recommend IVIG as maintenance therapy for MG patients [98, 112, 113].

Recommendations

Intravenous immunoglobulin is an effective treatment for acute exacerbations of MG and for short-term treatment of severe MG (Level A). IVIG is similar to PE regarding its effect. The treatment is safe for children, during pregnancy and for elderly patients with complicating disorders. There is insufficient evidence to recommend IVIG for chronic maintenance therapy in MG alone or in combination with other immunoactive drugs.

Post-polio syndrome

Post-polio syndrome is characterized by new muscle weakness, muscle atrophy, fatigue and pain developing several years after acute polio. Other potential causes of the new weakness have to be excluded [117, 118]. The prevalence of PPS in patients with previous polio is 20–60%. The prevalence of previous polio shows great variation according to geography. In Europe the last major epidemics occurred in the 1950s and mainly affected small children. Present prevalence of polio sequelae in most European countries is probably 50–200/100,000.

Post-polio syndrome is caused by an increased degeneration of enlarged motor units, and some motor neurones cannot maintain all their nerve terminals. Muscle overuse may be a contributory factor. Immunological and inflammatory signs have been reported in the cerebrospinal fluid and central nervous tissue [119].

There are two RCTs ($n = 155$ patients) of treatment with IVIG in PPS (Class I) [120, 121]. In addition, there is one open and uncontrolled study of 14 patients [122] and one case report [123] (Class IV). In the study with highest power, a significant increase of mean muscle strength of 8.3% was reported after two IVIG treatment cycles over 3 months. Physical activity and subjective vitality also differed significantly in favour of the IVIG group [121]. The smaller study of 20 patients and one-cycle IVIG found a significant improvement of pain but not of muscle strength and fatigue in the active treatment group [120]. The open study reported a positive effect on quality of life [122]. The report of an atypical case with rapid progression of muscle weakness described a marked improvement of muscle strength [123]. IVIG treatment reduced pro-inflammatory cytokines in the cerebrospinal fluid [119, 120].

Post-polio syndrome is a chronic condition. Although a modest IVIG effect has been described in the short term, nothing is known about its long-term effects. Responders and non-responders have not been defined. Any relationship between the clinical response to IVIG treatment and PPS severity, cerebrospinal fluid inflammatory changes and cerebrospinal fluid changes after IVIG is unknown. Optimal dose and IVIG cycle frequency has not been examined. Cost–benefit evaluation has not been performed. Non-IVIG interventions in PPS have recently been evaluated in an EFNS guideline article [117].

Recommendations

IVIG has a minor-to-moderate positive effect on muscle strength and some aspects of quality of life in PPS (Class I). As long as responding subgroups, long-term effects, dosing schedules and cost–benefit aspects are unknown, routine use of IVIG for PPS cannot be recommended (good practice point). However, in the very few patients with especially rapid progression of muscle weakness and atrophy, especially if there are indications of ongoing low-grade inflammation in the spinal cord, IVIG may be tried if a rigorous follow-up of muscle strength and quality of life can be undertaken (good practice point).

IVIG in multiple sclerosis

Four randomized double-blind studies have all shown a beneficial effect on disease activity in relapsing–remitting multiple sclerosis (RRMS) [124, 125, 126, 127]. All four studies have been rated as Class II due to limitations in methodology or size. IVIG 0.15–0.2 g/kg every 4 weeks

for 2 years showed a pronounced reduction in relapse rate in two placebo-controlled trials, 59% in a study by Fazekas et al. [125] and 63% in the study by Achion et al. [124]. In the largest 2-year study of 150 patients, IVIG showed a significant beneficial effect on the expanded disability status scale (EDSS) change from baseline compared with placebo ($P = 0.008$) [125]. A small study of two different doses of IVIG (0.2 or 0.4 g/kg every 4 weeks) showed a reduction in relapse rate compared with placebo, but no difference between the two IVIG doses [126]. A crossover study in RRMS patients showed a beneficial effect of IVIG 2 g/ kg every 4 weeks on new gadolinium-enhancing lesions in MRI compared with placebo [127].

A meta-analysis of four studies showed a significant reduction of the annual relapse rate (effect size divided by 0.5; $P = 0.00003$) and of disease progression (effect size divided by 0.25; $P = 0.04$) (Class I) [128].

Based on these studies IVIG was recommended as a second-line treatment in RRMS if s.c. or i.m. injectable therapies were not tolerated [129]. IVIG could not be included among first-line therapies, because of the limited evidence for clinical efficacy and because the optimum dose of IVIG had not been established.

Recently, the prevention of relapses with IVIG trial (PRIVIG) re-evaluating the effects of IVIG given 0.2 and 0.4 g/kg monthly failed to show an effect on the proportion of relapse-free patients and MRI activity in a placebo-controlled study of 127 patients with RRMS [130]. Thus, this trial failed to support earlier observations of a beneficial effect of IVIG in RRMS.

In a study of 91 patients with clinically isolated syndromes, IVIG significantly reduced the risk of conversion to clinically definite MS ($P = 0.03$) and reduced new T2 lesions in MRI compared with placebo (Class II) [131].

In secondary progressive MS, a large placebo-controlled trial of IVIG 1 g/kg monthly in 318 patients failed to show any beneficial effect on relapse rate, deterioration in EDSS and change in lesion volume of T2-weighted images (Class I). The only beneficial effect was a reduction in brain atrophy [132]. Very recently, however, a placebo-controlled trial of IVIG 0.4 g/kg monthly for 2 years in 231 patients with either primary progressive MS ($n = 34$) or secondary progressive MS ($n = 197$) showed a borderline significant delay in time to sustained progression on EDSS ($P = 0.04$), although the effect was limited to patients with primary progressive MS (Class II) [133].

Small studies with historical controls suggested that IVIG might reduce the relapse rate following childbirth (Class IV) [134, 135, 136].

Two studies of 76 and 19 patients with acute exacerbations showed that IVIG had no effect on recovery from acute relapses when given as add-on to i.v. methylprednisolone (Class II studies) [137, 138]. Chronic deficits in visual acuity or persistent stable muscular weakness were not affected by IVIG compared with placebo (Class I) [139, 140, 141].

Recommendations

The negative results of the PRIVIG study challenge recommendations for IVIG as a second-line treatment for RRMS. However, IVIG could still be considered as a second- or third-line therapy in RRMS if conventional immunomodulatory therapies are not tolerated because of side-effects or concomitant diseases (Level B), and in particular in pregnancy where other therapies may not be used (good practice point). IVIG cannot be recommended for treatment in secondary progressive MS (Level A). IVIG does not seem to have any beneficial effect as an add-on therapy to methylprednisolone for acute exacerbations (Level B) and cannot be recommended as treatment for chronic symptoms in MS (Level A). In clinically isolated syndromes and in primary progressive MS there is insufficient evidence to make any recommendations.

Other demyelinating diseases of the central nervous system

Neuromyelitis optica, also called Devic's disease, is a demyelinating disease of the spinal cord and optic nerves which may manifest as recurrent attacks and tends to have a poor prognosis. There is only one case-type study suggesting that monthly IVIG was associated with cessation of relapses (Class IV) [142].

Balo's concentric sclerosis is a severe demyelinating disease with poor prognosis. There is a case report suggesting that IVIG (0.4 g/kg/daily for 5 days) and interferon-β-1a given postpartum may result in partial neurological improvement (Class IV) [143].

Acute-disseminated encephalomyelitis (ADEM) is a monophasic immune-mediated demyelinating disease of the central nervous system and is associated with significant morbidity and mortality. Controlled studies on therapy in ADEM are not available. Standard treatment is high-dose steroids. The use of IVIG (0.4 g/kg/day for 5

days or 1 g/kg/2 days) has been reported in case reports and small series suggesting that IVIG may have favourable effects when used as an initial therapy in both adults and children (Class IV) [144, 145, 146, 147, 148]. IVIG may have beneficial effects also as second-line therapy (Class IV) [149, 150, 151, 152], especially in patients who cannot receive or fail to respond to steroids (Class IV) [153, 154, 155] or in patients with peripheral nervous system involvement and steroid failure (Class IV). Alternatively, combination therapy by steroids and IVIG (Class IV) [156, 157, 158, 159, 160, 161] or steroids, IVIG and PE were suggested to have favourable effects, especially if given early in the course of disease (Class IV) [162, 163].

Recommendations

IVIG may have a favourable effect in the treatment of ADEM and therefore it should be tried (0.4 g/kg/day for 4–5 consecutive days) in patients who fail to respond to high-dose steroids (good practice point). The cycles may be repeated. PE could also be considered in patients who do not respond to high-dose steroids.

Stiff-person syndrome

Published data are available on one randomized, double-blind, placebo-controlled, crossover trial (Class I) [164], one national experts opinion (Class IV) [113], three non-controlled studies (Class IV) [165, 166, 167], two case series (Class IV) [168, 169], 16 case reports (Class IV) and five adequately powered systematic review of prospective randomized controlled clinical trials (Class I) [170, 171, 172, 173, 174].

The randomized trial [164] enrolled 16 SPS patients who were treated with 2 g/kg IVIG, divided in two consecutive daily doses of 1 g/kg, or placebo for 3 months. After a washout period of 1 month, the patients crossed over to the alternative therapy for a further 3 months. All patients were followed for at least 3 months after the infusions. The results of the trial showed a significant decline of the stiffness scores in the IVIG-randomized patients from month 1 through 4, and rebound when they crossed to placebo. The scores in the placebo-randomized group remained constant from month 1 to 4 and dropped significantly after crossing to IVIG. Eleven of 16 patients who received IVIG became able to walk unassisted. The duration of benefit varied from 6–12 weeks to up to 1 year. The serum titres of anti-GAD antibody declined after IVIG, but not after placebo. This study has demonstrated that IVIG is a safe and effective therapy for patients with SPS.

According to uncontrolled studies IVIG improved the quality of life in six patients with SPS [165] and resulted in substantial objective improvement in two groups, each composed of three patients with SPS [166, 167]. Two case-series showed clinical improvement in five of six patients treated with IVIG [168, 169].

Recommendations

In patients with SPS incompletely responding to diazepam and/or baclofen and with significant disability requiring a cane or a walker due to truncal stiffness and frequent falls, the recommendation is to use IVIG (2 g/kg for 2–5 days) (Level A, based on Class I).

Drug-resistant infantile epilepsy

Drug-resistant infantile epilepsy (DRIE) includes such diseases as Landau-Kleffner syndrome (LKS), West syndrome, Lennox-Gastaut syndrome, severe myoclonic epilepsy and RE which typically manifest in childhood or adolescence and are characterized by epilepsy and progressive neurological dysfunction. Standard treatment of RE consists of anti-epileptic drugs, high-dose steroids or PE. Surgical treatment also may be considered. Case studies and small series have reported that some patients with RE respond in some measure to treatment with IVIG (Class IV) [175, 176].

Approximately 100 patients with West syndrome or Lennox-Gastaut syndrome have been treated with IVIG with widely varying results [176, 177]. The treatment has resulted in a reduction in the number of seizures with improvement in the EEG in about half the cases. The positive effects were noted a few days to several weeks to months after treatment. Relapses have been common.

Successful use of IVIG as the initial monotherapy in LKS has been reported in case studies [178, 179] and after initial therapy by steroids [180] or antiepileptic drugs and steroids [181, 182] in few patients [183].

Case studies on the use of IVIG in RE have suggested that monthly IVIG therapy (0.4 g/kg for 5 days at 4-week intervals followed by monthly maintenance IVIG) may ameliorate disease in patients who are refractory to antiepileptic drugs [184] or steroids and PE [185].

Recommendation

IVIG seems to have a favourable effect in RE and may be tried in selected patients who are refractory to other therapies (good practice point). IVIG has been administered at doses of 0.4 g/kg/day for 4–5 consecutive days; the cycles may be repeated after 2–6 weeks.

Side-effects of IVIG

Side-effects in PE and IVIG therapy have been reported in several studies (20–24). They reported more instances of pneumonia, atelectasis, thrombosis and haemodynamic difficulties related to PE than IVIG. The incidents related to IVIG included hypotension, dyspnoea, fever and haematuria, nausea or vomiting, meningism, exacerbation of chronic renal failure, possible myocardial infarction and painful erythema at the infusion site. The side-effects of IVIG in the treatment of neurological autoimmune diseases have been studied prospectively during 84 treatment courses with a total 341 infusions under routine clinical conditions [186]. Headache occurred during 30% of treatment courses. Severe adverse events leading to discontinuation of the treatment were noted in approximately 4% of all treatment courses. They included thrombosis of the jugular vein, allergic reaction and retrosternal pressure. The changes in blood laboratory findings included abnormalities of liver enzymes, changes for leucocytes, erythrocytes, haematocrit, haemoglobin, alanine aminotransferase and aspartateamino transferase. None of these laboratory changes was clinically significant. Based on these data IVIG can generally be regarded as a relatively safe treatment. However, to avoid these complications careful monitoring of laboratory findings, including full blood count, liver enzymes and renal functions, should be mandatory [186].

Conflicts of interest

Irina Elovaara has lectured on IVIG and participated in a trial on efficacy of IVIG in exacerbations of MS sponsored by Baxter.

None of the other Task Force members reported any conflict of interest.

References

1. Brainin, M, Barnes, M, Baron, JC, *et al.* Guidance for the preparation of neurological management guidelines by EFNS scientific task forces – revised recommendations 2004. *Eur J Neurol* 2004; **11**:577–81.

2. Kazatchkine, MD, Kaveri, SV. Immunomodulation of autoimmune and inflammatory diseases with intravenous immune globulin. *N Engl J Med*, 2001; **345**:747–55.

3. Masson, PL. Elimination of infectious antigens and increase of IgG catabolism as possible modes of action of IVIG. *J Autoimmun*, 1993; **6**:683–9.

4. Asakura, K, Miller, DJ, Murray, K, *et al.* Monoclonal autoantibody SCH94.03, which promotes central nervous system remyelination, recognizes an antigen on the surface of oligodendrocytes. *J Neurosci Res*, 1996; **43**:273–81.

5. Ciric, B, Van Keulen, V, Paz Soldan, M, *et al.* Antibody-mediated remyelination operates through mechanism independent of immunomodulation. *J Neuroimmunol* 2004; **146**:153–61.

6. Asakura, K, Pogulis, RJ, Pease, LR, Rodriguez, M. A monoclonal autoantibody which promotes central nervous system remyelination is highly polyreactive to multiple known and novel antigens. *J Neuroimmunol*, 1996; **65**: 11–19.

7. Miller, DJ, Rodriguez, M. A monoclonal autoantibody that promotes central nervous system remyelination in a model of multiple sclerosis is a natural autoantibody encoded by germline immunoglobulin genes. *J Immunol* 1995; **154**:2460–9.

8. Stangel, M, Compston, A, Scolding, NJ. Oligodendroglia are protected from antibody-mediated complement injury by normal immunoglobulins ('IVIG'). *J Neuroimmunol* 2000; **103**:195–201.

9. Stangel, M, Compston, DAS, Scolding, NJ. Polyclonal immunoglobulins for intravenous use do not influence the behaviour of cultured oligodendrocytes. *J Neuroimmunol*, 1999; **96**:228–33.

10. Aktas, O, Waiczies, S, Grieger, U, *et al.* Polyspecific immunoglobulins (IVIG) suppress proliferation of human (auto)antigen-specific T cells without inducing apoptosis. *J Neuroimmunol* 2001; **114**:160–7.

11. Prasad, NK, Papoff, G, Zeuner, A, *et al.* Therapeutic preparations of normal polyspecific IgG (IVIG) induce apoptosis in human lymphocytes and monocytes: a novel mechanism of action of IVIG involving the Fas apoptotic pathway. *J Immunol* 1998; **161**:3781–90.

12. Yuki, N, Miyagi, F. Possible mechanism of intravenous immunoglobulin treatment on anti-GM1 antibody-mediated neuropathies. *J Neurol Sci* 1996; **139**:160–2.

13. Buchwald, B, Ahangari, R, Weishaupt, A, Toyka, KV. Intravenous immunoglobulins neutralize blocking antibodies in Guillain-Barré syndrome. *Ann Neurol*, 2002; **51**:673–80.

14. Basta, M, Dalakas, MC. High-dose intravenous immunoglobulin exerts its beneficial effect in patients with dermatomyositis by blocking endomysial deposition of activated complement fragments. *J Clin Invest* 1994; **94**:1729–35.

15. Winer, JB, Hughes, RAC, Osmond, C. A prospective study of acute idiopathic neuropathy. I. Clinical features and their prognostic value. *J Neurol Neurosurg Psychiatry* 1988; **51**:605–12.

16. Brettle, RP, Gross, M, Legg, NJ, *et al.* Treatment of acute polyneuropathy by plasma exchange. *Lancet* 1978; **2**:1100.

17. The Guillain-Barré Syndrome Study Group Plasmapheresis and acute Guillain-Barré syndrome. *Neurology*, 1985; **35**:1096–104.

18. Consensus Conference The utility of therapeutic plasmapheresis for neurological disorders. NIH Consensus Development. *JAMA* 1986; **256**:1333–7.

19. Kleyweg, RP, Van der Meche', FGA, Meulstee, J. Treatment of Guillain-Barré syndrome with high-dose gammaglobulin. *Neurology* 1988; **38**:1639–41.

20. Van der Meché, FGA, Schmitz, PIM, The Dutch Guillain-Barré Study Group. A randomized trial comparing intravenous immune globulin and plasma exchange in Guillain-Barré syndrome. *N Engl J Med* 1992; **326**: 1123–9.

21. Bril, V, Ilse, WK, Pearce, R, *et al.* Pilot trial of immunoglobulin versus plasma exchange in patients with Guillain-Barré syndrome. *Neurology* 1996; **46**:100–3.

22. Plasma Exchange/Sandoglobulin Guillain-Barré Syndrome Trial Group. Randomised trial of plasma exchange, intravenous immunoglobulin, and combined treatments in Guillain-Barré syndrome. *Lancet* 1997; **349**:225–30.

23. Nomura, K, Hamaguchi, K, Hattori, T, *et al.* A randomized controlled trial comparing intravenous immunoglobulin and plasmapheresis in Guillain-Barré syndrome. *Neurol Ther* 2001; **18**:69–81.

24. Diener, HC, Haupt, WF, Kloss, TM, *et al.* A preliminary, randomized, multicenter study comparing intravenous immunoglobulin, plasma exchange, and immune adsorption in Guillain-Barré syndrome. *Eur Neurol* 2001; **46**:107–9.

25. Raphael, JC, Chevret, S, Harboun, M, *et al.* Intravenous immune globulins in patients with Guillain-Barré syndrome and contraindications to plasma exchange: 3 days versus 6 days. *J Neurol Neurosurg Psychiatry* 2001; **71**:235–8.

26. Gürses, N, Uysal, S, Cetinkaya, F, *et al.* Intravenous immunoglobulin treatment in children with Guillain-Barré syndrome. *Scand J Infect Dis* 1995; **27**:241–3.

27. Wang, R, Feng, A, Sun, W. Wen, Z. Intravenous immunoglobulin in children with Guillain-Barré syndrome. *J Appl Clin Pediatr* 2001; **16**:223–4.

28. Korinthenberg, R, Schessl, J, Kirschner, J, Möntning, JS. Intravenous immunoglobulin in the treatment of childhood Guillain-Barré syndrome. *Pediatrics* 2005; **116**:8–14.

29. Kanra, G, Ozon, A, Vajsar, J , *et al.* Intravenous immunoglobulin treatment in children with Guillain-Barré syndrome. *European Journal of Paediatric Neurology* 1997; **1**: 7–12.

30. van Koningsveld, R, Schmitz, PIM, Van der Meché, FGA, *et al.* Effect of methylprednisolone when added to standard treatment with intravenous immunoglobulin for Guillain-Barré syndrome: randomised trial. *Lancet* 2004; **363**: 192–6.

31. Hughes, RAC. Treatment of Guillain-Barré syndrome with corticosteroids: lack of benefit? *Lancet* 2004; **363**:181.

32. Hughes, RAC, Cornblath, DR. Guillain-Barré syndrome. *Lancet* 2005; **366**:1653–66.

33. Jacobs, BC, Van Doorn, PA, Schmitz, PI, *et al.* Campylobacter jejuni infections and anti-GM1 antibodies in Guillain-Barré syndrome. *Ann Neurol* 1996; **40**:181–7.

34. Yuki, N, Ang, CW, Koga, M, *et al.* Clinical features and response to treatment in Guillain-Barré syndrome associated with antibodies to GM1b ganglioside. *Ann Neurol* 2000; **47**:314–21.

35. Kuwabara, S, Mori, M, Ogawara, K,*et al.* Indicators of rapid clinical recovery in Guillain-Barré syndrome. *J Neurol Neurosurg Psychiatry* 2001; **70**:560–2.

36. Ruts, L, van Koningsveld, R, Van Doorn, PA. Distinguishing acute-onset CIDP from Guillain-Barré syndrome with treatment-related fluctuations. *Neurology* 2005; **65**: 138–40.

37. Hughes, RAC, Swan, AV, Raphael, JC. Immunotherapy for Guillain-Barré syndrome: a systematic review. *Brain* 2007; **130**:2245–57.

38. Dyck, PJ, Litchy, WJ, Kratz, KM, *et al.* A plasma exchange versus immune globulin infusion trial in chronic inflammatory demyelinating polyradiculoneuropathy. *Ann Neurol* 1994; **36**:838–45.

39. van Schaik, IN, Winer, JB, de Haan, R, Vermeulen, M. Intravenous immunoglobulin for chronic inflammatory demyelinating polyradiculoneuropathy. *Cochrane Database Syst Rev* 2004; **2**:CD001797.

40. Hahn, AF, Bolton, CF, Zochodne, DW, Feasby, TE. Intravenous immunoglobulin treatment in chronic inflammatory demyelinating polyneuropathy. A doubleblind,

41. Hughes, RA, Bensa, S, Willison, HJ, *et al.* Randomized controlled trial of intravenous immunoglobulin versus oral prednisolone in chronic inflammatory demyelinating polyradiculoneuropathy. *Ann Neurol* 2001; **50**: 195–201.

42. Mendell, JR, Barohn, RJ, Freimer, ML, *et al.* Randomized controlled trial of IVIG in untreated chronic inflammatory demyelinating polyradiculoneuropathy. *Neurology* 2001; **56**:445–9.

43. Thompson, N, Choudhary, PP, Hughes, RAC, Quinlivan, RM, A novel trial design to study the effect of intravenous immunoglobulin in chronic inflammatory demyelinating polyradiculoneuropathy *J Neurol* 1996; **243**:280–5.

44. Vermeulen, M, Van Doorn, PA, Brand, A, *et al.* Intravenous immunoglobulin treatment in patients with chronic inflammatory demyelinating polyneuropathy. *J Neurol Neurosurg Psychiatry* 1993; **56**:36–9.

45. Hughes, RA, Donofrio, P, Bril, V, *et al.* Intravenous immune globulin (10% caprylate-chromatography purified) for the treatment of chronic inflammatory demyelinating polyradiculoneuropathy (ICE study): a randomised placebo-controlled trial. *Lancet Neurol* 2008; **7**:136–44.

46. Hughes, RAC, Bouche, P, Cornblath, DR, *et al.* EFNS/ PNS guideline on management of chronic inflammatory demyelinating polyradiculoneuropathy. Report of a joint task force of the European Federation of Neurological Societies and the Peripheral Nerve Society. *Eur J Neurol* 2006; **13**:326–32.

47. Donaghy, M, Mills, KR, Boniface, SJ, *et al.* Pure motor demyelinating neuropathy: deterioration after steroid treatment and improvement with intravenous immunoglobulin. *J Neurol Neurosurg Psychiatry* 1994; **57**: 778–83.

48. Van Doorn, PA, Dippel, DWJ, Vermeulen, M. Longterm iv immunoglobulin treatment in chronic inflammatory demyelinating polyneuropathy. *J Peripher Nerv Syst* 2007; **12**(Suppl.):89.

49. Nobile-Orazio, E. Multifocal motor neuropathy. *J Neuroimmunol* 2001; **115**:4–18.

50. Carpo, M, Cappellari, A, Mora, G, *et al.* Deterioration of multifocal motor neuropathy after plasma exchange. *Neurology* 1998; **50**:1480–2.

51. Claus, D, Specht, S, Zieschang, M. Plasmapheresis in multifocal motor neuropathy: a case report. *J Neurol Neurosurg Psychiatry* 2000; **68**:533–5.

52. Van den Berg, LH, Lokhorst, H, Wokke, JH. Pulsed highdose dexamethasone is not effective in patients with multifocal motor neuropathy [comment]. *Neurology* 1997; **48**:1135.

placebo-controlled, cross-over study. *Brain* 1996; **119**: 1067–77.

53. van Schaik, IN, Van den Berg, LH, de Haan, R, Vermeulen, M. Intravenous immunoglobuline for multifocal motor neuropathy. *Cochrane Database Syst Rev* 2005; **2**: CD004429.

54. Azulay, JP, Blin, O, Pouget, J, *et al.* Intravenous immuno-globulin treatment in patients with motor neuron syn-dromes associated with anti-GM1 antibodies: a double-blind, placebo-controlled study. *Neurology* 1994; **44**:429–32.

55. Federico, P, Zochodne, DW, Hahn, AF, *et al.* Multifocal motor neuropathy improved by IVIG: randomized, double-blind, placebo-controlled study. *Neurology* 2000; **55**:1256–62.

56. Léger, JM, Chassande, B, Musset, L, *et al.* Intravenous immunoglobulin therapy in multifocal motor neuropathy: a double-blind, placebo-controlled study. *Brain* 2001; **124**:145–53.

57. Van den Berg, LH, Kerkhoff, H, Oey, PL, *et al.* Treatment of multifocal motor neuropathy with high dose intrave-nous immunoglobulins: a double-blind, placebo-controlled study. *J Neurol Neurosurg Psychiatry* 1995; **59**:248–52.

58. Van den Berg-Vos, RM, Franssen, H, Wokke, JHJ, *et al.* Multifocal motor neuropathy: diagnostic criteria that predict the response to immunoglobulin treatment. *Ann Neurol* 2000; **48**:919–26.

59. Léger, JM, Viala, K, Cancalon, F, *et al.* Intravenous immu-noglobulin as short- and long-term therapy of multifocal motor neuropathy: a retrospective study of response to IVIG and of its predictive criteria in 40 patients. *J Neurol Neurosurg Psychiatry* 2008; **79**:93–6.

60. Terenghi, F, Cappellari, A, Bersano, A, *et al.* How long is IVIG effective in multifocal motor neuropathy? *Neurology* 2004; **62**:666–8.

61. Van den Berg, LH, Franssen, H, Wokke, JHJ. The longterm effect of intravenous immunoglobulin treatment in multi-focal motor neuropathy. *Brain* 1998; **121**:421–8.

62. Vucic, S, Black, KR, Chong, PST, Cros, D. Multifocal motor neuropathy. Decrease in conduction blocks and reinnerva-tion with long-term IVIG. *Neurology* 2004; **63**:1264–9.

63. van Schaik, IN, Bouche, P, Illa, I, *et al.* EFNS/PNS guideline on management of multifocal motor neuropathy. Report of a joint task force of the European Federation of Neurological Societies and the Peripheral Nerve Society. *Eur J Neurol* 2006; **13**:802–8.

64. Kelly, JJ, Kyle, RA, O'Brien, PC, Dyck, PJ. Prevalence of monoclonal protein in peripheral neuropathy. *Neurology* 1981; **31**:1480–3.

65. Latov, N. Pathogenesis and therapy of neuropathies associ-ated with monoclonal gammopathies. *Ann Neurol* 1995; **37**(**S1**):S32–S42.

66. Nobile-Orazio, E, Manfredini, E, Carpo, M, *et al.* Frequency and clinical correlates of anti-neural IgM antibodies in neuropathy associated with IgM monoclonal gammopathy. *Ann Neurol* 1994; **36**:416–24.

67. Dalakas, MC, Quarles, RH, Farrer, RG, *et al.* A controlled study of intravenous immunoglobulin in demyelinating neuropathy with IgM gammopathy. *Ann Neurol* 1996; **40**:792–5.

68. Comi, G, Roveri, L, Swan, A, *et al.* A randomised controlled trial of intravenous immunoglobulin in IgM paraprotein associated demyelinating neuropathy. *J Neurol* 2002; **249**: 1370–7.

69. Mariette, X, Chastang, C, Louboutin, JP, *et al.* A ran-domised clinical trial comparing interferon-α and intrave-nous immunoglobulin in polyneuropathy associated with monoclonal IgM. *J Neurol Neurosurg Psychiatry* 1997; **63**: 28–34.

70. Lunn, MPT, Nobile-Orazio, E. Immunotherapy for IgM anti-myelin-associated glycoprotein paraprotein-associated peripheral neuropathies. *Cochrane Database Syst Rev* 2006; **2**:CD002827.

71. Cook, D, Dalakas, MC, Galdi, A, *et al.* High-dose intrave-nous immunoglobulin in the treatment of demyelinating neuropathy associated with monoclonal gammopathy. *Neurology* 1990; **40**:212–14.

72. Leger, JM, Ben Younes-Chennoufi, A, Chassande, B, *et al.* Human immunoglobulin treatment of multifocal motor neuropathy and polyneuropathy associated with mono-clonal gammopathy. *J Neurol Neurosurg Psychiatry* 1994; **57**(Suppl.):46–9.

73. Ellie, E, Vital, A, Steck, A, *et al.* Neuropathy associated with 'benign' anti-myelin-associated glycoprotein IgM gam-mopathy: clinical, immunological, neurophysiological pathological findings and response to treatment in 33 cases. *J Neurol* 1996; **243**:34–43.

74. Gorson, KC, Allam, G, Ropper, AH. Chronic inflammatory demyelinating polyneuropathy: clinical features and response to treatment in 67 consecutive patients with and without a monoclonal gammopathy. *Neurology* 1997; **48**: 321–8.

75. Nobile-Orazio, E, Meucci, N, Baldini, L, *et al.* Long-term prognosis of neuropathy associated with anti-MAG IgM M-proteins and its relationship to immune therapies. *Brain* 2000; **123**:710–17.

76. Gorson, KC, Ropper, AH, Weinberg, DH, Weinstein, R. Treatment experience in patients with anti-myelin-associated glycoprotein neuropathy. *Muscle Nerve* 2001; **24**:778–86.

77. Hadden, RDM, Nobile-Orazio, E, Sommer, C, *et al.* Paraproteinaemic demyelinating neuropathy, in *European Handbook of Neurological Management* (eds R Hughes, M Brainin, NE Gilhus) 2006; Blackwell Publishing, pp. 362–75.

78. Gorson, KC, Ropper, AH, Weinberg, DH, Weinstein, R. Efficacy of intravenous immunoglobulin in patients with IgG monoclonal gammopathy and polyneuropathy. *Arch Neurol* 2002; **59**:766–72.

79. Nobile-Orazio, E, Casellato, C, Di Troia, A. Neuropathies associated with IgG and IgA monoclonal gammopathy. *Rev Neuro (Paris)* 2002; **158**:979–87.

80. Allen, D, Lunn, MPT, Niermeijer, J, Nobile-Orazio, E. Treatment for IgG and IgA paraproteinaemic neuropathy. *Cochrane Database Syst Rev* 2007; **1**:CD005376.

81. Bain, PG, Motomura, M, Newsom-Davis, J, *et al.* Effects of intravenous immunoglobulin on muscle weakness and calcium-channel autoantibodies in the Lambert-Eaton myasthenic syndrome. *Neurology* 1996; **47**:678–83.

82. Maddison, P, Newsom-Davis, J. Treatment for Lambert-Eaton myasthenic syndrome. *Cochrane Database Syst Rev* 2005; **2**:CD003279.

83. Alessi, G, De Reuck, J, De Bleecker, J, Vancayzeele, S. Successful immunoglobulin treatment in a patient with neuromyotonia. *Clin Neurol Neurosurg* 2000; **102**:173–5.

84. Ishii, A, Hayashi, A, Ohkoshi, N, *et al.* Clinical evaluation of plasma exchange and high dose intravenous immunoglobulin in a patient with Isaacs' syndrome. *J Neurol Neurosurg Psychiatry* 1994; **57**:840–2.

85. Mitchell, WG, Davalos-Gonzalez, Y, Brumm, VL, *et al.* Opsoclonus-ataxia caused by childhood neuroblastoma: developmental and neurologic sequelae. *Pediatrics* 2002; **109**:86–98.

86. Bataller, L, Graus, F, Saiz, A, *et al.* Clinical outcome in adult onset idiopathic or paraneoplastic opsoclonusmyoclonus. *Brain* 2001; **2**:437–43.

87. Keime-Guibert, F, Graus, F, Fleury, A, *et al.* Treatment of paraneoplastic neurological syndromes with antineuronal antibodies (Anti-Hu, anti-Yo) with a combination of immunoglobulins, cyclophosphamide, and methylprednisolone. *J Neurol Neurosurg Psychiatry* 2000; **68**:479–82.

88. Dalakas, MC, Illa, I, Dambrosia, JM, *et al.* A controlled trial of high-dose intravenous immune globulin infusions as treatment for dermatomyositis. *N Engl J Med* 1993; **329**:1993–2000.

89. Al-Mayouf, SM, Laxer, RM, Schneider, R, *et al.* Intravenous immunoglobulin therapy for juvenile dermatomyositis – efficacy and safety. *J Rheumatol* 2000; **27**:2498–503.

90. Sansome, A, Dubowitz, V. Intravenous immunoglobulin in juvenile dermatomyositis – four-year review of nine cases. *Arch Dis Child* 1995; **72**:25–8.

91. Tsai, MJ, Lai, CC, Lin, SC, *et al.* Intravenous immunoglobulin therapy in juvenile dermatomyositis. *Zhonghua Min Guo Xiao Er Ke Yi Xue Hui Za Zhi* 1997; **38**:111–15.

92. Cherin, P, Piette, JC, Wechsler, B, *et al.* Intravenous gamma globulin as first line therapy in polymyositis and dermato-

myositis: an open study in 11 adult patients. *J Rheumatol* 1994; **21**:1092–7.

93. Danieli, MG, Malcangi, G, Palmieri, C, *et al.* Cyclosporin A and intravenous immunoglobulin treatment in polymyositis/dermatomyositis. *Ann Rheum Dis* 2002; **61**:37–41.

94. Dalakas, MC, Sonies, B, Dambrosia, J, *et al.* Treatment of inclusion-body myositis with IVIG: a double-blind, placebo-controlled study. *Neurology* 1997; **48**:712–16.

95. Walter, MC, Lochmuller, H, Toepfer, M, *et al.* High-dose immunoglobulin therapy in sporadic inclusion body myositis: a double-blind, placebo-controlled study. *J Neurol* 2000; **247**:22–8.

96. Dalakas, MC, Koffman, B, Fujii, M, *et al.* A controlled study of intravenous immunoglobulin combined with prednisone in the treatment of IBM. *Neurology* 2001; **56**:323–7.

97. Cherin, P, Pelletier, S, Teixeira, A, *et al.* Results and long-term follow up of intravenous immunoglobulin infusions in chronic, refractory polymyositis: an open study with thirty-five adult patients. *Arthritis Rheum* 2002; **46**:467–74.

98. Skeie, GO, Apostolski, S, Evoli, A, *et al.* Guidelines for the treatment of autoimmune neuromuscular transmission disorders. *Eur J Neurol* 2006; **13**:691–9.

99. Gajdos, P, Chevret, S, Clair, B, et al. Clinical trial of plasma exchange and high-dose intravenous immunoglobulin in myasthenia gravis. *Ann Neurol* 1997; **41**:789–96.

100. Gajdos, P, Tranchant, C, Clair, B, *et al.* Treatment of myasthenia gravis exacerbation with intravenous immunoglobulin – a randomized double-blind clinical trial. *Arch Neurol* 2005; **62**:1689–93.

101. Zinman, L, Ng, E, Bril, V. IV immunoglobulin in patients with myasthenia gravis – a randomized controlled trial. *Neurology* 2007; **68**:837–41.

102. Ronager, J, Ravnborg, M, Hermansen, I, Vorstrup, S. Immunoglobulin treatment versus plasma exchange in patients with chronic moderate to severe myasthenia gravis. *Artif Organs* 2001; **25**:967–73.

103. Wolfe, GI, Barohn, RJ, Foster, BM, *et al.* Randomized, controlled trial of intravenous immunoglobulin in myasthenia gravis. *Muscle Nerve* 2002; **26**:549–52.

104. Arsura, EL, Bick, A, Brunner, NG, et al. High-dose intravenous immunoglobulin in the management of myasthenia-gravis. *Arch Intern Med* 1986; **146**:1365–8.

105. Cosi, V, Lombardi, M, Piccolo, G, Erbetta, A. Treatment of myasthenia gravis with high-dose intravenous immunoglobulin. *Acta Neurol Scand* 1991; **84**:81–4.

106. Evoli, A, Palmisani, MT, Bartoccioni, E, *et al.* High-dose intravenous immunoglobulin in myasthenia- gravis. *Ital J Neurol Sci* 1993; **14**:233–7.

107. Perez-Nellar, J, Dominguez, AM, Llorens-Figueroa, JA, et al. A comparative study of intravenous immunoglobulin and plasmapheresis preoperatively in myasthenia. *Rev Neurol* 2001; **33**:413–16.

108. Qureshi, AI, Choudhry, MA, Akbar, MS, et al. Plasma exchange versus intravenous immunoglobulin treatment in myasthenic crisis. *Neurology* 1999; **52**:629–32.

109. Zeitler, H, Ulrich-Merzenich, G, Hoffmann, L, et al. Long-term effects of a multimodal approach including immunoadsorption for the treatment of myasthenic crisis. *Artif Organs* 2006; **30**:597–605.

110. Hain, B, Hanisch, F, Deschauer, M. Seronegative myasthenia with antibodies against muscle-specific tyrosine kinase. *Nervenarzt* 2004; **75**:362.

111. Takahashi, H, Kawaguchi, N, Nemoto, Y, Hattori, T. High-dose intravenous immunoglobulin for the treatment of MUSK antibody-positive seronegative myasthenia gravis. *J Neurol Sci* 2006; **247**:239–41.

112. Gajdos, P, Chevret, S, Toyka, K. Intravenous immunoglobulin for myasthenia gravis. *Cochrane Database Syst Rev* 2006; **2**.

113. Feasby, T, Banwell, B, Benstead, T, et al. Guidelines on the use of intravenous immune globulin for neurologic conditions. *Transfus Med* 2007; **21**(Suppl. 1):S57–S107.

114. Achiron, A, Barak, Y, Miron, S, Sarova-Pinhas, I. Immunoglobulin treatment in refractory myasthenia gravis. *Muscle Nerve* 2001; **23**:551–5.

115. Hilkevich, O, Drory, VE, Chapman, J, Korczyn, AD. The use of intravenous immunoglobulin as maintenance therapy in myasthenia gravis. *Clin Neuropharmacol* 2001; **24**:173–6.

116. Wegner, B, Ahmed, I. Intravenous immunoglobulin monotherapy in long-term treatment of myasthenia gravis. *Clin Neurol Neurosurg* 2002; **105**:3–8.

117. Farbu, E, Gilhus, NE, Barnes, MP, et al. EFNS guideline on diagnosis and management of post-polio syndrome. Report of an EFNS task force. *European J Neurol* 2006; **13**: 795–801.

118. Halstead, LS. Assessment and differential diagnosis for post-polio syndrome. *Orthopedics* 1991; **14**:1209–17.

119. Gonzalez, H, Khademi, M, Andersson, M, et al. Prior poliomyelitis – IVIG treatment reduces proinflammatory cytokine production. *J Neuroimmunol* 2004; **150**:139–44.

120. Farbu, E, Rekand, T, Vik-Mo, E, et al. Post-polio syndrome patients treated with intravenous immunoglobulin: a double-blinded randomized controlled pilot study. *Eur J Neurol* 2007; **14**:60–5.

121. Gonzalez, H, Sunnerhagen, KS, Sjoberg, I, et al. Intravenous immunoglobulin for post-polio syndrome: a randomised controlled trial. *Lancet Neurol* 2006; **5**:493–500.

122. Kaponides, G, Gonzalez, H, Olsson, T, Borg, K. Effect of intravenous immunoglobulin in patients with post-polio syndrome – an uncontrolled pilot study. *J Rehabil Med 2006* 2006; **38**:138–40.

123. Farbu, E, Rekand, T, Gilhus, NE, et al. Intravenous immunoglobulin in postpolio syndrome. *Tidsskr Nor Laegeforen* 2004; **124**:2357–8.

124. Achiron, A, Gabbay, U, Gilad, R, et al. Intravenous immunoglobulin treatment in multiple sclerosis. Effect on relapses. *Neurology* 1998; **50**:398–402.

125. Fazekas, F, Deisenhammer, F, Strasser Fuchs, S, et al. Randomised placebo-controlled trial of monthly intravenous immunoglobulin therapy in relapsing-remitting multiple sclerosis. Austrian Immunoglobulin in Multiple Sclerosis Study Group. *Lancet* 1997; **349**:589–93.

126. Lewanska, M, Zajdal, MS, Selmaj, K. No difference in efficacy of two different doses of intarvenous immunoglobulins in MS: clinical and MRI assessment. *Eur J Neurol* 2002; **9**:565–72.

127. Sorensen, PS, Wanscher, B, Jensen, CV, et al. Intravenous immunoglobulin G reduces MRI activity in relapsing multiple sclerosis. *Neurology* 1998; **50**:1273–81.

128. Sorensen, PS, Fazekas, F, Lee, M. Intravenous immunoglobulin G for the treatment of relapsing-remitting multiple sclerosis: a meta-analysis. *Eur J Neurol* 2002; **9**: 557–63.

129. Rieckmann, P, Toyka, KV, Bassetti, C, et al. Escalating immunotherapy of multiple sclerosis – new aspects and practical application. *J Neurol* 2004; **251**:1329–39.

130. Fazekas, F, Strasser-Fuchs, S, Hommes, OR. Intravenous immunoglobulin in MS: promise or failure? *J Neurol Sci* 2007; **259**:61–6.

131. Achiron, A, Kishner, I, Sarova-Pinhas, I, et al. Intravenous immunoglobulin treatment following the first demyelinating event suggestive of multiple sclerosis: a randomized, double-blind, placebo-controlled trial. *Arch Neurol* 2004; **61**:1515–20.

132. Hommes, OR, Sorensen, PS, Fazekas, F, et al. Intravenous immunoglobulin in secondary progressive multiple sclerosis: randomised placebo-controlled trial. *Lancet* 2004; **364**:1149–56.

133. Pohlau, D, Przuntek, H, Sailer, M, et al. Intravenous immunoglobulin in primary and secondary chronic progressive multiple sclerosis: a randomized placebo-controlled multicentre study. *Mult Scler* 2007; **13**: 1107–17.

134. Achiron, A, Rotstein, Z, Noy, S, et al. Intravenous immunoglobulin treatment in the prevention of childbirth-associated acute exacerbations in multiple sclerosis: a pilot study. *J Neurol* 1996; **243**:25–8.

135. Haas, J. High dose IVIG in the postpartum period for prevention of exacerbations in MS. *Mult Scler* 2000; **6**(Suppl. 2):S18–S20.

136. Haas, J, Hommes, OR. A dose comparison study of IVIG in postpartum relapsing-remitting multiple sclerosis. *Mult Scler* 2007; **13**:900–8.

137. Sorensen, PS, Haas, J, Sellebjerg, F, *et al.* IV immunoglobulins as add-on treatment to methylprednisolone for acute relapses in MS. *Neurology* 2004; **63**:2028–33.

138. Visser, LH, Beekman, R, Tijssen, CC, *et al.* A randomized, double-blind, placebo-controlled pilot study of i.v. immune globulins in combination with i.v. methylprednisolone in the treatment of relapses in patients with MS. *Mult Scler* 2004; **10**:89–91.

139. Noseworthy, JH, O'Brien, PC, Weinshenker, BG, *et al.* IV immunoglobulin does not reverse established weakness in MS. *Neurology* 2000; **55**:1135–43.

140. Noseworthy, JH, O'Brien, PC, Petterson, TM, *et al.* A randomized trial of intravenous immunoglobulin in inflammatory demyelinating optic neuritis. *Neurology* 2001; **56**:1514–22.

141. Stangel, M, Boegner, F, Klatt, CH, *et al.* Placebo-controlled pilot trial to study the remyelinating potential of intravenous immunoglobulins in multiple sclerosis. *J Neurol Neurosurg Psychiatry* 2000; **68**:89–92.

142. Bakker, J, Metz, L. Devic's neuromyelitis optica treated with intravenous gamma globulin (IVIG). *Can J Neurol Sci* 2004; **31**:265–7.

143. Airas, L, Kurki, T, Erjanti, H, Marttila, RJ. Successful pregnancy of a patients with Balo's concentric sclerosis. *Mult Scler* 2005; **11**:346–48.

144. Nishikawa, M, Ichiyama, T, Hayashi, T, *et al.* Intravenous immunoglobulin therapy in acute disseminated encephalomyelitis. *Pediatr Neurol* 1999; **21**:583–6.

145. Finsterer, J, Grass, R, Stöllberger, C, Mamoli, B. Immunoglobulins in acute parainfectious disseminated encephalomyelitis. *Clin Pharmacol* 1998; **21**:256–61.

146. Revel-Viik, S, Hurvitz, H, Klar, A, *et al.* Recurrent acute disseminated encephalomyelitis associated with acute cytomegalovirus and Epstein- Barr virus infection. *J Child Neurol* 2000; **15**:421–4.

147. Ünay, B, Sarici, Ü, Bulakbaği, N, *et al.* Intravenous immunoglobulin therapy in acute disseminated encephalomyelitis associated with hepatitis A infection. *Pediatr Int* 2004; **46**:171–3.

148. Yokoyama, T, Sakurai, M, Aota, Y, *et al.* An adult case of acute disseminated encephalomyelitis accompanied with measles infection. *Intern Med* 2005; **44**:1204–5.

149. Sahlas, DJ, Miller, SP, Guerin, M, *et al.* Treatment of acute disseminated encephalomyelitis with intravenous immunoglobulin. *Neurology* 2000; **54**:1370–2.

150. Kleinman, M, Brunquell, P. Acute disseminated encephalomyelitis: response to intravenous immunoglobulin. *J Child Neurol* 1995; **10**:481–3.

151. Hahn, JS, Siegler, DJ, Enzmann, D. Intravenous gammaglobulin therapy in recurrent acute disseminated encephalomyelitis. *Neurology* 1996; **46**:1173–4.

152. Andersen, JB, Rasmussen, LH, Herning, M, Parregaard, A. Dramatic improvement of severe acute disseminated encephalomyelitis after treatment with intravenous immunoglobulin in a three-year-old boy. *Dev Med Child Neurol* 2001; **43**:136–40.

153. Marchioni, E, Marinou-Aktipi, K, Uggetti, C, *et al.* Effectiveness of intravenous immunoglobulin treatment in adult patients with steroid-resistant monophasic or recurrent acute disseminated encephalomyelitis. *J Neurol* 2002; **249**:100–4.

154. Chandra, SR, Kalpana, D, Anilkumar, TV, *et al.* Acute disseminated encephalomyelitis following leptospirosis. *J Assoc Physicians India* 2004; **52**:327–9.

155. Marchioni, E, Ravaglia, S, Piccolo, G, *et al.* Postinfectious inflammatory disorders: subgroups based on prospective follow-up. *Neurology* 2005; **65**:1057–65.

156. Strassberg, R, Schonfeld, T, Weitz, R, *et al.* Improvement of atypical acute disseminated encephalomyelitis with steroids and intravenous immunoglobulins. *Pediatr Neurol* 2002; **24**:139–43.

157. Au, WY, Lie, AKW, Cheung, RTF, *et al.* Acute disseminated encephalomyelitis after para-influenza infection post bone marrow transplantation. *Leuk Lymphoma* 2002; **43**:455–7.

158. Krishna Murthy, SN, Faden, HS, Cohen, ME, Bakshi, R. Acute disseminated encephalomyelitis in children. *Pediatrics* 2002; **110**:e1–e7.

159. Nakamura, N, Nokura, K, Zettsu, T, *et al.* Neurologic complication associated with influenza vaccination: two adult cases. *Intern Med* 2003; **42**:191–4.

160. Sonmez, FM, Odemis, E, Ahmetoglu, A, Ayvaz, A. Brainstem encephalitis and acute disseminated encephalomyelitis following mumps. *Pediatr Neurol* 2004; **30**:132–4.

161. Bangsgaard, R, Larsen, VA, Milea, D. Isolated bilateral optic neuritis in acute disseminated encephalomyelitis. *Acta Ophthalmol Scand* 2006; **84**:815–17.

162. Lu, RP, Keilson, G. Combination regimen of methylprednisolone, IVIG immunoglobulin and plasmapheresis early in the treatment of acute disseminated encephalomyelitis. *J Clin Apheresis* 2006; **21**:260–5.

163. Khurana, DS, Melvin, JJ, Kothare, SV, *et al.* Acute disseminated encephalomyelitis in children: discordant neurologic and neuroimaging abnormalities and response toplasmapheresis. *Pediatrics* 2005; **116**:431–6.

164. Dalakas, MC, Fujii, M, Li, M, *et al.* High-dose intravenous immune globulin for stiff person syndrome. *N Engl J Med* 2001; **345**,:1870–6.

165. Gerschlager, W, Brown, P. Effect of treatment with intravenous immunoglobulin on quality of life in patients with stiff-person syndrome. *Mov Disord* 2002; **17**:590–3.

166. Amato, AA, Corman, EW, Kissel, JT. Treatment of stiff-man syndrome with intravenous immunoglobulin. *Neurology* 1994; **44**:1652–74.

167. Karlson, EW, Sudarsky, L, Ruderman, E, *et al.* Treatment of stiff-man syndrome with intravenous immune globulin. *Arthritis Rheum* 1994; **37**:915–18.

168. Cantiniaux, S, Azulay, JP, Boucraut, J, *et al.* Stiff man syndrome: clinical forms, treatment and clinical course. *Rev Neurol (Paris)* 2006; **162**:832–9.

169. Vieregge, P, Branczyk, B, Berrnet, W, *et al.* Stiff-man syndrome. Report of 4 cases. *Nervenarzt* 1994; **65**:712–17.

170. Gurcan, HM, Ahmed, AR. Efficacy of various intravenous immunoglobulin therapy protocols in autoimmune and chronic inflammatory disorders. *Ann Pharmacother* 2007; **41**:812–23.

171. Gold, R, Strangel, M, Dalakas, MC. Drug insight: the use of intravenous immunoglobulin in neurology-therapeutic considerations and practical issues. *Nat Clin Pract.Neurol* 2007; **3**:36–44.

172. Fergusson, D, Hutton, B, Sharma, M, *et al.* Use of intravenous immunoglobulin for treatment of neurological conditions: a systematic review. *Transfusion* 2005; **45**:1640–57.

173. Dalakas, MC. The use of intravenous immunoglobulin in the treatment of autoimmune neuromuscular diseases: evidence-based indications and safety profile. *Pharmacol Ther* 2004; **102**:177–93.

174. Dalakas, MC. Intravenous immunoglobulin in autoimmune neuromuscular diseases. *JAMA* 2004; **291**:2367–75.

175. Villani, F, Avanzini, G. The use of immunoglobulins in the treatment of human epilepsy. *Neurol Sci* 2002; **23** (Suppl. 1):s33–s37.

176. Billiau An, D, Witters, P, Ceulemans, B, *et al.* Intravevous immunoglobulins in refractory childhood-onset epilepsy: effects on seizure frequency, EEG activity and cerebrospinal fluid cytokine profile. *Epilepsia* 2007; **48**:1739–49.

177. Cavazzuti, GB. Infantile encephalopathies. *Neurol Sci* 2003; **24**:S244–S245.

178. Mikati, MA, Saab, R. Successful use of intravenous immunoglobilin as initial monotherapy in Landau- Kleffner syndrome. *Epilepsia* 2000; **41**:880–6.

179. Mikati, M, Saab, R, Fayad, MN, Choueiri, RN. Efficacy of intravenous immunoglobulin in Landau-Kleffner syndrome. *Pediatr Neurol* 2002; **26**,:298–300.

180. Lagae, LG, Silberstein, J, Gillis, PL, Caesaer, PJ. Successful use of intravenous immunoglobulins in Landau-Kleffner syndrome. *Pediatr Neurol* 1998; **18**:165–8.

181. Fayad, MN, Choueiri, R, Mikati, M. Landau-Kleffner syndrome: consistent response to repeared intravenous gamma-globulin doses: a case report. *Epilepsia* 1997; **38**:489–94.

182. Tütüncüoğlu, S, Serdaroğlu, G, Kadioğlu, B. Landau-Kleffner syndrome beginning with stuttering: case report. *J Child Neurol* 2002; **17**:785–8.

183. Mikati, MA, Shamseddine, AN. Management of Landau-Kleffner syndrome. *Pediatr Drugs* 2005; **7**:377–89.

184. Topcu, M, Turanlt, G, Aynact, FM, *et al.* Rasmussen's encephalitis in childhood. *Childs Nerv Syst* 1999; **15**:395–403.

185. Villani, F, Spreafico, R, Farina, L, *et al.* Positive response to immunomodulatory therapy in an adult patient with Rasmussen's encephalitis. *Neurology* 2001; **56**:248–50.

186. Stangel, M, Kiefer, R, Pette, M, *et al.* Side effects of intravenous immunoglobulin in autoimmune neurological diseases. *J Neurol* 2003; **250**:818–21.

CHAPTER 10

Sleep disorders in neurodegenerative disorders and stroke

P. Jennum,[1] J. Santamaria Cano,[2] C. Bassetti,[3] P. Clarenbach,[4] B. Högl,[5] J. Mathis,[6] R. Poirrier,[7] K. Sonka,[8] E. Svanborg,[9] L. Dolenc Grosel,[10] D. Kaynak,[11] M. Kruger,[12] A. Papavasiliou[13] and Z. Zahariev[14]

[1]Glostrup Hospital, University of Copenhagen, Denmark; [2]Neurology Service, Hospital Clinic of Barcelona, Spain; [3]University Hospital Zurich, Switzerland; [4]Evangelisches Johannes-Krankenhaus, Germany; [5]Medical University of Innsbruck, Austria; [6]University Hospital, Inselspital, 3010 Bern; [7]CHU Sart Tilman, Liège, Belgium; [8]Charles University of Prague, Czech Republic; [9]Division of Clinical Neurophysiology, Linköping, Sweden; [10]Division of Neurology, University Medical Centre, Ljubljana, Slovenia; [11]Sleep Disorders Unit, Faculty of Medicine, Dokuz Eylu l University, Izmir, Turkey; [12]Hôpital de la Ville, Luxembourg; [13]Palia Pendeli Children's Hospital, Athens, Greece; [14]High Medical School, Plovdiv, Bulgaria

Objectives

1. To review the different sleep disorders occurring in degenerative neurological diseases and stroke.
2. To review the different methods of sleep evaluation available in these patients.
3. To report the evidence supporting the hypothesis that the evaluation and treatment of sleep disorders in patients with degenerative neurological disorders and stroke improve the management of these diseases.

Background

Sleep is an active process generated and modulated by a complex set of neural systems located mainly in the hypothalamus, brain stem and thalamus. Sleep is altered in many neurological diseases due to several mechanisms: lesions of the brain areas that control sleep and wakefulness, lesions or diseases that produce pain, reduced mobility or treatments. Excessive daytime sleepiness (EDS), sleep fragmentation, insomnia, sleep-disordered breathing (SDB), nocturnal behavioural phenomena such as rapid eye movement (REM) sleep behaviour disorder or nocturnal seizures, restless leg syndrome and periodic leg movements (PLMs) are common symptoms and findings in neurological disorders Sleep disorders may precede and influence disease course of life in neurological diseases involving daytime functioning, quality of life, morbidity and mortality.

Diagnostic and treatment procedures and treatment of sleep disorders have developed considerably in recent

European Handbook of Neurological Management: Volume 2, Second Edition. Edited by Nils Erik Gilhus, Michael P. Barnes, Michael Brainin.

years. There are thus increased opportunities for management of sleep disorders in neurological diseases.

The current guidelines focus on *neurodegenerative disorders* and *stroke* with an emphasis on *sleep breathing disorders* in neurological disease and are an update from a former review [1] in accordance with the European Federation of Neurological Societies (EFNS) guidelines [2].

The chapter covers three main areas:
1. Tauopathies (Alzheimer's disease, progressive supranuclear palsy and corticobasal degeneration)
2. Synucleinopathies (Parkinson's disease, multiple system atrophy and dementia with Lewy bodies)
3. Stroke, amyotrophic lateral sclerosis (ALS), myotonic dystrophy, myasthenia gravis and spinocerebellar ataxias.

Search strategy

A literature search included PubMed and the Cochrane library. These were searched until 2009, or as much of this range as possible, looking for the different sleep disorders and symptoms in each of the most frequent or relevant degenerative neurological disorders and stroke. Language is restricted to European languages. Studies considered for inclusion were, when possible, randomized controlled trials of adult patients, in any setting, suffering a neurodegenerative disorder (motor neuron disease, Parkinson's disease, Alzheimer's disease) or stroke. There had to be an explicit complaint of insomnia, parasomnia or hypersomnia in study participants. We also included observational studies. Abstracts were selected by the chairmen and independently inspected by individual members of the Task Force; full papers were obtained where necessary. A classification of the different studies according to evidence levels for therapeutic interventions and diagnostic measures will be done in accordance with the guidance [2]. The panel will discuss what possible diagnostic tests and health-care interventions could be recommended in each particular disease.

Method for reaching consensus

Where there was uncertainty further discussion was sought by the panel. Data extraction and quality assessments were undertaken independently by the panel reviewers.

Sleep disorders

Classification of sleep disorders

The International Classification, version 2 (ICSD-2), lists 95 sleep disorders [3]. The ISCD-2 has eight major categories:
1. Insomnias
2. Sleep-related breathing disorders (SBDs)
3. Hypersomnias not due to a sleep-related breathing disorder
4. Circadian rhythm sleep disorders
5. Parasomnias
6. Sleep-related movement disorders
7. Isolated symptoms
8. Other sleep disorders.

In the following pages only a selected number of the sleep disorders related to neurological diseases are mentioned.

Insomnia

Insomnias are defined by a complaint of repeated difficulties with sleep initiation, sleep maintenance, duration, consolidation or quality that occurs despite adequate time and opportunity for sleep, and the result in some form of daytime impairment.

Insomnias can be divided into acute and chronic forms. The acute form, also termed 'adjustment insomnia', can usually be attributed to a well-defined circumstance, whereas chronic insomnia is often a consequence of conditional (psychophysiological) or idiopathic disorders, or found in patients with psychiatric, medical or neurological disorders. The last may be due either to degeneration or dysfunction of the central nervous system areas involved in sleep regulation or to motor or sensory symptoms produced by the disease (pain, reduced nocturnal mobility, nocturnal motor activity, etc.) that lower the threshold for arousal from sleep. Finally insomnia may be caused by the alerting effects of the drugs used in the treatment of neurological diseases.

Sleep-disordered breathing

These disorders are characterized by disordered breathing during sleep. A uniform syndrome recommendation was suggested in 1999 by the American Academy of Sleep Medicine [4], which is included in ICSD-2:
1. Obstructive sleep apnoea syndromes (OSAS)
2. Central sleep apnoea–hypopnoea syndrome (CSAHS)

3. Cheyne–Stokes breathing syndrome (CSBS) and sleep-related hypoventilation/hypoxaemic syndromes (SHVSs).

For a more thorough review of SDB we refer to the previous EFNS guideline [1]

Excessive daytime sleepiness not due to a sleep-related breathing disorder

Hypersomnia (EDS) is defined by the inability to stay fully alert and awake during the day, resulting in unintended lapses into sleep. EDS should be separated from fatigue, which refers to physical or mental weariness. The most common disorders in this group are narcolepsy, idiopathic hypersomnia, insufficient sleep and the use of sedating medication. EDS is also commonly reported in patients with neurological disease, including neurodegeneration, post-stroke, inflammation, tumour, injury or brain trauma, and may be caused by degeneration of sleep/wake centres, sleep fragmentation or medication. Hypersomnia in a narrow sense is describing a prolonged major sleep episode, usually beyond 10 hours. This phenomenon is typical in 'idiopathic hypersomnia with prolonged sleep time' but is also reported in 'non-organic hypersomnia' (ISCD-2). The diagnostic work-up should always consider the possibility of sleep insufficiency syndrome or poor sleep hygiene.

Circadian rhythm disorders

Circadian rhythm disorders are defined as a misalignment between the patient's sleep pattern and the pattern that is desired or regarded as the societal norm. Most of the conditions observed in this group are associated with external factors such as shift work, jet lag or social habits, but, in relation to neurological diseases, conditions that destruct the neural input to the suprachiasmatic nucleus (e.g. complete bilateral retinal, optic nerve, chiasms or hypothalamic lesions) may induce a condition that resembles circadian disorders.

Parasomnias

Parasomnias are undesirable sensorimotor events that appear exclusively during sleep. Parasomnias are disorders of arousal, partial arousal and sleep stage transition. These disorders do not primarily cause a complaint of insomnia or excessive sleepiness, but frequently involve abnormal behaviours during sleep. Many of the disorders are common in children, but some are also present in

adults. Parasomnias are subdivided into the following groups:

1. Disorders of arousal from non-REM (NREM) sleep: confusional arousal, sleep walking and sleep terror
2. Parasomnias usually associated with REM sleep: REM sleep behaviour disorder (RBD), recurrent isolated sleep paralysis and nightmare disorder
3. Other parasomnias, e.g. enuresis, sleep-related groaning (catathrenia), exploding head syndrome, sleep-related hallucinations and eating disorders.

Of these parasomnias, RBD has a particular relationship to neurodegenerative diseases.

REM sleep behaviour disorder

This disorder is characterized by vigorous movements occurring during REM sleep associated with abnormal absence of the physiological muscle atonia and increased phasic electromyographic (EMG) activity during REM sleep [5–7]. The following are diagnostic criteria:

1. Presence of REM sleep without atonia: the EMG finding of excessive amounts of sustained or intermittent elevation of fragmented EMG tone or excessive phasic submental or (upper or lower extremity) EMG twitching.
2. At least one of the following is present:
   (a) sleep-related injuries, potentially injurious or disruptive behaviours by history
   (b) abnormal REM sleep behaviours documented during polysomnographic monitoring.
3. Absence of EEG epileptiform activity during REM sleep unless an RBD can be clearly distinguished from any concurrent REM sleep-related seizure disorder.
4. The sleep disturbance is not better explained by another sleep disorder, medical or neurological disorder, mental disorder, and medication use or substance use disorder.

The patient and anyone sharing the bed can be injured. RBD is observed in most patients with multiple system atrophy (MSA), dementia with Lewy bodies (DLB) and in a significant proportion of patients with Parkinson's disease. RBD is also commonly observed in diffuse Lewy body and Machado–Joseph disease (MJD) [8–19]. Patients with an isolated RBD have a significant risk of developing Parkinson's disease, DLB or MSA, especially if other brain-stem manifestations, such as reduced smell, depression and mild cognitive impairment or incontinence, are present [5, 11, 20]. Occurrence of hallucinations in Parkinson's disease is related to the presence of an RBD [8]. Reduced striatal dopamine transporters have been observed in these patients [21]. RBDs are strongly linked to narcolepsy with cataplexy, especially in patients with hypocretin deficiency [22] and are further observed in a number of other diseases such as stroke and multiple sclerosis. A confident diagnosis relies on a full polysomnographic (PSG) recording which included EMG and electro-oculographic recording with adequate polygraphic measures of relevant physiological measures, preferably with synchronized audiovisual recording.

There is a need for further clarification of the EMG abnormalities in RBD, with special emphasis on muscle tone and motor activity (number of movements, duration, intensity) and their relationship to sleep stages. These are currently undergoing clarification and evaluation.

Sleep-related movement disorders

Sleep-related movement disorders are characterized by relatively simple, usually stereotypical, movements that disturb sleep to complex movements of different intensity, duration and periodicities or lack of it. Periodic limb movements (PLMs), restless legs syndrome (RLS), bruxism, leg cramps, rhythmic movement disorders and other sleep-related movement disorders are classified under this group. Of these RLSs and PLM are of particular interest in patients with neurodegenerative disorders. Of special focus is subdivision into different types of stage-dependent movements during sleep, as observed in most neurodegenerative disorders, RBDs and patients with narcolepsy with cataplexy. This area is currently undergoing clarification and evaluation.

Sleep disorders associated with neurological disease

Tauopathies

Patients with progressive supranuclear palsy (PSP), Alzheimer's disease and corticobasal degeneration (CBD) may complain of significant sleep-related circadian disturbances, sleep–wake and daytime problems [6, 23–29]. Sleep–wake disturbances and disruption are commonly observed in Alzheimer's disease, with daytime sleep, sleep attack and episodes of micro-sleep.

Insomnia (sleep fragmentation, difficulties maintaining sleep) is common, as are nocturnal wandering, nocturnal confusion, 'sundowning' psychosis and nocturia.

EDS, sleep attacks and episodes of micro-sleep during the daytime may be associated with cognitive problems.

Sleep-related disorders such as RBDs, RLS, PLMs, nocturnal complex and dystonic movements, and cramps may occur in PSP and CBD but are rare in Alzheimer's disease.

Sleep breathing disorders are common in Alzheimer's disease and associated with disease progression and poorer prognosis; however, the clinical significance of diagnosing and treating them in this group of patients is questionable.

Recommendations

Sleep disorders are commonly observed in patients with tauopathies, and there should be increased awareness of these disorders. It is recommended that a detailed medical history of sleep disorders be performed in tauopathies, i.e. insomnia, EDS, motor and dreaming activity, and SBDs. PSG recording, preferably with audiovisual recording, is suggested for the diagnosis, especially when RBDs and/or SBDs are the suspected disorders (level C).

Synucleinopathies

Parkinson's disease, MSA and DLB are often associated with major sleep–wake disorders [14, 15, 28, 30–39]:
• Parkinson's disease-related motor symptoms, including nocturnal akinesia, early morning dystonia, painful cramps, tremor and difficulties turning in bed
• Treatment-related nocturnal disturbances (e.g. insomnia, confusion, hallucinations and motor disturbances)
• Sleep-related symptoms such as hallucinations and vivid dreams (nightmares), insomnia (sleep fragmentation, difficulties maintaining sleep), nocturia, psychosis and panic attack
• EDS, sleep attacks and episodes of micro-sleep during waking hours
• Sleep-related disorders including RBDs, RLS, PLMs, nocturnal dystonic movements, cramps and SDB. Presence of RBDs in Parkinson's disease is associated with cognitive and autonomic changes.

Laryngeal stridor and OSA are commonly observed in MSA patients, which is associated with a poorer prognosis. Continuous positive airway pressure (CPAP) may improve respiration and prognosis (class III).

> **Recommendations**
>
> Most patients with synucleinopathies experience one or more sleep disorders. It is recommended that a detailed medical history of sleep disorders be performed in synucleinopathies, i.e. insomnia, EDS, motor and dreaming activity and SBD PSG recording, preferably with audiovisual recording, is suggested for the diagnosis especially when RBDs and/or SBDs are suspected (level B).

Other symptoms

Stroke

Patients with strokes, primarily infarctions, may suffer from several sleep disorders and disturbances. Their occurrence and manifestations may vary depending on the specific neurological deficits [40–51]:

1. SBDs, especially OSA and nocturnal oxygen desaturations, have been found commonly (>50%) in patients with acute stroke as well as after neurological recovery. OSA is a risk factor for stroke and coexisting OSA in stroke patients may increase restroke risk. Presence of SDB, especially OSA, may worsen the prognosis and increase the stroke recurrence risk. SDB may be provoked by stroke, especially after damage to the respiratory centres in the brain stem or bulbar/pseudobulbar paralysis due to brain-stem lesions. Pre-existing sleep apnoea before stroke may present a risk factor for stroke, with co-morbid obesity, diabetes, coronary artery disease and hypertension, and other cerebrovascular risk factors. There are several haemodynamic changes in sleep apnoea that may play a role in the pathogenesis of stroke development. Stroke and SBDs are both common and associated with significant morbidity and mortality.

2. CPAP treatment of OSA may reduce the risk of cardio- and cerebrovascular complications (class I) and potential re-stroke, but the compliance is poor to moderate compared with compliance in OSA non-stroke patients (level B).

Sleepiness and fatigue are commonly reported in patients after a stroke and are often disabling symptoms.

Other sleep disorders such as insomnia, RBDs and periodic limb movement in sleep may be observed as part of or after stroke.

> **Recommendations**
>
> Sleep disorders, especially SDB, occur often in stroke patients. Screening for SDB and other sleep disorders is recommended as part of the stroke evaluation programme especially in ischaemic stroke patients (level A).

Motor neuron, motor end-plate and muscle diseases

Sleep-disordered breathing is observed in several neuromuscular diseases including muscular dystrophy, myotonic dystrophy, myasthenia gravis, ALS and postpolio syndrome. Although there may be differences, some general observations can be made. Hypoxaemia, especially during REM sleep, is commonly found. Severity is correlated to respiratory strength, and sleep-related hypoventilation is usually non-obstructive [52, 53].

Patients with ALS and other severe motor neuron diseases have progressive motor deterioration with progressive respiratory insufficiency. This may manifest primarily during sleep when the motor drive is reduced. This is especially true for patients with the bulbar form of ALS or involvement of the C3–5 anterior horn [54, 55]. The prognosis is closely related to respiratory muscle strength [56]. Of note, sudden nocturnal death occurs often during sleep. Respiratory indices such as low nocturnal oxygen saturation are associated with poorer prognosis [57, 58]. Patients with diaphragmatic involvement may have significantly reduced REM sleep [59]. The primary SBD in patients with ALS – as in other neuromuscular diseases – is therefore a sleep hypoventilation syndrome (SHVS), whereas OSAs are rare [54].

Management of these patients should therefore include relevant questions about symptoms susceptive for SBDs. Common symptoms of nocturnal hypoventilations may include insomnia, headache and daytime somnolence [60].

Oximetry has been suggested for the identification and screening of sleep-related hypoventilation in patients with ALS; the value is limited to identification of nocturnal desaturations which may occur during NREM and REM sleep [58, 61, 62]. Care should be taken because the partial pressure of carbon dioxide (PCO_2) may increase before desaturations are observed, especially in patients with additional chronic obstructive lung disease. Nocturnal oximetry has been suggested as valuable for screening and evaluation of the treatment effect [54, 58]. There is no validation of the diagnostic yield for a full PSG, respiratory polygraphy and nocturnal oximetry in these patients. It is, however, important to identify early symptoms of respiratory failure in sleep, because these patients are able to compensate their hypercapnia during wakefulness for a long time. This is the point at which you should bring in regular measurement of respiratory parameters [63–67].

Recommendations

SDB often occurs in patients with motor neuron, motor end-plate and muscle diseases, and should be considered in all patients. Minimum evaluation should include PSG, eventually combined with additional CO_2 analysis, and then supplied with serial polygraphy or oximetry measures for the identification of sleep-related hypoventilation during the disease course (level B).

Genetic neurodegenerative disorders

Other neurodegenerative disorders of genetic cause may present several sleep disturbances. Individuals with SCA-3 (Machado–Joseph disease) may also complain of RLS, PLMs, vocal fold paralysis and RBDs [9, 10, 12, 68, 69]. In patients with Huntington's disease the involuntary movements tend to diminish during sleep [70]. Sleep disturbances, including disturbed sleep pattern with increased sleep-onset latency, reduced sleep efficiency, frequent nocturnal awakenings and more time spent awake with less slow wave sleep, have been reported. These abnormalities correlate in part with duration of illness, severity of clinical symptoms and degree of atrophy of the caudate nucleus [71]. The sleep phenotype of Huntington's disease may also insomnia, advanced sleep phase, PLMs, RBDs and reduced REM sleep, but not narcolepsy. Reduced REM sleep may precede chorea. Mutant huntingtin may exert an effect on REM sleep and motor control during sleep [72]. However, other studies have not reported specific sleep disorders in Huntington's disease patients [73].

Recommendations

Sleep disorders occur in several genetic neurological diseases. The patients should be questioned and further evaluation of these disorders should rely on a clinical judgement (level C).

Management of sleep disorders in neurological diseases

Diagnostic techniques in sleep disorders

Diagnostic procedures for sleep diagnosis include: PSG, partial time polysomnography, partial polygraphy (or respiratory polygraphy [RP]) and limited channel polygraphy – oximetry determining arterial oxygen saturation or SaO_2/pulse and actimetry. Daytime sleepiness may be evaluated with the multiple sleep latency test (MSLT) or maintenance of wakefulness test (MWT) [74–81]. Many of the tests are increasingly easy to perform in- or outside hospital due to technological advantages. Consequently the diagnostic procedures may be performed more easily as part of the diagnostic programme for neurology patients. An overview of these tests is presented in Table 10.1.

Treatment of SDB in neurological diseases
Treatment of OSAs

1. CPAP is a well-documented treatment for moderate and severe OSA (apnoea–hypopnoea index [AHI] ≥15/h) and improves nocturnal respiratory abnormalities, daytime function and cognitive problems [82–87] (class I). There is no significant difference with regard to treatment effect or changes in subjective variables between fixed pressure CPAP and autoadjusted CPAP [88, 89] (class I).

2. CPAP and bilevel PAP (bi-PAP) is potentially useful in patients with SBD in stroke [41, 42], despite of negative report [90]. The evidence, however, whether this influences quality of life, daytime symptoms, rehabilitation, morbidity and mortality is limited, which needs further clarification [51] (class II).

Severe SBDs including laryngeal stridor in patients with MSA may be treated with CPAP/bi-level PAP. Recent studies suggest that treatment with CPAP in MSA patients with laryngeal stridor showed high CPAP tolerance, no recurrence of stridor, no major side effects and subjective improvement in sleep quality, and increases the survival time for MSA patients without stridor [31, 91]. CPAP is therefore an effective non-invasive long-term therapy for nocturnal stridor (level C) and may prevent worsening of stridor under increasing dopaminergic dosages.

Table 10.1 Methods for the diagnosis of sleep disorders in neurological diseases.

Type of polysomnography	Definition	Indication	Advantage/Disadvantage
Routine	Multi-channel EEG, EOG, submental EMG, ECG, respiration, ±tibial EMG	Routine screening for sleep disorders: SBD, PLM, chronic insomnia	Golden standard. May be performed in- or outside hospital. Standard method
Extended	Routine PSG + extra physiological channels, e.g. EMG, intraoesophageal pressure, CO_2	Special indications: oesophageal reflux, myoclonias, etc. Depends on selected channels	Moderately expensive, time-consuming, staff demanding
Video	PSG + video recording	Motor and behavioural phenomena during sleep	A video signal is present. Full physiological recording. Includes audiovisual channels
Full EEG-PSG	Full 10–20 EEG + PSG	Motor and behavioural disturbances for differential diagnosis of epilepsies	Full diagnostic procedures are obtained. The difference between the methods is primarily the number of EEG channels. Expensive, time-consuming, staff demanding
Multiple sleep latency test (MSLT)	Multiple (four or more) trials per day of PSG determination of sleep latencies of intended sleep	Central hypersomnias including narcolepsy, distinction between tiredness and EDS. Supportive for EDS in neurological diseases	Supportive for the diagnosis of hypersomnia and narcolepsy/sensitive to foregoing sleep loss and discontinuation of REM sleep-inhibiting drugs
Maintenance of wakefulness test (MWT)	Multiple (four or more) trials per day of PSG determination of sleep latencies of intended sleep inhibition	Determination of ability to stay awake	Supportive for wakefulness capabilities, useful for driving ability and treatment effects.
Partial channel polygraphy			
Respiratory polygraphy	Monitoring of respiration + SaO_2 ± cardiac measures, e.g. pulse	OSAs	Easy, inexpensive. Moderate–good sensitivity and specificity for OSAs; the validity for other SBD is not present
Oximetry	Monitoring of SaO_2	Monitoring or screening for severe SBD	Easy, inexpensive. Low sensitivity and specificity for SBD. Exclusion of SDB not possible
Actigraphy	Determination of motor activity (days–months)	Sleep–wake disturbances	Inexpensive. Limited clinical usefulness

EDS, excessive daytime sleepiness; EEG, electroencephalography; EMG, electromyography; EOG, electro-oculography; OSA, obstructive sleep apnoea; PLM, periodic limb movement; PSG, polysomnography; REM, rapid eye movement; SaO_2, arterial oxygen saturation; SBD, sleep-related breathing disorder; SDB, sleep-disordered breathing.

In some patients, e.g. neuromuscular disorder patients, CPAP may be difficult to accept and bi-PAP may be used [92] (class IV).

There is evidence to suggest that oral appliance (OA) use improves subjective sleepiness and SDB compared with controls in patients with OSAs without neurological diseases (level B). Nasal continuous positive airway pressure (nCPAP) is apparently more effective in improving SDB than OA use (level B). There are no data regarding the use of oral appliances in patients with neurological diseases, which is why caution should be employed in OA use in patients with OSAs [93, 94] (level C).

Surgical treatment has limited effect on OSA [95, 96] (class III). There are no studies suggesting that surgery in the upper airway has any effect on OSAs in patients with neurological diseases.

Drug treatments have no positive effect on OSAs [97] (class II). There is no study available to indicate that medication has any treatment effect on OSAs in patients with neurological diseases.

Although some patients with OSAs present with increased weight and a negative lifestyle profile (tobacco, alcohol, physical activity), no controlled studies have evaluated the effect of intervention on these factors [98] (class IV). No studies have addressed the effect of lifestyle interventions on OSAs in patients with neurological diseases.

Treatment of central sleep apnoea–hypopnoea syndrome

Case series have shown that CPAP treatment does not influence the CO_2 response in CSAHS, despite a reduction in apnoeas, increase in PaO_2 and reduction in subjective sleepiness [99–101] (class IV). Probably due to the rareness of the disease, there are no randomized studies with regard to CSAHS and its treatment. Drug treatment with acetazolamide and theophylline has furthermore been suggested [102], but the evidence for their use is poor (class IV).

Treatment of Cheyne–Stokes breathing syndrome

Initially, CPAP was used in patients with central apnoea/CSBS and cardiac insufficiency [103–106], but in recent years adaptive ventilation has been found effective, probably by an increased preload in patients with significant cardiac failure, reducing the respiratory abnormalities,

although the long-term prognosis is not known [107, 108] (class IV). A recent randomized controlled study suggests that the use of non-invasive adaptive ventilation may improve daytime function and respiratory and cardiac measures [109] (class II). The experience with the use of adaptive ventilation, CPAP or bi-PAP in patients with Cheyne–Stokes respiration due to central respiratory failure, e.g. brain-stem lesions, is sparse and the evidence level is poor (class C).

Treatment of sleep hypoventilation syndrome

Treatment includes nasal intermittent positive pressure ventilation (NIPPV) with bi-PAP, variable PAP (VPAP), non-invasive volumetric ventilation, and eventually invasive ventilation, under control of nocturnal respiratory parameters [110] (class IV). CPAP is not the primary treatment, as the motor effort is mostly reduced in these patients, which may lead to worsening of the SBD. NIPPV may reduce sleep disturbances, increase cognitive function, and prolong the period to tracheostomy [111, 112] (class IV). Current evidence about the therapeutic benefit of mechanical ventilation is weak, but consistent, suggesting alleviation of the symptoms of chronic hypoventilation in the short-term. Evidence from a single randomized trial of non-invasive ventilation with a limited number of participants suggests a prolonged survival and improved quality of life in people with ALS, especially among those with minor bulbar involvement, but not in patients with severe bulbar impairment [113, 114] (class III).

Follow-up

Although there is no evidence when and how follow-up of treatment with CPAP and NIPPV should be executed, we recommend regular follow-up of the treatment with control of compliance and treatment effect (class IV).

Ethical aspects

Treatment of patients with severe neurological diseases such as ALS and MSA with NIPPV include medical and ethical problems that should be addressed. Adequate involvement of the patients and family, and the treatment, its use and limitations, should be carefully discussed early in the course of the disease. It is important to clarify the limitations of the treatment and the discussion should include careful debate about whether such treatment should be offered, initiation, the need for a tracheostomy, whether invasive ventilation should be offered and discontinuation [115, 116].

Drug treatment of EDS in neurological diseases

Several groups of patients with neurological diseases commonly complain of EDS. The aetiology may be secondary to the neurological disease, medication (dopaminergic or benzodiazepine drugs) or consequence of concomitant sleep disorders such as sleep apnoea, nocturnal motor phenomena, etc. In patients in whom these factors cannot be modified, stimulants such as methylphenidate or modafinil may be used as symptomatic therapy. Modafinil was primarily introduced to treat EDS in narcolepsy [117–122]. Case studies [123, 124] and double-blind controlled studies [125, 126] suggest that modafinil reduces EDS in Parkinson's patients (class B-II) despite the fact that Ondo's study did not prove any long-term effect of modafinil in Parkinson's disease [127]. Modafinil has also been suggested in ALS [128] and post-stroke depression [129, 130] but there are no controlled studies (class IV). Furthermore, modafinil has been used for treatment of residual EDS in OSAs undergoing CPAP treatment without neurological co-morbidity [131]. There is some evidence that other centrally acting drugs such as methylphenidate may have similar effects [132], but there is no comparison between modafinil and methylphenidate. EDS in Parkinson's disease was successfully reduced by sodium oxybate [133] (class II).

Other drug and non-pharmacological treatment of sleep disorders in neurological diseases

Treatment of sleep disorders in neurodegenerative diseases is often complex and may involve different strategies. Parkinson's disease-related motor symptoms can be treated with long-acting dopamine agonists (DAs) to obtain continuous DA-receptor stimulation during the night. On the other hand, nocturnal disturbances may be related to treatment and, therefore, continued monitoring of treatment effect should be offered.

Some sleep disorders, such as RLS and PLMs, may be controlled by DA agents, and others, such as insomnia and EDS, may be improved by reducing dopaminergic stimulation (class IV).

Clonazepam or donepezil, possibly prescribed with melatonin, has been suggested based on case series for the treatment of RBDs. No controlled studies are available [35, 39].

Patients with dementias often present circadian disturbances that may be relieved by melatonin and light therapy [134–150] (class IV).

In selected cases treatment with hypnotics is mentioned as useful, but the evidence is limited and care should be taken for chronic use, the risk of falls, daytime sedation, confusion and worsening of the SDB in elderly people.

Good practice points

1. Patients with neurological diseases often have significant sleep disorders that affect sleep and daytime function with increased morbidity and even mortality. Many of these disorders are treatable. Therefore, increased awareness should be directed to sleep disorders in patients with neurodegenerative, cerebrovascular and neuromuscular diseases. Despite this, there are limited number of studies with high evidence level.

2. A PSG is a diagnostic minimum for the diagnoses of sleep disorders in patients with neurological diseases.

3. In patients with nocturnal motor and/behaviour manifestations, a full video-PSG/video-EEG–PSG is recommended

4. RP has a moderate sensitivity and specificity in the diagnosis of OSAs without neurological diseases, but its value for diagnosis of other SBDs or in neurology patients with suspected OSAs has not been evaluated compared with the gold standard PSG. Consequently, RP may be used as a method for detecting OSA, but its value for the use for SDB in patients with neurological diseases needs further validation.

5. Oximetry has a poor sensitivity–specificity for the identification of OSAs in patients without neurological diseases. Oximetry cannot differentiate between obstructive and central sleep apnoea or is insufficient to identify stridor. Oximetry alone is not recommended for the diagnosis of SDB in neurological disorders.

6. Patients with SBDs and muscle weakness and cardiac or pulmonary co-morbidity may present a sleep hypoventilation syndrome, which manifests early as increased CO_2. $PaCO_2$ should be measured in such cases during sleep recordings.

7. Fixed pressure CPAP/auto-adjusted CPAP is the most effective treatment of OSAs. This probably also includes patients with OSAs and neurological diseases. However, there is a need for further evaluation of the effect of CPAP in patients with OSAs and neurological diseases.

8. Bi-PAP/variable PAP, NIPPV and volumetric ventilation are useful for SBD-like central apnoeas, Cheyne–Stokes breathing and alveolar hypoventilation.

9. There is a clear need for further studies focusing on the diagnostic procedures and treatment modalities in neurology patients with sleep disorders.

Conflicts of interest

None reported.

References

1. Jennum, P, Santamaria, J, Clarenbach, P, *et al*. Report of an EFNS task force on management of sleep disorders in neurological disease (degenerative neurological disorders and stroke). *Eur J Neurol* 2007; **14**:1189–2005.

2. Brainin, M, Barnes, M, Baron, JC, *et al*. Guidance for the preparation of neurological management guidelines by EFNS scientific task forces–revised recommendations 2004. *Eur J Neurol* 2004; **11**:577–81.

3. American Academy of Sleep Medicine: International Classification of Sleep Disorders. *Diagnostic and Coding Manual*, 2nd edn. Westchester, IL: American Academy of Sleep Medicine, 2005.

4. American Academy of Sleep Medicine Task Force. Sleep-related breathing disorders in adults: recommendations for syndrome definition and measurement techniques in clinical research. The Report of an American Academy of Sleep Medicine Task Force. *Sleep* 1999c; **22**:667–89.

5. Schenck, CH, Bundlie, SR, Mahowald, MW. Delayed emergence of a parkinsonian disorder in 38% of 29 older men initially diagnosed with idiopathic rapid eye movement sleep behaviour disorder. *Neurology* 1996; **46**:388–93.

6. Schenck, CH, Mahowald, MW, Anderson, ML, Silber, MH, Boeve, BF, Parisi, JE. Lewy body variant of Alzheimer's disease (AD) identified by postmortem ubiquitin staining in a previously reported case of AD associated with REM sleep behavior disorder. *Biol Psychiatry* 1997; **42**:527–8.

7. Schenck, CH, Mahowald, MW. REM sleep behavior disorder: clinical, developmental, and neuroscience perspectives 16 years after its formal identification in SLEEP. *Sleep* 2002; **25**:120–38.

8. Onofrj, M, Thomas, A, D'Andreamatteo, G, *et al*. Incidence of RBD and hallucination in patients affected by Parkinson's disease: 8-year follow-up. *Neurol Sci* 2002; **23**(suppl 2):S91–4.

9. Friedman, JH, Fernandez, HH, Sudarsky, LR. REM behavior disorder and excessive daytime somnolence in Machado-Joseph disease (SCA-3). *Mov Disord* 2003; **18**: 1520–2.

10. Iranzo, A, Munoz, E, Santamaria, J, Vilaseca, I, Mila, M, Tolosa, E. REM sleep behavior disorder and vocal cord paralysis in Machado-Joseph disease. *Mov Disord* 2003; **18**:1179–83.

11. Iranzo, A, Molinuevo, JL, Santamaria, J, *et al*. Rapid-eye-movement sleep behaviour disorder as an early marker for a neurodegenerative disorder: a descriptive study. *Lancet Neurol* 2006; **5**:572–7.

12. Syed, BH, Rye, DB, Singh, G. REM sleep behavior disorder and SCA-3 (Machado-Joseph disease). *Neurology* 2003; **60**:148.

13. Uchiyama, M, Isse, K, Tanaka, K, *et al*. Incidental Lewy body disease in a patient with REM sleep behavior disorder. *Neurology* 1995; **45**:709–12.

14. Boeve, BF, Silber, MH, Ferman, TJ, Lucas, JA, Parisi, JE. Association of REM sleep behavior disorder and neurodegenerative disease may reflect an underlying synucleinopathy. *Mov Disord* 2001; **16**:622–30.

15. Boeve, BF, Silber, MH, Ferman, TJ. REM sleep behavior disorder in Parkinson's disease and dementia with Lewy bodies. *J Geriatr Psychiatry Neurol* 2004; **17**:146–57.

16. Turner, RS. Idiopathic rapid eye movement sleep behavior disorder is a harbinger of dementia with Lewy bodies. *J Geriatr Psychiatry Neurol* 2002; **15**:195–9.

17. De Cock, VC, Vidilhet, M, Leu, S, *et al*. Restoration of normal motor control in Parkinson's disease during REM sleep. *Brain* 2007a; **130**:450–6.

18. De Cock, VC, Lannuzel, A, Verhaeghe, S, *et al*. REM sleep behavior disorder in patients with guadeloupean parkinsonism, a tauopathy. *Sleep* 2007b; **30**:1026–32.

19. Iranzo, A, Santamaria, J, Tolosa, E. The clinical and pathophysiological relevance of REM sleep behavior disorder in neurodegenerative diseases. *Sleep Med Rev* 2009; **13**: 385–401.

20. Postuma, RB, Gagnon, JF, Vendette, M, *et al*. Quantifying the risk of neurodegenerative disease in idiopathic REM sleep behavior disorder. *Neurology* 2009; **72**:1296–300.

21. Eisensehr, I, Linke, R, Tatsch, K, *et al*. Increased muscle activity during rapid eye movement sleep correlates with decrease of striatal presynaptic dopamine transporters. IPT and IBZM SPECT imaging in subclinical and clinically manifest idiopathic REM sleep behavior disorder, Parkinson's disease, and controls. *Sleep* 2003; **26**:507–12.

22. Knudsen, S, Gammeltoft, S, Jennum, P. The association between hypocretin-1 deficiency, cataplexy, and REM Sleep Behaviour Disorder (RBD) in narcolepsy. *Brain* 2010; **133**: 568–79. in press.

23. De Bruin, VS, Machado, C, Howard, RS, Hirsch, NP, Lees, AJ. Nocturnal and respiratory disturbances in Steele–Richardson–Olszewski syndrome (progressive supranuclear palsy). *Postgrad Med J* 1996; **72**:293–6.

24. Pareja, JA, Caminero, AB, Masa, JF, Dobato, JL. A first case of progressive supranuclear palsy and pre-clinical REM sleep behavior disorder presenting as inhibition of speech during wakefulness and somniloquy with phasic muscle twitching during REM sleep. *Neurologia* 1996; **11**:304–6.

25. Kimura, K, Tachibana, N, Aso, T, Kimura, J, Shibasaki, H. Subclinical REM sleep behavior disorder in a patient with corticobasal degeneration. *Sleep* 1997; **20**:891–4.

26. Janssens, JP, Pautex, S, Hilleret, H, Michel, JP. Sleep disordered breathing in the elderly. *Aging (Milano)* 2000; **12**:417–29.

27. Volicer, L, Harper, DG, Manning, BC, Goldstein, R, Satlin, A. Sundowning and circadian rhythms in Alzheimer's disease. *Am J Psychiatry* 2001; **158**:704–11.

28. Ferman, TJ, Smith, GE, Boeve, BF, *et al*. DLB fluctuations: specific features that reliably differentiate DLB from AD and normal aging. *Neurology* 2004; **62**:181–7.

29. Reynolds, CF, III, Kupfer, DJ, Taska, LS, *et al*. Sleep apnea in Alzheimer's dementia: correlation with mental deterioration. *J Clin Psychiatry* 1985b; **46**:257–61.

30. Silber, MH, Levine, S. Stridor and death in multiple system atrophy 10. *Mov Disord* 2000; **15**:699–704.

31. Iranzo, A, Santamaria, J, Tolosa, E. Continuous positive air pressure eliminates nocturnal stridor in multiple system atrophy. Barcelona Multiple System Atrophy Study Group. *Lancet* 2000; **356**:1329–30.

32. Ferman, TJ, Boeve, BF, Smith, GE, *et al*. Dementia with Lewy bodies may present as dementia and REM sleep behavior disorder without parkinsonism or hallucinations. *J Int Neuropsychol Soc* 2002; **8**:907–14.

33. Gilman, S, Chervin, RD, Koeppe, RA, *et al*. Obstructive sleep apnea is related to a thalamic cholinergic deficit in MSA. *Neurology* 2003a; **61**:35–9.

34. Gilman, S, Koeppe, RA, Chervin, RD, *et al*. REM sleep behavior disorder is related to striatal monoaminergic deficit in MSA. *Neurology* 2003; **61**:29–34.

35. Massironi, G, Galluzzi, S, Frisoni, GB. Drug treatment of REM sleep behavior disorders in dementia with Lewy bodies. *Int Psychogeriatr* 2003; **15**:377–83.

36. Yamaguchi, M, Arai, K, Asahina, M, Hattori, T. Laryngeal stridor in multiple system atrophy. *Eur Neurol* 2003; **49**:154–9.

37. Barone, P, Amboni, M, Vitale, C, Bonavita, V. Treatment of nocturnal disturbances and excessive daytime sleepiness in Parkinson's disease. *Neurology* 2004; **63**(**8** suppl 3): S35–8.

38. Vendette, M, Gagnon, JF, Décary, A, *et al*. REM sleep behavior disorder predicts cognitive impairment in Parkinson disease without dementia. *Neurology* 2007; **69**:1843–9.

39. Boeve, BF, Silber, MH, Ferman, TJ. Melatonin for treatment of REM sleep behavior disorder in neurologic disorders: results in 14 patients. *Sleep Med* 2003; **4**:281–4.

40. Bassetti, C, Mathis, J, Gugger, M, Lovblad, KO, Hess, CW. Hypersomnia following paramedian thalamic stroke: a report of 12 patients. *Ann Neurol* 1996; **39**:471–80.

41. Harbison, J, Ford, GA, Gibson, GJ. Nasal continuous positive airway pressure for sleep apnoea following stroke. *Eur Respir J* 2002a; **19**:1216–17.

42. Harbison, J, Ford, GA, James, OF, Gibson, GJ. Sleep-disordered breathing following acute stroke. *QJM* 2002b; **95**:741–7.

43. Cherkassky, T, Oksenberg, A, Froom, P, Ring, H. Sleep-related breathing disorders and rehabilitation outcome of stroke patients: a prospective study. *Am J Phys Med Rehabil* 2003; **82**:452–5.

44. McArdle, N, Riha, RL, Vennelle, M, *et al*. Sleep-disordered breathing as a risk factor for cerebrovascular disease: a case-control study in patients with transient ischemic attacks. *Stroke* 2003; **34**:2916–21.

45. Nachtmann, A, Stang, A, Wang, YM, Wondzinski, E, Thilmann, AF. Association of obstructive sleep apnea and stenotic artery disease in ischemic stroke patients. *Atherosclerosis* 2003; **169**:301–7.

46. Palomaki, H, Berg, A, Meririnne, E, *et al*. Complaints of poststroke insomnia and its treatment with mianserin. *Cerebrovasc Dis* 2003; **15**(**1–2**):56–62.

47. Kang, SY, Sohn, YH, Lee, IK, Kim, JS. Unilateral periodic limb movement in sleep after supratentorial cerebral infarction. *Parkinsonism Relat Disord* 2004; **10**: 429–31.

48. Mohsenin, V. Is sleep apnea a risk factor for stroke? A critical analysis. *Minerva Med* 2004; **95**(**4**):291–305.

49. Parra, O, Arboix, A, Montserrat, JM, Quinto, L, Bechich, S, Garcia-Eroles, L. Sleep-related breathing disorders: impact on mortality of cerebrovascular disease. *Eur Respir J* 2004; **24**:267–72.

50. Brown, DL, Chervin, RD, Hickenbottom, SL, Langa, KM, Morgenstern, LB. Screening for obstructive sleep apnea in stroke patients: a cost-effectiveness analysis. *Stroke* 2005; **36**:1291–3.

51. Hermann, DL, Basetti, C. Sleep-related breathing and sleep-wake disturbances in ischemic stroke. *Neurology* 2009; **73**:1313–22.

52. Hukins, CA, Hillman, DR. Daytime predictors of sleep hypoventilation in Duchenne muscular dystrophy. *Am J Respir Crit Care Med* 2000; **161**:166–70.

53. Dedrick, DL, Brown, LK. Obstructive sleep apnea syndrome complicating oculopharyngeal muscular dystrophy. *Chest* 2004; **125**:334–6.

54. Ferguson, KA, Strong, MJ, Ahmad, D, George, CF. Sleep-disordered breathing in amyotrophic lateral sclerosis. *Chest* 1996; **110**:664–9.

55. Kimura, K, Tachibana, N, Kimura, J, Shibasaki, H. Sleep-disordered breathing at an early stage of amyotrophic lateral sclerosis. *J Neurol Sci* 1999; **164**:37–43.

56. Lyall, RA, Donaldson, N, Polkey, MI, Leigh, PN, Moxham, J. Respiratory muscle strength and ventilatory failure in amyotrophic lateral sclerosis. *Brain* 2001; **124**(Pt 10): 2000–13.

57. Velasco, R, Salachas, F, Munerati, E, *et al.* Nocturnal oximetry in patients with amyotrophic lateral sclerosis: role in predicting survival. *Rev Neurol (Paris)* 2002; **158**(5 Pt 1):575–8.

58. Pinto, A, de Carvalho, M, Evangelista, T, Lopes, A, Sales-Luis, L. Nocturnal pulse oximetry: a new approach to establish the appropriate time for non-invasive ventilation in ALS patients. *Amyotroph Lateral Scler Other Motor Neuron Disord* 2003; **4**:31–5.

59. Arnulf, I, Similowski, T, Salachas, F, *et al.* Sleep disorders and diaphragmatic function in patients with amyotrophic lateral sclerosis. *Am J Respir Crit Care Med* 2000; **161** (3 Pt 1):849–56.

60. Takekawa, H, Kubo, J, Miyamoto, T, Miyamoto, M,. Hirata, K. Amyotrophic lateral sclerosis associated with insomnia and the aggravation of sleep-disordered breathing. *Psychiatry Clin Neurosci* 2001; **55**:263–4.

61. Elman, LB, Siderowf, AD, McCluskey, LF. Nocturnal oximetry: utility in the respiratory management of amyotrophic lateral sclerosis. *Am J Phys Med Rehabil* 2003; **82**: 866–70.

62. Bach, JR, Bianchi, C, Aufiero, E Oximetry and indications for tracheotomy for amyotrophic lateral sclerosis. *Chest* 2004; **126**:1502–7.

63. Budweiser, S, Murbeth, RE, Jorres, RA, Heinemann, F, Pfeifer, M Predictors of long-term survival in patients with restrictive thoracic disorders and chronic respiratory failure undergoing non-invasive home ventilation. *Respirology* 2007; **12**:551–9.

64. Ragette, R, Mellies, U, Schwake, C, Voit, T, Teschler, H Patterns and predictors of sleep disordered breathing in primary myopathies. *Thorax* 2002; **57**:724–8.

65. Storre, JH, Steurer, B, Kabitz, H, Dreher, M, Windisch, W Transcutaneous PCO2 monitoring during initiation of noninvasive ventilation. *Chest* 2007; **132**:1810–16.

66. Ward, S, Chatwin, M, Heather, S, Simonds, AK Randomised controlled trial of non-invasive ventilation (NIV) for nocturnal hypoventilation in neuromuscular and chest wall disease patients with daytime normocapnia. *Thorax* 2005; **60**:1019–24.

67. Fauroux, B, Lofaso, F Non-invasive mechanical ventilation: when to start for what benefit? *Thorax* 2005; **60**:979–80.

68. Schols, L, Haan, J, Riess, O, Amoiridis, G, Przuntek, H Sleep disturbance in spinocerebellar ataxias: is the SCA3 mutation a cause of restless legs syndrome? *Neurology* 1998; **51**:1603–7.

69. Fukutake, T, Shinotoh, H, Nishino, H, *et al.* Homozygous Machado-Joseph disease presenting as REM sleep behaviour disorder and prominent psychiatric symptoms. *Eur J Neurol* 2002; **9**:97–100.

70. Fish, DR, Sawyers, D, Allen, PJ, Blackie, JD, Lees, AJ, Marsden, CD The effect of sleep on the dyskinetic movements of Parkinson's disease, Gilles de la Tourette syndrome, Huntington's disease, and torsion dystonia. *Arch Neurol* 1991; **48**:210–14.

71. Wiegand, M, Moller, AA, Lauer, CJ, *et al.* Nocturnal sleep in Huntington's disease. *J Neurol* 1991; **238**:203–8.

72. Arnulf, I, Nielsen, J, Lohmann, E, *et al.* Rapid eye movement sleep disturbances in Huntington disease. *Arch Neurol* 2008; **65**:482–8.

73. Emser, W, Brenner, M, Stober, T, Schimrigk, K Changes in nocturnal sleep in Huntington's and Parkinson's disease. *J Neurol* 1988; **235**:177–9.

74. Carvalho, BS, Waterhouse, J, Edwards, B, Simons, R, Reilly, T The use of actimetry to assess changes to the rest-activity cycle. *Chronobiol Int* 2003; **20**:1039–59.

75. Chesson, AL Jr, Ferber, RA, Fry, JM, *et al.* The indications for polysomnography and related procedures. *Sleep* 1997; **20**:423–87.

76. Chesson, AL Jr, Wise, M, Davila, D, *et al.* Practice parameters for the treatment of restless legs syndrome and periodic limb movement disorder. An American Academy of Sleep Medicine Report. Standards of Practice Committee of the American Academy of Sleep Medicine. *Sleep* 1999; **22**:961–8.

77. Chesson, AL Jr, Berry, RB, Pack, A Practice parameters for the use of portable monitoring devices in the investigation of suspected obstructive sleep apnea in adults. *Sleep* 2003; **26**:907–13.

78. Hayward, P News from the European Neurological Society meeting. *Lancet Neurol* 2004; **3**:449.

79. Johns, MW Sensitivity and specificity of the multiple sleep latency test (MSLT), the maintenance of wakefulness test and the Epworth sleepiness scale: failure of the MSLT as a gold standard. *J Sleep Res* 2000; **9**:5–11.

80. Le Bon, O, Hoffmann, G, Tecco, J, *et al.* Mild to moderate sleep respiratory events: one negative night may not be enough. *Chest* 2000; **118**:353–9.

81. Middelkoop, HA, van Dam, EM, Smilde-van den Doel, DA, Van Dijk, G 45-hour continuous quintuple-site actimetry: relations between trunk and limb movements and effects of circadian sleep-wake rhythmicity. *Psychophysiology* 1997; **34**:199–203.

82. Wright, J, Johns, R, Watt, I, Melville, A, Sheldon, T Health effects of obstructive sleep apnoea and the effectiveness of continuous positive airways pressure: a systematic review of the research evidence. *BMJ* 1997; **314**:851–60.

83. Douglas, NJ Systematic review of the efficacy of nasal CPAP. *Thorax* 1998; **53**(5):414–15.

84. McMahon, JP, Foresman, BH, Chisholm, RC The influence of CPAP on the neurobehavioral performance of patients with obstructive sleep apnea hypopnea syndrome: a systematic review. *WMJ* 2003; **102**:36–43.

85. Sanchez, AI, Martinez, P, Miro, E, Bardwell, WA, Buela-Casal, G CPAP and behavioral therapies in patients with obstructive sleep apnea: effects on daytime sleepiness, mood, and cognitive function. *Sleep Med Rev* 2009; **13**:223–33.

86. McDaid, C, Griffin, S, Weatherly, H, *et al.* Continuous positive airway pressure devices for the treatment of obstructive sleep apnoea-hypopnoea syndrome: a systematic review and economic analysis. *Health Technol Assess* 2009; **13**:iii–xiv. 1.

87. Giles, TL, Lasserson, TJ, Smith, BH, White, J, Wright, J, Cates, CJ Continuous positive airways pressure for obstructive sleep apnoea in adults. *Cochrane Database Syst Rev* 2006;(3):CD001106.

88. Berry, RB, Parish, JM, Hartse, KM The use of auto-titrating continuous positive airway pressure for treatment of adult obstructive sleep apnea. An American Academy of Sleep Medicine review. *Sleep* 2002; **25**:148–73.

89. Noseda, A, Andre, S, Potmans, V, Kentos, M, de Maertelaer, V, Hoffmann, G CPAP with algorithm-based versus titrated pressure: a randomized study. *Sleep Med* 2009; **10**:988–92.

90. Hsu, CY, Vennelle, M, Li, HY, *et al.* Sleep-disordered breathing after stroke: a randomised controlled trial of continuous positive airway pressure. *J Neurol Neurosurg Psychiatry* 2006; **77**:1143–9.

91. Iranzo, A, Santamaria, J, Tolosa, E, *et al.* Long-term effect of CPAP in the treatment of nocturnal stridor in multiple system atrophy. *Neurology* 2004; **63**:930–2.

92. Randerath, WJ, Galetke, W, Ruhle, KH Auto-adjusting CPAP based on impedance versus bilevel pressure in difficult-to-treat sleep apnea syndrome: a prospective randomized crossover study. *Med Sci Monit* 2003; **9**:CR353–8.

93. Lim, J, Lasserson, TJ, Fleetham, J, Wright, J Oral appliances for obstructive sleep apnoea. *Cochrane Database Syst Rev* 2003; (4):CD004435.

94. Cohen, R Limited evidence supports use of oral appliances in obstructive sleep apnoea. *Evid Based Dent* 2004; **5**:76.

95. Bridgman, SA, Dunn, KM Surgery for obstructive sleep apnoea. *Cochrane Database Syst Rev* 2000;(2):CD001004.

96. Sundaram, S, Bridgman, SA, Lim, J, Lasserson, TJ Surgery for obstructive sleep apnoea. *Cochrane Database Syst Rev* 2005; (4):CD001004.

97. Smith, I, Lasserson, T, Wright, J Drug treatments for obstructive sleep apnoea. *Cochrane Database Syst Rev* 2002; (2):CD003002.

98. Shneerson, J, Wright, J Lifestyle modification for obstructive sleep apnoea. *Cochrane Database Syst Rev* 2001; (1):CD002875.

99. Yu, L, Huang, XZ, Wu, QY Management of nocturnal nasal mask continuous positive airway pressure in central hypoventilation in patients with respiratory diseases. *Zhonghua Jie He He Hu Xi Za Zhi* 1994; **17**(1):38–40.

100. Hommura, F, Nishimura, M, Oguri, M, *et al.* Continuous versus bilevel positive airway pressure in a patient with idiopathic central sleep apnea. *Am J Respir Crit Care Med* 1997; **155**:1482–5.

101. Verbraecken, J, Willemen, M, Wittesaele, W, Van de Heyning, P, De Backer, W Short-term CPAP does not influence the increased CO_ drive in idiopathic central sleep apnea. *Monaldi Arch Chest Dis* 2002; **57**:10–18.

102. American Thoracic Society. Idiopathic congenital central hypoventilation syndrome: diagnosis and management. American Thoracic Society. *Am J Respir Crit Care Med* 1999b; **160**:368–73.

103. Bradley, TD Hemodynamic and sympathoinhibitory effects of nasal CPAP in congestive heart failure. *Sleep* 1996; **19**:S232–5.

104. Granton, JT, Naughton, MT, Benard, DC, Liu, PP, Goldstein, RS, Bradley, TD CPAP improves inspiratory muscle strength in patients with heart failure and central sleep apnea. *Am J Respir Crit Care Med* 1996; **153**:277–82.

105. Sin, DD, Logan, AG, Fitzgerald, FS, Liu, PP, Bradley, TD Effects of continuous positive airway pressure on cardiovascular outcomes in heart failure patients with and without Cheyne-Stokes respiration. *Circulation* 2000; **102**: 61–6.

106. Krachman, SL, Crocetti, J, Berger, TJ, Chatila, W, Eisen, HJ, D'Alonzo, GE Effects of nasal continuous positive airway pressure on oxygen body stores in patients with Cheyne-Stokes respiration and congestive heart failure. *Chest* 2003; **123**:59–66.

107. Teschler, H, Dohring, J, Wang, YM, Berthon-Jones, M Adaptive pressure support servo-ventilation: a novel treatment for Cheyne-Stokes respiration in heart failure. *Am J Respir Crit Care Med* 2001; **164**:614–19.

108. Arzt, M, Floras, JS, Logan, AG, *et al.*, CANPAP Investigators. Suppression of central sleep apnea by continuous positive airway pressure and transplant-free survival in heart failure: a post hoc analysis of the Canadian Continuous Positive Airway Pressure for Patients with Central Sleep Apnea and Heart Failure Trial (CANPAP). *Circulation* 2007; **115**:3173–80.

109. Pepperell, JC, Maskell, NA, Jones, *et al.* A randomized controlled trial of adaptive ventilation for Cheyne-Stokes breathing in heart failure. *Am J Respir Crit Care Med* 2003; **168**:1109–14.

110. Gonzalez, MM, Parreira, VF, Rodenstein, DO Non-invasive ventilation and sleep. *Sleep Med Rev* 2002; **6**:29–44.

111. Newsom-Davis, IC, Lyall, RA, Leigh, PN, Moxham, J, Goldstein, LH The effect of non-invasive positive pressure ventilation (NIPPV) on cognitive function in amyotrophic lateral sclerosis (ALS): a prospective study. *J Neurol Neurosurg Psychiatry* 2001; **71**:482–7.

112. Butz, M, Wollinsky, KH, Wiedemuth-Catrinescu, U, *et al.* Longitudinal effects of noninvasive positive-pressure ventilation in patients with amyotrophic lateral sclerosis. *Am J Phys Med Rehabil* 2003; **82**:597–604.

113. Annane, D, Orlikowski, D, Chevret, S, Chevrolet, JC, Raphael, JC Nocturnal mechanical ventilation for chronic hypoventilation in patients with neuromuscular and chest wall disorders. *Cochrane Database Syst Rev* 2007; (**4**):CD001941.

114. Radunovic, A, Annane, D, Jewitt, K, Mustfa, N Mechanical ventilation for amyotrophic lateral sclerosis/motor neuron disease. *Cochrane Database Syst Rev* 2009; (**4**): CD004427.

115. Bourke, SC, Gibson, GJ Non-invasive ventilation in ALS: current practice and future role. *Amyotroph Lateral Scler Other Motor Neuron Disord* 2004; **5**:67–71.

116. Mast, KR, Salama, M, Silverman, GK, Arnold, RM End-of-life content in treatment guidelines for life-limiting diseases. *J Palliat Med* 2004; **7**:754–73.

117. Besset, A, Chetrit, M, Carlander, B, Billiard, M Use of modafinil in the treatment of narcolepsy: a long term follow-up study. *Neurophysiol Clin* 1996; **26**:60–6.

118. Narcolepsy Multicenter Study Group. Randomized trial of modafinil for the treatment of pathological somnolence in narcolepsy. US Modafinil in Narcolepsy Multicenter Study Group. *Ann Neurol* 1998; **43**:88–97.

119. Narcolepsy Multicenter Study Group. Randomized trial of modafinil as a treatment for the excessive daytime somnolence of narcolepsy: US Modafinil in Narcolepsy Multicenter Study Group. *Neurology* 2000; **54**:1166–75.

120. Mitler, MM, Harsh, J, Hirshkowitz, M, Guilleminault, C Long-term efficacy and safety of modafinil (PROVIGIL((R)

121. Moldofsky, H, Broughton, RJ, Hill, JD A randomized trial of the long-term, continued efficacy and safety of modafinil in narcolepsy. *Sleep Med* 2000; **1**:109–16.

122. Schwartz, JR, Nelson, MT, Schwartz, ER, Hughes, RJ Effects of modafinil on wakefulness and executive function in patients with narcolepsy experiencing late-day sleepiness. *Clin Neuropharmacol* 2004; **27**:74–9.

123. Rabinstein, A, Shulman, LM, Weiner, WJ Modafinil for the treatment of excessive daytime sleepiness in Parkinson's disease: a case report. *Parkinsonism Relat Disord* 2001; **7**: 287–8.

124. Nieves, AV, Lang, AE Treatment of excessive daytime sleepiness in patients with Parkinson's disease with modafinil. *Clin Neuropharmacol* 2002; **25**:111–14.

125. Hogl, B, Saletu, M, Brandauer, E, *et al.* Modafinil for the treatment of daytime sleepiness in Parkinson's disease: a double-blind, randomized, crossover, placebo-controlled polygraphic trial. *Sleep* 2002; **25**:905–9.

126. Adler, CH, Caviness, JN, Hentz, JG, Lind, M, Tiede, J Randomized trial of modafinil for treating subjective daytime sleepiness in patients with Parkinson's disease. *Mov Disord* 2003; **18**:287–93.

127. Ondo, WG, Fayle, R, Atassi, F, Jankovic, J Modafinil for daytime somnolence in Parkinson's disease: double blind, placebo controlled parallel trial. *Neurol Neurosurg Psychiatry* 2005; **76**:1636–9.

128. Sternbach, H Adjunctive modafinil in ALS. *J Neuropsychiatry Clin Neurosci* 2002; **14**:239.

129. Smith, BW Modafinil for treatment of cognitive side effects of antiepileptic drugs in a patient with seizures and stroke. *Epilepsy Behav* 2003; **4**:352–3.

130. Sugden, SG, Bourgeois, JA Modafinil monotherapy in post-stroke depression. *Psychosomatics* 2004; **45**:80–1.

131. Kingshott, RN, Vennelle, M, Coleman, EL, Engleman, HM, Mackay, TW, Douglas, NJ Randomized, double-blind, placebo-controlled crossover trial of modafinil in the treatment of residual excessive daytime sleepiness in the sleep apnea/hypopnea syndrome. *Am J Respir Crit Care Med* 2001; **163**:918–23.

132. Morgenthaler, TI, Kapur, VK, Brown, T, *et al.* Practice parameters for the treatment of narcolepsy and other hypersomnias of central origin. Standards of Practice Committee of the American Academy of Sleep Medicine. *Sleep* 2007; **30**:1705–11.

133. Ondo, WG, Perkins, T, Swick, T, *et al.* Sodium oxybate for excessive daytime sleepiness in Parkinson disease: an open-label polysomnographic study. *Arch Neurol* 2008; **65**: 1337–40.

134. Mishima, K, Okawa, M, Hishikawa, Y, Hozumi, S, Hori, H, Takahashi, K Morning bright light therapy for sleep and behavior disorders in elderly patients with dementia. *Acta Psychiatr Scand* 1994; **89**:1–7.

135. Mishima, K, Hishikawa, Y, Okawa, M Randomized, dim light controlled, crossover test of morning bright light therapy for rest-activity rhythm disorders in patients with vascular dementia and dementia of Alzheimer's type. *Chronobiol Int* 1998; **15**:647–54.

136. Mishima, K, Okawa, M, Hozumi, S, Hishikawa, Y Supplementary administration of artificial bright light and melatonin as potent treatment for disorganized circadian rest-activity and dysfunctional autonomic and neuroendocrine systems in institutionalized demented elderly persons. *Chronobiol Int* 2000; **17**:419–32.

137. Lovell, BB, Ancoli-Israel, S, Gevirtz, R Effect of bright light treatment on agitated behavior in institutionalized elderly subjects. *Psychiatry Res* 1995; **57**:7–12.

138. McGaffigan, S, Bliwise, DL The treatment of sundowning. A selective review of pharmacological and nonpharmacological studies. *Drugs Aging* 1997; **10**:10–17.

139. Van Someren, EJ, Kessler, A, Mirmiran, M, Swaab, DF Indirect bright light improves circadian rest-activity rhythm disturbances in demented patients. *Biol Psychiatry* 1997; **41**:955–63.

140. Okumoto, Y, Koyama, E, Matsubara, H, Nakano, T, Nakamura, R Sleep improvement by light in a demented aged individual. *Psychiatry Clin Neurosci* 1998; **52**:194–6.

141. Koyama, E, Matsubara, H, Nakano, T Bright light treatment for sleep-wake disturbances in aged individuals with dementia. *Psychiatry Clin Neurosci* 1999; **53**:227–9.

142. Lyketsos, CG, Lindell, VL, Baker, A, Steele, C A randomized, controlled trial of bright light therapy for agitated behaviors in dementia patients residing in long-term care. *Int J Geriatr Psychiatry* 1999; **14**:520–5.

143. Yamadera, H, Ito, T, Suzuki, H, Asayama, K, Ito, R, Endo, S Effects of bright light on cognitive and sleep-wake (circadian) rhythm disturbances in Alzheimer-type dementia. *Psychiatry Clin Neurosci* 2000; **54**:352–3.

144. Haffmans, PM, Sival, RC, Lucius, SA, Cats, Q, van Gelder, L Bright light therapy and melatonin in motor restless behaviour in dementia: a placebo-controlled study. *Int J Geriatr Psychiatry* 2001; **16**:106–10.

145. Sheehan, B, Keene, J Sunlight levels and behavioural disturbance in dementia. *Int J Geriatr Psychiatry* 2002; **17**:784–5.

146. Fetveit, A, Skjerve, A, Bjorvatn, B Bright light treatment improves sleep in institutionalised elderly – an open trial. *Int J Geriatr Psychiatry* 2003; **18**:520–6.

147. Fontana, GP, Krauchi, K, Cajochen, C, *et al.* Dawn-dusk simulation light therapy of disturbed circadian rest-activity cycles in demented elderly. *Exp Gerontol* 2003; **38** (**1–2**):207–16.

148. Luijpen, MW, Scherder, EJ, Van Someren, EJ, Swaab, DF, Sergeant, JA Non-pharmacological interventions in cognitively impaired and demented patients–a comparison with cholinesterase inhibitors. *Rev Neurosci* 2003; **14**: 343–68.

149. Skjerve, A, Bjorvatn, B, Holsten, F Light therapy for behavioural and psychological symptoms of dementia. *Int J Geriatr Psychiatry* 2004; **19**:516–22.

150. Sutherland, D, Woodward, Y, Byrne, J, Allen, H, Burns, A The use of light therapy to lower agitation in people with dementia. *Nurs Times* 2004; **100**:32–4.

CHAPTER 11

Management of community-acquired bacterial meningitis

A. Chaudhuri,[1] P. Martinez-Martin,[2] P. G. E. Kennedy,[3] R. Andrew Seaton,[4] P. Portegie,s[5] M. Bojar[6] and I. Steiner[7]

[1]Essex Centre for Neurological Sciences, Queen's Hospital, Romford, UK; [2]National Centre for Epidemiology, Carlos III Institute of Health, Madrid, Spain; [3]Division of Clinical Neurosciences, University of Glasgow, Glasgow, UK; [4]Brownlee Centre, Gartnavel General Hospital, Glasgow, UK; [5]OLVG Hospital, Amsterdam, The Netherlands; [6]Charles University Prague 2nd Medical School, University Hospital Motol, Prague, Czech Republic; [7]Hadassah University Hospital, Jerusalem, Israel

Objectives

The primary objective of this guideline is to assist neurologists with the diagnosis and treatment of community-acquired acute bacterial meningitis (ABM) in older children and adults based on literature evidence and expert consensus. Here, we propose diagnosis and treatment of ABM as soon as possible, and a target time of no longer than 3 h from door-to-first antibiotic therapy, based on secured diagnosis supported by clinical and cerebrospinal fluid (CSF) findings. The management of hospital-acquired ABM and chronic meningitis, including tuberculous meningitis, is not considered.

Search strategy and selection criteria

Data for this guideline were identified by searches of Medline, EMBASE, the Cochrane databases and references from relevant articles. Search terms used were (alone and in combination): bacterial meningitis, meningococcal meningitis, pneumococcal meningitis, Listeria meningitis and meningoencephalitis, lumbar puncture (LP), CSF, treatment for meningitis, antibiotic, dexamethasone and vaccine. For determining the levels of evidence for therapeutic interventions, the EFNS guideline was followed [1] (Supplementary Material online, Table S1). Only research papers published in English were considered. Limitations of the search strategy include non-randomized clinical data, lack of sensitivity and specificity, small numbers of cohorts and case-control studies.

Background

Acute bacterial meningitis is a life-threatening neurological emergency. Its estimated annual incidence is 2–5/100,000 people in the Western world and may be 10 times as high in the less developed countries [1 online]. ABM is one of the top 10 causes of infection-related deaths worldwide [2 online] and 30–50% of its survivors have permanent neurological sequelae [3, 4 online]. The causative organism of ABM can be reliably predicted by the age of the patient, predisposing factors, underlying diseases and immunological competence. *Streptococcus pneumoniae* and

European Handbook of Neurological Management: Volume 2, Second Edition. Edited by Nils Erik Gilhus, Michael P. Barnes, Michael Brainin.
© 2012 Blackwell Publishing Ltd. Published 2012 by Blackwell Publishing Ltd.

Neisseria meningitidis are the two most common aetiological agents of ABM in immunocompetent infants (> 4 weeks) and children, as well as in adults, comprising nearly 80% of all cases, followed by *Listeria monocytogenes* and staphylococci (Table S2). Gram-negative bacilli (*Escherichia coli*, *Klebsiella*, *Enterobacter* and *Pseudomonas aeruginosa*) contribute to <10% of the cases. *Haemophilus influenzae* meningitis caused by the capsular b strains (Hib) was the leading cause of meningitis in infants and younger children, but has become rare after universal Hib immunization with an emerging trend of *H. influenzae* meningitis caused by uncapsulated strains. In immunocompromised patients, the most common agents causing ABM are *S. pneumoniae*, *L. monocytogenes* and Gram-negative bacilli, including *Ps. aeruginosa*. Mixed bacterial infection with more than one agent typically accounts for 1% of all cases of ABM and is seen in patients who are immunosuppressed, have skull fracture or externally communicating dural fistula, parameningeal source of infection (otitis and sinusitis) and previous neurosurgery. Nosocomial bacterial meningitis is often caused by staphylococci (aureus and albus, including methicillin-resistant strains) and Gram-negative bacilli. Enterobacteriaceae are the most common aetiological agents of bacterial meningitis following neurosurgical procedures. The present guideline does not address the treatment of nosocomial meningitis and neonatal meningitis.

S. pneumoniae has emerged as the single most common cause of community-acquired bacterial meningitis after postnatal life both in the developed and developing countries [5, 6 online]. *S. pneumoniae* is susceptible to penicillins and cephalosporins, although emergence of penicillin- and cephalosporin-resistant *S. pneumoniae* has increased in recent years [7, 8, 9 online]. However, in children as well as in adults, the severity of disease and the outcome of meningitis caused by penicillin-sensitive *S. pneumoniae* are similar to those caused by the penicillin-resistant strains [10, 11 online].

Early management of ABM

Early diagnosis and effective antibiotic treatment remain the cornerstone of successful management of ABM. An understanding of the pathophysiological 'timetable' of ABM [2], summarized in Table 11.1, is essential for its successful and timely management.

Clinical features of ABM

The suspicion of ABM is critically dependent on the early recognition of the meningitis syndrome. In a Dutch study of adults presenting with community-acquired ABM, the

Table 11.1 Time line of ABM [2].

Early events			Intermediate events	Late events
Pathophysiology				
Phase 1	Phase 2	Phase 3		
Release of pro-inflammatory cytokines from bacterial invasion and consequent inflammation of subarachnoid space	Subpial encephalopathy induced by cytokines and other chemical Mediators	Breakdown in the blood-brain-barrier, transendothelial emigration of leukocytes and development of cerebral oedema	Impaired CBF, rising intracranial pressure and vasculitis	Focal neuronal injury
Clincal				
Fever, headache	Meningism, confusion, reduced CSF glucose	Impaired consciousness, elevated CSF pressure, increased CSF protein, focal symptoms	Obtundation, seizures, focal neurological symptoms and/signs (e.g. cranial nerve palsies)	Paralysis, cognitive impairment coma, possibly death in untreated cases

Table 11.2 Differential diagnosis of acute bacterial meningitis.

Other infective meningitis and meningoencephalitis (viral,
   tuberculous, fungal, leptospiral and primary amoebic)
Viral encephalitis
Brain abscess
Spinal epidural abscess (cervical)
Parameningeal infection (cranial osteomyelitis, subdural
   empyema)
Aseptic meningitis (e.g., SLE, Behcet's, sarcoidosis)
Chemical meningitis (e.g., after human IVIG therapy,
   subarachnoid haemorrhage)

sensitivity of the classic triad of fever, neck stiffness and altered mental status was found to be low, but almost all patients with ABM had at least two of the four symptoms of headache, fever, neck stiffness and altered mental status [3]. In children, irritability, refusal to eat, vomiting and seizures are often early symptoms. The level of consciousness in ABM is variable and may range from drowsiness, confusion, stupor to coma.

Differential diagnosis

A high index of suspicion is required for the diagnosis of ABM and a list of common differential diagnosis is provided in Table 11.2.

Initial management

Examination of CSF by LP is an indisputable and indispensable part of assessment of patients who present with symptoms and signs of meningitis unless the procedure is contraindicated for reasons of clinical safety. Treatment in ABM will be initiated in the hospital setting for the majority of cases, and after the diagnosis of bacterial meningitis is confirmed by the CSF formula obtained by LP. However, there will be situations where antibiotic treatment may have to be commenced on suspicion before it is possible to confirm the diagnosis of ABM by CSF examination. This could occur in a primary care setting where transfer to a secondary care unit is likely to take some time. Even in hospitalized patients, CSF analysis may be delayed for clinical or logistic reasons. There are no randomized controlled trials to determine the

outcome of bacterial meningitis based on timing of administration of the antibiotic. There are no prospective case-control studies of the potential benefit of pre-hospital antibiotic treatment. The evidence is conflicting between countries, and pooled analysis of the published results did not confirm the perceived advantage of pre-hospital antibiotic treatment in ABM, which may relate to differences in sample size and reporting bias [11 online]. In a case-control study of 158 children (age 0–16 years) with suspected meningococcal disease, pre-hospital treatment by general practitioners with parenteral penicillin was associated with an increased odds ratios for death (7.4, 95% confidence interval [CI] 1.5–37.7) and complications in survivors (5.0, CI 1.7–15.0) [4]. The adverse outcome from pre-hospital antibiotic therapy was interpreted as indicative of more severe disease in these cases and lack of supportive treatment before hospital admission. A recent multivariate regression analysis of a retrospective case study of 119 adults with ABM showed that time from presentation to antibiotic administration of >6 h was associated with an adjusted 8.4 times increased risk of death (95% CI 1.7–40.9) [5]. Absence of the classical triad of meningitis and delay in the diagnosis–treatment sequence (transfer to institution, CT scan before LP, antibiotics) were associated with the door-to-antibiotic time of >6 h in this study. Delay in antibiotic administration beyond 3 h and penicillin resistance were two major risk factors associated with adverse outcome in adults with severe pneumococcal meningitis [12 online]. Despite the relative paucity of controlled studies on the timing of antibiotics administration to the outcome of ABM, available data point to a cut-off period of 3–6 h, beyond which there is a significant increase in mortality.

In patients attending hospital, antibiotic treatment for ABM should be considered before CSF analysis only if LP is contraindicated (Table 11.3) or the facility for rapid brain imaging (CT scan) prior to LP is not immediately available. A normal CT scan in a patient with clinical manifestations of cerebral herniation does not guarantee absence of risk from the procedure of LP [13, 14, 15, 16 online]. In all cases of ABM, blood cultures must be obtained before any treatment is administered. The time taken for antibiotic therapy ideally should coincide with, or occur immediately before, the administration of adjunctive dexamethasone therapy for suspected pneumococcal and *H. influenzae* meningitis. The choice of

Table 11.3 Contraindications for lumbar puncture in suspected acute bacterial meningitis.

Absolute (lumbar puncture is not to be recommended)
Signs of raised intracranial pressure (papilloedema, decrebrate posturing)
Local skin infection in needle track
Evidence of obstructive hydrocephalus, cerebral oedema or herniation in CT (or MR) scan of brain
Relative (appropriate therapeutic measures and/or investigations are indicated before lumbar puncture)
Sepsis or hypotension (systolic blood pressure < 100 mmHg, diastolic blood pressure < 60 mmHg): patients should be stabilized first
Coagulation disorder (disseminated intravascular coagulopathy, platelet count < 50,000/mm^3, therapeutic use of warfarin): appropriate correction first
Presence of focal neurological deficit, especially when posterior fossa lesion is suspected
Glasgow coma score of 8 or less
Epileptic seizures
In all these cases, a CT (or MR) scan of brain should be the first step. Isolated single cranial nerve palsy without papilloedema does not necessarily contraindicate LP without brain imaging.

antibiotic in ABM may be influenced by a number of factors, including the patient's age, systemic symptoms and local pattern of bacterial resistance. A recent Cochrane database review, however, found no clinically important difference between the third-generation cephalosporins (ceftriaxone or cefotaxime) and conventional antibiotics (penicillin, ampicillin–chloramphenicol or chloramphenicol) as the empirical therapy in the treatment of ABM [6].

Investigations in ABM

The primary purpose of investigations in ABM is to confirm the diagnosis and identify the causal bacteria. The recommended specific laboratory tests for patients with suspected ABM are listed in Table 11.4. In uncomplicated meningitis, plain CT and MR scans are often normal. Contrast scans may show abnormal enhancement of basal cisterns and subarachnoid space (involving

Recommendation

The Task Force recommends (Figure 11.1) that all patients with suspected ABM should be hospitalized as soon as possible (Class III, Level A). Treatment of patients with suspected ABM should be considered as an emergency and fast-tracked for rapid assessment and treatment. We propose the following timeline for management of ABM: admission to hospital within first 90 min of making contact with the health service; and assessment and treatment commenced within 60 min of hospital admission, and no longer than 3 h after contact with the health service (Class IV, Level C).

Pre-hospital antibiotic treatment should be initiated only for patients with strong suspicion of disseminated meningococcal infection (meningococcemia) due to the unpredictable risk of early circulatory collapse from adrenocortical necrosis (Waterhouse– Fredrichsen syndrome). For other patients, rapid preadmission antibiotic therapy should be considered only if a delay >90 min in hospital transfer is anticipated (Class III, Level C).

LP and CSF analysis is the specific investigation required for diagnosis and management of ABM. Therefore, if diagnosis of bacterial meningitis is suspected and there are no clinical contraindications, LP should be performed as soon as safely possible (Class III, Level C).

In patients with symptoms and signs suggestive of raised intracranial pressure or with high risk of cerebral herniations following LP (imaging evidence of intracranial mass lesion,

obstructive hydrocephalus or midline shift), diagnostic LP should be postponed (Class I, Level A).

In a patient with suspected ABM in whom LP is delayed or postponed, antibiotic therapy should be commenced immediately after collecting a blood sample for culture. Intravenous (i.v.) or intramuscular (i.m.) benzyl penicillin, or i.v. cefotaxime or ceftriaxone should be administered for ABM and may be commenced immediately (Class III, Level A).

In patients with a known history of severe β-lactam allergy, vancomycin should be administered as the alternative for pneumococcal meningitis and chloramphenicol for meningococcal meningitis (Class IV, Level C).

In regions with known or suspected penicillin-resistant strains of pneumococcus, high-dose vancomycin should be used in combination with a third-generation cephalosporin (Class IV, Level C).

Patients with risk factors for Listerial meningitis (old age, immunosuppression and/or signs of rhombencephalitis) should receive i.v. amoxicillin in addition to a third-generation cephalosporin as the   empirical treatment of ABM initially (Class IV, Level C).

Dexamethasone in high doses may be appropriate as an adjunctive therapy and should be given shortly before or with the first dose of antibiotics (see Adjunctive therapy on ABM).

All ABM patients should be managed as medical emergencies and, when available, treated in a neurological intensive care unit.

Table 11.4 Laboratory investigations in acute bacterial meningitis (ABM).

Blood (the 3 Cs)
Culture
Cell count
C-reactive protein (CRP)
Cerebrospinal fluid (CSF)
Opening pressure (always raised in ABM)
Appearance
Cell count
Biochemistry:
Glucose, and the ratio of blood glucose (obtained before
    lumbar puncture)
Protein
Optional:lactate, ferritin, chloride, lactate dehydrogenase (LDH)
Microbiology
Gram stain, culture
Others: counterimmunoelectrophoresis (CIE), radioimmunoassay
    (RIA), latex particle agglutination (LPA), enzyme-linked
    immunosorbent assay (ELISA), polymerase chain reaction
    (PCR)
Body fluid culture
Petechial fluid, sputum, secretions from oropharynx, nose and
    ear

convexity, falx, tentorium, base of the brain) because of the presence of inflammatory exudates [17, 18, 19 online]; some MRI methods may have high sensitivity [20 online].

An increased CSF-opening pressure, high polymorphonuclear leukocytes count and raised protein concentration, together with a decreased CSF:plasma ratio of glucose (< 0.3) are characteristic findings supportive of ABM (Table 11.5). Listerial meningitis may have CSF findings identical to chronic tuberculous or fungal meningitis [22, 23, 24, 25 online].

The identification of the causal bacteria depends on staining (Table S3) and culture of CSF, which should always be tested in freshly obtained samples. Gram stain is used most widely and has the best predictive value, but is probably less sensitive.

Identification of bacteria in CSF staining depends on both the bacterial concentration and the specific organism [30 online]. The percentage of positive cultures (sensitivity) is variable and ranges from 50% to 90% for ABM [23, 24, 31 online]. A variable percentage of 'positive' cultures is due to contaminating organisms but these are not responsible for the meningeal infection [31 online]. In patients with ABM, the probability of a negative CSF

Table 11.5 Comparison of cerebrospinal fluid findings (CSF) of meningitis.

	Acute bacterial meningitis	Viral meningitis/ meningo-encephalitis	Chronic meningitis (tuberculous meningitis)	Normal CSF
Characteristics	Turbid, cloudy, purulent	Clear	Clear, cloudy	Clear
Opening pressure (mm H2O)	>180	>180	>180	180 (upper limit)[a]
WBC count (cells/mm3)	1000–10000	5–1000	25–500[b]	0–5 (0–30 in newborns)
Neutrophils (%)	>60[c]	<20	<50[c]	0–15
Protein (g/l)	>0.5	<1.0	>0.5	0.15–0.5
Glucose (mM)	<2.5	2.5–4.5	<2.5	2.5–4.5
CSF/blood glucose ratio	<0.3	>0.5	<0.5	0.6

[a]It may reach 250 mm H_2O in obese adults [w21].
[b]Higher cellularity in tuberculous meningitis has been occasionally observed in immunocompetent and BCG-vaccinated subjects soon after the initiation of anti-tuberculous therapy.
[c]Neutrophilic response in tuberculous meningitis is known with acute onset and in HIV patients. Lymphocytic pleocytosis in ABM is seen in cases who have already been partially treated with antibiotics.
ABM, acute bacterial meningitis.

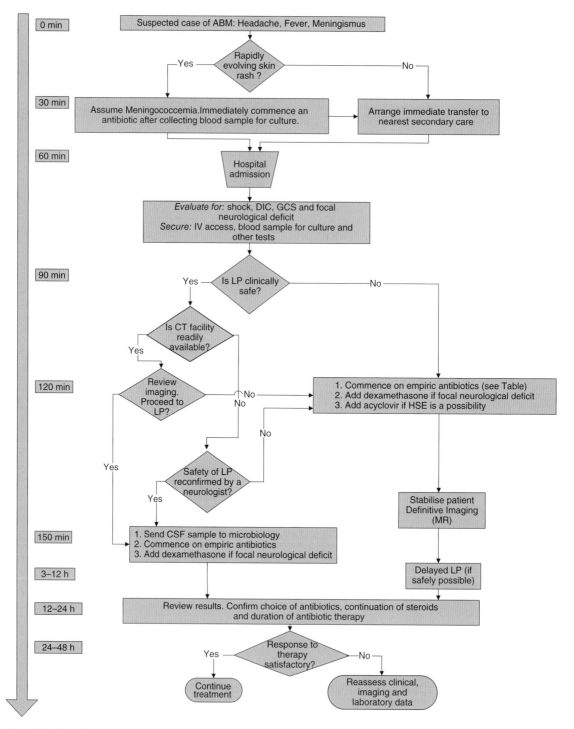

Figure 11.1 Flow chart of emergency management of patients with suspected bacterial meningitis. ABM, acute bacterial meningitis; DIC, disseminated intravascular coagulation; GCS, Glasgow Coma Scale; HSE, herpes simplex encephalitis; LP, lumbar puncture.

culture in previously treated patients is increased compared with non-treated patients (odds ratio 16; 95% CI 1.45–764.68; $P = 0.01$) [32 online]. In ABM, the likelihood of diagnostic yield in CSF microbiology is highest before antibiotic treatment. Three other supportive and indirect diagnostic markers of ABM are: (a) elevated serum C-reactive protein (quantified) in children [33 online] (sensitivity: 96%, specificity: 93%, negative predictive value: 99%); (b) increased CSF lactate [34, 35 online] (sensitivity: 86–90%, specificity: 55–98%, positive predictive value: 19–96%, negative predictive value: 94–98%); and (c) high CSF ferritin [36, 37, 38 online] (sensitivity: 92–96%, specificity: 81–100%).

Several rapid methods for detecting components of bacteria in CSF have been based on bacterial antigen detection, counter-immunoelectrophoresis, coagglutination, latex agglutination and ELISA. The average efficacy of these tests is sensitivity: 60–90%, specificity: 90–100%, predictive positive value: 60– 85%, predictive negative value: 80–95% [39, 40, 41, 42, 43 online]. Currently available PCR methods have a sensitivity of 87–100% and specificity of 98– 100% [44, 45, 46, 47, 48 online], and detect *H. influenzae*, *N. meningitidis*, *S. pneumoniae* and *L. monocytogenes* in CSF. Fluorescence *in situ* hybridization (FISH) is less sensitive, but may be useful for identification of bacteria in CSF samples in some cases [49 online].

CSF analysis may have to be repeated during the course of ABM in certain situations: partially treated cases, uncertain diagnosis, poor clinical response in the absence of other causes, vancomycin-treated patients receiving dexamethasone, Gram-negative bacillary meningitis, meningitis complicating CSF shunt and for intrathecal antibiotic therapy.

Specific antibiotic treatment

Clinical outcome in bacterial meningitis is directly related to concentrations of bacteria and bacterial antigens in the CSF [50, 51 online]. Within the first 48 h of appropriate antibiotic therapy, CSF cultures invariably become sterile in pyogenic meningitis [51 online]. In children with ABM, CSF sterilization of meningococci occurs within 2 h and pneumococci by 4 h. Third-generation cephalosporins are widely regarded as the standard of care in the management of bacterial meningitis in both adults

and children [52, 53, 54, 55 online]. Ceftriaxone and cefotaxime have been compared with meropenem in licensing studies which were randomized but not controlled in adults and children. Efficacy was found to be similar [55 online].

Choice of treatment

Third-generation cephalosporins are the established agents of choice in Europe and North America for pneumococcal meningitis [52, 53, 54 online]. When penicillin or cephalosporin resistance is possible, vancomycin should be combined with a third-generation cephalosporin. The combination has not been evaluated in randomized trials. Although there have been concerns regarding the penetration of vancomycin across the blood–brain barrier, when corticosteroids are used, a prospective study of 14 patients treated with vancomycin, ceftriaxone and dexamethasone confirmed therapeutic CSF concentration of vancomycin (7.2 mg/l; corresponding serum concentration 25.2 mg/l) at 72 h [7]. Rifampicin penetrates the blood–brain barrier well and an animal model reduces early mortality in pneumococcal meningitis [56 online]. It therefore should be considered in addition to vancomycin. If confirmed or strongly suspected (presence of the characteristic rash), meningococcal meningitis should be treated with benzyl penicillin a third-generation cephalosporin or chloramphenicol if there is a history of life-threatening β-lactam allergy. Listeria is intrinsically resistant to the cephalosporins and suspected Listerial meningitis should be treated with high-dose i.v. ampicillin or amoxicillin usually in conjunction with i.v. gentamicin (1–2 mg/kg 8 h) for the first 7–10 days which is synergistic in vivo, or with high-dose IV cotrimoxazole when there is history of penicillin allergy [52, 54, 57 online]. The doses for common antibiotics in children are provided in Table S4.

There are no randomized controlled trials on the treatment of staphylococcal meningitis which is usually nosocomial (e.g., shunt infection). Linezolid has been used successfully in a number of case reports and pharmacokinetics are persuasive and may be an option for the treatment of methicillin-resistant staphylococcal meningitis and ventriculitis [58 online]. Lizezolid, however, must be used with caution because of adverse events and drug interactions, particularly in intensive care when vasoactive agents are used. The use of intrathecal or intraventricular antibiotics is to be considered in patients who fail conventional treatment. Intraventricular vancomycin may achieve better CSF concentration as compared with the intravenous route and the addition of intrathecal or intraventricular aminoglycosides as an additional agent is an option for patients with Gram-negative bacillary meningitis who do not respond well to monotherapy.

Recommendation

Initial antibiotic treatment of ABM should be parenteral (Class I, Level A).

Antibiotic therapy in suspected ABM

Ceftriaxone 2 g 12–24 hourly or cefotaxime 2 g 6–8 hourly (Class III, Level B).

Alternative therapy: Meropenem 2 g 8 hourly (Class III, Level C) or chloramphenicol 1 g 6 hourly.

If penicillin- or cephalosporin-resistant pneumococcus is suspected, use ceftriaxone or cefotaxime plus vancomycin 60 mg/kg/24 h (adjusted for creatinine clearance) after loading dose of 15 mg/kg (Class IV, Level A). Ampicillin/amoxicillin 2 g 4 hourly if listeria is suspected (Class IV, Level A).

Pathogen specific therapy

1. Penicillin-sensitive pneumococcal meningitis (and other sensitive streptococcal species); benzyl penicillin 250,000 U/kg/day (equivalent to 2.4 g 4 hourly) (Class IV, Level A) or ampicillin/amoxicillin 2 g 4 hourly or ceftriaxone 2 g 12 hourly or cefotaxime 2 g 6–8 hourly.

Alternative therapy: meropenem 2 g 8 hourly (Class IV, Level C) or vancomycin 60 mg/kg/24 hourly as continuous infusion (adjusted for creatinine clearance) after 15 mg/kg loading dose aiming for serum levels of 15–25 mg/l) plus rifampicin 600 mg 12 hourly (Class IV, Level C) or moxifloxacin 400 mg daily (Class IV, Level C).
2. Pneumococcus with reduced susceptibility to penicillin or cephalosporins; ceftriaxone or cefotaxime plus vancomycin ± rifampicin (Class IV).

Alternative therapy: moxifloxacin, meropenem or linezolid 600 mg combined with rifampicin (Class IV).
3. Meningococcal meningitis: benzyl penicillin or ceftriaxone or cefotaxime (Class IV).

Alternative therapy: meropenem, chloramphenicol or moxifloxacin (Class IV, Level C).
4. *Haemophilus infuenzae* type B: ceftriaxone or cefotaxime (Class IV, Level C).

Alternative therapy: IV Chloramphenicol–ampicillin/amoxicillin (Class IV, Level C).
5. Listerial meningitis: ampicillin or amoxicillin 2 g 4 hourly ± gentamicin 1–2 mg 8 hourly for the first 7–10 days (Class IV, Level C).

Alternative therapy: trimethoprim–sulfamethoxazole 10–20 mg/kg 6–12 hourly or meropenem (Class IV).
6. Staphylococcal species: Flucloxacillin 2 g 4 hourly [IV] or vancomycin if penicillin allergy is suspected (Class IV). Rifampicin should also be considered in addition to either agent, and linezolid for methicillin-resistant staphylococcal meningitis (Class IV, Level C).
7. Gram-negative enterobacteriaceae: ceftriaxone or cefotaxime or meropenem.
8. Pseudomonal meningitis: meropenem ± gentamicin.

Duration of therapy

The optimum duration of therapy in ABM is not known. In a prospective, observational study of meningococcal disease in adults from New Zealand, which had a majority of cases with meningitis, a 3-day course of i.v. benzyl penicillin was successful [59 online]. Among children with uncomplicated ABM, 7 days of ceftriaxone was found to be equivalent to 10 days in India [60 online] and 4 days was found to be equivalent to 7 days in Chile [61 online]. In a Swiss multicentre study in children, a short course of therapy (7 days or less) was equivalent to 8–12 days of treatment with ceftriaxone [62 online]. Two single doses of intramuscular oily chloramphenicol separated by 48 h were found in African children to be equivalent to 8 days' parenteral ampicillin [63 online]. In the absence of controlled clinical trials in adults, the recommended duration of antibiotic therapy in ABM is based on current standards of practice and in most cases with early and uncomplicated ABM, the shorter range of therapy would be appropriate.

> **Recommendations**
>
> - Unspecified bacterial meningitis 10–14 days (Class IV, Level C).
> - Pneumococcal meningitis 10–14 days (Class IV, Level A).
> - Meningococcal meningitis 5–7 days (Class IV, Level A).
> - Hib meningitis 7–14 days (Class IV, Level B).
> - Listerial meningitis 21 days (Class IV, Level B).
> - Gram-negative bacillary and pseudomonal meningitis: 21–28 days (Class IV, Level B).

Monitoring treatment

In general, if clinical condition does not improve by 48 h after commencing appropriate antibiotics (and dexamethasone when indicated), the following considerations should be given:
- raised intracranial pressure from cerebral oedema or obstructive hydrocephalus;
- vascular complications (arteritis or venous sinus thrombosis);
- inappropriate antibiotic;
- poor antibiotic penetration (e.g., vancomycin if the patient is on dexamethasone);
- wrong diagnosis;
- epileptic seizures (e.g., non-convulsive status);
- metabolic complications (e.g., SIADH);
- persistence of source of primary infection (e.g., pneumonia, bacterial endocarditis, mastoiditis or otitis).

Risk scores for unfavourable outcome in ABM have been recently validated in adults [8] and children [9] and may be useful as prognostic tools. In a retrospective study, a disturbed level of consciousness and higher age at the time of admission were found to be risk factors for developing hydrocephalus in the early phase of ABM [64 online]. A CT or MR scan of the brain can identify areas of ischemia or infarction, brain abscess, subdural empyema, signs of venous sinus thrombosis, hydrocephalus and ventriculitis (Class III, Level B).

Adjunctive therapy of ABM

Corticosteroids

Of all the adjunctive treatments in ABM, only corticosteroids have been properly evaluated in clinical trials. The rationale for using corticosteroids was that the treatment would attenuate subarachnoid space inflammation and vasogenic oedema in meningitis which may have potentially serious and damaging effects [2]. In 1988, published results of two double-blind, placebo-controlled trials of dexamethasone as an adjunctive treatment of bacterial meningitis in infants and older children showed convincing benefit from steroid therapy (decreased incidence of sensorineural hearing loss in the treated children with Hib meningitis) [65 online]. In two subsequent trials in paediatric patients, dexamethasone given before or with the first dose of antibiotic significantly reduced one or more neurological sequelae [66, 67 online]. In 1997, a meta-analysis of all randomized clinical trials since 1988 using dexamethasone as an adjunctive therapy in bacterial meningitis concluded that steroid treatment benefited Hib meningitis and, when commenced with or before parenteral antibiotics, showed benefit for children with pneumococcal meningitis [68 online].

A large, prospective, open trial of dexamethasone in adults showed a benefit of dexamethasone therapy in a subgroup of patients with pneumococcal meningitis [69 online]. Another multi-centre double-blind, randomized trial of dexamethasone treatment for severe bacterial meningitis in adults proved inconclusive because the trial was stopped prematurely due to the emergence of penicillin-resistant *S. pneumoniae* [70 online]. A placebo-controlled, double-blind trial of dexamethasone in 40 adult patients from India concluded that steroid treatment reduced neurological complications because of meningitis, but secondary fever, gastrointestinal manifestations and neuropsychiatric symptoms were common side-effects in the treated group [71 online].

Results of a double-blind, placebo-controlled, randomized European trial of dexamethasone in 301 adult patients with ABM showed that early steroid use (before or with the first dose of antibiotics) is associated with improved survival and significantly better outcome in these patients as measured by the Glasgow Outcome Scale at 8 weeks [10]. The benefit was by far most convincing in patients with pneumococcal meningitis who were given dexamethasone (10 mg 6 hourly for the first 4 days) beginning before or with the first dose of the antibiotic. The benefit of adjuvant dexamethasone in this trial was not undermined by an increase in the incidence of severe neurological disability in patients who survived, or by any serious steroid-induced complications.

The positive outcome of the European dexamethasone trial in adult bacterial meningitis contrasted sharply with the results of a randomized controlled trial of adjuvant dexamethasone in 598 children with bacterial meningitis from Malawi [72 online]. The Malawi trial failed to demonstrate any treatment benefit in terms of survival or neurological outcome. A recently published trial of dexamethasone in adult patients with bacterial meningitis from Malawi [73 online] reached very similar conclusions. In this trial, mortality was exceptionally high in both groups of patients receiving dexamethasone (56% of 233 patients) or placebo (53% of 232 patients) at 40 days and there was no difference in disability rates or hearing loss between these groups at 6 months. Nearly 90% patients in this study were seropositive for HIV infection. The results of the Vietnamese trial of dexamethasone in bacterial meningitis [74 online] was, however, more favourable for the steroid-treated patients with proven ABM. In this trial, 435 subjects >14 years of age were randomly assigned to receive 0.4 mg/kg of dexamethasone ($n = 217$) or placebo ($n = 218$) every 12 h for 4 days commencing shortly before the administration of antibiotics in most cases with meningitis caused by *S. suis* (which is similar to *S. pneumoniae*).

Taken together, results of these trials confirm the earlier view [2] that longer use (4 days) of dexamethasone in pharmacological doses is not appropriate if patients are thought to be immunocompromised or have a tentative diagnosis of ABM unsupported by appropriate investigations. The role of dexamethasone as an adjunctive therapy in ABM is clearly maximal in those who are not significantly immunosuppressed and have a confirmed microbiological diagnosis of ABM. In the context of the bacterial aetiology of ABM, evidence confirms its therapeutic benefit in cases with pneumococcal and Hib meningitis. Wider use of high-dose dexamethasone in ABM because of other bacterial aetiologies is currently proposed [75, 76 online], but its therapeutic benefit is not conclusive across all groups of patients.

Recommendation

- Adjuvant dexamethasone is recommended with or shortly before the first parenteral dose of antibiotic in all previously well and non-immunosuppressed adults with pneumococcal meningitis at a dose of 10 mg/6 h for 4 days (Class I, Level A)

and children at a dose of 0.15 mg/kg every 6 h for 4 days for Hib and pneumococcal meningitis (Class I, Level A).

- In all patients with clinically suspected pneumococcal or Hib meningitis (early focal neurological signs), we recommend that dexamethasone is given with the first dose of empirical antibiotic therapy as above (Class IV, Level C).

- In ABM because of other bacterial aetiology, routine use of high dose dexamethasone is not presently recommended (Class I, Level A).

- If dexamethasone was initiated on clinical suspicion of ABM, which was subsequently shown to be inaccurate by CSF microbiology, the treatment should be promptly withdrawn.

- There is insufficient evidence to recommend the use of dexamethasone in pharmacological doses after antibiotic therapy has begun. Dose and duration of therapy with corticosteroids in such cases should be guided by specific clinical indications in individual patients (e.g., physiological doses of steroids in cases of adrenal insufficiency because of meningococcaemia, pharmacological doses of steroids for raised intracranial pressure).

- By reducing subarachnoid space inflammation and blood–brain barrier permeability, steroids may reduce CSF penetration of antibiotics and patients receiving vancomycin for penicillin-resistant pneumococcal meningitis require close clinical and CSF monitoring.

Other symptomatic and adjunctive therapies

Circulatory shock as part of severe sepsis or in meningococcaemia should be handled in a neurointensive care unit. Treatment should consist of a 30° head-up position, head midline, minimal suction, deep sedation, normo- or moderate hypothermia and strict avoidance of hypercapnia [11]. Head elevation and hyperosmolar agents are recommended for the management of cerebral oedema but have not been systematically evaluated in the context of bacterial meningitis. As a hyperosmolar agent, 20% mannitol may be given intravenously either as a bolus injection of 1 g/kg over 10–15 min, repeated at 4–6 h intervals, or in smaller but frequent doses (0.25 mg/kg every 2–3 h), to maintain a target serum osmolality of 315–320 mOsm/l (Class IV, Level C). CSF pressure monitoring may be helpful in cases where CSF drainage (ventricular) is under consideration for obstructive hydrocephalus, and the decision to perform the procedure should be based on patient's level of consciousness and the degree of ventricular dilatation visualized in brain imaging (CT or MRI) (Class IV, Level C). Seizures are frequent in ABM and are associated with severe inflammation, structural brain lesion and pneumococcal meningitis, may increase mortality [12] and should be treated with a parenteral anticonvulsant, such as phenytoin (fosphenytoin) (Class III). Prophylactic anti-coagulation to prevent deep vein thrombosis may be considered in patients who do not have coagulaopathy and are considered to be at a high risk of deep vein thrombosis (e.g., due to obesity or recent hip surgery). Heparin was considered beneficial in a retrospective study of patients with septic cavernous sinus thrombosis [77 online]; however, experience with therapeutic anticoagulation for venous sinus thrombosis in ABM is limited and is best reserved for patients who deteriorate neurologically because of venous sinus thrombosis and require close monitoring of coagulation profile and brain imaging (Class IV, Level C).

Managing complications of ABM

Death in bacterial meningitis may occur within the first 48 h and sometimes even before the diagnosis is made. In a review of the autopsy data, it was noted that deaths because of *N. meningitidis* often occurred within 12–24 h of the first symptoms [78 online]. Delayed neurological sequelae may occur in 20–40% of patients. Audiological complications have been reported in over a third of children with bacterial meningitis, mostly because of *H. influenzae*. Cognitive dysfunction, behavioural changes, seizures and motor impairment are common complications of meningitis in adults and in children. Some survivors have permanent visual impairment caused by optic atrophy from opticochiasmatic arachnoiditis, persistent hydrocephalus or as a result of cortical blindness from arterial infarction involving the occipital lobes. The range of post-meningitic motor deficits includes unilateral or bilateral hemiparesis, weakness of eye movements, spastic paraparesis with sensory loss from spinal cord damage and, rarely, a tabetic syndrome because of the involvement of lumbosacral nerve roots. Growth retardation and arrest of mental development are delayed complications of bacterial meningitis seen in children. The range of complications in pneumococcal meningitis is particularly severe. Austrian syndrome is a severe condition of invasive pneumococcal disease characterized by

meningitis, endocarditis and pneumonia and carries a high mortality rate. A recent study in adults has drawn attention to problems such as myelitis and subarachnoid bleeding and higher incidences of cerebrovascular lesions (22% arterial and 9% venous strokes) [13]. Chronic fatigue, depression and sleep disorders are significantly higher among the survivors of meningitis and a smaller proportion of patients may present with epilepsy in later years (Table S5).

> ### Recommendations
>
> - All survivors of ABM should be offered access to a neurology service.
> - Audiometry is recommended in recovering patients with suspected hearing impairment.
> - Seizures in patients with ABM may be early (acute symptomatic epilepsy) or delayed, appearing after several months or years. Long-term antiepileptic drug therapy is recommended in patients with late-onset seizures. For patients with acute symptomatic seizures, antiepileptic drug therapy may be withdrawn after 1 year in the absence of seizure recurrence and structural brain (cortical) injury as visualized in brain imaging.
> - Driving restriction in adults may apply if they had seizures or have functional impairment such as visual field defect and limb weakness.

Prevention of secondary cases of ABM

It is the responsibility of the diagnosing clinician to inform the local public health authorities of any case of suspected invasive meningococcal infection. Asymptomatic carriers of *N. meningitidis* may pass the organism via droplet/close contact spread to others, usually a household member or a close ('kissing') contact, who, in turn may become a carrier or may develop invasive infection. Secondary cases in close contacts occur at a rate of about 2–4/1,000 [79 online]. Asymptomatic carriers are the target of chemoprophylaxis. A meta-analysis of retrospective, uncontrolled observational studies of chemoprophylaxis with rifampicin, minocycline, sulphonamide or ciprofloxacin vs. no chemoprophylaxis demonstrated a reduction of 89% risk in secondary household cases with about 200 contacts needed to be treated to prevent one further case [80 online]. In Nordic countries, antibiotic therapy with 7 days of oral penicillin is recommended in addition to chemoprophylaxis for household contacts of <15 years to treat early or incubating infection which may be unaffected by chemoprophylaxis alone [81 online]. As benzyl penicillin does not eradicate carriage, all patients with meningococcal infection who have not received a third-generation cephalosporin should receive further antibiotic prophylaxis with either rifampicin for 2 days or with a single dose of ciprofloxacin or ceftriaxone. If vaccine-preventable strains are implicated (serotypes A or C) in the outbreak setting, vaccination should be given to all unvaccinated households or close contacts. Patients at risk of primary meningococcal infection, including travellers to endemic areas, the immunosuppressed and the asplenic should be offered primary immunization. The polysaccharide–protein conjugated meningococcal type C vaccine is highly effective at preventing serotype C infections and is part of the standard childhood immunization schedule in much of Europe [82 online].

Primary prevention of pneumococcal disease in general with the pneumococcal vaccine should be offered to all immunosuppressed and asplenic patients and to those with chronic pulmonary, renal, hepatic or cardiac disease or those aged over 65 years, those with a cochlear implant, previous basal skull fracture, *in situ* CSF shunt or CSF leak. Asplenic or hyposplenic individuals (e.g., those with sickle cell disease) are also at risk of invasive disease. In at-risk individuals, vaccination may be repeated at 5-yearly intervals. Although Hib very rarely causes meningitis in adults, if this does occur, all household members should have their vaccination status evaluated. Prophylaxis with rifampicin is recommended and unimmunized children should be vaccinated against Hib.

Recommendations

- All cases of suspected meningococcal or Hib meningitis should be reported urgently to the local public health authorities (Class IV, Level C).
- Chemoprophylaxis with oral rifampicin (600 mg 12 hourly for 48 h), ciprofloxacin (500 mg single dose) or ceftriaxone (i.v. or i.m. injection of a single 1 g dose) should be given to those adults with meningococcal infection who were treated without a third-generation cephalosporin (Class IV, Level C).
- Chemoprophylaxis with rifampicin, ciprofloxacin or ceftriaxone should be given to household or close contacts

of patients with suspected or proven meningococcal or haemophilus infection (Class IV, Level C).
- A therapeutic 7-day course of phenoxymethyl penicillin or amoxicillin should be considered in addition to chemoprophylaxis for any household or close contact of a patient with meningococcal disease aged < 15 years (Class IV, Level C).
- Chemoprophylaxis for meningococcal meningitis is rarely indicated for healthcare workers and is only recommended in situations where there has been mouth to mouth contact or direct exposure to infectious droplets from a patient with meningococcal disease (Class IV, Level C).
- Immunization with meningococcal or *H. influenzae* type B vaccine should be considered in the public health management of an outbreak (Class IV, Level C).
- Primary vaccination against *N. meningitidis* and *H. influenzae* type B infection should be given to all at-risk groups (Class IV, Level C).
- Vaccination against *N. meningitides* type C and *H. influenzae* type B should be given to all children as part of the normal childhood immunization schedule (Class IV, Level C).

Supplementary material

A full (unabridged) version of this chapter is available online at www.blackwell-synergy.com/doi/abs/10.1111/j.1468-1331.2008.02193.x (this link will take you to the article abstract. Blackwell is not responsible for the content or functionality of any supplementary materials supplied by the authors. Any queries (other than missing material) should be directed to the corresponding author.)

References

1. Brainin, M, Barnes, M, Baron, JC, *et al.* Guidance for the preparation of neurological management guidelines by EFNS scientific task forces – revised recommendations 2004. *Eur J Neurol* 2004; **11**:1–6.
2. Chaudhuri, A. Adjuvant dexamethasone use in acute bacterial meningitis. *Lancet Neurol* 2004; **3**:54–61.
3. Van de Beek, D, de Gans, J, Spanjaard, L, *et al.* Clinical features and prognostic factors in adults with bacterial meningitis. *N Engl J Med* 2004; **351**:1849–59.
4. Harnden, A, Ninis, N, Thompson, M, *et al.* Parenteral penicillin for children with meningococcal disease before hospital admission: case-control study. *Br Med J* 2006; **332**: 1295–8.

5. Proulx, N, Frechette, D, Toye, B, *et al.* Delays in the administration of antibiotics are associated with mortality from acute bacterial meninigitis. *QJM* 2005; **98**:291–8.

6. Prasad, K, Kumar, A, Gupta, PK, Singhal, T. Third generation cephalosporins versus conventional antibiotics for treating acute bacterial meningitis. *Cochrane Database Syst Rev* 2004; **2**:CD001832.

7. Richard, JD, Wolff, M, Lachareade, JC, *et al.* Levels of vancomycin in cerebrospinal fluid of adult patients receiving adjunctive corticosteroids to treat pneumococcal meningitis: a prospective multicentre observation study. *Clin Infect Dis* 2007; **44**:250–5.

8. Weisfelt, M, van de Beek, D, Spanjaard, L, *et al.* A risk score for unfavourable outcome in adults with bacterial meningitis. *Ann Neurol* 2008; **63**:90–7.

9. Dubos, F, De la Rocque, F, Levy, C, *et al.* Sensitivity of the bacterial meningitis score in 889 children with bacterial meningitis. *J Paediatr* 2008; **152**:378–82.

10. de Gans, J, van de Beck, D. Dexamethasone in adults with bacterial meningitis. *N Engl J Med* 2002; **347**:1549–56.

11. Nadel, S, Kroll, JS. Diagnosis and management of meningococcal disease: the need for centralized care. *FEMS Microbiol Rev* 2007; **31**:71–83.

12. Zoons, E, Weisfelt, M, de Gans, J. *et al.* Seizures in adults with bacterial meningitis. *Neurology* 2008; **7**:2109–15. doi:10.1212/ 01.wnl.0000288178.91614.5d.

13. Kastenbauer, S, Pfister, HW. Pneumococcal meningitis in adults: spectrum of complications and prognostic factors in a series of 87 cases. *Brain* 2003; **126**:1015–25.

CHAPTER 12

Diagnosis and management of European lyme neuroborreliosis

Åse Mygland,[1,2] Unn Ljøstad,[1] Volker Fingerle,[3] Tobias Rupprecht,[4] Erich Schmutzhard[5] and Israel Steiner[6]

[1]Sørlandet Sykehus, Kristiansand, Norway; [2]University of Bergen, Bergen, Norway; [3]Bavarian Health and Food Safety Authority, Oberschleißheim, Germany; [4]Ludwig-Maximilians University, Munich, Germany; [5]Medical University Innsbruck, Austria; [6]Hadassah University Hospital, Mount Scopus, Jerusalem, Israel

Introduction

Lyme neuroborreliosis (LNB) is an infectious disorder of the nervous system caused by tick–borne spirochetes of the *Borrelia burgdorferi* (*Bb*) sensu lato complex. Clinical features of LNB are diverse and differ in European and American patients, most probably due to different bacteria species.

Laboratory confirmation of LNB is hampered by the low yield of culture and of polymerase chain reaction (PCR) examination of cerebrospinal fluid (CSF) [1, 2]. Presence of *Bb* specific antibodies in the CSF with evidence of intrathecal production is the traditional diagnostic gold standard, but has limitations, such as low sensitivity in the very early phase of the disease [3, 4, 5] and persistence for years after eradication of the infection [6, 7]. Several other, more or less validated, laboratory tests have been developed to improve diagnosis.

LNB should be treated with antibiotics to achieve rapid resolution of symptoms and, theoretically, to avoid spread and persistence of infection. The choice of the best antibiotic, the preferred mode of administration and the duration of treatment are still debated issues. The purpose of this guideline is to present evidence-based recommendations for diagnostic evaluation and management of European LNB.

The analytic process

Data were collected by searching Medline, EMBASE, the Cochrane databases and other evidence-based guidelines and reviews, including the practice parameters proposed by the American Academy of Neurology [8] and The Infectious Diseases Society of America (IDSA) guidelines [9]. The search terms 'Lyme disease' and 'Lyme neuroborreliosis' were cross-referenced with encephalopathy, meningitis, peripheral nervous system disease, peripheral facial palsy, laboratory test, diagnosis and treatment. For determining levels of evidence the EFNS guidelines were used [10]. Review articles and book chapters were included if they were considered to provide comprehensive reviews of the topic. The final choice of literature and the references included were based on our judgement of their relevance to this subject. Two authors independently assessed the quality of treatment trials. Recommendations were reached by consensus of all Task Force participants by a modified Delphi method, and

European Handbook of Neurological Management: Volume 2, Second Edition. Edited by Nils Erik Gilhus, Michael P. Barnes, Michael Brainin.
© 2012 Blackwell Publishing Ltd. Published 2012 by Blackwell Publishing Ltd.

were also based on our own awareness and clinical experience. Where there was lack of evidence but consensus was clear we have stated our opinion as good practice points.

Diagnostic evaluation

Clinical features of Lyme neuroborreliosis

Neurological symptoms usually occur 1–12 (mostly 4–6) weeks after the tick bite, mainly between July and December. Only 40–50% of the patients can recall a tick bite and 20–30% report a local skin infection (erythema migrans) (stage I) [11, 12]. More than 95% can be classified as early LNB (stage II), defined as signs and symptoms lasting <6 months. Less than 5% have late LNB (stage III) with duration between 6 months and several years [12]. The natural course of early LNB is often self-limiting [13], whereas late LNB has a chronic course, which probably reflects persistent survival of bacteria in nervous tissue.

Early LNB

Peripheral nervous system (PNS)

The most common manifestation of early LNB (Table 12.1) in Europe is a painful meningoradiculitis (Bannwarth's syndrome). The clinical hallmarks of Bannwarth's syndrome are radicular pain in 86% of patients and paresis in 61% [3]. The pain is generally described as being of a type never experienced before. Its intensity and localization may vary from day to day and typically is worse at night. The paresis may affect muscles innervated by cranial nerves (especially the facial nerve,

less often the abducens or the oculomotor nerves), the abdominal wall or the limbs. Headache occurs in about 43%, but a prominent headache without radicular pain or paresis is rare in adults. Apart from Bannwarth's syndrome and lymphocytic meningitis, other peripheral neurological manifestations (in 5–10% of the patients) are plexus neuritis and mononeuritis multiplex.

Central nervous system (CNS)

Involvement is rare, but patients may present with myelitis or encephalitis. Clinical manifestations (e.g., confusion, cerebellar ataxia, opsoclonus-myoclonus, ocular flutter, apraxia, hemiparesis or parkinson-like symptoms) have been associated with *Bb* infection [14]. Poliomyelitis-like syndromes [15] and acute stroke-like symptoms due to cerebral vasculitis [16] are rare and have been documented only in single-case reports.

Late LNB (Table 12.1)

Late neurological manifestations are also entitled chronic neuroborreliosis.

PNS manifestations

Manifestations may consist of mononeuropathy, radiculopathy and polyneuropathy [17, 18]. In Europe, late polyneuropathy has only been observed in combination with acrodermatitis chronica atrophicans (ACA) [19] – the typical dermatological manifestation during late stage III of borrelia infection – while isolated cases of distal symmetric polyneuropathy due to a borrelial infection have been reported in American patients [20]. It is of note that a causative relationship between polyneuropathy and borrelia infection cannot be based on the sole detection of *Bb* specific antibodies in patients with polyneuropathy as those antibodies can also be found in 5–25% of healthy persons [21].

CNS manifestations

These include cerebral vasculitis and chronic progressive Lyme encephalitis or encephalomyelitis with tetraspastic syndrome, spastic-ataxic gait disorder and disturbed micturition [18].

Differences between European and American LNB

Unlike the European Lyme disease, the North American disorder is characterized by erythema migrans, arthritis

---

Table 12.1 Classification of LNB.

Early LNB
Neurological symptoms for less than 6 months:
- with symptoms confined to PNS (cranial nerves, spinal roots, or peripheral nerves) (Bannwarth syndrome)
- with CNS manifestations

Late LNB
Neurological symptoms for more than 6 months
- with PNS manifestations
- with CNS manifestations

and meningitis. It is usually deficient of painful radicular symptoms, other cranial nerve involvement (other than the facial nerve) and ACA.

Paediatric LNB

The most common manifestations of LNB in European children are acute facial nerve palsy (in 55%), other cranial nerve palsies and lymphocytic meningitis (in 27%) [22, 23]. Small children may present with nonspecific symptoms, such as loss of appetite and fatigue. CNS symptoms are rare, but children with early LNB may present with acute myelitis [24], acute hemiparesis [25], opsoclonus-myoclonus [26] or ataxia [27]. Late LNB with chronic hemiparesis has also been reported [25].

Laboratory tests

CSF – inflammatory parameters

European LNB is associated with an elevated cell count in the CSF, typically 10–1,000 leucocytes/mm^3 [12], mainly lymphocytes and plasma cells. A substantial number of patients have elevated CSF protein and oligoclonal IgG bands [12]. Patients with ACA-associated polyneuropathy often have normal CSF findings. A normal cell count is otherwise rare, but is sometimes present [5], especially in the very early stage, in immunosuppressed individuals and possibly in rare cases of LNB caused by the species *Borrelia afzelii* [5, 28]. In such cases, the bacterial pathogen has to be identified by culture or PCR in order to confirm the clinical diagnosis.

Microscope-based assays

Bb can be seen directly in liquid patient material (e.g., CSF) by applying dark-field microscopy or after staining histological sections [29, 30, 31] (Class IV), but sensitivity and specificity are low [31]. Focus floating microscopy was recently described as a sensitive method for detection of *Bb* in skin biopsies [32] (Class IV).

Recommendations

There is not enough evidence to recommend any of these microscope-based assays as a routine diagnostic tool.

PCR

There are numerous PCR protocols for detection of *Bb* DNA in clinical specimens [1, 33, 34]. Due to lack of a gold standard method and lack of large comparative studies it is impossible to recommend a specific PCR protocol. Diagnostic sensitivity of PCR in CSF for early LNB is 10–30% (median). In blood it is even lower [35], and PCR studies in urine are contradictory [1, 33, 36, 37, 38]. In late LNB, sensitivity of PCR is extremely low.

Analytic specificity of PCR (the ability to identify exclusively *Bb* DNA rather than similar DNA) is 98–100%, provided precautions are taken to avoid contaminations and amplified products are specified by an appropriate method (e.g., sequencing) [1, 33, 35, 39]. There are no studies of diagnostic specificity (the ability to correctly identify a person without active infection with a negative test).

Recommendation

PCR on CSF samples has a low sensitivity, but may be useful in very early LNB with a negative antibody index or in patients with immunodeficiency (good practice point). Due to low sensitivity and unknown specificity, PCR cannot be recommended as a diagnostic method in patients with chronic symptoms or for follow-up of therapy.

Cultivation

Bb can be recovered from CSF, skin or blood using modified Kelly medium at 30–34°C [40, 41, 42, 43]. Cultures should be monitored for up to 12 weeks due to the spirochete's slow growth *in vitro* (7–>20h). Since microscopic detection of *Bb* can lead to false-positive readings, spirochete-like structures need to be confirmed as *Bb* by PCR or staining with specific monoclonal antibodies [39, 44]. The sensitivity is 10–30% in CSF in early LNB, 50–70% in skin biopsies and <10% in blood (erythema migrans).

Recommendation

Due to its low sensitivity, slow growth and restriction to a few specialized laboratories, culture of *Bb* is limited to special indications, such as atypical clinical presentation or patients with immune deficiencies (good practice point).

Bb-specific antibodies in serum and CSF

Bb-specific antibodies in serum can be detected with an IgG and IgM differentiating enzyme-linked immuno-sorbent assay (ELISA) using sonified whole Borrelia, recombinant antigens or single antigens (e.g., VlsE or the C6 peptide) [45–49]. Many laboratories use a two-step approach where sera that are positive in the ELISA screening assay are subjected to immunoblot (IB) for confirmation [39, 50, 51, 52]. As a confirmatory test, the IB should have an analytic specificity of at least 95%. Diagnostic sensitivity of ELISA screening assays in early LNB is 70–90%, and for late LNB (only IgG since IgM is not diagnostic for late disease) it is >90–100% [45, 46, 47, 48, 49] (Class III and one Class II).

The diagnostic specificity of serum antibody tests are low since seropositivity in the normal population ranges from 5 to >20% [21, 47]. IgM might be false-positive due to oligoclonal stimulation, and IgG and IgM antibodies may persist for years after successful therapy [6, 7]. The diagnostic specificity of C6 ELISA was 61% in one Class II study [47]. Immunoblot (IB) used alone or after a negative ELISA is reported by many laboratories to have a very low specificity. A two-step approach, using WB as a confirmatory assay only on sera positive in ELISA, increases the diagnostic specificity according to a Class III study [52].

To prove intrathecal production of *Bb*-specific antibodies, calculations that consider blood–CSF barrier dysfunctions (antibody index; AI) based on quantitative ELISA are used. Intrathecally produced IgM antibodies show a high sensitivity in LNB of short duration, especially in children [5, 53, 54]. However, false-positive IgM reactivity has been observed in EBV meningitis [53]. In some cases antibodies are detectable in CSF while serum is negative [53]. A positive AI may persist for years after successful therapy [6, 7].

Diagnostic sensitivity of the AI is about 80% in LNB of short duration (<6 weeks) [3, 4] and nearly 100% in LNB of longer duration [4, 5, 39] (Class III). Diagnostic specificity was 63% in one Class II study [55].

Recommendation

Antibody tests for serum (ELISA or ELISA followed by IB if ELISA is positive [good practice point]) and CSF (AI) are useful in the diagnosis of LNB (Level B), but are hampered by a low sensitivity in patients with symptom duration of <6 weeks, and by low specificity if judged without other criteria. Due to low specificity, antibody results can only be interpreted together with clinical data and CSF inflammation parameters. Therefore, antibody testing should only be undertaken in patients with symptoms suggestive of LNB.

Chemokine CXCL13

Recent studies have suggested that the B-cell attracting chemokine CXCL13 is reliably increased in the CSF of patients with well-defined, early LNB [38, 55, 56, 57]. In one Class II study the diagnostic sensitivity of a CXCL13 ELISA in the CSF was 100% in early LNB, the specificity was 63% and it was normalized in 82% four months after treatment [55]. The test might be helpful in seronegative patients during early disease, and for control of therapy.

Recommendation

There is not enough evidence to recommend CXCL13 test as a routine diagnostic tool or in follow-up after treatment.

Antigen detection

Assays for antigen detection have been used to detect *Bb* antigens in CSF and in urine samples [58, 59, 60]. Limitations include low sensitivity and poor specificity and reproducibility [61, 62].

Recommendation

There is not enough evidence to recommend antigen detection assays as a routine diagnostic tool or in follow-up after treatment.

Detection of antibodies that bind in circulating immune complexes

Sequestration of specific antibodies in immune complexes has been suggested as an important factor for seronegativity in early Lyme borreliosis [63, 64, 65, 66]. Results from studies measuring antibodies from dissociated immune complexes are contradictory [63, 67]. Detection of immune complexes might be helpful in seronegative patients during early disease.

Lymphocyte transformation test (LTT)

The aim of LTT is to detect active *Bb* infection by testing the cellular immune response. Activation of patient-derived lymphocytes is measured after incubation with Borrelia antigens. Results of studies are contradictory and, moreover, there is no relevant study that allows assessment of diagnostic sensitivity and specificity of the tests that are promulgated for diagnosis of Lyme borreliosis [68, 69, 70, 71, 72].

Cyst formation

So called cysts, spheroblasts or L-forms of *Bb* can be induced *in vitro* by stressors such as high temperature or change in pH [73, 74, 75, 76]. Whether, or to what extent, such forms may have significance for pathogenesis or for the diagnosis of LNB is uncertain.

CD57+/CD3- lymphocyte subpopulation

There is one study reporting a decreased level of a CD57+/CD3- lymphocyte subpopulation in patients with nonspecific symptoms suffering from chronic Lyme [77]. However, the case group was poorly defined and the controls inappropriately chosen. Another study found no association between CD57+ and post-Lyme disease symptoms [78].

Table 12.2 Suggested case definitions for Lyme neuroborreliosis.

Definite neuroborreliosis[*] All three criteria fulfilled	Possible neuroborreliosis[**] Two criteria fulfilled
Neurological symptoms suggestive of Lyme neuroborreliosis without other obvious causes	
CSF pleocytosis	
Intrathecal *Bb* antibody production	

[*]These criteria apply to all subclasses of LNB except for late LNB with polyneuropathy where the following should be fulfilled for definite diagnosis: (a) peripheral neuropathy; (b) ACA; (c) *Bb* specific antibodies in serum.
[**]If criterion 3 is lacking; after a duration of 6 weeks, there have to be found *Bb* specific IgG antibodies in the serum.

Diagnostic criteria

LNB poses a clinical diagnostic challenge. In view of the variable presentations, diagnostic criteria rooted in a combination of clinical and laboratory findings are necessary. Unfortunately, such criteria based on international consensus do not exist. In Europe, detection of intrathecal synthesis of *Bb* specific antibodies – a positive *Bb* antibody index (AI) – is considered necessary for the diagnosis [79], but its sensitivity can be as low as 55% [4, 5, 80, 81, 82, 83, 84]. American criteria do not require a positive *Bb* AI [85].

We recommend (good practice point) the following criteria for definite and possible LNB (Table 12.2).

Definite LNB: The following three criteria are fulfilled: 1) neurological symptoms suggestive of LNB (with other causes excluded); 2) CSF pleocytosis; and 3) *Bb* specific antibodies in CSF (produced intrathecally).

Possible LNB: Two of the above mentioned three criteria are fulfilled. If criterion 3 is lacking after 6 weeks, *Bb*-specific antibodies have to be found in the serum.

These criteria apply to all subclasses of LNB, except for late LNB with polyneuropathy where the following should be fulfilled for a definite diagnosis: 1) peripheral neuropathy; 2) clinical diagnosis of ACA; and 3) *Bb*-specific antibodies in serum.

Treatment

Early LNB with symptoms confined to the PNS and meninges
Effective agents
In 1983 two Class IV, small case-series indicated the effect of high-dose intravenous (i.v.) penicillin [86, 87]. Several Class III and IV studies have reported response to 10–28 day courses of i.v. penicillin (20 million U daily), i.v. ceftriaxone (2 g or 4 g daily), i.v. cefotaxime (3 g × 2 or 2 g × 3 daily) and oral doxycycline (200 mg daily for 2 days and 100 mg daily for 8 days) [14, 88, 89, 90, 91] (Table 12.3). Intravenous ceftriaxone, cefotaxime and penicillin seem to have similar efficacy [88, 90, 91] (Class III). First-generation cephalosporins were ineffective *in vitro* against *Bb* in an American study [98]. There are not enough data to support the use of the following: metronidazole, trimetoprim-sulfamethoxazole, fluconazole, isoniazid, combinations of antibiotics or steroids.

Oral vs. intravenous administration of antibiotics
Oral doxycycline has a good CSF penetration and gives CSF concentrations above the minimum inhibitory concentration [99]. Several Class III studies have shown that oral doxycycline has similar short- and long-term efficacy as have various parenteral regimens [89, 92, 93, 94, 95, 96]. A recent Norwegian Class I study of 102 LNB patients showed that oral doxycycline (200 mg daily for 14 days) was non-inferior compared with i.v. ceftriaxone (2 g daily for 14 days) [11].

Duration of treatment
The occurrence of persistent residual symptoms after standard antibiotic therapy has led to speculation about surviving bacteria and the need for longer treatment duration. There are no Class I comparisons of different

treatment durations. In most European treatment studies the duration ranged from 10 to 14 days (Table 12.3), and in a few studies for up to 28 days. A case-series reported excellent or good response in 90% of patients with disseminated Lyme (including neuroborreliosis) after treatment with oral cefixime or i.v. ceftriaxone for 14 days followed by oral amoxicillin for 100 days [97] (Class IV). However, a Finnish Class II study showed no benefit of extended treatment [100]. In this study, 152 patients with disseminated Lyme disease, including 62 with neuroborreliosis, were randomized to treatment of 3 weeks with i.v. ceftriaxone followed by either oral amoxicillin (2 g b.i.d.) or placebo for 100 days. At 1-year follow-up the groups were similar, with about 90% having excellent or good outcome.

Recommendations
Adult patients with definite or possible early LNB with symptoms confined to the meninges, cranial nerves, nerve roots or peripheral nerves (Bannwarth syndrome) should be offered a single, 14-day course of antibiotic treatment:
- Oral doxycycline, i.v. ceftriaxone, i.v. penicillin are i.v. cefotaxime are all effective and safe treatments (Level B).
- Oral doxycycline (200 mg daily) and i.v. ceftriaxone (2 g daily) for 14 days are equally effective (Level A). The advantages of doxycycline are the oral route of administration and the lower costs. Doxycycline is relatively contraindicated during pregnancy or lactation.

Early LNB with CNS symptoms
Whether early LNB with CNS manifestations (encephalitis, myelitis or vasculitis) should be treated differently from Bannwarth syndrome is uncertain. Case studies suggest good recovery with i.v. ceftriaxone for 2–3 weeks [15, 101, 102, 103, 104] (Class IV). In a Swedish Slovenian comparative study of i.v. ceftriaxone and oral doxycycline 2 of 29 patients in the ceftriaxone group and 3 of 36 in the doxycycline group had encephalitis. All patients were reported to improve after treatment [95] (Class III).

Recommendations
Adult patients with definite or possible early LNB with CNS manifestations (myelitis, encephalitis, vasculitis) should be treated with i.v. ceftriaxone (2 g daily) for 14 days (not enough evidence: good practice point).

Table 12.3 Inclusion criteria and clinical outcome results of treatment trials for adult Lyme neuroborreliosis.

First author, year	Inclusion criteria	Response criteria	Disease duration*	Treatment	Response rate	Remarks
Dattwyler, 1988 [88]	Physician observed EM or ELISA and two organ manifestations	Absence of arthritis, neurophysiologic findings and encephalopathy	35 mo 28 mo 29 mo 39 mo	i.v. penicillin 10 d vs. i.v. Ceftriaxone 2g 14 d and i.v. Ceftriaxone 2g vs. i.v. Ceftriaxone 4g	5/10 12/13 13/14 14/17	Half the patients had received oral antibiotics. Class III
Kohlhepp,1989 [14]	ELISA and three of: TB/EM, radicular pain, radiculitis, arthritis/carditis/neurological findings, meningitis, cranial neuritis	Complete recovery at 12 mo	4 mo 5 mo	i.v. doxycycline 10 d (n = 39) vs. i.v. penicillin 10 d (n = 36)	2/3 in both groups	10 patients were retreated. Class III
Pfister, 1989 [90]	Bannwarth syndrome or meningitis with TB or EM and ELISA	Normal neurological findings at 7.7 mo	29 d 24 d	i.v. penicillin 10 d vs. i.v. cefotaxime 10 d	8/10 9/11	Class III
Hassler, 1990 [89]	ELISA and arthritis, neuropathy or ACA lasting at least 6 mo	Absence of symptoms within 6 mo and persisting remission in 24 mo	>6 mo	i.v. cefotaxime 8–10 d vs. i.v. penicillin 8–10 d	44/69 25/66 $P = 0.002$	Class III
Logigian, 1990 [17]	Previously signs of LD, neurological symptoms >3 mo and immunity to *Bb*	Neurological improvement at 6 mo	12 mo	i.v. ceftriaxone 14 d	17/27	Half of the patients had received oral or i.v. antibiotics. Class IV
Pfister,1991 [91]	Bannwarth syndrome or meningitis with ELISA	Normal neurological findings at mean 8.1 mo after therapy	33 d 32 d (median)	i.v. ceftriaxone 10 d vs. i.v. cefotaxime 10 d	8/12 9/15	Class III
Karlsson, 1994 [92]	Meningoradiculitis, encephalomyelitis or chronic meningitis and CSF pleocytosis and positive ELISA or cultivation	Complete recovery at 12 mo	3.5 w 4 w (median)	i.v. penicillin 14 d vs. oral doxycycline 14 d	18/21 27/30	2 patients were retreated. Class III
Dotevall,1999 [93]	Facial palsy, CSF pleocytosis and ELISA or EM	Complete recovery at 6 mo	23 d	Oral doxycycline 9–17 d	26/29	Class IV
Karkkonen, 2001 [94]	Bannwarth syndrome or encephalomyelitis, CSF pleocytosis and ELISA or EM	Complete recovery at 1 year and Improvement at 1 year	4 w (median)	Oral doxycycline 10–28 d	56/69 69/69	6 patients were retreated. Class IV

continued

165

Table 12.3 continued

First author, year	Inclusion criteria	Response criteria	Disease duration[*]	Treatment	Response rate	Remarks
Borg, 2005 [95]	Clinical neuroborreliosis, CSF pleocytosis and one of: EM, intrathecal antibody production, isolation of Borrelia or seroconversion	Complete recovery at 6 mo	21 d 28 d (median)	i.v. ceftriaxone 10–14 d vs. Oral doxycycline 10–14 d	23/29 26/36	Class III
Ogrinc, 2006 [96]	Neurological symptoms, no CSF pleocytosis, ELISA or EM	Clinical improvement at 12 mo	18 mo (median)	Oral doxycycline 28 d (n = 23) vs. i.v. ceftriaxone 14 d + PO doxycycline 14 d (n = 23)	74% 70%	Class III
Dattwyler, 2005 [88]	Objective organ manifestations of at least 3 mo duration, EM or exposure to endemic area and ELISA and WB	Complete recovery/ treatment failures	>3 mo	i.v. ceftriaxone 14 d (n = 65) vs. i.v. ceftriaxone 28 d (n = 43)	76%/6% 70%/0%	Many dropouts. Half of the patients had received oral antibiotics. Class III
Oksi, 2007 [97]	Clinical disseminated Lyme borreliosis (of which 62 neuroborreliosis) confirmed by ELISA, PCR or culture	VAS < 30	?	i.v. ceftriaxone 21 d followed by oral amoxicillin in 100 d vs. placebo in 100 d	49/52 47/54	Class II
Ljøstad, 2008 [11]	Neurological symptoms and one of: CSF pleocytosis, intrathecal antibody production or ACA	Improvement on a composite clinical score at 4 mo	10 w 8 w	Oral doxycycline 14 d (n = 54) vs. i.v. Ceftriaxone (n = 48)	4.5 units 4.4 units P = 0.84	Class I

d = days, w = weeks, mo = months, ACA = acrodermatitis chronica atrophicans, ELISA = Bb antibodies detected by ELISA method, EM = erythema migrans, i.v.=I ntravenous, LD = Lyme disease, TB = tick bite, VAS = visual analogue scale, WB = Bb antibodies detected by Western blot

[*] Pre-treatment disease duration

166

Late LNB

Effective agents

There are no randomized treatment studies of European late LNB. Small subgroup analyses and case studies indicate the effect of i.v. ceftriaxone (2 g daily) given for to 2–4 weeks, or i.v. penicillin (20 million U daily for 10 days) or doxycycline (200 mg daily) [16, 91, 101, 105] (Class IV). An American study showed better effect of ceftriaxone than penicillin [88] (Class III). There are not enough data to support the use of steroids alone or in combination with antibiotics.

Oral vs. intravenous administration of antibiotics

Subgroup analysis of 10 patients with late LNB in a Class I comparative Norwegian study showed equal improvement after 14 days of oral doxycycline as after 14 days of i.v. ceftriaxone [11] (Class III). In a Swedish study of late LNB with peripheral neuropathy and ACA, improvement of neurological symptoms was similar in the 26 patients who received oral doxycycline for 3 weeks as in 21 who received i.v. penicillin for 2 weeks followed by oral doxycycline for 2 weeks [19] (Class III).

A European open-label study of late Lyme borreliosis (defined as nonspecific CNS symptoms but without CSF pleocytosis or other neurological findings, and therefore not convincing LNB) showed similar improvement rates 6 months after treatment with 4 weeks of oral doxycycline vs. 2 weeks of i.v. ceftriaxone followed by 2 weeks of oral doxycycline (59% vs. 67%) [96] (Class III).

Duration of treatment

There are no comparative controlled studies of treatment length in European late LNB. A recent American open-label randomized comparison (Class III) of 14 days vs. 28 days treatment with ceftriaxone (2 g daily) for late Lyme borreliosis (143 patients, of whom a third with neurological symptoms) showed similar cure rates (76% and 70%, respectively) after 1 year, and there were more discontinuations due to adverse events in the 28-day group [106]. Another series (Class IV) of late LNB showed disappearance of symptoms in 69 of 79 (87%) after a 100-day regimen with various antibiotics, whereas 14 days with ceftriaxone cured 4 of 13 (31%) [107].

Recommendations

- Adult patients with definite or possible late LNB with peripheral neuropathy and ACA should be treated with oral doxycycline (200 mg daily) or i.v. ceftriaxone (2 g daily) for 3 weeks (not enough evidence: good practice point).
- Adult patients with definite or possible late LNB with CNS manifestations (myelitis, encephalitis, vasculitis) should be treated with i.v. ceftriaxone (2 g daily) for 3 weeks (not enough evidence: clinical practice point).

Clinical course after treatment

Most studies report marked improvement of demonstrable neurological abnormalities within weeks to a few months after 10–14 days' antibiotic treatment. Symptoms and mild pleocytosis may however persist for several months. Relapses or treatment failures (defined as loss of significant improvement) are very rare.

Disabling neurological sequelae were found in 12% of patients after 12 months' follow-up [108], and in 5% after 33 months' follow-up [3]. They were more frequent in patients with CNS manifestations or long duration of symptoms before treatment [8, 10, 24, 41, 43, 52] (Class III). Persistent or new subjective complaints (concentration or memory problems, headache, fatigue, myalgias and paraesthesiae) may be more common [109, 110] (Class IV). When taking both objective and subjective complaints into consideration, complete recovery was achieved in 41% of patients after 4 months [11], in 61–72% after 6–9 months [95, 108], in 50–70% after 12 months [14, 108, 110] and in 50–90% after 5 years [92, 108, 109, 110]. However, the studies are hampered by ill-defined outcome measures and lack of control groups. One Swedish study found persistent complaints 2.5 years post-treatment in 50% of patients who had experienced neuroborreliosis as compared to 16% in control patients who had experienced erythema migrans [111].

Post-Lyme disease syndrome

If subjective complaints or symptoms (fatigue, paraesthesiae, difficulty in sleeping, cognitive impairment, headache, arthralgia, myalgia) persist for more than 6 months after standard treatment of LNB or other clearly defined

Lyme disease manifestations, the condition is often termed post-Lyme disease syndrome (PLDS) [112].

American trials have demonstrated that additional prolonged antimicrobial treatment is ineffective in PLDS [113–116] . A regimen of i.v. ceftriaxone for 30 days followed by 60 days of oral doxycycline was no more beneficial than placebo on health-related quality of life as measured by SF-36 [115] (Class I) or cognitive functioning [114] (Class II) in 78 seropositive and 51 seronegative PLDS patients. Of note, placebo-treated patients had a 36% improvement on SF-36 scores. Another Class I study [116] of 55 patients randomized to receive a 28-day course of i.v. ceftriaxone or i.v. placebo showed a higher reduction in fatigue score in the ceftriaxone group after 6 months follow-up, but the groups did not differ in the other primary endpoint (mental speed) or in secondary endpoints (e.g., a scale for fatigue and pain, SF 36, self-reported depression and various cognitive functions). Four severe adverse events occurred: one case of anaphylaxis (the ceftriaxone group) and three cases of sepsis (the placebo group). The effect on fatigue may have been due to the placebo effect since more patients in the ceftriaxone group guessed their correct assignment. In the most recent study [113] (Class I), a small selection of PLDS patients with objective memory impairment (encephalopathy) were randomized to 10 weeks of i.v. ceftriaxone (23 patients) or placebo (14 patients), and compared with 18 healthy control patients. At week 12 there was a moderate improvement on a calculated aggregate of neuropsychological measures in favour of the ceftriaxone-treated patients, but the effect was not sustained to week 24.

Recommendations

Antibiotic therapy has no impact on PLDS (Level A).

Paediatric neuroborreliosis

One Austrian Class II study suggests similar effect of 14 days i.v. penicillin as compared to 14 days i.v. ceftriaxone in acute paediatric LNB [117]. Several European Class III and IV studies suggest good response to 10–14-day

courses of i.v. penicillin, ceftriaxone, cefotaxime and oral doxycycline [3, 53, 118, 119]. There are no data to suggest a better response to i.v. than oral treatment. However, in most countries doxycycline is not recommended in children under 8 years of age since it may cause staining of the teeth. Nevertheless, recent data suggest that this may be less common than previously thought and that it can be prevented by avoiding sunlight [120, 121]. There are no data to suggest treatment duration longer than 14 days in paediatric patients with CNS manifestations or late LNB.

As in adults, 11–22% of paediatric LNB patients have neurological sequelae (mostly facial palsy) after treatment [23, 119]. In a recent prospective follow-up study of 177 Swedish children evaluated for LNB, persisting unspecific symptoms (mainly headache and fatigue) at 6 months were not more frequent in patients than in controls. Another Swedish series of 203 children with LNB treated for 10 days with i.v. penicillin (53), ceftriaxone (109), cefotaxime (19) or oral doxycycline (22) showed resolution of symptoms and signs in 58% by the end of treatment in 92% by two months and in 100% by 6 months [119] (Class IV).

In an American study of 43 children with facial palsy attributable to Lyme and treated with i.v. ceftriaxone (16%) or oral doxycycline or amoxicillin (84%), 79% reported to be cured after an average of 49 months' follow-up. The frequency of self-reported problems with normal daily activities was similar in patients and age-matched controls [122].

Recommendations

Paediatric patients with definite or possible early LNB with symptoms confined to the meninges, cranial nerves, nerve roots or peripheral nerves (Bannwarth syndrome) should be offered a single 14-day course of antibiotic treatment:

- Oral doxycycline i.v. penicillin, i.v. ceftriaxone or i.v. cefotaxime are effective and safe treatments (Level B).

- Oral doxycycline (200 mg daily) and i.v. ceftriaxone (2 g daily) for 14 days are equally effective (Level B). The advantages of doxycycline are the oral route of administration and lower costs. Doxycycline is contraindicated in those < 8 years (in some countries 9 years).

- Paediatric patients with CNS manifestations (myelitis, encephalitis, vasculitis) should be treated with i.v. ceftriaxone (2 g daily) for 14 days (not enough evidence: good practice point).

Conflicts of interest

Åse Mygland, Unn Ljøstad, Tobias Rupprecht, Volker Fingerle and Israel Steiner have no conflicts of interest.

Erich Schmutzhard has received fees or grants from Novo Nordisk, Bayer, Actelion, KCI and ALSIUS.

Acknowledgement

The authors would like to extend warm thanks to Professor Peter Kennedy, former chair of this EFNS Infection Panel, for his leadership in conceiving and setting up the original Neuroborreliosis Task Force.

References

1. Aguero-Rosenfeld, ME, Wang, G, Schwartz, I, Wormser, GP. Diagnosis of Lyme borreliosis. *Clin Microbiol Rev* 2005; **18**:484–509.

2. Lebech, AM, Hansen, K, Brandrup, F, *et al.* Diagnostic value of PCR for detection of *Borrelia burgdorferi* DNA in clinical specimens from patients with erythema migrans and Lyme neuroborreliosis. *Mol Diagn* 2000; **5**:139–50.

3. Hansen, K, Lebech, AM. The clinical and epidemiological profile of Lyme neuroborreliosis in Denmark 1985–1990. A prospective study of 187 patients with *Borrelia burgdorferi* specific intrathecal antibody production. *Brain* 1992; **115** (Pt 2):399–423.

4. Ljøstad, U, Skarpaas, T, Mygland, A. Clinical usefulness of intrathecal antibody testing in acute Lyme neuroborreliosis. *Eur J Neurol* 2007; **14**:873–6.

5. Blanc, F, Jaulhac, B, Fleury, M, *et al.* Relevance of the antibody index to diagnose Lyme neuroborreliosis among seropositive patients. *Neurology* 2007; **69**:953–8.

6. Hammers-Berggren, S, Hansen, K, Lebech, AM, Karlsson, M. *Borrelia burgdorferi*-specific intrathecal antibody production in neuroborreliosis: a follow-up study. *Neurology* 1993; **43**:169–75.

7. Kruger, H, Reuss, K, Pulz, M, *et al.* Meningoradiculitis and encephalomyelitis due to *Borrelia burgdorferi*: a follow-up study of 72 patients over 27 years. *J Neurol* 1989; **236**: 322–8.

8. Halperin, JJ, Shapiro, ED, Logigian, E, *et al.* Practice parameter: treatment of nervous system Lyme disease (an evidence-based review): report of the Quality Standards Subcommittee of the American Academy of Neurology. *Neurology* 2007; **69**:91–102.

9. Wormser, GP, Dattwyler, RJ, Shapiro, ED, *et al.* The clinical assessment, treatment, and prevention of Lyme disease, human granulocytic anaplasmosis, and babesiosis: clinical practice guidelines by the Infectious Diseases Society of America. *Clin Infect Dis* 2006; **43**:1089–134.

10. Brainin, M, Barnes, M, Baron, JC, *et al.* Guidance for the preparation of neurological management guidelines by EFNS scientific task forces – revised recommendations 2004. *Eur J Neurol* 2004; **11**:577–81.

11. Ljøstad, U, Skogvoll, E, Eikeland, R, *et al.* Oral doxycycline versus intravenous ceftriaxone for European Lyme neuroborreliosis: a multicentre, non-inferiority, double-blind, randomised trial. *Lancet Neurol* 2008; **7**:690–5.

12. Oschmann, P, Dorndorf, W, Hornig, C, *et al.* Stages and syndromes of neuroborreliosis. *J Neurol* 1998; **245**: 262–72.

13. Kruger, H, Kohlhepp, W, Konig, S. Follow-up of antibiotically treated and untreated neuroborreliosis. *Acta Neurol Scand* 1990; **82**:59–67.

14. Kohlhepp, W, Oschmann, P, Mertens, HG. Treatment of Lyme borreliosis. Randomized comparison of doxycycline and penicillin G. *J Neurol* 1989; **236**:464–9.

15. Charles, V, Duprez, TP, Kabamba, B, *et al.* Poliomyelitis-like syndrome with matching magnetic resonance features in a case of Lyme neuroborreliosis. *J Neurol Neurosurg Psychiatry* 2007; **78**:1160–1.

16. Topakian, R, Stieglbauer, K, Nussbaumer, K, Aichner, FT. Cerebral vasculitis and stroke in Lyme neuroborreliosis. Two case reports and review of current knowledge. *Cerebrovasc Dis* 2008; **26**:455–61.

17. Logigian, EL, Kaplan, RF, Steere, AC. Chronic neurologic manifestations of Lyme disease. *N Engl J Med* 1990; **323**: 1438–44.

18. Pfister, HW, Rupprecht, TA. Clinical aspects of neuroborreliosis and post-Lyme disease syndrome in adult patients. *Int J Med Microbiol* 2006; **296**(Suppl. 40):11–16.

19. Kindstrand, E, Nilsson, BY, Hovmark, A, *et al.* Peripheral neuropathy in acrodermatitis chronica atrophicans – a late Borrelia manifestation. *Acta Neurol Scand* 1997; **95**: 338–45.

20. Halperin, J, Luft, BJ, Volkman, DJ, Dattwyler, RJ. Lyme neuroborreliosis. Peripheral nervous system manifestations. *Brain* 1990; **113**:1207–21.

21. Mygland, A, Skarpaas, T, Ljøstad, U. Chronic polyneuropathy and Lyme disease. *Eur J Neurol* 2006; **13**:1213–15.

22. Christen, HJ. Lyme neuroborreliosis in children. *Ann Med* 1996; **28**:235–40.

23. Skogman, BH, Croner, S, Nordwall, M, *et al.* Lyme neuroborreliosis in children: a prospective study of clinical features, prognosis, and outcome. *Pediatr Infect Dis J* 2008; **27**:1089–94.

24. Huisman, TA, Wohlrab, G, Nadal, D, *et al.* Unusual presentations of neuroborreliosis (Lyme disease) in childhood. *J Comput Assist Tomogr* 1999; **23**:39–42.

25. Wilke, M, Eiffert, H, Christen, HJ, Hanefeld, F. Primarily chronic and cerebrovascular course of Lyme neuroborreliosis: case reports and literature review. *Arch Dis Child* 2000; **83**:67–71.

26. Vukelic, D, Bozinovic, D, Morovic, M, *et al.* Opsoclonus-myoclonus syndrome in a child with neuroborreliosis. *J Infect* 2000; **40**:189–91.

27. Ylitalo, V, Hagberg, BA. Progressive ataxia in Swedish children: a re-evaluation study. *Acta Neurol Scand* 1994; **89**:299–302.

28. Strle, F, Ruzic-Sabljic, E, Cimperman, J, *et al.* Comparison of findings for patients with Borrelia garinii and Borrelia afzelii isolated from cerebrospinal fluid. *Clin Infect Dis* 2006; **43**:704–10.

29. Marcus, LC, Steere, AC, Duray, PH, *et al.* Fatal pancarditis in a patient with coexistent Lyme disease and babesiosis. Demonstration of spirochetes in the myocardium. *Ann Intern Med* 1985; **103**:374–6.

30. Reimers, CD, de Koning, J, Neubert, U, *et al.* Borrelia burgdorferi myositis: report of eight patients. *J Neurol* 1993; **240**:278–83.

31. Aberer, E, Duray, PH. Morphology of *Borrelia burgdorferi*: structural patterns of cultured borreliae in relation to staining methods. *J Clin Microbiol* 1991; **2:** 764–72.

32. Zelger, B, Eisendle, K, Mensing, C, Zelger, B. Detection of spirochetal micro-organisms by focus-floating microscopy in necrobiotic xanthogranuloma. *J Am Acad Dermatol* 2007; **57**:1026–30.

33. Dumler, JS. Molecular diagnosis of Lyme disease: review and meta-analysis. *Mol Diagn* 2001; **6**:1–11.

34. Schmidt, BL. PCR in laboratory diagnosis of human *Borrelia burgdorferi* infections. *Clin Microbiol Rev* 1997; **10**:185–201.

35. Cerar, T, Ogrinc, K, Cimperman, J, *et al.* Validation of cultivation and PCR methods for diagnosis of Lyme neuroborreliosis. *J Clin Microbiol* 2008; **46**:3375–9.

36. Rauter, C, Mueller, M, Diterich, I, *et al.* Critical evaluation of urine-based PCR assay for diagnosis of Lyme borreliosis. *Clin Diagn Lab Immunol* 2005; **12**:910–17.

37. Brettschneider, S, Bruckbauer, H, Klugbauer, N, Hofmann, H. Diagnostic value of PCR for detection of *Borrelia burgdorferi* in skin biopsy and urine samples from patients with skin borreliosis. *J Clin Microbiol* 1998; **36**:2658–65.

38. Goodman, JL, Jurkovich, P, Kramber, JM, Johnson, RC. Molecular detection of persistent *Borrelia burgdorferi* in the urine of patients with active Lyme disease. *Infect Immun* 1991; **59**:269–78.

39. Wilske, B, Fingerle, V, Schulte-Spechtel, U. Microbiological and serological diagnosis of Lyme borreliosis. *FEMS Immunol Med Microbiol* 2007; **49**:13–21.

40. Arnez, M, Ruzic-Sabljic, E, Ahcan, J, *et al.* Isolation of *Borrelia burgdorferi* sensu lato from blood of children with solitary erythema migrans. *Pediatr Infect Dis J* 2001; **20**:251–5.

41. Barbour, AG. Isolation and cultivation of Lyme disease spirochetes. *Yale J Biol Med* 1984; **57**:521–5.

42. Preac, MV, Wilske, B, Schierz, G, *et al.* Repeated isolation of spirochetes from the cerebrospinal fluid of a patient with meningoradiculitis Bannwarth. *Eur J Clin Microbiol* 1984; **3**:564–5.

43. Zore, A, Ruzic-Sabljic, E, Maraspin, V, *et al.* Sensitivity of culture and polymerase chain reaction for the etiologic diagnosis of erythema migrans. *Wien Klin Wochenschr* 2002; **114**:606–9.

44. Greene, RT, Walker, RL, Greene, CE. Pseudospirochetes in animal blood being cultured for *Borrelia burgdorferi*. *J Vet Diagn Invest* 1991; **3**:350–2.

45. Panelius, J, Lahdenne, P, Saxen, H, *et al.* Diagnosis of Lyme neuroborreliosis with antibodies to recombinant proteins DbpA, BBK32, and OspC, and VlsE IR6 peptide. *J Neurol* 2003; **250**:1318–27.

46. Riesbeck, K, Hammas, B. Comparison of an automated Borrelia indirect chemiluminescent immunoassay (CLIA) with a VlsE/C6 ELISA and Immunoblot. *Eur J Clin Microbiol Infect Dis* 2007; **26**:517–19.

47. Skarpaas, T, Ljostad, U, Sobye, M., Mygland, A. Sensitivity and specificity of a commercial C6 peptide enzyme immuno assay in diagnosis of acute Lyme neuroborreliosis. *Eur J Clin Microbiol Infect Dis* 2007; **26**:675–7.

48. Tjernberg, I, Schon, T, Ernerudh, J, *et al.* C6-peptide serology as a diagnostic tool in neuroborreliosis. *APMIS* 2008; **116**:393–9.

49. Vermeersch, P, Resseler, S, Nackers, E, Lagrou, K. The C6 Lyme antibody test has low sensitivity for antibody detection in cerebrospinal fluid. *Diagn Microbiol Infect Dis* 2009; **64**(3):347–9.

50. Centers for Disease Control and Prevention (CDC). Recommendations for test performance and interpretation from the Second National Conference on Serologic Diagnosis of Lyme Disease. *MMWR Morb Mortal Wkly Rep* 1995; **44**:590–591.

51. Brouqui, P, Bacellar, F, Baranton, G, *et al.* Guidelines for the diagnosis of tick-borne bacterial diseases in Europe. *Clin Microbiol Infect* 2004; **10**:1108–32.

52. Johnson, BJ, Robbins, KE, Bailey, RE, *et al.* Serodiagnosis of Lyme disease: accuracy of a two-step approach using a flagella-based ELISA and immunoblotting. *J Infect Dis* 1996; **174**:346–53.

53. Christen, HJ, Hanefeld, F, Eiffert, H, Thomssen, R. Epidemiology and clinical manifestations of Lyme borreliosis in childhood. A prospective multicentre study with

special regard to neuroborreliosis. *Acta Paediatr Suppl* 1993; **386**:1–75.

54. Hansen, K, Lebech, AM. Lyme neuroborreliosis: a new sensitive diagnostic assay for intrathecal synthesis of *Borrelia burgdorferi* – specific immunoglobulin G, A, and M. *Ann Neurol* 1991; **30**:197–205.

55. Ljostad, U, Mygland, A. CSF B – lymphocyte chemoattractant (CXCL13) in the early diagnosis of acute Lyme neuroborreliosis. *J Neurol* 2008; **255**:732–7.

56. Rupprecht, TA, Pfister, HW, Angele, B, *et al.* The chemokine CXCL13 (BLC): a putative diagnostic marker for neuroborreliosis. *Neurology* 2005; **65**:448–50.

57. Rupprecht, TA, Kirschning, CJ, Popp, B, *et al.* Borrelia garinii induces CXCL13 production in human monocytes through Toll-like receptor 2. *Infect Immun* 2007; **75**:4351–6.

58. Coyle, PK, Schutzer, SE, Deng, Z, *et al.* Detection of *Borrelia burgdorferi*-specific antigen in antibody-negative cerebrospinal fluid in neurologic Lyme disease. *Neurology* 1995; **45**:2010–15.

59. Dorward, DW, Schwan, TG, Garon, CF. Immune capture and detection of *Borrelia burgdorferi* antigens in urine, blood, or tissues from infected ticks, mice, dogs, and humans. *J Clin Microbiol* 1991; **29**:1162–70.

60. Hyde, FW, Johnson, RC, White, TJ, Shelburne, CE. Detection of antigens in urine of mice and humans infected with *Borrelia burgdorferi*, etiologic agent of Lyme disease. *J Clin Microbiol* 1989; **27**:58–61.

61. Klempner, MS, Schmid, CH, Hu, L, *et al.* Intralaboratory reliability of serologic and urine testing for Lyme disease. *Am J Med* 2001; **110**:217–19.

62. Burkot, TR, Patrican, L, Piesman, J. Field trial of an outer surface protein A (OspA) antigen-capture enzyme-linked immunosorbent assay (ELISA) to detect *Borrelia burgdorferi* in Ixodes scapularis. *Am J Trop Med Hyg* 1994; **50**:354–8.

63. Brunner, M, Sigal, LH. Use of serum immune complexes in a new test that accurately confirms early Lyme disease and active infection with *Borrelia burgdorferi*. *J Clin Microbiol* 2001; **39**:3213–21.

64. Coyle, PK, Schutzer, SE, Belman, AL, *et al.* Cerebrospinal fluid immune complexes in patients exposed to *Borrelia burgdorferi*: detection of Borrelia-specific and nonspecific complexes. *Ann Neurol* 1990; **28**:739–44.

65. Hardin, JA, Steere, AC, Malawista, SE. Immune complexes and the evolution of Lyme arthritis. Dissemination and localization of abnormal C1q binding activity. *N Engl J Med* 1979; **301**:1358–63.

66. Schutzer, SE, Coyle, PK, Belman, AL, *et al.* Sequestration of antibody to *Borrelia burgdorferi* in immune complexes in seronegative Lyme disease. *Lancet* 1990; **335**:312–15.

67. Marques, AR, Hornung, RL, Dally, L, Philipp, MT. Detection of immune complexes is not independent of detection of antibodies in Lyme disease patients and does not confirm active infection with *Borrelia burgdorferi*. *Clin Diagn Lab Immunol* 2005; **12**:1036–40.

68. Dressler, F, Yoshinari, NH, Steere, AC. The T-cell proliferative assay in the diagnosis of Lyme disease. *Ann Intern Med* 1991; **115**:533–9.

69. Huppertz, HI, Mosbauer, S, Busch, DH, Karch, H. Lymphoproliferative responses to *Borrelia burgdorferi* in the diagnosis of Lyme arthritis in children and adolescents. *Eur J Pediatr* 1996; **155**:297–302.

70. Krause, A, Rensing, A, Kalden, JR, Burmester, GR. Cellular immune response to *Borrelia burgdorferi* in patients with Lyme borreliosis. *Behring Inst Mitt* 1991; **88**:52–8.

71. Kruger, H, Pulz, M, Martin, R, Sticht-Groh, V. Long-term persistence of specific T- and B-lymphocyte responses to *Borrelia burgdorferi* following untreated neuroborreliosis. *Infection* 1990; **18**:263–7.

72. Valentine-Thon, E, Ilsemann, K, Sandkamp, M. A novel lymphocyte transformation test (LTT-MELISA) for Lyme borreliosis. *Diagn Microbiol Infect Dis* 2007; **57**:27–34.

73. Alban, PS, Johnson, PW, Nelson, DR. Serum-starvation-induced changes in protein synthesis and morphology of Borrelia burgdorferi. *Microbiology* 2000; **146**(Pt 1): 119–27.

74. Brorson, O, Brorson, SH. Transformation of cystic forms of *Borrelia burgdorferi* to normal, mobile spirochetes. *Infection* 1997; **25**:240–6.

75. Gruntar, I, Malovrh, T, Murgia, R, Cinco, M. Conversion of Borrelia garinii cystic forms to motile spirochetes in vivo. *APMIS* 2001; **109**,:383–8.

76. Murgia, R, Cinco, M. Induction of cystic forms by different stress conditions in *Borrelia burgdorferi*. *APMIS* 2004; **112**:57–62.

77. Stricker, RB, Winger, EE. Decreased CD57 lymphocyte subset in patients with chronic Lyme disease. *Immunol Lett* 2001; **76**:43–8.

78. Marques, A, Brown, MR, Fleisher, TA. Natural killer cell counts are not different between patients with post-Lyme disease syndrome and controls. *Clin Vaccine Immunol* 2009; **16**:1249–50.

79. Stanek, G, O'Connell, S, Cimmino, M, *et al.* European Union Concerted Action on Risk Assessment in Lyme Borreliosis: clinical case definitions for Lyme borreliosis. *Wien Klin Wochenschr* 1996; **108**:741–7.

80. Hansen, K, Cruz, M, Link, H. Oligoclonal *Borrelia burgdorferi*-specific IgG antibodies in cerebrospinal fluid in Lyme neuroborreliosis. *J Infect Dis* 1990; **161**: 1194–202.

81. Picha, D, Moravcova, L, Zdarsky, E, Benes, J. Clinical comparison of immunoblot and antibody index for detection of intrathecal synthesis of specific antibodies in Lyme neuroborreliosis. *Eur J Clin Microbiol Infect Dis* 2000; **19**:805–6.

82. Steere, AC, Berardi, VP, Weeks, KE, *et al*. Evaluation of the intrathecal antibody response to *Borrelia burgdorferi* as a diagnostic test for Lyme neuroborreliosis. *J Infect Dis* 1990; **161**:1203–9.

83. Stiernstedt, GT, Granstrom, M, Hederstedt, B, Skoldenberg, B. Diagnosis of spirochetal meningitis by enzyme-linked immunosorbent assay and indirect immunofluorescence assay in serum and cerebrospinal fluid. *J Clin Microbiol* 1985; **21**:819–25.

84. Tumani, H, Nolker, G, Reiber, H. Relevance of cerebrospinal fluid variables for early diagnosis of neuroborreliosis. *Neurology* 1995; **45**:1663–70.

85. Centers for Disease Control and Prevention (CDC). Case definitions for infectious conditions under public health surveillance. Centers for Disease Control and Prevention. *MMWR Recomm Rep* 1997; **46**:1–55.

86. Skoldenberg, B, Stiernstedt, G, Garde, A, *et al*. Chronic meningitis caused by a penicillin-sensitive microorganism? *Lancet* 1983; **2**:75–8.

87. Steere, AC, Pachner, AR, Malawista, SE. Neurologic abnormalities of Lyme disease: successful treatment with high-dose intravenous penicillin. *Ann Intern Med* 1983; **99**:767–72.

88. Dattwyler, RJ, Halperin, JJ, Volkman, DJ, Luft, BJ. Treatment of late Lyme borreliosis – randomised comparison of ceftriaxone and penicillin. *Lancet* 1988; **1**:1191–4.

89. Hassler, D, Zoller, L, Haude, M. Cefotaxime versus penicillin in the late stage of Lyme disease – prospective, randomized therapeutic study. *Infection* 1990; **18**:16–20.

90. Pfister, HW, Preac-Mursic, V, Wilske, B, Einhaupl, KM. Cefotaxime vs penicillin G for acute neurologic manifestations in Lyme borreliosis. A prospective randomized study. *Arch Neurol* 1989; **46**:1190–4.

91. Pfister, HW, Preac-Mursic, V, Wilske, B, *et al*. Randomized comparison of ceftriaxone and cefotaxime in Lyme neuroborreliosis. *J Infect Dis* 1991; **163**:311–18.

92. Karlsson, M, Hammers-Berggren, S, Lindquist, L, *et al*. Comparison of intravenous penicillin G and oral doxycycline for treatment of Lyme neuroborreliosis. *Neurology* 1994; **44**:1203–7.

93. Dotevall, L, Hagberg, L. Successful oral doxycycline treatment of Lyme disease-associated facial palsy and meningitis. *Clin Infect Dis* 1999; **28**:569–74.

94. Karkkonen, K, Stiernstedt, SH, Karlsson, M. Follow-up of patients treated with oral doxycycline for Lyme neuroborreliosis. *Scand J Infect Dis* 2001; **33**:259–62.

95. Borg, R, Dotevall, L, Hagberg, L, *et al*. Intravenous ceftriaxone compared with oral doxycycline for the treatment of Lyme neuroborreliosis. *Scand J Infect Dis* 2005; **37**:449–54.

96. Ogrinc, K, Logar, M, Lotric-Furlan, S, *et al*. Doxycycline versus ceftriaxone for the treatment of patients with chronic Lyme borreliosis. *Wien Klin Wochenschr* 2006; **118**:696–701.

97. Oksi, J, Nikoskelainen, J, Viljanen, MK. Comparison of oral cefixime and intravenous ceftriaxone followed by oral amoxicillin in disseminated Lyme borreliosis. *Eur J Clin Microbiol Infect Dis* 1998; **17**:715–19.

98. Agger, WA, Callister, SM, Jobe, DA. *In vitro* susceptibilities of *Borrelia burgdorferi* to five oral cephalosporins and ceftriaxone. *Antimicrob Agents Chemother* 1992; **36**:1788–90.

99. Karlsson, M, Hammers, S, Nilsson-Ehle, I, *et al*. Concentrations of doxycycline and penicillin G in sera and cerebrospinal fluid of patients treated for neuroborreliosis. *Antimicrob Agents Chemother* 1996; **40**:1104–7.

100. Oksi, J, Nikoskelainen, J, Hiekkanen, H, *et al*. Duration of antibiotic treatment in disseminated Lyme borreliosis: a double-blind, randomized, placebo-controlled, multicenter clinical study. *Eur J Clin Microbiol Infect Dis* 2007; **26**:571–81.

101. May, EF, Jabbari, B. Stroke in neuroborreliosis. *Stroke* 1990; **21**:1232–5.

102. Peter, L, Jung, J, Tilikete, C, *et al*. Opsoclonus-myoclonus as a manifestation of Lyme disease. *J Neurol Neurosurg Psychiatry* 2006; **77**:1090–1.

103. Skeie, GO, Eldoen, G, Skeie, BS, *et al*. Opsoclonus myoclonus syndrome in two cases with neuroborreliosis. *Eur J Neurol* 2007; **14**:e1–e2.

104. Gyllenborg, J, Milea, D. Ocular flutter as the first manifestation of Lyme disease. *Neurology* 2009; **72**:291.

105. Kindstrand, E, Nilsson, BY, Hovmark, A, *et al*. Peripheral neuropathy in acrodermatitis chronica atrophicans – effect of treatment. *Acta Neurol Scand* 2002; **106**:253–7.

106. Dattwyler, R.J., Wormser, G.P., Rush, T.J., *et al*. A comparison of two treatment regimens of ceftriaxone in late Lyme disease. *Wien Klin Wochenschr* 2005; **117**:393–7.

107. Wahlberg, P, Granlund, H, Nyman, D, *et al*. Treatment of late Lyme borreliosis. *J Infect* 1994; **29**:255–61.

108. Berglund, J, Stjernberg, L, Ornstein, K, *et al*. 5-year Follow-up study of patients with neuroborreliosis. *Scand J Infect Dis* 2002; **34**:421–5.

109. Ljostad, U, Mygland, A, Skarpaas, T. Neuroborreliosis in Vest-Agder. *Tidsskr Nor Laegeforen* 2003; **123**:610–13.

110. Treib, J, Fernandez, A, Haass, A, *et al*. Clinical and serologic follow-up in patients with neuroborreliosis. *Neurology* 1998; **51**:1489–91.

111. Vrethem, M, Hellblom, L, Widlund, M, *et al*. Chronic symptoms are common in patients with neuroborreliosis – a questionnaire follow-up study. *Acta Neurol Scand* 2002; **106**:205–8.

112. Feder, HM, Jr, Johnson, BJ, O'Connell, S, *et al*. A critical appraisal of 'chronic Lyme disease'. *N Engl J Med* 2007; **357**:1422–30.

113. Fallon, BA, Keilp, JG, Corbera, KM, *et al*. A randomized, placebo-controlled trial of repeated IV antibiotic therapy for Lyme encephalopathy. *Neurology* 2008; **70**:992–1003.

114. Kaplan, RF, Trevino, RP, Johnson, GM, *et al*. Cognitive function in post-treatment Lyme disease: do additional antibiotics help? *Neurology* 2003; **60**:1916–22.

115. Klempner, MS, Hu, LT, Evans, J, *et al*. Two controlled trials of antibiotic treatment in patients with persistent symptoms and a history of Lyme disease. *N Engl J Med* 2001; **345**:85–92.

116. Krupp, LB, Hyman, LG, Grimson, R, *et al*. Study and treatment of post-Lyme disease (STOP-LD): a randomized double masked clinical trial. *Neurology* 2003; **60**: 1923–30.

117. Mullegger, RR, Millner, MM, Stanek, G, Spork, KD. Penicillin G sodium and ceftriaxone in the treatment of neuroborreliosis in children – a prospective study. *Infection* 1991; **19**:279–83.

118. Krbkova, L, Stanek, G. Therapy of Lyme borreliosis in children. *Infection* 1996; **24**:170–3.

119. Thorstrand, C, Belfrage, E, Bennet, R, *et al*. Successful treatment of neuroborreliosis with ten day regimens. *Pediatr Infect Dis J* 2002; **21**:1142–5.

120. Ayaslioglu, E, Erkek, E, Oba, AA, Cebecioglu, E. Doxycycline-induced staining of permanent adult dentition. *Aust Dent J* 2005; **50**:273–5.

121. Volovitz, B, Shkap, R, Amir, J, *et al*. Absence of tooth staining with doxycycline treatment in young children. *Clin Pediatr (Phila)*, 2007; **46**:121–6.

122. Vazquez, M, Sparrow, SS, Shapiro, ED. Long-term neuropsychologic and health outcomes of children with facial nerve palsy attributable to Lyme disease. *Pediatrics* 2003; **112**:e93–e97.

CHAPTER 13

Disease-specific cerebrospinal fluid investigations

F. Deisenhammer,[1] R. Egg,[1] G. Giovannoni,[2] B. Hemmer,[3] A. Petzold,[4] F. Sellebjerg,[5] C. Teunissen[6] and H. Tumani[7]

[1]Innsbruck Medical University, Innsbruck, Austria; [2]Barts and The London School of Medicine and Dentistry, London, UK; [3]Technische Universität München, Munich, Germany; [4]University College London, London, UK; [5]Copenhagen University Hospital, Copenhagen, Denmark; [6]VUmc, Amsterdam, The Netherlands; [7]Universität Ulm, Ulm, Germany

Introduction

Investigation of the cerebrospinal fluid (CSF) in neurological diseases has a long history and a small number of molecules have become the standard repertoire in routine CSF work-up such as total protein, glucose, cell count and differentiation, as well as quantitative and qualitative detection of immunoglobulins [1]. In recent years, the search for biomarkers – a characteristic that is objectively measured and evaluated as an indicator of normal biological, pathogenic or pharmacological responses to a therapeutic intervention, as defined by the Biomarkers Definition Working Group [2] – in body fluids, including the CSF, has increased substantially. In addition to the guidelines on routine CSF investigations [1], we wanted to evaluate newer CSF markers with respect to their disease specificity or prognostic relevance.

Search strategy

Tau protein, amyloid β, 14-3-3 and myelin basic protein

PubMed was searched up to January 2008 for keywords including 'CSF', 'tau', 'amyloid', '14-3-3', 'myelin basic

protein' and 'mbp', which yielded 1785 hits. Only papers in English and relating to adult clinical neurology were considered for further analysis.

Hypocretin

A Medline search using the search terms cerebrospinal fluid (CSF), narcolepsy, sleep disorder, hypocretin and orexin was conducted. The search was limited to the time between 1 January 1980 and 1 May 2008. The key words were cross-referenced as follows: ('cerebrospinal fluid' or 'CSF') AND ('hypocretin or orexin') AND ('narcolepsy OR sleep disorder OR cataplexy'). The search returned 73 documents. Abstracts that did not primarily deal with human sleep disorders, case reports, reviews, comments and original articles that were not published in English were excluded. The remaining 13 articles were further analysed.

β₂-Transferrin

Using (Cerebrospinal fluid OR CSF) and (beta 2 transferrin) and (otorrhea OR otorrhoea OR rhinorrhoea OR rhinorrhea) NOT beta trace resulted in 60 abstracts. Reviews and reports not dealing with diagnostic issues or with fluids other than CSF were excluded resulting in 42 articles.

Beta trace protein (prostaglandin D synthase)

(Beta-trace protein OR Prostaglandin D Synthase) and (otorrhea OR otorrhoea OR rhinorrhoea OR rhinorrhea) NOT beta 2 transferrin resulted in 16 abstracts.

Vascular endothelial growth factor

PubMed Search for ('VEGF' OR 'vascular endothelial growth factor') AND 'CSF'; limits: 1980 until May 2008, language German or English, reports on humans resulted in 51 abstracts. Of those four reviews, 21 papers not related to diagnostic VEGF testing in CSF, and four paediatric reports were excluded. The remaining 22 papers were included for evaluation.

Neurofilaments

PubMed was searched up to January 2008 for keywords including CSF, neurofilament (Nf) and patients, which yielded 91 hits. Articles dealing with adult patients were included (children excluded). Articles excluded were: articles focusing on anti-Nf antibodies, serum analysis only, animal studies, reviews, case reports or method description, rather than biomarker investigation in patients, animal studies and articles that were not in English.

Evidence was classified as class I–IV and recommendations as level A–C according to the scheme agreed for the European Federation of Neurological Societies (EFNS) guidelines [3], with class I and level A being the strongest classes of evidence/recommendation.

At a conference held in March 2006, various potential CSF biomarkers and methods of detection were discussed by the members of the taskforce, including CSF proteomics, markers of axonal damage focusing on different subsets of Nfs, neurotransmitters, autoantibodies, anti-neural antibodies, ferritin, amyloid β (Aβ), tau and hyperphosphorylated tau, 14-3-3 protein, myelin basic protein, sulfatid, β_2-transferrin, VEGF and S-100. Of those, only the markers discussed below were felt to be sufficiently relevant to receive further attention for the current report.

The Cochrane database and guideline papers of the American Academy of Neurology (AAN) were searched for all above topics. No relevant publication was found.

CSF markers recommended for use in clinical routine

Tau protein and amyloid β peptide

Tau proteins are microtubule-associated proteins important for the maintenance of axonal microtubules. Hyperphosporylated tau (P-tau) is present in neuritic tangles in Alzheimer's disease (AD). Amyloid β (Aβ) peptides are derived from cleavage of the amyloid precursor protein by β- and γ-secretases, resulting in the $A\beta_{1-40}$ and $A\beta_{1-42}$ peptide fragments. $A\beta_{1-42}$ has a strong tendency to aggregate, and is a major component of amyloid plaques in AD. Increased CSF concentrations of tau and P-tau, and low CSF concentrations of $A\beta_{1-42}$ are typical findings in AD, have been reviewed by a task force of the World Federation of Societies of Biological Psychiatry, and have been incorporated in the latest research criteria for the diagnosis of AD [4–7]. Tau proteins and Aβ peptides can be easily measured by commercially available sandwich ELISA (enzyme-linked immunosorbent assay), but Aβ measurements should be interpreted with some caution (see below).

At a specificity of 90%, the sensitivity for AD according to clinical criteria of the most commonly used tau immunoassay is approximately 80%, and the sensitivity of $A\beta_{1-42}$ is 80–90% (class I) [4]. The sensitivity for the diagnosis of AD of P-tau assays, based on immunoassays recognizing tau phosphorylated on different serine and threonine residues, is more variable (class II) [4, 8, 9]. The combination of tau and $A\beta_{1-42}$ has been assessed in several studies, and has been found to give a high sensitivity and specificity against normal ageing and psychiatric disorders, whereas the specificity against other diseases is lower (class II) [10, 11]. Increases in tau and low $A\beta_{1-42}$ concentrations are also found in stroke, trauma and other diseases with a neurodegenerative component (Table 13.1). However, at least for stroke, P-tau levels have been reported as being normal [35, 36]. P-tau may provide better specificity against dementia with Lewy bodies and frontotemporal dementia, but the phosphorylation sites providing the best discrimination may differ from one disease to another [46–50]. Low concentrations of $A\beta_{1-42}$ and dramatic increases in tau without a similarly strong increase in P-tau, is observed in CJD (class I) [51–59]. In contrast, tau and P-tau increase in parallel in variant CJD

Table 13.1 Summary of studies of total tau and amyloid β_{1-42} (Aβ_{1-42}) peptide in cerebrospinal fluid in diseases other than Alzheimer's disease dementia.

Disease and results	Evidence classification	Reference
Multiple sclerosis (MS)		
Increase in tau and P-tau in MS	Class II	[12–16]
Normal tau in most MS patients	Class II	[17]
Dementia with Lewy bodies (LBD)		
Lower Aβ_{1-42} in LBD	Class II	[10, 18]
Increase in tau in LBD	Class III	[19, 20]
Normal tau and Aβ_{1-42} in LBD	Class II	[21]
Lower Aβ_{1-42} and increased tau in LBD	Class II	[22, 23]
Semantic dementia (SD)		
Increase in tau in SD	Class III	[24]
Frontotemporal dementia (FD)		
Increase in tau in FD	Class III	[19, 20]
Increase in tau in FD	Class II	[25]
Increase in tau, decrease in Aβ_{1-42}	Class II	[26]
Low Aβ_{1-42} in FD	Class III	[27]
Parkinson's disease (PD)		
Lower Aβ_{1-42} to Aβ_{1-37} ratio in Parkinson's disease (PD) with dementia	Class III	[28]
Normal Aβ_{1-42} in PD	Class II	[29]
Lower Aβ_{1-42} and higher tau in PD with dementia, intermediate values in PD	Class II	[30]
Low Aβ_{1-42} in PD	Class III	[27]
Multiple system atrophy (MSA)		
Higher tau in MSA than in PD	Class II	[31]
Higher tau in MSA than in idiopathic cerebellar ataxia	Class II	[32]
Low Aβ_{1-42} in MSA	Class II	[29]
Corticobasal degeneration (CBD) and progressive supranuclear palsy (PSP)		
Higher tau in CBD than in PSP	Class II	[20, 33]
Normal Aβ_{1-42} in PSP	Class II	[29]
Low Aβ_{1-42} in CBD and PSP	Class III	[34]
Vascular dementia (VD) and stroke		
Increase in tau in VD	Class II	[10]
Increase in tau in stroke	Class II	[35]
Increase in tau, low Aβ_{1-42} and normal P181-tau in VD	Class II	[36, 37]
Increase in tau, normal Aβ_{1-42} and normal P181-tau in VD	Class II	[37]
Neuromuscular diseases		
Increased tau in amyotrophic lateral sclerosis	Class II	[38]
Low Aβ_{1-42} in ALS	Class III	[27]
Increased tau in Guillain–Barré syndrome, correlation with prognosis	Class II	[39]
AIDS–dementia complex (ADC)		
Low Aβ_{1-42} and high tau in ADC	Class II	[40]
Head injury		
Increased tau in head injury	Class III	[41, 42]
Decreased Aβ_{1-42} in head injury	Class III	[41, 43]
Normal pressure hydrocephalus (NPH)		
Low tau, P-tau and Aβ_{1-42} in NPH	Class II	[44]
Increased tau in NPH	Class III	[20, 45]

(class III) [60]. The discrimination between different tau and Aβ isoforms in CSF may be useful for discrimination between different disease processes, but larger studies are needed to address this in detail [28, 61–64].

A special indication for CSF studies is the identification of patients with mild cognitive impairment with CSF findings typical of AD [4], because there is class I evidence that such patients may be at increased risk of progression to AD [65–74]. When interpreting the results of $A\beta_{1-42}$ measurements, it should be taken into account that concentrations may decrease after glucocorticoid treatment (class III) [75] and show pronounced diurnal fluctuations [76], and erroneously low values of $A\beta_{1-42}$ are found if the CSF is not sampled and handled optimally [77–79]. Indeed, freezing and prolonged storage impair the discriminatory value of ELISA measurements of Aβ [80]. Furthermore, age-dependent reference values should be used for tau measurements, whereas $A\beta_{1-42}$ values are independent of age. In one study, the reference value for $A\beta_{1-42}$ was above 500 ng/l; for tau the reference value was <300 ng/l in patients in the age range 21–50 years, <450 ng/l in the range 51–70 years and <500 ng/l in the range 71–93 years [81].

Recommendation

In studies assessing the sensitivity and specificity of CSF markers for AD, the diagnosis has not been confirmed neuropathologically. $A\beta_{1-42}$ values should be interpreted with some caution. There is, however, evidence that tau, P-tau and $A\beta_{1-42}$ measurements have high sensitivity and specificity for discriminating AD against normal ageing, and may identify patients with mild cognitive impairment at increased risk of progression to AD (level A rating). The last finding is of clear importance if therapies affecting the disease course of AD become available in the future.

14-3-3 protein

14-3-3 is a ubiquitous protein with the highest concentrations found in the brain [82]. Mostly, it is determined qualitatively by western blot techniques, although a quantitative ELISA method is available. An initial study showed the presence of 14-3-3 in CSF from 96% of 71 patients with CJD (class II) [83]. In a prospective study including 805 patients with neuropathologically confirmed CJD, the sensitivity of a positive 14-3-3 test was 94%, the specificity 84%, and the 14-3-3 test was superior

to EEG studies (class I) [84]. High sensitivity and specificity of 14-3-3 has also been found in other studies (class I) [85–89]. Increases in 14-3-3 protein are less frequent in new variant CJD (class III) [90], familial forms of spongiform encephalopathies and infrequent subtypes of CJD (class III) [87, 91, 92]. Furthermore, increases in 14-3-3 protein are less frequent early and late in the course of sporadic CJD and early in the course of iatrogenic (growth hormone-induced) CJD (class III) [12, 46, 74]. Positive results of the 14-3-3 test have also been reported in other dementias, cerebrovascular disease, metabolic and hypoxic encephalopathies, brain metastases and CNS infections (class III) [59, 83, 86, 89, 93, 94]. The detection of 14-3-3 in CSF has been reported to indicate a poor prognosis in patients with transverse myelitis, clinically isolated syndromes suggestive of multiple sclerosis (class II) [95–97]; another study did not confirm these findings (class III) [98].

Recommendation

The detection of 14-3-3 has been reported to have a high sensitivity (94%) and specificity (84%) for the diagnosis of CJD in patients with clinical findings suggestive of this disease, but 14-3-3 can also be detected in CSF from patients with more common diseases (level A rating).

Hypocretin-1 (orexin-1) levels in narcolepsy

Human narcolepsy is a sleep disorder that affects up to 0.5% of the population. It is characterized by hypersomnia, cataplexia, sleep paralysis and hypnagogic hallucinations [99]. The full spectrum of symptoms occurs only in a minority of patients. The disease is strongly associated with the HLA allele DQB1*0602. Based on animal models it is believed that narcolepsy is caused by a dysfunction of the hypocretin-1 (orexin-1) neurotransmitter system in the posterior and lateral hypothalamus. In human narcolepsy, CSF hypocretin-1 (orexin-1) levels were reported to be low or absent. Thirteen studies were used to evaluate the role of CSF hypocretin-1 (orexin-1) in sleep disorders. Three studies were excluded from the analysis because of low patient numbers or lack of control groups [100–102]. The study Mignot *et al.* included patients from two previous studies, which were therefore also excluded from the analysis [103, 104]. In all studies

Table 13.2 Summary of the results from hypcretin-1/orexin-1 levels in narcolepsy[a].

Sensitivity (%)		Prevalence in controls[a] (%)				
With cataplexy	Without cataplexy	ND including SD[b]	ND without SD[c]	Cut-off (pg/ml)	Class of evidence	Reference
69.3[d] (137)	14.3 (21)	1.7 (228)	0% (47)[e]	110	III[f]	[105]
91.7 (48)	40 (15)	0 (10)	0% (50)[g]	110	II	[106]
81.8 (9)	0 (5)	8.3 (12)	nd	194	III	[107]
70.6 (17)	0 (9)	nd	0% (15)[h]	200	IV	[108]
100 (14)	100 (10)	0 (24)[g]	nd	100	IV	[109]
88.5 (26)	11.1 (9)	0 (103)	nd	110	II	[110]
66.0 (47)	0 (7)	0[i] (10)	nd	209 pg/dl	II	[111]

All hypcretin-1/orexin-1 measurements were performed by radioimmunoassay; numbers in parentheses refer to total number of investigated individuals.
[a]100% minus these figures result in specificities.
[b]Neurological disease including other sleep disorders.
[c]Neurological disease without sleep disorders.
[d]including patients with atypical cataplexia.
[e]patients who had no sleep disorder.
[f]samples were included before in other studies.
[g]neurological diseases and pregnant women.
[h]patients who underwent back surgery.
[i]idiopathic hypersomnia.

hypocretin-1 (orexin-1) levels in CSF were measured by radioimmunoassay (RIA). Cut-off points ranged from 202 pg/ml to 110 pg/ml. In most patients who had narcolepsy with cataplexy orexin/hypocretin concentrations were low (sensitivities between 66% and 100%), in most patients even below the detection limit of 40 pg/ml of the RIA (Table 13.2). This was in particular true for patients with HLA-DQB1*0602 status [102]. Low levels of hypocretin-1 (orexin-1) were also found in a minority of patients who had narcolepsy without cataplexy and other neurological disease (specificities between 92% and 100%) [112].

Recommendation

Based on three class II and several class III and IV studies, hypocretin-1 (orexin-1) levels of <110 pg/ml in CSF can be classified as a diagnostic biomarker for narcolepsy with cataplexy (level A recommendation, in compliance with the International Classification of Sleep Disorders). The value of measuring hypocretin-1 (orexin-1) in CSF of other sleep disorders is controversial.

β_2-Transferrin

Transferrin is a polypeptide of the β-globulin family, which is involved in ferrous ion transport. β_2-Transferrin (synonyms: asialotransferrin, tau fraction) is a transferrin form without sialic acid side chains. In healthy human beings β_2-transferrin has only been demonstrated in CSF, perilymph and aqueous humour of the eye, but not in serum [113, 114]. In patients with chronic liver diseases [115, 116], inborn error of glycoprotein metabolism [117] and people with a genetic variant of transferrin [115, 118, 119] β_2-transferrin can be also found in the blood.

Due to shortcomings of earlier methods (high-resolution electrophoresis) [120, 121] an isoelectric pH-focusing method was developed followed by immunofixation and silver staining, for which as little as 5 μg total protein is necessary (class III). Various sources of error in use of β_2-transferrin analysis for diagnosing CSF leaks were described [122], such as transferrin isoforms especially in saliva with electrophoretic mobility similar to that of β_2-transferrin (class IV) [123].

In combination with other methods such as high-resolution computed tomography (HRCT) the detection of β_2-transferrin in CSF-contaminated nasal discharges and blood was able to confirm oto- and rhinorrhoea of different aetiologies [120, 121, 124–131] (all class III, except one class IV) and used to monitor patients after surgical reconstruction of the frontal skull base (class III) [132]. The test sensitivity varied between 79% and 100% (class III) [131, 133, 134] at a specificity of about 95% (class III) [134]. Venous blood sampled at the same time as CSF may exclude false-positive results due to inborn errors of glycoprotein metabolism, genetic variants of transferrin or chronic liver disease (class IV) [118, 129].

Recommendation

Measurement of β_2-transferrin in combination with CT of the scull detects CSF contamination in oto- and rhinorrhoea with high sensitivity (79–100%) at a specificity of 95% (level B recommendation).

Beta-trace protein or β-TP (prostaglandin D synthase)

β-TP (molecular mass 25 kDa) is one of the most abundant locally synthesized proteins in the CSF [135, 136]. Based on amino acid sequencing, it has been identified as prostaglandin D synthase (PGDS) which is a member of the lipocalin superfamily composed of various secretory lipophilic ligand-carrier proteins [137]. Within the central nervous system, β-TP has been localized by immunohistochemistry and *in situ* hybridization mainly in choroid plexus and leptomeninges [138]. Concentrations of β-TP in CSF ranged between 8 and 40 mg/l (age dependent) and between 0.4 and 1.5 mg/l in serum. As a result of its relatively high CSF concentration β-TP has been explored for the diagnosis of oto- and rhinorrhoea [139–141].

For quantitative nephelometric analysis, a sample volume of at least 5 μl is needed which is diluted with a dilution buffer to a total volume of 500 μl. The detection range of the assay is between 0.25 and 15.8 mg/l, and the detection limit is at 2.5 mg/l. The test requires <15 min, having the advantage of intraoperative use and repeated frequent testing, e.g. evaluation of treatment success of CSF fistula repair [142].

Highest sensitivities and specificities as well as accuracy values were reported using a cut-off value of 1.31–6.00 mg/l [140, 143, 144] (Table 13.3, twice class II, one class III study). In addition, a secretion/serum ratio of β-TP has been introduced with a normal range below 1.57, yielding 100% specificity [145]. A cut-point at 1.11 mg/l for β-TP gave the best trade-off between high sensitivity and high specificity when including the secretion/serum ratio [139]. In direct comparison to β_2-transferrin the sensitivity and specificity values to detect CSF contamination in oto- and rhinorrhoea were similar (class II) [139, 140].

A limitation of the β-TP assay is that, in patients with renal insufficiency and bacterial meningitis, levels may substantially increase in serum and decrease in CSF, respectively. Hence, its use in such instances should be associated with cautious interpretation of the results.

Table 13.3 Different cut-off values have been evaluated for diagnostic accuracy of cerebrospinal fluid (CSF) fistula (beta-trace protein).

Sensitivity (%)	Specificity (%)	Rhino-/ otorrhoea cut-off[a]	Normal nasal secretion, mean, (range)[a]	Serum mean, (range)[a]	CSF mean, (range)[a]	Class of evidence	Reference
92	100	>6 (n = 33)	0.9 (n = 107)	0.5 (n = 34)	11.1 (n = 20)	II	[143]
Not reported	Not reported	>0.35 (n = 20)	0.016 (0.0–0.12) (n = 29)	0.6 (0.38–0–86) (n = 132)	18.4 (9.4–29.2) (n = 132)	III	[144]
93	100	>1.31 (n = 53)	0.4 (0.22–1.69) (n = 160)	0.6 (0.12–1.44) (n = 116)	19.6 (11.5–32.6) (n = 19)	II	[140]

[a]All units of measurements are milligrams per litre.

CSF markers with a future potential to be used in clinical routine

Vascular endothelial growth factor

Vascular endothelial growth factor (VEGF) is a glycosylated homodimeric protein of approximately 45 kDa. It is produced by a broad range of cell types in response to stimuli such as hypoxia or tumour necrosis factor (TNF) α [146–150]. VEGF is selectively mitogenic for endothelial cells and plays a fundamental role in both normal and abnormal angiogenesis [151]. VEGF can be measured with several commercially available sandwich ELISAs. As those tests use various capture reagents, the resulting 'normal' ranges of VEGF in CSF depend on the test used.

VEGF in CSF was suggested to determine prognosis in several malignancies. VEGF was negatively correlated with survival in patients with leptomeningeal metastases [152, 153] (class II) and astrocytic brain tumours [154, 155] (class III). Furthermore, it serves as a biological marker for the diagnosis and evaluation of treatment response in leptomeningeal metastases [156] (class III) (Table 13.4). VEGF is not detectable in lower-grade gliomas (grade 2) [158] (class III).

Studies investigating CSF VEGF in a number of other neurological conditions are summarized in Table 13.5, demonstrating a possible role in the pathogenesis of some diseases as well as some inconsistent findings.

CSF neurofilaments

Neurofilaments (Nfs) constitute the axonal cytoskeleton [177]. There are four Nf subunits: a light (NfL, 68 kDa), intermediate (NfM, 115 kDa) and heavy chain (NfH, 190–210 kDa) and also α-internexin. Nfs are released into the CSF after axonal damage. The normal upper reference rages for CSF NfH and NfL levels are presented in Table 13.6.

A comprehensive list of studies on NfL and NfH, including cut-off points and diagnostic sensitivity and specificity values, is summarized in Table 13.6. Reference values depend on many pre-analytical and analytical factors and vary between laboratories. It is therefore, strongly encouraged that each laboratory establish its own reference values.

Table 13.4 Vascular endothelial growth factor (VEGF) diagnostic sensitivity and specificity in leptomeningeal metastases.

Sensitivity (%)	Specificity (%)	Cut point (ng/ml)	Method/isoform	Class of evidence	Reference
100 ($n = 19$)	73	(log tPA index − 0.7229 × log VEGF index) <−0.18182	ELISA/121, 165		[157]
85 ($n = 53$)	100	>262	ELISA	II	[152]
73 ($n = 37$)	93	>100	ELISA/121, 165	II	[153]
51	98.3	>250			
100 ($n = 11$)	100	>633.1	ELISA/121, 165	III	[156]

Table 13.5 Vascular endothelial growth factor (VEGF) levels in studies not investigating leptomeningeal metastases.

Study population (N)	VEGF mean values (pg/ml)[a]	Control group	VEGF controls mean values (pg/ml)[a]	Method/ isoforms	Class of evidence	Reference
Meningitis						
Tuberculous (48)[b]	106[c]–144[c]	Various other forms of meningitis	5.7–80.1	ELISA/121, 165	II	[159, 160]
Eosinophilic (9)	568	None		ELISA/165	IV	[161]
Pneumococcal (10)	Below lod	Viral meningitis (10) non-inflammatory controls (10)	Slightly elevated below LOD	Protein array	III	[162]
Cryptococcal (95)	37.5[c] (geometric mean)	Spinal anaesthesia (17)	Below lod	ELISA/121, 165	II	[163]
Any bacterial (37)	30% above cut point (25 pg/ml)[c]	Viral meningitis (16)	Below lod	ELISA	III	[164]
HIV with CNS infection (8) HIV without CNS infection (19)	49.7 42.6	Non-inflammatory controls (35) HIV-negative CNS infection (18)	Below lod 43.7	ELISA	III	[165]
CNS glioma grade 2 (7)	Below lod	Controls unspecified (3)	Below lod	ELISA	III	[158]
CNS glioma grades 1 and 2 (7)	Median 7.2 ng/ml	Hydrocephalus (10)	Median 8.3 ng/ml	ELISA	Uncertain[d]	[154]
CNS glioma grades 3 and 4 (19)	17.6 ng/ml[c]					
CNS glioma grades 3 and 4 (27)	4.9 ng/mg of total protein	Various tumours (31)	0.006 ng/mg of total protein	Not stated	IV	[155]
Amyotrophic lateral sclerosis (105)[b]	Various ways of expressing VEGF levels (pg/ml, pg/l, IU)	Various groups including 'neurological' controls, neurodegenerative disorders, headache, radiculopathies, total n = 124	Ranging from significantly lower to equal to higher	ELISA/165	All class III	[166–170]
Pre-eclampsia (15)	6.6	Pregnant normal pressure	5.5	ELISA	III	[171]
Alzheimer disease (43)[b]	Below lod 500[c] (only versus vascular dementia)	'Healthy' controls (27) Vascular dementia (26)	Below lod 330	ELISA ELISA/165	III Uncertain[e]	[172, 173]
SAH (14)	90	'Healthy' controls (27)	130	ELISA/165	III, IV	[174, 175]
SAH (15)	0–2000	Non-SAH and 'healthy' controls (14)	13–19	ELISA		
POEMS syndrome (10)	6.8	Other neurological disease, GBS, CIDP (total 40)	3.0–9.1	ELISA/165	III	[176]

CNS, central nervous system; ELISA, enzyme-linked immunosorbent assay; lod, limit of detection; SAH, subarachnoid haemorrhage; VEGF, vascular endothelial growth factor.

[a] Unless stated otherwise.

[b] Total number derived from more than one study.

[c] Significant difference between study population and one or more control groups.

[d] uncertain because VEGF concentrations are 1000 times higher than in most other studies.

[e] uncertain because of unusually high levels in 'healthy' controls.

Table 13.6 Conditions in which increased neurofilament (Nf) has been shown.

Condition	NfH	Remarks	Sensitivity (%)	Specificity (%)	NfL	Remarks	Sensitivity	Specificity (%)	Level of evidence
Cut-off value	0.73 ng/ml [178]	Based on a reference population from a neurological hospital (n = 416)			Rosengren: 125 pg/l; <60 years: <0.25 ng/ml; 60–70: 0.38 ng/ml; 71–80: <0.75 ng/ml Norgren: 100 ng/l Van Geel: 40 ng/l	Population-based reference values (healthy volunteers)			
Condition in which neurofilament is increased									
ALS	[38, 178, 179]	Five times higher than in controls In upper motor symptoms two times higher than in lower motor symptoms	At cut-off of 0.73: 80% for ALS versus control ALS versus AD: 80	75% (ALS versus control) ALS versus AD: 97%	[180–182]	About 10 times increase in patients with upper motor symptoms. About two times increase in patients with lower motor symptoms	NA	NA	Class II
PD and MSA	[183, 184]	About three times elevated in MSA, not elevated in IPD	NfH: cut-off of 114.5: 83% for MSA-P versus IPD 77% for PSP from IPD (cut-off of 1.4 ng/ml)	87% for MSA versus IPD; 94% for PSP versus IPD	[184, 185]	About seven times elevated in MSA, not elevated in IPD	NfL: cut-off of 17.15: 83% for MSA-P versus IPD	90%	Class III
PSP	[183]	The ROC optimized cut-off level of 1.48 ng/ml is used for distinguishing patients with PSP from those with PD or CBD	76.5%	93.8%	[185]	NA	NA	NA	Class III

continued

Table 13.6 continued

Condition	NfH	Remarks	Sensitivity (%)	Specificity (%)	NfL	Remarks	Sensitivity	Specificity (%)	Level of evidence
MS	In most MS patients CSF NfH levels are within the normal reference range [178]	At a cut-off: 160pg/ml: sensitivity 34% and specificity 88% for conversion from CIS to RRMS [14] Contradictory results found by Lim [186] Relationship with progression Phophorylation rate eight times higher in severely disabled compared with mildly disabled patients [187] and also prognostic for deterioration at follow-up [188] NfH increases during follow-up [177]	NA	NA	[180, 189, 190] Not increased: [191]	2–10 times higher during relapses versus remission or SP [189, 190] R progression index: 0.29 ($P < 0.023$) [190]	78% for MS; 91% for relapse, 44% for remission, 48% for SP	92–100	Relationship with progression: class II
AD	[192, 193]	Using ROC optimized cut-off levels NfH higher in AD compared with controls Effect size 0.71 [194]	[192] 57.5	77.0	[180, 195–197]	Increased in AD and VD compared with controls In the meta-analysis the effect size distinguishing AD from controls was 1.27 with AD patients having the higher CSF NfL levels [194]	58–78%	28–77	Class II

continued

Disease	NfH References	NfH description			NfL References	NfL description			Class
FTLD	[193, 197]	NfH higher in FTLD compared with controls Effect size 0.74 [194]	NA		[193, 195, 197–199]	NfL higher in FTLD compared with controls Effect size was 1.38 [194]	82% to discriminate FTD from EAD in [193] contradictory to Pijnenburg et al.	70	Class II
VD	[192]	NfH is higher in VD then in AD	NA		[180, 195, 196, 200]	NfL Higher than in AD then in controls Effect size 1.24 [194]	85%	68	Class II
DLBD	[193]	Using ROC optimized cut-off levels. NfH higher in DLBD compared with late AD	89	28	[193]	Using ROC optimized cut-off levels NfH higher in DLBD compared with late AD	33%	82	Class III
Spinal cord injury	ND				[201]	5–450 times increased in acute cervical spine injury, and levels increase during 21 days after the injury	Cut-off of 125 ng/l, 100% sensitivity for acute spinal cord injury, 18% for whiplash	100	Class III
AIDS–dementia complex	ND				[202–206]	n = 8, three patients increased NfL after interruption No clinical signs, but f.u. time only 101 days Subclinical marker?	NA	86 [203]	Class II

Table 13.6 continued

Condition	NfH	Remarks	Sensitivity (%)	Specificity (%)	NfL	Remarks	Sensitivity	Specificity (%)	Level of evidence
SAH	[207–209]	Prognostic for outcome	Cut-off: highest value in survivors: 57–100% for unfavourable outcome	71–75	[180, 210, 211]	Lumbar CSF	Cut-off for unfavourable outcome: 6,400 ng/l: 100% sensitivity	50	Class I
NPH	ND				[44, 212–214]	Ten times increased compared to reference values	NA	NA	Class III
Binswanger's disease	ND				[212]	Four times increased compared with reference values.	NA	NA	Class III
GBS	[215]	A prognostic marker for poor outcome Not a diagnostic test	NA	NA	ND				Class III
Cardiac arrest	ND				[216]	Prognostic for axonal damage after cardiac arrest	Poor outcome (Glasgow Coma Scale): 75–92	80–100% for different cut-offs	Class III
HSV encephalitis relapse	ND				[217]	Higher during encephalitis relapse	NA	NA	Class III

AD, Alzheimer's disease; ALS, amyotrophic lateral sclerosis; CBD, corticobasal degeneration; CIS, clinically isolated syndrome; CSF, cerebrospinal fluid; DLBD, diffuse Lewy body disease; FTLD, frontotemporal lobar degeneration; f.u. follow up time; GBS, Guillain–Barré syndrome; HSV, herpes simplex virus; ICH, intracerebral hemorrhage; MMC, meningomyelocele; MS, multiple sclerosis; MSA, multiple system atrophy; NA, not available; ND, not done; NMO, neuromyelitis optica; ON, optic neuritis; PD, Parkinson's disease; PSP, progressive supranuclear palsy; ROC, receiver operating characteristic; RRMS, relapsing remitting multiple sclerosis; SAH, subarachnoid haemorrhage; VD, vascular dementia.

Neurofilaments are of prognostic value in subarachnoid haemorrhage (SAH). Increased levels of NfH and NfL in ventricular and lumbar CSF are related to poor outcome using the Glasgow Outcome Score (class I) [178, 207–209] [180, 210, 211]. In multiple sclerosis (MS), high CSF NfL levels were of prognostic value on a number of clinical outcome scales (class III) [189, 190]. The heavy chain of Nfs in CSF was also related to progression within the subsequent year in relapsing–remitting MS patients (class III) [187, 188, 191]. Moreover, CSF NfH levels in the CSF or plasma of patients with optic neuritis (ON) predicted the degree of permanent loss of visual function (class III) [186, 187]. Finally, CSF NfH levels were significantly higher in patients with neuromyelitis optica (NMO) which is consistent with the clinical experience of more severe disease and more extensive axonal loss in NMO than in MS (class III) [179].

In amyotrophic lateral sclerosis (ALS) patient's high CSF NfH levels were related to a more rapid clinical progression and with upper motor neuron symptoms (class II) [38, 181]. In the AIDS–dementia complex, elevated CSF NfL levels were shown to be a good secondary outcome measure in an antiretroviral treatment trial (class III) [202–206]. CSF Nf levels could discriminate different parkinsonian disorders. NfL and NfH levels were higher in patients with multisystem atrophy (MSA) compared with patients with Parkinson's disease (class II) [183–185].

A recent meta-analysis reviewing the value of CSF NfL and NfH in neurodegenerative dementia concluded that CSF NfL and NfH levels were increased in AD, frontotemporal lobar dementia (FTLD) and vascular dementia (class III) (see Table 13.6 for references and [178]). In comparison to CSF tau and $A\beta_{1-42}$ levels, the diagnostic accuracy of CSF NfL and NfH levels is lower.

Recommendations

CSF Nf levels can be used as a biomarker for neuronal death and axonal degeneration (level B rating). The prognostic value of CSF Nf levels is highest in acute conditions such as SAH, ALS, MSA, MS, acute ON and NMO (level B rating). There is further evidence from longitudinal studies that there is potential for CSF Nf to be used to monitor disease progression in SAH, MS and spinal cord injury (level B rating). As reference values depend on many preanalytical and analytical factors, laboratories should establish their own reference values.

Myelin basic protein

Myelin basic protein (MBP) is a major protein in central nervous system myelin, but constitutes a lesser proportion of myelin in the peripheral nervous system [218]. The CSF concentration of MBP increases with age (class I) [219], and many disease processes, even diseases affecting mainly peripheral nerve myelin, may show increases in the CSF concentration of MBP (class II) [220–223]. It is mostly measured by RIA, but ELISAs have also been developed. The CSF concentration of MBP is increased in MS (class I), where it is higher in relapses than in progression (class I), correlates with the severity of the relapse (class II), is higher in patients with multifocal relapses than in monofocal relapses (class III), and is higher in relapses with new symptoms than with the recurrence of previous symptoms (class III) [224–231]. Increased CSF concentrations of MBP in patients in clinical remission may be associated with an increased relapse risk and a lower risk of a benign disease course (class III) [232, 233].

The CSF concentration of MBP decreases in parallel with spontaneous remission of clinical symptoms and with the resolution of active brain lesions on gadolinium (Gd)-enhanced magnetic resonance imaging (MRI) after treatment with methylprednisolone (class III) [234, 235]. Increased CSF concentrations of MBP may indicate a better short-term response to treatment with methylprednisolone, but Gd-enhanced MRI studies are superior to MBP measurements in this respect (class III) [236, 237].

Recommendations

MBP immunoassays are technically demanding because the analyte exists both in free and lipid-bound forms and bound in immune complexes. This is often not considered in CSF research. Increased CSF concentrations of MBP are unspecific and can be found in a variety of diseases, not only in MS (level A rating). It is possible that MBP measurements could be of prognostic value in MS (level C rating).

Recommendations for future research

In general, disease-specific biomarkers for diagnostic, prognostic and monitoring purposes should be validated using established protocols [238, 239]. Furthermore, validation across laboratories is urgently needed for many biomarkers, as shown for Aβ and tau proteins [240]. With respect to $A\beta_{1-42}$, tau and P-tau, there is a need for evaluation of the precise predictive value of these methods in the differentiation between different neurodegenerative diseases, rather than as done for the discrimination between healthy ageing and patients with AD (incipient or definite). There seems to be a potential for assays recognizing different phosphoforms of tau in differential diagnosis, and this issue should be pursued in future studies.

Studies of 14-3-3 protein, $A\beta_{1-42}$, tau and P-tau may also be helpful as diagnostic aids in patients with suspected CJD, but, as CJD is a rare disorder, a very high diagnostic specificity against a wide spectrum of other diseases presenting with rapidly progressing dementia is necessary, and this issue needs to be investigated more thoroughly. The value of measuring hypocretin-1 (orexin-1) levels in CSF of patients with other sleep disorders needs to be addressed. A serum marker for narcolepsy with cataplexy would be helpful for early diagnosis and serial analysis during the course and treatment of the disease.

The diagnostic and prognostic value of VEGF in leptomeningeal metastases should be confirmed in a larger prospective study, specifically in cytology-negative patients. For patients with leptomeningeal metastases from haematological tumours more sensitive markers need to be explored. Regarding the Nf assays, standardization of the assays and variation among different laboratories should be investigated, in order to define reliable reference values. The use of Nfs in predicting neurological decline must be explored further. Further research should also focus on combining Nfs with other markers, because they will probably not be able to predict neurological decline with sufficient specificity and sensitivity as a stand-alone marker.

References

1. Deisenhammer, F, Bartos, A, Egg, R, et al. Guidelines on routine cerebrospinal fluid analysis. Report from an EFNS task force. *Eur J Neurol* 2006; **13**:913–22.

2. Biomarkers Definition Working Group. Biomarkers and surrogate endpoints: preferred definitions and conceptual framework. *Clin Pharmacol Ther* 2001; **69**:89–95.

3. Brainin, M, Barnes, M, Baron, JC, et al. Guidance for the preparation of neurological management guidelines by EFNS scientific task forces–revised recommendations 2004. *Eur J Neurol* 2004; **11**:577–81.

4. Blennow, K, Hampel, H. CSF markers for incipient Alzheimer's disease. *Lancet Neurol* 2003; **2**:605–613.

5. Dubois, B, Feldman, HH, Jacova, C, et al. Research criteria for the diagnosis of Alzheimer's disease: revising the NINCDS-ADRDA criteria. *Lancet Neurol* 2007; **6**: 734–46.

6. Sunderland, T, Linker, G, Mirza, N, et al. Decreased betaamyloid1- 42 and increased tau levels in cerebrospinal fluid of patients with Alzheimer disease. *JAMA* 2003; **289**: 2094–103.

7. Wiltfang, J, Lewczuk, P, Riederer, P, et al. Consensus paper of the WFSBP Task Force on Biological Markers of Dementia: the role of CSF and blood analysis in the early and differential diagnosis of dementia. *World J Biol Psychiatry* 2005; **6**:69–84.

8. Ishiguro, K, Ohno, H, Arai, H, et al. Phosphorylated tau in human cerebrospinal fluid is a diagnostic marker for Alzheimer's disease. *Neurosci Lett* 1999; **270**:91–4.

9. Itoh, N, Arai, H, Urakami, K, et al. Large-scale, multicenter study of cerebrospinal fluid tau protein phosphorylated at serine 199 for the antemortem diagnosis of Alzheimer's disease. *Ann Neurol* 2001; **50**:150–156.

10. Andreasen, N, Minthon, L, Davidsson, P, et al. Evaluation of CSF-tau and CSF-Abeta42 as diagnostic markers for Alzheimer disease in clinical practice. *Arch Neurol* 2001; **58**: 373–9.

11. Hulstaert, F, Blennow, K, Ivanoiu, A, et al. Improved discrimination of AD patients using beta-amyloid(1-42) and tau levels in CSF. *Neurology* 1999; **52**:1555–62.

12. Bartosik-Psujek, H, Stelmasiak, Z. The CSF levels of total-tau and phosphotau in patients with relapsing–remitting multiple sclerosis. *J Neural Transm* 2006; **113**:339–345.

13. Bartosik-Psujek, H, Archelos, JJ. Tau protein and 14-3-3 are elevated in the cerebrospinal fluid of patients with multiple sclerosis and correlate with intrathecal synthesis of IgG. *J Neurol* 2004; **251**:414–20.

14. Brettschneider, J, Petzold, A, Junker, A, Tumani, H. Axonal damage markers in the cerebrospinal fluid of patients with clinically isolated syndrome improve predicting conversion to definite multiple sclerosis. *Mult Scler* 2006; **12**:143–8.

15. Martinez-Yelamos, A, Saiz, A, Bas, J, Hernandez, JJ, Graus, F, Arbizu, T. Tau protein in cerebrospinal fluid: a possible marker of poor outcome in patients with early relapsing-remitting multiple sclerosis. *Neurosci Lett* 2004; **363**: 14–17.

16. Terzi, M, Birinci, A, Cetinkaya, E, Onar, MK. Cerebrospinal fluid total tau protein levels in patients with multiple sclerosis. *Acta Neurol Scand* 2007; **115**:325–30.

17. Guimaraes, I, Cardoso, MI, Sa, MJ. Tau protein seems not to be a useful routine clinical marker of axonal damage in multiple sclerosis. *Mult Scler*, 2006; **12**, 354–356.

18. Kanemaru, K, Kameda, N, Yamanouchi, H. Decreased CSF amyloid beta42 and normal tau levels in dementia with Lewy bodies. *Neurology* 2000; **54**:1875–6.

19. Arai, H, Morikawa, Y, Higuchi, M, *et al.* Cerebrospinal fluid tau levels in neurodegenerative diseases with distinct tau-related pathology. *Biochem Biophys Res Commun* 1997; **236**:262–4.

20. Shoji, M, Matsubara, E, Murakami, T, *et al.* Cerebrospinal fluid tau in dementia disorders: a large scale multicenter study by a Japanese study group. *Neurobiol Aging* 2002; **23**: 363–70.

21. Gomez-Tortosa, E, Gonzalo, I, Fanjul, S, *et al.* Cerebrospinal fluid markers in dementia with Lewy bodies compared with Alzheimer disease. *Arch Neurol* 2003; **60**:1218–22.

22. Mollenhauer, B, Cepek, L, Bibl, M, *et al.* Tau protein, Abeta42 and S-100B protein in cerebrospinal fluid of patients with dementia with Lewy bodies. *Dement Geriatr Cogn Disord* 2005; **19**:164–70.

23. Mollenhauer, B, Bibl, M, Wiltfang, J, *et al.* Total tau protein, phosphorylated tau (181p) protein, beta-amyloid(1-42), and beta-amyloid(1-40) in cerebrospinal fluid of patients with dementia with Lewy bodies. *Clin Chem Lab Med* 2006; **44**:192–5.

24. Andersen, C, Froelich, FS, Ostberg, P, Lannfelt, L, Wahlund, L. Tau protein in cerebrospinal fluid from semantic dementia patients. *Neurosci Lett* 2000; **294**:155–8.

25. Pijnenburg, YA, Schoonenboom, SN, Barkhof, F, *et al.* CSF biomarkers in frontotemporal lobar degeneration: relations with clinical characteristics, apolipoprotein E genotype, and neuroimaging. *J Neurol Neurosurg Psychiatry* 2006; **77**:246–8.

26. Riemenschneider, M, Wagenpfeil, S, Diehl, J, *et al.* Tau and Abeta42 protein in CSF of patients with frontotemporal degeneration. *Neurology* 2002; **58**:1622–8.

27. Sjogren, M, Davidsson, P, Wallin, A, *et al.* Decreased CSF-beta-amyloid 42 in Alzheimer's disease and amyotrophic lateral sclerosis may reflect mismetabolism of beta-amyloid induced by disparate mechanisms. *Dement Geriatr Cogn Disord* 2002; **13**:112–18.

28. Bibl, M, Mollenhauer, B, Esselmann, H, *et al.* CSF amyloid-beta-peptides in Alzheimer's disease, dementia with Lewy bodies and Parkinson's disease dementia. *Brain* 2006; **5**: 1177–87.

29. Holmberg, B, Johnels, B, Blennow, K, Rosengren, L. Cerebrospinal fluid Abeta42 is reduced in multiple system atrophy but normal in Parkinson's disease and progressive supranuclear palsy. *Mov Disord* 2003; **18**: 186–90.

30. Mollenhauer, B, Trenkwalder, C, von Ahsen, N, *et al.* Betaamlyoid 1-42 and Tau-protein in cerebrospinal fluid of patients with Parkinson's disease dementia. *Dement Geriatr Cogn Disord* 2006; **22**:200–8.

31. Abdo, WF, De, JD, Hendriks, JC, *et al.* Cerebrospinal fluid analysis differentiates multiple system atrophy from Parkinson's disease. *Mov Disord* 2004; **19**:571–9.

32. Abdo, WF, van de Warrenburg, BP, Munneke, M, *et al.* CSF analysis differentiates multiple-system atrophy from idiopathic late-onset cerebellar ataxia. *Neurology* 2006; **67**: 474–9.

33. Urakami, K, Mori, M, Wada, K, *et al.* A comparison of tau protein in cerebrospinal fluid between corticobasal degeneration and progressive supranuclear palsy. *Neurosci Lett* 1999; **259**:127–9.

34. Noguchi, M, Yoshita, M, Matsumoto, Y, Ono, K, Iwasa, K, Yamada, M. Decreased beta-amyloid peptide42 in cerebrospinal fluid of patients with progressive supranuclear palsy and corticobasal degeneration. *J Neurol Sci* 2005; **237**: 61–5.

35. Hesse, C, Rosengren, L, Vanmechelen, E, *et al.* Cerebrospinal fluid markers for Alzheimer's disease evaluated after acute ischemic stroke. *J Alzheimers Dis* 2000; **4**:199–206.

36. Nagga, K, Gottfries, J, Blennow, K, Marcusson, J. Cerebrospinal fluid phospho-tau, total tau and beta-amyloid(1-42) in the differentiation between Alzheimer's disease and vascular dementia. *Dement Geriatr Cogn Disord* 2002; **14**:183–90.

37. Stefani, A, Bernardini, S, Panella, M, *et al.* AD with subcortical white matter lesions and vascular dementia: CSF markers for differential diagnosis. *J Neurol Sci* 2005; **237**:83–8.

38. Brettschneider, J, Petzold, A, Sussmuth, SD, Ludolph, AC, Tumani, H. Axonal damage markers in cerebrospinal fluid are increased in ALS. *Neurology* 2006; **66**:852–6.

39. Jin, K, Takeda, A, Shiga, Y, *et al.* CSF tau protein: a new prognostic marker for Guillain–Barré syndrome. *Neurology* 2006; **67**:1470–2.

40. Brew, BJ, Pemberton, L, Blennow, K, Wallin, A, Hagberg, L. CSF amyloid beta42 and tau levels correlate with AIDS dementia complex. *Neurology* 2005; **65**:1490–2.

41. Franz, G, Beer, R, Kampfl, A, *et al.* Amyloid beta 1-42 and tau in cerebrospinal fluid after severe traumatic brain injury. *Neurology* 2003; **60**:1457–61.

42. Ost, M, Nylen, K, Csajbok, L, *et al.* Initial CSF total tau correlates with 1-year outcome in patients with traumatic brain injury. *Neurology* 2006; **67**:1600–4.

43. Kay, AD, Petzold, A, Kerr, M, Keir, G, Thompson, E, Nicoll, JA. Alterations in cerebrospinal fluid apolipoprotein E and amyloid beta-protein after traumatic brain injury. *J Neurotrauma* 2003; **20**:943–52.

44. Agren-Wilsson, A, Lekman, A, Sjoberg, W, et al. CSF biomarkers in the evaluation of idiopathic normal pressure hydrocephalus. *Acta Neurol Scand* 2007; **116**:333–9.

45. Kapaki, EN, Paraskevas, GP, Tzerakis, NG, et al. Cerebrospinal fluid tau, phospho-tau181 and beta-amyloid1- 42 in idiopathic normal pressure hydrocephalus: a discrimination from Alzheimer's disease. *Eur J Neurol* 2007; **14**:168–73.

46. Hampel, H, Buerger, K, Zinkowski, R, et al. Measurement of phosphorylated tau epitopes in the differential diagnosis of Alzheimer disease: a comparative cerebrospinal fluid study. *Arch Gen Psychiatry* 2004; **61**:95–102.

47. Parnetti, L, Lanari, A, Amici, S, Gallai, V, Vanmechelen, E, Hulstaert, F. CSF phosphorylated tau is a possible marker for discriminating Alzheimer's disease from dementia with Lewy bodies. Phospho-Tau International Study Group. *Neurol Sci* 2001; **22**:77–8.

48. Schoonenboom, NS, Pijnenburg, YA, Mulder, C, et al. Amyloid beta(1-42) and phosphorylated tau in CSF as markers for early-onset alzheimer disease. *Neurology* 2004; **62**:1580–4.

49. Vanderstichele, H, De, VK, Blennow, K, et al. Analytical performance and clinical utility of the INNOTEST PHOSPHO-TAU181P assay for discrimination between Alzheimer's disease and dementia with Lewy bodies. *Clin Chem Lab Med* 2006; **44**:1472–80.

50. Vanmechelen, E, Vanderstichele, H, Davidsson, P, et al. Quantification of tau phosphorylated at threonine 181 in human cerebrospinal fluid: a sandwich ELISA with a synthetic phosphopeptide for standardization. *Neurosci Lett* 2000; **285**:49–52.

51. Blennow, K, Johansson, A, Zetterberg, H. Diagnostic value of 14-3-3beta immunoblot and T-tau/P-tau ratio in clinically suspected Creutzfeldt–Jakob disease. *Int J Mol Med* 2005; **16**:1147–9.

52. Buerger, K, Otto, M, Teipel, SJ, et al. Dissociation between CSF total tau and tau protein phosphorylated at threonine 231 in Creutzfeldt–Jakob disease. *Neurobiol Aging* 2006; **27**:10–15.

53. Otto, M, Esselmann, H, Schulz-Shaeffer, W, et al. Decreased beta-amyloid1-42 in cerebrospinal fluid of patients with Creutzfeldt–Jakob disease. *Neurology* 2000; **54**:1099–102.

54. Otto, M, Wiltfang, J, Cepek, L, et al. Tau protein and 14- 3-3 protein in the differential diagnosis of Creutzfeldt–Jakob disease. *Neurology* 2002; **58**:192–7.

55. Riemenschneider, M, Wagenpfeil, S, Vanderstichele, H, et al. Phospho-tau/total tau ratio in cerebrospinal fluid discriminates Creutzfeldt-Jakob disease from other dementias. *Mol Psychiatry* 2003; **8**:343–7.

56. Satoh, K, Shirabe, S, Eguchi, H, et al. 14-3-3 protein, total tau and phosphorylated tau in cerebrospinal fluid of patients with Creutzfeldt-Jakob disease and neurodegenerative disease in Japan. *Cell Mol Neurobiol* 2006; **26**: 45–52.

57. Van Everbroeck, B, Green, AJ, Pals, P, Martin, JJ, Cras, P. Decreased levels of amyloid-beta 1-42 in cerebrospinal fluid of Creutzfeldt–Jakob disease patients. *J Alzheimers Dis* 1999; **1**:419–24.

58. Van Everbroeck, B, Green, AJ, Vanmechelen, E, et al. Phosphorylated tau in cerebrospinal fluid as a marker for Creutzfeldt-Jakob disease. *J Neurol Neurosurg Psychiatry* 2002; **73**:79–81.

59. Van Everbroeck, B, Quoilin, S, Boons, J, Martin, JJ, Cras, P. A prospective study of CSF markers in 250 patients with possible Creutzfeldt-Jakob disease. *J Neurol Neurosurg Psychiatry* 2003; **74**:1210–14.

60. Goodall, CA, Head, MW, Everington, D, et al. F phospho-tau concentrations in variant Creutzfeldt-Jakob disease: diagnostic and pathological implications. *J Neurol Neurosurg Psychiatry* 2006; **77**:89–91.

61. Bibl, M, Mollenhauer, B, Lewczuk, P, et al. Validation of amyloid-beta peptides in CSF diagnosis of neurodegenerative dementias. *Mol Psychiatry* 2007; **12**:671–80.

62. Bibl, M, Mollenhauer, B, Wolf, S, et al. Reduced CSF carboxy-terminally truncated Abeta peptides in frontotemporal lobe degenerations. *J Neural Transm* 2007; **114**: 621–8.

63. Borroni, B, Gardoni, F, Parnetti, L, et al. Pattern of Tau forms in CSF is altered in progressive supranuclear palsy. *Neurobiol Aging* 2009; **30**:34–40.

64. Mollenhauer, B, Bibl, M, Esselmann, H, et al. Tauopathies and synucleinopathies: do cerebrospinal fluid betaamyloid peptides reflect disease-specific pathogenesis? *J Neural Transm* 2007; **114**:919–27.

65. Andersson, C, Blennow, K, Almkvist, O, et al. Increasing CSF phospho-tau levels during cognitive decline and progression to dementia. *Neurobiol Aging* 2008; **29**:1466–73.

66. Buerger, K, Teipel, SJ, Zinkowski, R, et al. CSF tau protein phosphorylated at threonine 231 correlates with cognitive decline in MCI subjects. *Neurology* 2002; **59**:627–9.

67. Buerger, K, Ewers, M, Andreasen, N, et al. Phosphorylated tau predicts rate of cognitive decline in MCI subjects: a comparative CSF study. *Neurology* 2005; **65**:1502–3.

68. Ewers, M, Buerger, K, Teipel, SJ, et al. Multicenter assessment of CSF-phosphorylated tau for the prediction of conversion of MCI. *Neurology* 2007; **69**:2205–12.

69. Fagan, AM, Roe, CM, Xiong, C, Mintun, MA, Morris, JC, Holtzman, DM. Cerebrospinal fluid tau/beta-amyloid(42) ratio as a prediction of cognitive decline in nondemented older adults. *Arch Neurol* 2007; **64**:343–9.

70. Gustafson, DR, Skoog, I, Rosengren, L, Zetterberg, H, Blennow, K. Cerebrospinal fluid beta-amyloid 1-42 con-

centration may predict cognitive decline in older women. *J Neurol Neurosurg Psychiatry* 2007; **78**:461–4.

71. Riemenschneider, M, Lautenschlager, N, Wagenpfeil, S, Diehl, J, Drzezga, A, Kurz, A. Cerebrospinal fluid tau and beta-amyloid 42 proteins identify Alzheimer disease in subjects with mild cognitive impairment. *Arch Neurol* 2002; **59**:1729–34.

72. Schonknecht, P, Pantel, J, Kaiser, E, Thomann, P, Schroder, J. Increased tau protein differentiates mild cognitive impairment from geriatric depression and predicts conversion to dementia. *Neurosci Lett* 2007; **416**:39–42.

73. Stomrud, E, Hansson, O, Blennow, K, Minthon, L, Londos, E. Cerebrospinal fluid biomarkers predict decline in subjective cognitive function over 3 years in healthy elderly. *Dement Geriatr Cogn Disord* 2007; **24**:118–24.

74. Zetterberg, H, Wahlund, LO, Blennow, K. Cerebrospinal fluid markers for prediction of Alzheimer's disease. *Neurosci Lett* 2003; **352**:67–9.

75. Tokuda, T, Oide, T, Tamaoka, A, Ishii, K, Matsuno, S, Ikeda, S. Prednisolone (30–60 mg/day) for diseases other than AD decreases amyloid beta-peptides in CSF. *Neurology* 2002; **58**:1415–18.

76. Bateman, RJ, Wen, G, Morris, JC, Holtzman, DM. Fluctuations of CSF amyloid-beta levels: implications for a diagnostic and therapeutic biomarker. *Neurology* 2007; **68**:666–9.

77. Kaiser, E, Schonknecht, P, Thomann, PA, Hunt, A, Schroder, J. Influence of delayed CSF storage on concentrations of phospho-tau protein (181), total tau protein and beta-amyloid (1-42). *Neurosci Lett* 2007; **417**:193–5.

78. Lewczuk, P, Beck, G, Esselmann, H, *et al.* Effect of sample collection tubes on cerebrospinal fluid concentrations of tau proteins and amyloid beta peptides. *Clin Chem* 2006; **52**:332–4.

79. Schoonenboom, NS, Mulder, C, Vanderstichele, H, *et al.* Effects of processing and storage conditions on amyloid beta (1-42) and tau concentrations in cerebrospinal fluid: implications for use in clinical practice. *Clin Chem* 2005; **51**:189–95.

80. Bibl, M, Esselmann, H, Otto, M, *et al.* Cerebrospinal fluid amyloid beta peptide patterns in Alzheimer's disease patients and nondemented controls depend on sample pretreatment: indication of carrier-mediated epitope masking of amyloid beta peptides. *Electrophoresis* 2004; **25**: 2912–18.

81. Sjogren, M, Vanderstichele, H, Agren, H, *et al.* Tau and Abeta42 in cerebrospinal fluid from healthy adults 21–93 years of age: establishment of reference values. *Clin Chem* 2001; **47**:1776–81.

82. Boston, PF, Jackson, P, Thompson, RJ. Human 14-3-3 protein: radioimmunoassay, tissue distribution, and cere-

brospinal fluid levels in patients with neurological disorders. *J Neurochem* 1982; **38**:1475–82.

83. Hsich, G, Kenney, K, Gibbs, CJ, Lee, KH, Harrington, MG. The 14-3-3 brain protein in cerebrospinal fluid as a marker for transmissible spongiform encephalopathies. *N Engl J Med* 1996; **335**:924–30.

84. Zerr, I, Pocchiari, M, Collins, S, *et al.* Analysis of EEG and CSF 14-3-3 proteins as aids to the diagnosis of Creutzfeldt-Jakob disease. *Neurology* 2000; **55**:811–15.

85. Beaudry, P, Cohen, P, Brandel, JP, *et al.* 14-3-3 protein, neuron-specific enolase, and S-100 protein in cerebrospinal fluid of patients with Creutzfeldt–Jakob disease. *Dement Geriatr Cogn Disord* 1999; **10**:40–6.

86. Collins, S, Boyd, A, Fletcher, A, *et al.* Creutzfeldt–Jakob disease: diagnostic utility of 14-3-3 protein immunodetection in cerebrospinal fluid. *J Clin Neurosci* 2000; **7**:203–8.

87. Collins, SJ, Sanchez-Juan, P, Masters, CL, *et al.* Determinants of diagnostic investigation sensitivities across the clinical spectrum of sporadic Creutzfeldt–Jakob disease. *Brain* 2006; **9**:2278–87.

88. Kenney, K, Brechtel, C, Takahashi, H, Kurohara, K, Anderson, P, Gibbs, CJ, Jr. An enzyme-linked immunosorbent assay to quantify 14-3-3 proteins in the cerebrospinal fluid of suspected Creutzfeldt–Jakob disease patients. *Ann Neurol* 2000; **48**:395–8.

89. Lemstra, AW, van Meegen, MT, Vreyling, JP, *et al.* 14-3-3 testing in diagnosing Creutzfeldt-Jakob disease: a prospective study in 112 patients. *Neurology* 2000; **55**:514–16.

90. Green, AJ, Ramljak, S, Muller, WE, Knight, RS, Schroder, HC 14-3-3 in the cerebrospinal fluid of patients with variant and sporadic Creutzfeldt–Jakob disease measured using capture assay able to detect low levels of 14- 3-3 protein. *Neurosci Lett* 2002; **324**:57–60.

91. Zerr, I, Schulz-Schaeffer, WJ, Giese, A, *et al.* Current clinical diagnosis in Creutzfeldt–Jakob disease: identification of uncommon variants. *Ann Neurol* 2000; **48**:323–9.

92. Castellani, RJ, Colucci, M, Xie, Z, *et al.* Sensitivity of 14-3-3 protein test varies in subtypes of sporadic Creutzfeldt–Jakob disease. *Neurology* 2004; **63**:436–42.

93. Zerr, I, Bodemer, M, Gefeller, O, *et al.* Detection of 14-3-3 protein in the cerebrospinal fluid supports the diagnosis of Creutzfeldt–Jakob disease. *Ann Neurol* 1998; **43**:32–40.

94. Burkhard, PR, Sanchez, JC, Landis, T, Hochstrasser, DF. CSF detection of the 14-3-3 protein in unselected patients with dementia. *Neurology* 2001; **56**:1528–33.

95. Irani, DN, Kerr, DA 14-3-3 protein in the cerebrospinal fluid of patients with acute transverse myelitis. *Lancet* 2000; **355**:901.

96. Colucci, M, Roccatagliata, L, Capello, E, *et al.* The 14-3-3 protein in multiple sclerosis: a marker of disease severity. *Mult Scler* 2004; **10**:477–81.

97. Martinez-Yelamos, A, Rovira, A, Sanchez-Valle, R, et al. CSF 14-3-3 protein assay and MRI as prognostic markers in patients with a clinically isolated syndrome suggestive of MS. *J Neurol* 2004; **251**:1278–9.

98. de Seze, J, Peoc'h, K, Ferriby, D, Stojkovic, T, Laplanche, JL, Vermersch, P 14-3-3 Protein in the cerebrospinal fluid of patients with acute transverse myelitis and multiple sclerosis. *J Neurol* 2002; **249**:626–7.

99. Yasui, K, Inoue, Y, Kanbayashi, T, Nomura, T, Kusumi, M, Nakashima, K. CSF orexin levels of Parkinson's disease, dementia with Lewy bodies, progressive supranuclear palsy and corticobasal degeneration. *J Neurol Sci* 2006; **250**: 120–3.

100. Wurtman, RJ. Narcolepsy and the hypocretins. *Metabolism* 2006; **55**(10 suppl 2):S36–9.

101. Dohi, K, Nishino, S, Nakamachi, T, et al. CSF orexin A concentrations and expressions of the orexin-1 receptor in rat hippocampus after cardiac arrest. *Neuropeptides* 2006; **40**:245–50.

102. Oyama, K, Takahashi, T, Shoji, Y, et al. Niemann–Pick disease type C: cataplexy and hypocretin in cerebrospinal fluid. *Tohoku J Exp Med* 2006; **209**:263–7.

103. Grady, SP, Nishino, S, Czeisler, CA, Hepner, D, Scammell, TE. Diurnal variation in CSF orexin-A in healthy male subjects. *Sleep* 2006; **29**:295–7.

104. Baumann, CR, Khatami, R, Werth, E, Bassetti, CL. Hypocretin (orexin) deficiency predicts severe objective excessive daytime sleepiness in narcolepsy with cataplexy. *J Neurol Neurosurg Psychiatry* 2006; **77**:402–4.

105. Mignot, E, Lammers, GJ, Ripley, B, et al. The role of cerebrospinal fluid hypocretin measurement in the diagnosis of narcolepsy and other hypersomnias. *Arch Neurol*, 2002; **59**:1553–62.

106. Hong, SC, Lin, L, Jeong, JH, et al. A study of the diagnostic utility of HLA typing, CSF hypocretin-1 measurements, and MSLT testing for the diagnosis of narcolepsy in 163 Korean patients with unexplained excessive daytime sleepiness. *Sleep* 2006; **29**:1429–38.

107. Kanbayashi, T, Inoue, Y, Chiba, S, et al. CSF hypocretin-1 (orexin-A) concentrations in narcolepsy with and without cataplexy and idiopathic hypersomnia. *J Sleep Res* 2002; **11**:91–3.

108. Krahn, LE, Pankratz, VS, Oliver, L, Boeve, BF, Silber, MH. Hypocretin (orexin) levels in cerebrospinal fluid of patients with narcolepsy: relationship to cataplexy and HLA DQB1*0602 status. *Sleep* 2002; **25**:733–6.

109. Ebrahim, IO, Sharief, MK, de Lacy S, et al. Hypocretin (orexin) deficiency in narcolepsy and primary hypersomnia. *J Neurol Neurosurg Psychiatry* 2003; **74**:127–30.

110. Dauvilliers, Y, Baumann, CR, Carlander, B, et al. CSF hypocretin-1 levels in narcolepsy, Kleine-Levin syndrome,

and other hypersomnias and neurological conditions. *J Neurol Neurosurg Psychiatry* 2003; **74**:1667–73.

111. Heier, MS, Evsiukova, T, Vilming, S, Gjerstad, MD, Schrader, H, Gautvik, K. CSF hypocretin-1 levels and clinical profiles in narcolepsy and idiopathic CNS hypersomnia in Norway. *Sleep* 2007; **30**:969–73.

112. Gaus, SE, Lin, L, Mignot, E. CSF hypocretin levels are normal in Huntington's disease patients. *Sleep* 2005; **28**:1607–8.

113. Arrer, E, Oberascher, G, Gibitz, HJ. Protein distribution in the human perilymph. A comparative study between perilymph (post mortem), CSF and blood serum. *Acta Otolaryngol* 1988; **2**:117–23.

114. Arrer, E, Gibitz, HJ. Detection of beta 2-transferrin with agarose gel electrophoresis, immunofixation and silver staining in cerebrospinal fluid, secretions and other body fluids. *J Clin Chem Clin Biochem* 1987; **25**:113–16.

115. Stibler, H. Carbohydrate-deficient transferrin in serum: a new marker of potentially harmful alcohol consumption reviewed. *Clin Chem* 1991; **37**:2029–37.

116. Bell, H, Tallaksen, C, Sjaheim, T, et al. Serum carbohydrate-deficient transferrin as a marker of alcohol consumption in patients with chronic liver diseases. *Alcohol Clin Exp Res* 1993; **17**:246–52.

117. Kristiansson, B, Andersson, M, Tonnby, B, Hagberg, B. Disialotransferrin developmental deficiency syndrome. *Arch Dis Child* 1989; **64**:71–6.

118. Sloman, AJ, Kelly, RH. Transferrin allelic variants may cause false positives in the detection of cerebrospinal fluid fistulae. *Clin Chem* 1993; **39**:1444–5.

119. Jaeken, J, van Eijk, HG, van der Heul, C, Corbeel, L, Eeckels, R, Eggermont, E. Sialic acid-deficient serum and cerebrospinal fluid transferrin in a newly recognized genetic syndrome. *Clin Chim Acta* 1984; **144**:245–7.

120. Zaret, DL, Morrison, N, Gulbranson, R, Keren, DF. Immunofixation to quantify beta 2-transferrin in cerebrospinal fluid to detect leakage of cerebrospinal fluid from skull injury. *Clin Chem* 1992; **38**:1908–12.

121. Oberascher, G. Cerebrospinal fluid otorrhea–new trends in diagnosis. *Am J Otol* 1988; **9**:102–8.

122. Skedros, DG, Cass, SP, Hirsch, BE, Kelly, RH. Sources of error in use of beta-2 transferrin analysis for diagnosing perilymphatic and cerebral spinal fluid leaks. *Otolaryngol Head Neck Surg* 1993; **109**: 861–4.

123. Kelly, RH, Kelly, CM, Busis, SN. Factitious hearing loss and otorrhea in an adolescent boy. *Clin Chim Acta* 2000; **299**:205–9.

124. Nandapalan, V, Watson, ID, Swift, AC. Beta-2-transferrin and cerebrospinal fluid rhinorrhoea. *Clin Otolaryngol* 1996; **21**:259–64.

125. Roelandse, FW, van der Zwart, N, Didden, JH, van Loon, J, Souverijn, JH. Detection of CSF leakage by isoelectric focusing on polyacrylamide gel, direct immunofixation of transferrins, and silver staining. *Clin Chem* 1998; **44**: 351–3.

126. Normansell, DE, Stacy, EK, Booker, CF, Butler, TZ. Detection of beta-2 transferrin in otorrhea and rhinorrhea in a routine clinical laboratory setting. *Clin Diagn Lab Immunol* 1994; **1**:68–70.

127. Keir, G, Zeman, A, Brookes, G, Porter, M, Thompson, EJ. Immunoblotting of transferrin in the identification of cerebrospinal fluid otorrhoea and rhinorrhoea. *Ann Clin Biochem* 1992; **29**(Pt 2):210–13.

128. Ryall, RG, Peacock, MK, Simpson, DA. Usefulness of beta 2-transferrin assay in the detection of cerebrospinal fluid leaks following head injury. *J Neurosurg* 1992; **77**:737–9.

129. Bateman, N, Jones, NS. Rhinorrhoea feigning cerebrospinal fluid leak: nine illustrative cases. *J Laryngol Otol* 2000; **114**:462–4.

130. Warnecke, A, Averbeck, T, Wurster, U, Harmening, M, Lenarz, T, Stover, T. Diagnostic relevance of beta2- transferrin for the detection of cerebrospinal fluid fistulas. *Arch Otolaryngol Head Neck Surg* 2004; **130**:1178–84.

131. Oberascher, G 1988;A modern concept of cerebrospinal fluid diagnosis in oto- and rhinorrhea. *Rhinology*, **26**, 89–103.

132. Seidl, RO, Todt, I, Ernst, A. Reconstruction of traumatic skull base defects with alloplastic, resorbable fleece. *HNO* 2000; **48**:753–7.

133. Simmen, D, Bischoff, T, Schuknecht, B. Experiences with assessment of frontobasal defects, a diagnostic concept. *Laryngorhinootologie* 1997; **76**:583–7.

134. Skedros, DG, Cass, SP, Hirsch, BE, Kelly, RH. Beta-2 transferrin assay in clinical management of cerebral spinal fluid and perilymphatic fluid leaks. *J Otolaryngol* 1993; **22**: 341–4.

135. Tumani, H, Reiber, H, Nau, R, *et al.* Beta-trace protein concentration in cerebrospinal fluid is decreased in patients with bacterial meningitis. *Neurosci Lett* 1998; **242**:5–8.

136. Hochwald, GM, Pepe, AJ, Thorbecke, GJ. Trace proteins in biological fluids. IV. Physicochemical properties and sites of formation of gamma-trace and beta-trace proteins. *Proc Soc Exp Biol Med* 1967; **124**:961–6.

137. Urade, Y, Tanaka, T, Eguchi, N, *et al.* Structural and functional significance of cysteine residues of glutathione-independent prostaglandin D synthase. Identification of Cys65 as an essential thiol. *J Biol Chem* 1995; **270**:1422–8.

138. Blodorn, B, Mader, M, Urade, Y, Hayaishi, O, Felgenhauer, K, Bruck, W. Choroid plexus: the major site of mRNA expression for the beta-trace protein (prostaglandin D synthase) in human brain. *Neurosci Lett* 1996; **209**:117–20.

139. Bachmann-Harildstad, G. Diagnostic values of beta-2 transferrin and beta-trace protein as markers for cerebrospinal fluid fistula. *Rhinology* 2008; **46**:82–5.

140. Meco, C, Oberascher, G, Arrer, E, Moser, G, Albegger, K. Beta-trace protein test: new guidelines for the reliable diagnosis of cerebrospinal fluid fistula. *Otolaryngol Head Neck Surg* 2003; **129**:508–17.

141. Felgenhauer, K, Schadlich, HJ, Nekic, M. Beta traceprotein as marker for cerebrospinal fluid fistula. *Klin Wochenschr* 1987; **65**:764–8.

142. Meco, C, Arrer, E, Oberascher, G. Efficacy of cerebrospinal fluid fistula repair: sensitive quality control using the beta-trace protein test. *Am J Rhinol* 2007; **21**:729–36.

143. Petereit, HF, Bachmann, G, Nekic, M, Althaus, H, Pukrop, R. A new nephelometric assay for beta-trace protein (prostaglandin D synthase) as an indicator of liquorrhea. *J Neurol Neurosurg Psychiatry* 2001; **71**:347–51.

144. Reiber, H, Walther, K, Althaus, H. Beta-trace protein as sensitive marker for CSF rhinorrhea and CSF otorrhea. *Acta Neurol Scand* 2003; **108**:359–62.

145. Bachmann-Harildstad, G. Incidence of CSF fistula after paranasal sinus surgery: the Northern Norwegian experience. *Rhinology* 2007; **45**:305–7.

146. Inoue, T, Kibata, K, Suzuki, M, Nakamura, S, Motoda, R, Orita, K. Identification of a vascular endothelial growth factor (VEGF) antagonist, sFlt-1, from a human hematopoietic cell line NALM-16. *FEBS Lett* 2000; **469**:14–18.

147. Gaudry, M, Bregerie, O, Andrieu, V, El Benna, J, Pocidalo, MA, Hakim, J. Intracellular pool of vascular endothelial growth factor in human neutrophils. *Blood* 1997; **90**: 4153–61.

148. Perez-Ruiz, M, Ros, J, Morales-Ruiz, M, *et al.* Vascular endothelial growth factor production in peritoneal macrophages of cirrhotic patients: regulation by cytokines and bacterial lipopolysaccharide. *Hepatology* 1999; **29**:1057–63.

149. Xiong, M, Elson, G, Legarda, D, Leibovich, SJ. Production of vascular endothelial growth factor by murine macrophages: regulation by hypoxia, lactate, and the inducible nitric oxide synthase pathway. *Am J Pathol* 1998; **153**: 587–98.

150. Williams, B, Quinn-Baker, A, Gallacher, B. Serum and platelet-derived growth factor-induced expression of vascular permeability factor mRNA by human vascular smooth muscle cells in vitro. *Clin Sci (Lond)* 1995; **88**: 141–7.

151. Ferrara, N. Role of vascular endothelial growth factor in regulation of physiological angiogenesis. *Am J Physiol Cell Physiol* 2001; **280**:C1358–66.

152. Reijneveld, JC, Brandsma, D, Boogerd, W, *et al.* CSF levels of angiogenesis-related proteins in patients with leptomeningeal metastasis. *Neurology* 2005; **65**:1120–2.

153. Herrlinger, U, Wiendl, H, Renninger, M, Forschler, H, Dichgans, J, Weller, M. Vascular endothelial growth factor (VEGF) in leptomeningeal metastasis: diagnostic and prognostic value. *Br J Cancer* 2004; **91**:219–24.

154. Peles, E, Lidar, Z, Simon, AJ, Grossman, R, Nass, D, Ram, Z. Angiogenic factors in the cerebrospinal fluid of patients with astrocytic brain tumors. *Neurosurgery* 2004; **55**: 562–7.

155. Sampath, P, Weaver, CE, Sungarian, A, Cortez, S, Alderson, L, Stopa, EG. Cerebrospinal fluid (vascular endothelial growth factor) and serologic (recoverin) tumor markers for malignant glioma. *Cancer Control* 2004; **11**:174–80.

156. Stockhammer, G, Poewe, W, Burgstaller, S, *et al.* Vascular endothelial growth factor in CSF: a biological marker for carcinomatous meningitis. *Neurology* 2000; **54**: 1670–6.

157. van de Langerijt, B, Gijtenbeek, JM, de Reus, HP, *et al.* CSF levels of growth factors and plasminogen activators in leptomeningeal metastases. *Neurology* 2006; **67**:114–19.

158. Ribom, D, Larsson, A, Pietras, K, Smits, A. Growth factor analysis of low-grade glioma CSF: PDGF and VEGF are not detectable. *Neurol Sci* 2003; **24**:70–3.

159. Husain, N, Awasthi, S, Haris, M, Gupta, RK, Husain, M. Vascular endothelial growth factor as a marker of disease activity in neurotuberculosis. *J Infect* 2008; **56**:114–19.

160. Matsuyama, W, Hashiguchi, T, Umehara, F, *et al.* Expression of vascular endothelial growth factor in tuberculous meningitis. *J Neurol Sci* 2001; **186**:75–9.

161. Tsai, HC, Liu, YC, Lee, SS, Chen, ER, Yen, CM. Vascular endothelial growth factor is associated with blood brain barrier dysfunction in eosinophilic meningitis caused by *Angiostrongylus cantonensis* infection. *Am J Trop Med Hyg* 2007; **76**:592–5.

162. Kastenbauer, S, Angele, B, Sporer, B, Pfister, HW, Koedel, U. Patterns of protein expression in infectious meningitis: a cerebrospinal fluid protein array analysis. *J Neuroimmunol* 2005; **164**:134–9.

163. Coenjaerts, FE, van der Flier M, Mwinzi, PN, *et al.* Intrathecal production and secretion of vascular endothelial growth factor during cryptococcal meningitis. *J Infect Dis* 2004; **190**:1310–17.

164. van der Flier, M, Hoppenreijs, S, van Rensburg, AJ, *et al.* Vascular endothelial growth factor and blood-brain barrier disruption in tuberculous meningitis. *Pediatr Infect Dis J* 2004; **23**:608–13.

165. Sporer, B, Koedel, U, Paul, R, Eberle, J, Arendt, G, Pfister, HW. Vascular endothelial growth factor (VEGF) is increased in serum, but not in cerebrospinal fluid in HIV associated CNS diseases. *J Neurol Neurosurg Psychiatry* 2004; **75**:298–300.

166. Moreau, C, Devos, D, Brunaud-Danel, V, *et al.* Paradoxical response of VEGF expression to hypoxia in CSF of patients with ALS. *J Neurol Neurosurg Psychiatry* 2006; **77**:255–7.

167. Just, N, Moreau, C, Lassalle, P, *et al.* High erythropoietin and low vascular endothelial growth factor levels in cerebrospinal fluid from hypoxemic ALS patients suggest an abnormal response to hypoxia. *Neuromuscul Disord* 2007; **17**:169–73.

168. Nagata, T, Nagano, I, Shiote, M, *et al.* Elevation of MCP-1 and MCP-1/VEGF ratio in cerebrospinal fluid of amyotrophic lateral sclerosis patients. *Neurol Res* 2007; **29**: 772–6.

169. Devos, D, Moreau, C, Lassalle, P, *et al.* Low levels of the vascular endothelial growth factor in CSF from early ALS patients. *Neurology* 2004; **62**:2127–9.

170. Ilzecka, J. Cerebrospinal fluid vascular endothelial growth factor in patients with amyotrophic lateral sclerosis. *Clin Neurol Neurosurg* 2004; **106**:289–93.

171. Foyouzi, N, Norwitz, ER, Tsen, LC, Buhimschi, CS, Buhimschi, IA. Placental growth factor in the cerebrospinal fluid of women with preeclampsia. *Int J Gynaecol Obstet* 2006; **92**:32–7.

172. Blasko, I, Lederer, W, Oberbauer, H, *et al.* Measurement of thirteen biological markers in CSF of patients with Alzheimer's disease and other dementias. *Dement Geriatr Cogn Disord* 2006; **21**:9–15.

173. Tarkowski, E, Issa, R, Sjogren, M, *et al.* Increased intrathecal levels of the angiogenic factors VEGF and TGFbeta in Alzheimer's disease and vascular dementia. *Neurobiol Aging* 2002; **23**:237–43.

174. Scheufler, KM, Drevs, J, van Velthoven, V, *et al.* Implications of vascular endothelial growth factor, sFlt-1, and sTie-2 in plasma, serum and cerebrospinal fluid during cerebral ischemia in man. *J Cereb Blood Flow Metab* 2003; **23**: 99–110.

175. Borel, CO, McKee, A, Parra, A, *et al.* Possible role for vascular cell proliferation in cerebral vasospasm after subarachnoid hemorrhage. *Stroke* 2003; **34**:427–433.

176. Watanabe, O, Maruyama, I, Arimura, K, *et al.* Overproduction of vascular endothelial growth factor/ vascular permeability factor is causative in Crow-Fukase (POEMS) syndrome. *Muscle Nerve* 1998; **21**:1390–7.

177. Petzold, A. Neurofilament phosphoforms: surrogate markers for axonal injury, degeneration and loss. *J Neurol Sci* 2005; **233**:183–98.

178. Petzold, A, Baker, D, Pryce, G, Keir, G, Thompson, EJ, Giovannoni, G. Quantification of neurodegeneration by measurement of brain-specific proteins. *J Neuroimmunol* 2003; **138**:45–8.

179. Miyazawa, I, Nakashima, I, Petzold, A, Fujihara, K, Sato, S, Itoyama, Y. High CSF neurofilament heavy chain levels in neuromyelitis optica. *Neurology* 2007; **68**:865–7.

180. Norgren, N, Rosengren, L, Stigbrand, T. Elevated neurofilament levels in neurological diseases. *Brain Res* 2003; **987**:25–31.

181. Rosengren, LE, Karlsson, JE, Karlsson, JO, Persson, LI, Wikkelso, C. Patients with amyotrophic lateral sclerosis and other neurodegenerative diseases have increased levels of neurofilament protein in CSF. *J Neurochem* 1996; **67**:2013–18.

182. Zetterberg, H, Jacobsson, J, Rosengren, L, Blennow, K, Andersen, PM. Cerebrospinal fluid neurofilament light levels in amyotrophic lateral sclerosis: impact of SOD1 genotype. *Eur J Neurol* 2007; **14**:1329–33.

183. Brettschneider, J, Petzold, A, Sussmuth, SD, *et al.* Neurofilament heavy-chain NfH(SMI35) in cerebrospinal fluid supports the differential diagnosis of Parkinsonian syndromes. *Mov Disord* 2006; **21**:2224–7.

184. Abdo, WF, Bloem, BR, van Geel, WJ, Esselink, RA, Verbeek, MM. CSF neurofilament light chain and tau differentiate multiple system atrophy from Parkinson's disease. *Neurobiol Aging* 2007; **28**:742–7.

185. Holmberg, B, Rosengren, L, Karlsson, JE, Johnels, B. Increased cerebrospinal fluid levels of neurofilament protein in progressive supranuclear palsy and multiple system atrophy compared with Parkinson's disease. *Mov Disord* 1998; **13**:70–7.

186. Lim, ET, Grant, D, Pashenkov, M, *et al.* Cerebrospinal fluid levels of brain specific proteins in optic neuritis 2. *Mult Scler* 2004; **10**:261–5.

187. Petzold, A, Eikelenboom, MI, Keir, G, *et al.* The new global multiple sclerosis severity score (MSSS) correlates with axonal but not glial biomarkers. *Mult Scler* 2006; **12**:325–8.

188. Lim, ET, Sellebjerg, F, Jensen, CV, *et al.* Acute axonal damage predicts clinical outcome in patients with multiple sclerosis. *Mult Scler* 2005; **11**:532–6.

189. Malmestrom, C, Haghighi, S, Rosengren, L, Andersen, O, Lycke, J. Neurofilament light protein and glial fibrillary acidic protein as biological markers in MS. *Neurology* 2003; **61**:1720–5.

190. Norgren, N, Sundstrom, P, Svenningsson, A, Rosengren, L, Stigbrand, T, Gunnarsson, M. Neurofilament and glial fibrillary acidic protein in multiple sclerosis. *Neurology* 2004; **63**:1586–90.

191. Eikelenboom, MJ, Petzold, A, Lazeron, RH, *et al.* Multiple sclerosis: neurofilament light chain antibodies are correlated to cerebral atrophy. *Neurology* 2003; **60**:219–23.

192. Brettschneider, J, Petzold, A, Schottle, D, Claus, A, Riepe, M, Tumani, H. The neurofilament heavy chain (NfH) in

the cerebrospinal fluid diagnosis of Alzheimer's disease. *Dement Geriatr Cogn Disord* 2006; **6**:291–5.

193. de Jong, D, Jansen, RW, Pijnenburg, YA, *et al.* CSF neurofilament proteins in the differential diagnosis of dementia. *J Neurol Neurosurg Psychiatry* 2007; **78**:936–8.

194. Petzold, A, Keir, G, Warren, J, Fox, N, Rossor, MN. A systematic review and meta-analysis of CSF neurofilament protein levels as biomarkers in dementia. *Neurodegen Dis* 2007; **4**:185–94.

195. Rosengren, LE, Karlsson, JE, Sjogren, M, Blennow, K, Wallin, A. Neurofilament protein levels in CSF are increased in dementia. *Neurology* 1999; **52**:1090–3.

196. Sjogren, M, Blomberg, M, Jonsson, M, *et al.* Neurofilament protein in cerebrospinal fluid: a marker of white matter changes. *J Neurosci Res* 2001; **66**:510–16.

197. Pijnenburg, YA, Janssen, JC, Schoonenboom, NS, *et al.* CSF neurofilaments in frontotemporal dementia compared with early onset Alzheimer's disease and controls. *Dement Geriatr Cogn Disord* 2007; **23**:225–30.

198. Sjogren, M, Rosengren, L, Minthon, L, Davidsson, P, Blennow, K, Wallin, A. Cytoskeleton proteins in CSF distinguish frontotemporal dementia from AD. *Neurology* 2000; **54**:1960–4.

199. Sjogren, M, Wallin, A. Pathophysiological aspects of frontotemporal dementia–emphasis on cytoskeleton proteins and autoimmunity. *Mech Ageing Dev* 2001; **122**:1923–35.

200. Wallin, A, Sjogren, M. Cerebrospinal fluid cytoskeleton proteins in patients with subcortical white-matter dementia. *Mech Ageing Dev* 2001; **122**:1937–49.

201. Guez, M, Hildingsson, C, Rosengren, L, Karlsson, K, Toolanen, G. Nervous tissue damage markers in cerebrospinal fluid after cervical spine injuries and whiplash trauma. *J Neurotrauma* 2003; **20**:853–8.

202. Gisslen, M, Rosengren, L, Hagberg, L, Deeks, SG, Price, RW. Cerebrospinal fluid signs of neuronal damage after antiretroviral treatment interruption in HIV-1 infection. *AIDS Res Ther* 2005; **2**:6.

203. Hagberg, L, Fuchs, D, Rosengren, L, Gisslen, M. Intrathecal immune activation is associated with cerebrospinal fluid markers of neuronal destruction in AIDS patients. *J Neuroimmunol* 2000; **102**:51–5.

204. Gisslen, M, Hagberg, L, Brew, BJ, Cinque, P, Price, RW, Rosengren, L. Elevated cerebrospinal fluid neurofilament light protein concentrations predict the development of AIDS dementia complex. *J Infect Dis* 2007; **195**:1774–8.

205. Abdulle, S, Mellgren, A, Brew, BJ, *et al.* CSF neurofilament protein (NFL) – a marker of active HIV-related neurodegeneration. *J Neurol* 2007; **254**:1026–32.

206. Mellgren, A, Price, RW, Hagberg, L, Rosengren, L, Brew, BJ, Gisslen, M. Antiretroviral treatment reduces increased CSF

neurofilament protein (NFL) in HIV-1 infection. *Neurology* 2007; **69**:1536–41.

207. Petzold, A, Rejdak, K, Belli, A, *et al.* Axonal pathology in subarachnoid and intracerebral hemorrhage. *J Neurotrauma* 2005; **22**:407–14.

208. Lewis, SB, Wolper, RA, Miralia, L, Yang, C, Shaw, G. Detection of phosphorylated NF-H in the cerebrospinal fluid and blood of aneurysmal subarachnoid hemorrhage patients. *J Cereb Blood Flow Metab* 2008; **28**:1261–71.

209. Petzold, A, Keir, G, Kay, A, Kerr, M, Thompson, EJ. Axonal damage and outcome in subarachnoid haemorrhage. *J Neurol Neurosurg Psychiatry* 2006; **77**:753–9.

210. Nylen, K, Csajbok, LZ, Ost, M, *et al.* CSF -Neurofilament correlates with outcome after aneurysmal subarachnoid hemorrhage. *Neurosci Lett* 2006; **404**:132–6.

211. van Geel, WJ, Rosengren, LE, Verbeek, MM. An enzyme immunoassay to quantify neurofilament light chain in cerebrospinal fluid. *J Immunol Methods* 2005; **296**:179–85.

212. Tullberg, M, Hultin, L, Ekholm, S, Mansson, JE, Fredman, P, Wikkelso, C. White matter changes in normal pressure hydrocephalus and Binswanger disease: specificity, predictive value and correlations to axonal degeneration and demyelination. *Acta Neurol Scand* 2002; **105**:417–26.

213. Tisell, M, Tullberg, M, Mansson, JE, Fredman, P, Blennow, K, Wikkelso, C. Differences in cerebrospinal fluid dynamics do not affect the levels of biochemical markers in ventricular CSF from patients with aqueductal stenosis and idiopathic normal pressure hydrocephalus. *Eur J Neurol* 2004; **11**:17–23.

214. Tullberg, M, Blennow, K, Mansson, JE, Fredman, P, Tisell, M, Wikkelso, C. Ventricular cerebrospinal fluid neurofilament protein levels decrease in parallel with white matter pathology after shunt surgery in normal pressure hydrocephalus. *Eur J Neurol* 2007; **14**:248–54.

215. Petzold, A, Hinds, N, Murray, NM, *et al.* CSF neurofilament levels: a potential prognostic marker in Guillain–Barré syndrome. *Neurology* 2006; **67**:1071–3.

216. Rosen, H, Karlsson, JE, Rosengren, L. CSF levels of neurofilament is a valuable predictor of long-term outcome after cardiac arrest. *J Neurol Sci* 2004; **221**:19–24.

217. Skoldenberg, B, Aurelius, E, Hjalmarsson, A, *et al.* Incidence and pathogenesis of clinical relapse after herpes simplex encephalitis in adults. *J Neurol* 2006; **253**:163–70.

218. Baumann, N, Pham-Dinh, D. Biology of oligodendrocyte and myelin in the mammalian central nervous system. *Physiol Rev* 2001; **81**:871–927.

219. van Engelen, BG, Lamers, KJ, Gabreels, FJ, Wevers, RA, van Geel, WJ, Borm, GF. Age-related changes of neuron specific enolase, S-100 protein, and myelin basic protein concentrations in cerebrospinal fluid. *Clin Chem* 1992; **38**: 813–16.

220. Cornblath, DR, Griffin, JW, Tennekoon, GI. Immunoreactive myelin basic protein in cerebrospinal fluid of patients with peripheral neuropathies. *Ann Neurol* 1986; **20**:370–2.

221. Edstrom, S, Hanner, P, Andersen, O, Rosenhall, U, Vahlne, A, Karlsson, B. Elevated levels of myelin basic protein in CSF in relation to auditory brainstem responses in Bell's palsy. *Acta Otolaryngol* 1987; **103**:198–203.

222. Davies, L, McLeod, JG, Muir, A, Hensley, WJ. Diagnostic value of cerebrospinal fluid myelin basic protein in patients with neurological illness. *Clin Exp Neurol* 1987; **24**:5–10.

223. Lamers, KJ, van Engelen, BG, Gabreels, FJ, Hommes, OR, Borm, GF, Wevers, RA. Cerebrospinal neuron-specific enolase, S-100 and myelin basic protein in neurological disorders. *Acta Neurol Scand* 1995; **92**:247–51.

224. Cohen, SR, Herndon, RM, McKhann, GM. Radio-immunoassay of myelin basic protein in spinal fluid. An index of active demyelination. *N Engl J Med* 1976; **295**: 1455–7.

225. Noppe, M, Crols, R, Andries, D, Lowenthal, A. Determination in human cerebrospinal fluid of glial fibrillary acidic protein, S-100 and myelin basic protein as indices of nonspecific or specific central nervous tissue pathology. *Clin Chim Acta* 1986; **155**:143–50.

226. Whitaker, JN. Myelin encephalitogenic protein fragments in cerebrospinal fluid of persons with multiple sclerosis. *Neurology* 1977; **27**:911–20.

227. Thomson, AJ, Brazil, J, Feighery, C, *et al.* CSF myelin basic protein in multiple sclerosis. *Acta Neurol Scand* 1985; **72**:577–83.

228. Cohen, SR, Brune, MJ, Herndon, RM, McKhann, GM. Cerebrospinal fluid myelin basic protein and multiple sclerosis. *Adv Exp Med Biol* 1978; **100**:513–19.

229. Martin-Mondiere, C, Jacque, C, Delassalle, A, Cesaro, P, Carydakis, C, Degos, JD. Cerebrospinal myelin basic protein in multiple sclerosis. Identification of two groups of patients with acute exacerbation. *Arch Neurol* 1987; **44**: 276–8.

230. Sellebjerg, F, Jensen, CV, Christiansen, M. Intrathecal IgG synthesis and autoantibody-secreting cells in multiple sclerosis. *J Neuroimmunol* 2000; **2**:207–15.

231. Warren, KG, Catz, I, McPherson, TA. CSF myelin basic protein levels in acute optic neuritis and multiple sclerosis. *Can J Neurol Sci* 1983; **10**:235–8.

232. Thompson, AJ, Hutchinson, M, Brazil, J, Feighery, C, Martin, EA. A clinical and laboratory study of benign multiple sclerosis. *Q J Med* 1986; **58**:69–80.

233. Thompson, AJ, Brazil, J, Hutchinson, M, Feighery, C. Three possible laboratory indexes of disease activity in multiple sclerosis. *Neurology* 1987; **37**:515–19.

234. Barkhof, F, Frequin, ST, Hommes, OR, *et al.* A correlative triad of gadolinium-DTPA MRI, EDSS, and CSFMBP in

relapsing multiple sclerosis patients treated with high-dose intravenous methylprednisolone. *Neurology* 1992; **42**:63–7.

235. Sellebjerg, F, Christiansen, M, Jensen, J, Frederiksen, JL. Immunological effects of oral high-dose methylprednisolone in acute optic neuritis and multiple sclerosis. *Eur J Neurol* 2000; **7**:281–9.

236. Whitaker, JN, Layton, BA, Herman, PK, Kachelhofer, RD, Burgard, S, Bartolucci, AA. Correlation of myelin basic protein-like material in cerebrospinal fluid of multiple sclerosis patients with their response to glucocorticoid treatment. *Ann Neurol* 1993; **33**:10–17.

237. Sellebjerg, F, Jensen, CV, Larsson, HB, Frederiksen, JL. Gadolinium-enhanced magnetic resonance imaging pre-

dicts response to methylprednisolone in multiple sclerosis. *Mult Scler* 2003; **9**:102–7.

238. Bossuyt, PM, Reitsma, JB, Bruns, DE, *et al.* Towards complete and accurate reporting of studies of diagnostic accuracy: the STARD initiative. Standards for Reporting of Diagnostic Accuracy. *Clin Chem* 2003; **49**:1–6.

239. McShane, LM, Altman, DG, Sauerbrei, W, Taube, SE, Gion, M, Clark, GM. Reporting recommendations for tumour marker prognostic studies (REMARK). *Br J Cancer* 2005; **93**:387–91.

240. Lewczuk, P, Beck, G, Ganslandt, O, *et al.* International quality control survey of neurochemical dementia diagnostics. *Neurosci Lett* 2006; **409**:1–4.

CHAPTER 14

Neuroimaging in the management of motor neuron diseases

M. Filippi,[1] F. Agosta,[1] S. Abrahams,[2] F. Fazekas,[3] J. Grosskreutz,[4] S. Kalra,[5] J. Kassubek,[6] V. Silani,[7] M.R. Turner[8] and J.C. Masdeu[9]

[1]San Raffaele Scientific Institute, Vita-Salute San Raffaele University. Milan, Italy; [2]Euan MacDonald Centre, The University of Edinburgh, Edinburgh, UK; [3]Medical University of Graz, Graz, Austria; [4]Friedrich-Schiller-University Hospital Jena, Jena, Germany; [5]University of Alberta, Edmonton, Alberta, Canada; [6]University of Ulm, Ulm, Germany; [7]Università degli Studi di Milano, IRCCS Istituto Auxologico Italiano, Milan, Italy; [8]University of Oxford, Oxford, UK; [9]Clínica de la Universidad de Navarra, Pamplona, Spain

Background

The term motor neuron disease (MND) comprises a group of disorders involving preferential damage to upper (UMN) and/or lower (LMN) motor neurons. The clinical spectrum of MND is wide in adulthood, ranging from simultaneous involvement of UMN and LMN (classic amyotrophic lateral sclerosis [ALS], and 90% of all MND cases), a pure UMN syndrome (primary lateral sclerosis [PLS]), and an isolated LMN involvement (variously defined by the term progressive muscular atrophy [PMA]). A diagnosis of MND predominantly relies on the interpretation of clinical symptoms and signs, with the use of paraclinical and laboratory tests to exclude other causes [1, 2]. Indeed, the greatest contribution of neuroimaging to the diagnosis of MND so far has been its sensitivity to detect changes suggestive of alternative diagnoses [3].

Reliable objective biomarkers of both UMN and LMN involvement are critical for the early diagnosis and monitoring of disease progression in patients with MNDs.

Proton magnetic resonance spectroscopic imaging (^{1}H-MRSI) and diffusion tensor imaging (DTI) hold particular promise for the UMN lesion in this regard [3]. Moreover, it is recognized that ALS is characterized by an extramotor cerebral pathology that, to a variable extent, overlaps with the clinico-pathological features of fronto-temporal lobar degeneration (FTLD) [4]. The use of other neuroimaging techniques, such as positron emission tomography (PET) and functional magnetic resonance imaging (fMRI), have provided a more complete picture of this extramotor involvement and enabled functional changes to be studied in MNDs.

These guidelines comprise an objective appraisal of the evidence with regard to the utility of neuroimaging techniques in adult patients with MNDs, which ranges from diagnostic and monitoring aspects to the *in vivo* study of the pathobiology of MNDs. Consensus recommendations are given and graded according to the EFNS guidance regulations [5]. Where there was lack of evidence but consensus was reached, we have stated our opinion as good practice points.

European Handbook of Neurological Management: Volume 2, Second Edition. Edited by Nils Erik Gilhus, Michael P. Barnes, Michael Brainin.
© 2012 Blackwell Publishing Ltd. Published 2012 by Blackwell Publishing Ltd.

Aims of the European Federation of Neurological Societies (EFNS) Task Force

The objectives of the Task Force on Neuroimaging of Motor Neuron Disease are: 1) to provide guidelines for the application of conventional MRI for the diagnosis and monitoring of adult patients with MNDs in clinical practice; 2) to clarify the current status and clinical role of advanced neuroimaging techniques in MNDs; and 3) to investigate the role of neuroimaging for exploring differences in the patterns of brain involvement between sporadic and familial MND groups.

Search strategy

Data for this review were identified by searches of Medline for relevant articles from January 1965 to July 2009. The search terms 'amyotrophic lateral sclerosis', 'primary lateral sclerosis', 'progressive muscular atrophy', 'motor neuron disease', 'frontotemporal dementia AND motor neuron disease', 'frontotemporal dementia AND amyotrophic lateral sclerosis', 'superoxide dismutase-1', 'corticospinal tract', 'magnetic resonance imaging', 'atrophy', 'voxel-based morphometry', 'proton magnetic resonance spectroscopy', 'proton magnetic resonance spectroscopy imaging', 'diffusion weighted MRI', 'diffusion tensor MRI', 'diffusion tensor imaging', 'diffusion tensor imaging-based tractography', 'magnetization transfer MRI', 'positron emission tomography', 'functional MRI' and 'disability' were used. Using this strategy we identified 386 papers. We also searched reference lists of reports identified and selected those we judged relevant. Original papers, meta-analyses, review papers as well as guideline recommendations were reviewed. Only papers published in English were considered.

Methods for reaching consensus

MF and FA searched for relevant articles and prepared an initial draft. Consensus was reached by circulating drafts of the manuscript to the Task Force members and by discussion of the classification of evidence and recommendations.

Signal changes on conventional MRI in patients with sporadic MNDs

The revised criteria of the World Federation of Neurology Research Group on Motor Neuron Diseases [6] state that conventional MRI studies are not required in those cases that have a clinically definite disease with a bulbar or pseudobulbar onset. On the other hand, in patients with clinically probable or possible ALS, routine brain and/or spinal cord MRI can be useful in excluding several ALS mimic syndromes, including cerebral lesions (e.g., multiple sclerosis and cerebrovascular disease), skull base lesions, cervical spondylitic myelopathy, other myelopathy (e.g., foramen magnum lesions, intrinsic and extrinsic tumours, syringomyelia), conus lesions and thoraco-lumbar-sacral radiculopathy [7].

Corticospinal tract (CST) hyperintensities on T2-weighted, proton density (PD)-weighted, and fluid-attenuated inversion recovery (FLAIR) images are frequently found in MND patients [8, 9, 10, 11, 12, 13, 14, 15, 16, 17]. CST hyperintensities, which are best followed on coronal scans, have been reported mostly bilaterally and can be recognized in the caudal portion of the posterior limb of the internal capsule. They typically extend downward to the ventral portion of the brainstem and less consistently upward through the corona radiata. Such lesions may occur more often in younger patients with greater disability [13]. It is not yet clear which may be the more sensitive MR sequence to detect CST hyperintensities in MND patients. Three studies have found PD-weighted images as more reliable than T2-weighted images [9, 18, 19], whereas two other groups showed the opposite [16, 20]. Finally, other studies reported that CST signal abnormalities in ALS are better detected with FLAIR imaging [11]. In patients with MND, increased T2 signal intensity has also been described in extramotor frontotemporal regions [21, 22].

Increased CST signal intensity has also been described in healthy individuals [14] and, strikingly, after hepatic transplantation [23]. Thus, CST hyperintensity is considered nonspecific for MNDs overall. Furthermore, the reported frequency of conventional MRI abnormalities in ALS patients is very heterogeneous, ranging from 15% to 76%. However, most of the studies used a dichotomous approach (present/absent) to interrogate the signal abnormality of the CST and this may have contributed to the reduced sensitivity of conventional MRI. In contrast, Cheung *et al.* evaluated the spatial extent of CST signal changes and reported the highest MRI sensitivity for detecting CST abnormality [9]. In a recent study in ALS and PLS patients, the combined application of T2-weighted, PD-weighted and FLAIR images reached a sensitivity of ~62% [19]. It is interesting to note that in PLS patients the sensitivity was higher (~78%), while in 'possible' or 'probable laboratory-supported' ALS patients (according to the revised El Escorial criteria [24]), the sensitivity of conventional MRI dropped significantly, to ~21% [19]. Finally, CST signal changes on FLAIR images increase with disease duration, but do not correlate with clinical scores [11].

In ALS patients, the precentral cortex can present a low signal intensity (hypointense rim) on T2-weighted images [9, 12, 13, 15, 16, 25]. This so-called ribbon-like hypointensity is sharply contrasted by the hyperintense signal of cerebrospinal fluid in the adjacent sulci.

T2-weighted [15, 26] or T1-weighted [16] hyperintensities of the anterolateral columns of the cervical cord have been observed in ALS patients, with higher specificity than signal changes of brain MR scans [15, 26]. T1-hyperintensity of the anterolateral cervical cord has been associated with younger patients and rapid disease progression [16].

Recommendations

- All patients suspected of having a MND, where a plausible alternative unifying neuroanatomical explanation exists, should undergo an MRI of the brain, whole cord or both depending on the clinical presentation (Class IV, good practice point) [2].

- The detection of CST hyperintensities on T2-weighted, PD-weighted and FLAIR imaging and a T2-hypointense rim in the precentral gyrus can support a pre-existing suspicion of ALS (Class IV, good practice point). However, considering the low sensitivity and specificity of such abnormalities and the weak correlation with clinical findings, the specific search of these abnormalities for the purpose of making a firm diagnosis of ALS is not recommended (Class IV, good practice point).

Advanced neuroimaging techniques in patients with sporadic MNDs

Atrophy

In ALS patients compared to controls, reduced brain parenchymal fraction (BPF) has been reported in two studies [27, 28]. It is remarkable that atrophy could only be appreciated in the analysis of BPF, defined as the proportion of brain parenchymal volume normalized to total intracranial volume, whereas neither the calculation of normalized brain volume [28] nor the absolute volume measurements in non-normalized three-dimensional MR images [29, 30] revealed significant group differences. This highlights the fact that global atrophy is relatively mild in ALS and regional differences may be more important. Lower whole-brain volume has been recently demonstrated in a group of PLS patients relative to controls [31].

With respect to the regional distribution of brain atrophy, the pattern and extent of volume loss vary among studies. Differences in image pre-processing and statistical analysis, as well as in the clinical characteristics of the cohorts of patients studied, may contribute to explain this variability. This is particularly relevant in relation to the cognitive status of the patients. Indeed, a significant proportion of patients with ALS (perhaps up to 50%) have cognitive or behavioural dysfunction due to coexisting FTLD [4]. Furthermore, a small subset of patients meets criteria for frontotemporal dementia (ALS-FTD). Some studies have included patients with an ALS-FTD syndrome, while others restrict their sample to non-demented patients with or without cognitive impairment. Cross-sectional MRI studies did not reach firm conclusions regarding the presence of motor/premotor cortical atrophy in ALS, since this was found by some authors [22, 27, 32, 33, 34, 35, 36, 37], but not by others [28, 29, 38, 39]. Although some MRI studies in PLS patients failed to show consistent precentral atrophy by visual assessment [40, 41], central atrophy has been noted in PLS [20], and moreover in the same study striking parietal region atrophy was noted in nearly half the cases of ALS [20]. A recent investigation using an automated analysis programme demonstrated significant atrophy of the precentral cortex in PLS patients, which was associated with disease severity [31]. In ALS patients with no cognitive impairment, voxel-based morphometry (VBM) studies consistently found regional grey matter (GM) loss which extends beyond the motor cortex to the frontotemporal and parietal regions [27, 28, 29, 32, 33, 34, 35, 36]. In non-demented ALS patients a trend was also observed with reduced amygdala size in the patient group compared with controls [30]. A significant correlation between disease severity and GM atrophy was found only in one study [33].

In ALS patients, white matter (WM) tissue loss along the CST has been observed in two studies [27, 29]. Ellis et al. [29] demonstrated WM tissue loss extending bilaterally from the precentral gyrus into the internal capsule and brainstem in patients with bulbar onset only. Extramotor WM atrophy, which included the anterior (prefrontal) corpus callosum, cerebellum and frontotemporal and occipital regions [27, 39], was also found; however, this was not confirmed by other authors [33, 34, 36]. Corpus callosum atrophy has been reported in PLS patients [31].

Studies investigating the cognitive status of the patients have revealed that ALS-FTD patients when compared to controls show a pattern of GM atrophy that involves motor/premotor cortices bilaterally, several prefrontal regions, superior temporal gyri, both temporal poles and left thalamus [34]. Most of the frontal regions were significantly more atrophied in the ALS-FTD group than in the ALS group [34]. Compared with cognitively normal patients, ALS patients with even sub-threshold variants of cognitive or behavioural impairment (i.e., not meeting criteria for dementia) demonstrated reduced GM in frontal, parietal and limbic lobes [42]. In cognitively impaired ALS patients, the performance on measures requiring action knowledge correlated with cortical atrophy in premotor and prefrontal cortex, while that on measures requiring object knowledge was associated with prefrontal cortex atrophy [35]. Only one study reported greater WM tissue loss in frontotemporal regions in cognitively impaired (non-demented) ALS patients compared with those with no evidence of cognitive impairment. Such tissue loss was associated with cognitive deficits on verbal fluency, although less extensive WM changes were also revealed in cognitively intact ALS patients [39].

A few longitudinal studies have attempted to assess quantitatively the dynamics of brain atrophy in patients with ALS [43, 44]. The first study showed that 16 ALS patients with no evidence of cognitive impairment experienced progression of GM atrophy in the left premotor cortex and right basal ganglia over <1 year [43]. Patients with rapidly progressing ALS showed greater GM atrophy in motor and extramotor frontal regions compared to non-rapidly progressing cases [43]. In a second study, significant longitudinal cortical atrophy in motor and premotor areas after about 5 months was found in four patients with ALS-FTD compared with controls [44].

Compared with controls, ALS patients demonstrated a decreased cervical cord cross-sectional area [45]. However, this finding was not confirmed by a second study [46]. A longitudinal study showed a significant development of cord atrophy over a 9-month follow-up [47].

^{1}H-MRSI

Nearly all ^{1}H-MRSI studies in ALS have demonstrated that either N-acetylaspartate (NAA) concentrations [48, 49, 50] or NAA:creatine (Cr) [50, 51, 52, 53, 54], NAA:choline (Cho) [51, 55] and NAA:Cr+Cho [54] ratios are reduced in the motor cortex of these patients. The reduction of the NAA:Cr ratio in the motor cortex was found to vary from 5% to 32% [50, 52, 53, 54, 56, 57]. NAA:Cho is reduced more than NAA:Cr in the motor cortex in those studies that measured both [51, 55, 56, 58, 59, 60, 61]. NAA:Cr and NAA:Cho ratios are reduced along the length of the intracranial CST from the motor cortex to the cerebral peduncle, however this reduction is most significant rostrally in the precentral gyrus and corona radiata [59]. Nevertheless, ^{1}H-MRSI changes in the brainstem have also been reported in ALS patients, with the greatest decrease of the NA (NAA+N acetylaspartylglutamate):Cr ratio in the pons and upper medulla of patients with prominent UMN or bulbar signs [62]. The finding of reduced NAA concentrations or NAA ratios were confirmed by cross-sectional studies performed at 3.0 T [58, 61, 63].

^{1}H-MRSI studies reported significant correlations between motor cortex NAA concentrations (or its ratios defined above) and disease severity (revised ALS Functional Rating Scale score [50, 61, 64]), the Norris limb scale [65], UMN signs [66] and maximum finger tapping rate [54]. Ellis et al. showed that bulbar onset patients have a lower NAA:Cho+Cr ratio in the motor cortex compared with limb onset patients. In a multiparametric study, T2 hypointensity of the motor cortex and bulbar onset were associated independently with the degree of NAA loss [49]. In a prospective ^{1}H-MRSI study of patients with probable or definite ALS, a multivariate analysis showed reduced survival for individuals with lower NAA:Cho, older age and shorter symptom duration [63]. Patients with NAA:Cho < 2.11 had a survival of 19.4 vs. 31.9 months of the others [63].

In ALS patients, decreased NAA:Cr ratios have been observed in premotor regions, primary sensory cortex and extramotor frontal regions, with relative sparing of the parietal lobe [53, 65]. Decreased frontal NAA:Cr ratio correlated with cognitive dysfunction [65]. Strong *et al.* [67] showed that ALS patients with bulbar onset and greater cognitive impairment compared to those with limb onset had a decrease in the NAA:Cr ratio in the cingulate gyrus.

Myo-inositol (mI), a spectroscopic marker for glial activity, was found to be increased in the motor cortex of ALS patients [51, 68]. Increased mI levels were associated with motor cortex hypointensity on T2-weighted images [68]. The NAA:mI ratio may provide better sensitivity and specificity for detecting disease than the other metabolite ratios, shown by a cross-sectional study of ALS patients using a magnetic field strength of 3.0 T [63]. In this study, decreased NAA:Cr and increased Ins:Cr had high sensitivity but low specificity, and decreased NAA:Cho had low sensitivity but high specificity; while the NAA:Ins ratio had moderate sensitivity (71%), the highest specificity (93%) and the best sensitivity and specificity profile among the four metabolite ratios [63].

Two studies in patients with PMA found normal NAA levels in the motor cortex [40, 48]. However, more recently a modest reduction in NAA:Cr ratio was found in 9 PMA patients relative to controls [50], and abnormal ^{1}H-MRSI was found in 63% of 27 patients with PMA [66]. Reasons for this variability may include different sample size and methodology (i.e., single-voxel vs. multi-voxel ^{1}H-MRSI) among studies. In two studies including PLS patients, mean NAA:Cr values were significantly different relative to control subjects [40, 50]: when the optimal cut-off was set (2.5), NAA:Cr values were found to be abnormal in 67% of patients.

^{1}H-MRSI studies with an adequate follow-up are scarce. Moreover, study designs consisted of a relatively short follow-up period of no more than 15 months, with assessment at variable observation points. Together with the variety of image analysis used, this makes comparisons between studies very difficult. One longitudinal study investigated ^{1}H-MRSI changes in 9 ALS patients: in the most affected motor cortex, NAA:Cr and NAA:Cho+Cr ratios decreased significantly after 1 month, while no significant changes were found in the least symptomatic of the two sides of the motor cortex after 3 months [60]. Other follow-up studies showed similar results [55, 69, 70]. In one study, changes of metabolite ratios were significantly correlated with progression of disease severity

[55]. However, one prospective study using multivoxel ^{1}H-MRSI in 30 patients with ALS did not confirm these findings [50]. Rule *et al.* found a significant decrease of NAA levels outside the motor cortex after 9 months [70]. These findings were not confirmed by another study where no longitudinal NAA, Cre and Cho concentration changes were detected in extramotor regions [60]. There is minimal experience of treatment effects on ^{1}H-MRSI measures in ALS. Kalra *et al.* reported an increase of NAA:Cr ratio in the motor cortex of ALS patients after only a short course of treatment with riluzole [57, 71]. No effect on ^{1}H-MRSI metrics was seen with treatment with gabapentin [72] or brain-derived neurotrophic factor [73].

Diffusion tensor imaging

Region of interest (ROI)-based DTI studies reported consistently decreased fractional anisotropy (FA) values along the CST in ALS patients [74, 75, 76, 77, 78, 79, 80, 81]. FA shows a downward linear trend from the cerebral peduncles to the pyramids [76]. Patients with bulbar onset may have the most marked FA decrease [75]. Decreased FA was found to be related to disease severity [61, 74, 75, 79], as well as to clinical [75, 77] and electrophysiological [78] measures of UMN degeneration in ALS patients. However, these findings were not confirmed by other studies [50, 76, 80]. Increased mean diffusivity (MD) along the CST, which was associated with disease duration [74, 75], was reported by some studies [75, 76, 77], but not by others [79].

Using DTI-based tractography, lower mean FA was demonstrated in the CST of ALS patients with rapid disease progression compared to controls [82]. A strong correlation was found between disease progression rate and left CST structural connectivity measures [82]. DTI-based tractography has also been shown to be helpful in guiding the placement of ROIs on the CST [83, 84] and the corticobulbar tract [83] in these patients.

MRI studies that employed a voxel-based approach to investigate differences in FA between ALS patients and controls reported that ALS patients show a decrease of FA values not only in the CST, but also in regions outside the 'classic' motor network [32, 85, 86, 87, 88]. FA decrease was found in the corpus callosum [32, 85, 85, 87, 88], the premotor WM [85, 87, 88], the prefrontal WM [85, 87, 88] and the temporal WM [87, 88]. One study did not confirm extramotor FA changes in ALS [77]. A few studies have investigated the regional patterns of MD changes in ALS patients and found increased MD in the corpus callosum and in several frontal and temporal WM regions compared to controls [32, 88].

PMA patients have been shown to have subclinical UMN involvement in a neuropathological study [89]. In one DTI study [79], patients with PMA had FA values in the posterior limb of the internal capsule that were similar to those of patients with UMN signs. A voxel-based DTI study of patients with ALS and PMA [86] showed decreased FA values along the CST in both groups relative to controls [86]; all patients with PMA later developed ALS, suggesting that DTI may be a marker for early and clinically silent UMN involvement [86]. In contrast, another study found no FA changes in the CST of patients with PMA [74]. However, this latter study used more stringent criteria for the diagnosis of PMA (i.e., the presence of a pure LMN syndrome and areflexia for at least two years after diagnosis [74]), which was not the case for the other studies [79, 86]. The only voxel-based DTI study investigating differences in FA between PLS and ALS patients [85] showed that PLS patients had lower FA than ALS patients in the body of the corpus callosum and in the WM adjacent to the right primary motor cortex, while ALS patients had reduced FA compared with PLS patients in the WM adjacent to the superior frontal gyrus [85]. Significant correlations were found between disease progression rate and 1) FA in WM adjacent to the primary motor cortex in PLS, and 2) FA along the CST and in the body of the corpus callosum in ALS [85].

Longitudinal DTI studies of ALS patients produced conflicting results [43, 50, 87, 90], since only one study of 7 ALS patients reported a significant progression of brain damage, which was moderately correlated with the concomitant worsening of disability [87], while others did not [47, 50, 90].

More recently, DTI has been successfully used to grade the extent of cervical cord damage associated with ALS [45]. Compared with controls, patients with ALS had significantly lower FA of the cervical cord, while MD did not differ between the two groups [45]. A strong correlation was found between cord FA and disease severity [45]. After a mean follow-up of 9 months [47] these patients showed a significant decrease of cord FA and a significant increase of cord MD [47]. In the same patient group,

brain CST DTI metrics remained stable over time and did not correlate with cord damage [47].

Magnetization transfer (MT) MRI

In one preliminary study using T1-weighted MT contrast-enhanced images, hyperintensity along the CST was found in 80% of patients with ALS [91]. Two of the three reports on quantitative MT MRI in ALS showed a reduction of the MT ratio in the CST from 2.6% [92] to 20% [93] compared to controls. The other study did not find any difference between patients and controls [19]. It is not yet clear that this technique offers any significant advantages over DTI.

Functional imaging

In MND patients with UMN signs, activation PET studies using ^{18}F-fluoro-2-deoxyglucose demonstrated reduced regional cerebral metabolic rates (rCMRGlc) throughout the cerebral hemispheres [94, 95], which was marked in the sensorimotor cortex and putamen [95]. The degree of glucose hypometabolism has been correlated with disease duration [94]. In contrast, PMA patients appeared to have normal or near-normal rCMRGlc relative to controls [94]. At rest, a marked reduction of regional cerebral blood flow (rCBF) as measured by PET tracer H_2 ^{15}O was found in the primary sensorimotor cortex and the adjacent premotor, parietal and insular cortices from ALS patients [96, 97]. During a motor activation task, rCBF was significantly reduced in the medial prefrontal cortex, anterior cingulate gyrus and parahippocampal gyrus in these patients relative to controls [96, 97]. rCBF changes were not seen in patients with PMA [98].

Patients with ALS have decreased glucose uptake in the frontal lobe, and some have additional abnormalities in the temporal, parietal and right thalamic regions [94, 95]. One study linked the glucose hypometabolism of the frontal lobes to ALS-associated neuropsychological deficits [99]. Non-demented ALS patients with decreased verbal fluency scores also have reduced rCBF of the prefrontal cortex, premotor cortex, bilateral insular cortex and thalamus compared to those patients who were cognitively intact using a verbal fluency activation paradigm [100, 101].

Using ligand-based PET, a reduction of cortical ^{11}C-flumazenil binding has been detected in the motor/premotor [102–104] and extramotor [102] cortical regions of patients with ALS. Poorer performance on verbal fluency correlated with decreased ^{11}C-flumazenil binding in frontotemporal regions, while poorer performance on a confrontation naming test correlated with decreased binding in the left middle frontal gyrus and cuneus [105]. One PET study with ^{11}C-WAY100635, which binds selectively to the 5-hydroxytryptamine (5-HT) 1A receptor on cortical pyramidal neurons, revealed marked binding reductions in the precentral and cingulate gyri, and frontotemporal regions of ALS patients [106]. Such reduced 5-HT1A receptor binding was also seen in similar areas in FTD patients [107]. Microglial activation may have a role in ALS pathogenesis [108] and has been detected using PET *in vivo* in ALS patients [109]: significantly increased [11]C(R)-PK11195 binding was found in the motor cortex, pons, prefrontal cortex and thalamus, with a significant correlation between binding in the motor cortex and clinical UMN signs [109]. Increased uptake rate of [11]C(L)-deprenyl, which allows to localize astrocytosis *in vivo*, was demonstrated in ALS patients in the pons and global WM [110].

fMRI studies have superseded activation PET in the investigation of patterns of cortical recruitment in MNDs [111] and have the advantage of wider accessibility, noninvasive study and lack of ionizing radiation. During motor tasks, fMRI has consistently demonstrated an increased activation of the contralateral sensorimotor cortex, supplementary motor area, basal ganglia and cerebellum [112, 113, 114, 115]. Increased sensorimotor activation was also reported in the hemisphere ipsilateral to the movement [114]. Furthermore, ALS patients showed motor-associated reduced activation in the prefrontal cortex [115]. One study demonstrated movement-associated decreased cortical responses of the contralateral sensorimotor cortex, premotor area, supplementary motor area and posterior parietal cortex and relatively increased responses of the putamen in ALS patients relative to controls [116]. The difficulty to control task performance in ALS patients may be responsible for the variability of motor fMRI studies. More recently, during a motor imagery task, patients with ALS showed a reduced activation of the left inferior parietal lobule, anterior cingulate gyrus and prefrontal cortex [117]. In ALS, the analysis of the resting state fMRI demonstrated not only sensorimotor network changes in the premotor cortex, but also a reduced activation of the default mode network [118].

In ALS patients relative to controls, a letter fluency fMRI task revealed significantly impaired activation in frontal, parietal and temporal lobes [119]. A confrontation naming fMRI task also revealed impaired activation of a prefrontal region (including Broca's area) and areas of the temporal, parietal and occipital lobes [119]. This pattern of dysfunction corresponded to the presence of cognitive deficits on both letter fluency and confrontation naming [119].

Recommendations

1. At present, advanced neuroimaging techniques do not have a role in the diagnosis or routine monitoring of MNDs (Class IV, good practice point).

2. Quantitative measurements of brain atrophy in clinical practice continue to be considered at a preliminary stage of development (Class IV, good practice point), as they need to be standardized in terms of acquisition and post-processing, and validated further in the context of longitudinal and normative studies.

3. Measurement of cervical cord area is a promising tool to monitor MND evolution (Class IV, good practice point). At present, however, such an approach showed differences at group level only in a single study and does not permit inferences at an individual level.

4. Brain and cord atrophy should be included as secondary end-points in disease-modifying agent trials of MNDs, in order to further elucidate the mechanisms responsible for disability in these conditions.

5. Monitoring NAA levels in the primary motor cortex and CST may be useful in the evaluation of MND progression and response to treatment (Class IV, good practice point).

6. DTI holds promise in the assessment of UMN damage before clinical symptoms of CST involvement become apparent (Class IV, good practice point).

7. The contribution of DTI and ^{1}H-MRSI in multicentre studies requires further evaluation. It is strongly advisable to incorporate measures derived from these techniques into new clinical trials as exploratory outcomes to gain additional insights into disease pathophysiology and into the value of these techniques in the assessment of MNDs.

8. fMRI can be useful in the assessment of cognitive network abnormalities in MND patients (Class IV, good practice point), and should be considered first-line over activation PET studies for this purpose at present.

9. Ligand-based PET still has potential to generate new as well as test existing hypotheses relating to receptor changes within MND pathogenesis, but it will require the development of novel, robust ligands through investment in radiochemistry.

Neuroimaging in patients with familial MND

Mitsumoto *et al.* showed reduced FA values in the CST at the level of the internal capsule in six patients with familial ALS relative to controls [50]. Decreased FA values have been reported in the posterior limb of the internal capsule in eight asymptomatic members of a large Chinese family with autosomal dominant familial ALS with a known superoxide dismutase 1 (SOD1) mutation relative to controls [120].

Neuroimaging studies provide evidence for different patterns of cortical neuronal vulnerability in patients homozygous for the D90A (homD90A) mutation of the SOD1 gene vs. sporadic ALS, which may explain the slower rate of disease progression in most familial cases. A VBM study showed that GM atrophy in the homD90A group was more pronounced in the frontal lobes, while the sporadic ALS group showed areas of atrophy mainly confined to motor and premotor cortices bilaterally [121]. Six patients with homD90A SOD1 ALS showed less extensive WM changes (i.e., decreased FA values) in motor and extramotor pathways compared to patients with sporadic ALS, despite similar disease severity [122]. In homD90A SOD1 ALS patients, FA values correlated with clinical measures of severity and UMN involvement [122]. Using ^{11}Cflumazenil PET, a less extensive and more frontal pattern of reduced binding was observed among patients with homD90A SOD1 compared with patients with sporadic ALS and similar disability [103, 104]. Finally, 11 homD90A SOD1 patients demonstrated significantly less reduction in the cortical binding of ^{11}C-WAY100635 than a group of patients with sporadic ALS of similar disability [123].

The presence of a thin corpus callosum – the so-called 'ears of the lynx' abnormality (i.e., the frontal horn region bears a remarkable resemblance to the ears of a lynx, with the areas of abnormal signal reminiscent of the tufts of hair crowning the tips of the ears of this animal) – in the forceps minor of the corpus callosum has been linked to the presence of a mutation in the SPG11 gene on chromosome 15, which is associated with a spastic paraparesis condition which can enter in the differential diagnosis of MNDs [124]. Mutations of the Senataxin gene are associated with autosomal dominant juvenile ALS (ALS4) and autosomal recessive ataxia-ocular apraxia 2 (AOA2). In a two-generation family, whose affected individuals had a clinical phenotype combining typical features of AOA2 and ALS4, MRI revealed severe cerebellar atrophy [125].

Recommendations

1. DTI may be useful in the assessment of UMN damage in asymptomatic members of family with familial ALS (Class IV, good practice point).

2. The presence of a thin corpus callosum ('ears of the lynx' abnormality) in the forceps minor of the corpus callosum should raise the suspicion of a hereditary spastic paraparesis in an otherwise appropriate clinical context (Class IV, good practice point).

3. Neuroimaging techniques need to be further applied in familial ALS with mutations of newly identified genes (e.g., angiogenin gene, TAR DNA binding protein [TDP-43] gene, fused in sarcoma/translated in liposarcoma [FUS/TLS] gene).

Abbreviations

5-hydroxytryptamine 1A receptor: 5-HT1A; amyotrophic lateral sclerosis: ALS; amyotrophic lateral sclerosis with frontotemporal dementia: ALS-FTD; ataxia-ocular apraxia 2: AOA2; brain parenchymal fraction: BPF; choline: Cho; corticospinal tract: CST; creatine: Cr; diffusion tensor imaging: DTI; fluid-attenuated inversion recovery: FLAIR; fractional anisotropy: FA; frontotemporal lobar degeneration: FTLD; functional magnetic resonance imaging: fMRI; fused in sarcoma/translated in liposarcoma gene: FUS/TLS; good clinical practice point: GCPP; grey matter: GM; homozygous for the D90A mutation: homD90A; mean diffusivity: MD; lower motor neuron: LMN; motor neuron disease: MND; myo-inositol: mI; N-acetylaspartate: NAA; positron emission tomography: PET; primary lateral sclerosis: PLS, progressive muscular atrophy: PMA; proton density: PD; proton magnetic resonance spectroscopic imaging: 1H-MRSI; region of interest: ROI; regional cerebral blood flow: rCBF; regional cerebral metabolic rates: rCMRGlc; superoxide dismutase 1: SOD1; TAR DNA binding protein gene: TDP-43; upper motor neuron: UMN; voxel-based morphometry: VBM; white matter: WM.

Conflicts of interest

Members of this Task Force have no conflicts of interest related to the recommendations given in this chapter.

References

1. Leigh, PN, Abrahams, S, Al-Chalabi, A, *et al.* The management of motor neurone disease. *J Neurol Neurosurg Psychiatry* 2003; **74**(Suppl. 4):iv32–iv47.

2. Andersen, PM, Borasio, GD, Dengler, R, *et al.* EFNS task force on management of amyotrophic lateral sclerosis: guidelines for diagnosing and clinical care of patients and relatives. *Eur J Neurol* 2005; **12**:921–38.

3. Turner, MR, Kiernan, MC, Leigh, PN, Talbot, K. Biomarkers in amyotrophic lateral sclerosis. *Lancet Neurol* 2009; **8**:94–109.

4. Phukan, J, Pender, NP, Hardiman, O. Cognitive impairment in amyotrophic lateral sclerosis. *Lancet Neurol* 2007; **6**:994–1003.

5. Brainin, M, Barnes, M, Baron, JC, *et al.* Guidance for the preparation of neurological management guidelines by EFNS scientific task forces – revised recommendations 2004. *Eur J Neurol* 2004; **11**:577–81.

6. Brooks, BR, Miller, RG, Swash, M, Munsat, TL. El Escorial revisited: revised criteria for the diagnosis of amyotrophic lateral sclerosis. *Amyotroph Lateral Scler Other Motor Neuron Disord* 2000; **1**:293–9.

7. Kato, S, Shaw, P, Wood-Allum, C, *et al.* Amyotrophic lateral sclerosis, in *Neurodegeneration: The Molecular Pathology of Dementia and Movement Disorders* (ed. DW Dickson), 2003; ISN Neuropath Press, pp. 350–71.

8. Abe, K, Fujimura, H, Kobayashi, Y, *et al.* Degeneration of the pyramidal tracts in patients with amyotrophic lateral sclerosis. A premortem and postmortem magnetic resonance imaging study. *J Neuroimaging* 1997; **7**:208–12.

9. Cheung, G, Gawel, MJ, Cooper, PW, *et al.* Amyotrophic lateral sclerosis: correlation of clinical and MR imaging findings. *Radiology* 1995; **194**:263–70.

10. Goodin, DS, Rowley, HA, Olney, RK. Magnetic resonance imaging in amyotrophic lateral sclerosis. *Ann Neurol* 1988; **23**:418–20.

11. Hecht, MJ, Fellner, F, Fellner, C, *et al.* MRI-FLAIR images of the head show corticospinal tract alterations in ALS patients more frequently than T2-, T1- and proton-density-weighted images. *J Neurol Sci* 2001; **186**:37–44.

12. Hecht, MJ, Fellner, F, Fellner, C, *et al.* Hyperintense and hypointense MRI signals of the precentral gyrus and corticospinal tract in ALS: a follow-up examination including FLAIR images. *J Neurol Sci* 2002; **199**:59–65.

13. Ishikawa, K, Nagura, H, Yokota, T, Yamanouchi, H. Signal loss in the motor cortex on magnetic resonance images in amyotrophic lateral sclerosis. *Ann Neurol* 1993; **33**:218–22.

14. Mirowitz, S, Sartor, K, Gado, M, Torack, R. Focal signal-intensity variations in the posterior internal capsule: normal MR findings and distinction from pathologic findings. *Radiology* 1989; **172**:535–9.

15. Thorpe, JW, Moseley, IF, Hawkes, CH, *et al.* Brain and spinal cord MRI in motor neuron disease. *J Neurol Neurosurg Psychiatry* 1996; **61**:314–17.

16. Waragai, M. MRI and clinical features in amyotrophic lateral sclerosis. *Neuroradiology* 1997; **39**:847–51.

17. Basak, M, Erturk, M, Oflazoglu, B, *et al.* Magnetic resonance imaging in amyotrophic lateral sclerosis. *Acta Neurol Scand* 2002; **105**, 395–9.

18. Hofmann, E, Ochs, G, Pelzl, A, Warmuth-Metz, M. The corticospinal tract in amyotrophic lateral sclerosis: an MRI study. *Neuroradiology* 1998; **40**:71–5.

19. Charil, A, Corbo, M, Filippi, M. *et al.* Structural and metabolic changes in the brain of patients with upper motor neuron disorders: a multiparametric MRI study. *Amyotroph Lateral Scler* 2009; **10**:269–79.

20. Peretti-Viton, P, Azulay, JP, Trefouret, S, *et al.* MRI of the intracranial corticospinal tracts in amyotrophic and primary lateral sclerosis. *Neuroradiology* 1999; **41**:744–9.

21. Andreadou, E, Sgouropoulos, P, Varelas, P, *et al.* Subcortical frontal lesions on MRI in patients with motor neurone disease. *Neuroradiology* 1998; **40**:298–302.

22. Kato, S, Hayashi, H, Yagishita, A. Involvement of the frontotemporal lobe and limbic system in amyotrophic lateral sclerosis: as assessed by serial computed tomography and magnetic resonance imaging. *J Neurol Sci* 1993; **116**, 52–8.

23. Turner, MR. Reversible diffusion MRI abnormalities and transient mutism after liver transplantation. *Neurology* 2005; **64**:177; author reply 177.

24. Brooks, BR. El Escorial World Federation of Neurology criteria for the diagnosis of amyotrophic lateral sclerosis. Subcommittee on Motor Neuron Diseases/Amyotrophic Lateral Sclerosis of the World Federation of Neurology Research Group on Neuromuscular Diseases and the El Escorial 'Clinical limits of amyotrophic lateral sclerosis' workshop contributors. *J Neurol Sci* 1994; **124** (Suppl.): 96–107.

25. Oba, H, Araki, T, Ohtomo, K, *et al.* Amyotrophic lateral sclerosis: T2 shortening in motor cortex at MR imaging. *Radiology* 1993; **189**:843–6.

26. Terao, S, Sobue, G, Yasuda, T, *et al.* Magnetic resonance imaging of the corticospinal tracts in amyotrophic lateral sclerosis. *J Neurol Sci* 1995; **133**:66–72.

27. Kassubek, J, Unrath, A, Huppertz, HJ, *et al.* Global brain atrophy and corticospinal tract alterations in ALS, as investigated by voxel-based morphometry of 3-D MRI. *Amyotroph Lateral Scler Other Motor Neuron Disord* 2005; **6**:213–20.

28. Mezzapesa, DM, Ceccarelli, A, Dicuonzo, F, *et al*. Whole-brain and regional brain atrophy in amyotrophic lateral sclerosis. *AJNR Am J Neuroradiol* 2007; **28**: 255–9.

29. Ellis, CM, Suckling, J, Amaro, E, Jr, *et al*. Volumetric analysis reveals corticospinal tract degeneration and extramotor involvement in ALS. *Neurology* 2001; **57**:1571–8.

30. Pinkhardt, EH, van Elst, LT, Ludolph, AC, Kassubek, J. Amygdala size in amyotrophic lateral sclerosis without dementia: an in vivo study using MRI volumetry. *BMC Neurol* 2006; **6**:48.

31. Tartaglia, MC., Laluz, V, Rowe, A, *et al*. Brain atrophy in primary lateral sclerosis. *Neurology* 2009; **72**:1236–41.

32. Agosta, F, Pagani, E, Rocca, MA, *et al*. Voxel-based morphometry study of brain volumetry and diffusivity in amyotrophic lateral sclerosis patients with mild disability. *Hum Brain Mapp* 2007; **28**:1430–8.

33. Grosskreutz, J, Kaufmann, J, Fradrich, J, *et al*. Widespread sensorimotor and frontal cortical atrophy in Amyotrophic Lateral Sclerosis. *BMC Neurol* 2006; **6**:17.

34. Chang, JL, Lomen-Hoerth, C, Murphy, J, *et al*. A voxel-based morphometry study of patterns of brain atrophy in ALS and ALS/FTLD. *Neurology* 2005; **65**:75–80.

35. Grossman, M, Anderson, C, Khan, A, *et al*. Impaired action knowledge in amyotrophic lateral sclerosis. *Neurology* 2008; **71**:1396–1401.

36. Thivard, L, Pradat, PF, Lehericy, S, *et al*. Diffusion tensor imaging and voxel based morphometry study in amyotrophic lateral sclerosis: relationships with motor disability. *J Neurol Neurosurg Psychiatry* 2007; **78**:889–92.

37. Roccatagliata, L, Bonzano, L, Mancardi, G, *et al*. Detection of motor cortex thinning and corticospinal tract involvement by quantitative MRI in amyotrophic lateral sclerosis. *Amyotroph Lateral Scler* 2009; **10**:47–52.

38. Kiernan, JA, Hudson, AJ. Frontal lobe atrophy in motor neuron diseases. *Brain* 1994; **117**(Pt 4):747–57.

39. Abrahams, S, Goldstein, LH, Suckling, J, *et al*. Frontotemporal white matter changes in amyotrophic lateral sclerosis. *J Neurol* 2005; **252**:321–31.

40. Chan, S, Shungu, DC, Douglas-Akinwande, A, *et al*. Motor neuron diseases: comparison of single-voxel proton MR spectroscopy of the motor cortex with MR imaging of the brain. *Radiology* 1999; **212**:763–9.

41. Le Forestier, N, Maisonobe, T, Piquard, A, *et al*. Does primary lateral sclerosis exist? A study of 20 patients and a review of the literature. *Brain* 2001; **124**:1989–9.

42. Murphy, JM, Henry, RG, Langmore, S, *et al*. Continuum of frontal lobe impairment in amyotrophic lateral sclerosis. *Arch Neurol* 2007; **64**:530–4.

43. Agosta, F, Gorno-Tempini, ML, Pagani, E, *et al*. Longitudinal assessment of grey matter contraction in amyotrophic lateral sclerosis: a tensor based morphometry study. *Amyotroph Lateral Scler* 2009; **10**:168–74.

44. Avants, B, Khan, A, McCluskey, L, *et al*. Longitudinal cortical atrophy in amyotrophic lateral sclerosis with fronto-temporal dementia. *Arch Neurol* 2009; **66**:138–9.

45. Valsasina, P, Agosta, F, Benedetti, B, *et al*. Diffusion anisotropy of the cervical cord is strictly associated with disability in amyotrophic lateral sclerosis. *J Neurol Neurosurg Psychiatry* 2007; **78**:480–4.

46. Sperfeld, AD, Bretschneider, V, Flaith, L, *et al*. MR-pathologic comparison of the upper spinal cord in different motor neuron diseases. *Eur Neurol* 2005; **53**:74–7.

47. Agosta, F, Rocca, MA, Valsasina, P, *et al*. A longitudinal diffusion tensor MRI study of the cervical cord and brain in amyotrophic lateral sclerosis patients. *J Neurol Neurosurg Psychiatry* 2009; **80**:53–5.

48. Gredal, O, Rosenbaum, S, Topp, S, *et al*. Quantification of brain metabolites in amyotrophic lateral sclerosis by localized proton magnetic resonance spectroscopy. *Neurology* 1997; **48**:878–81.

49. Sarchielli, P, Pelliccioli, GP, Tarducci, R, *et al*. Magnetic resonance imaging and 1H-magnetic resonance spectroscopy in amyotrophic lateral sclerosis. *Neuroradiology* 2001; **43**:189–97.

50. Mitsumoto, H, Ulug, AM, Pullman, SL, *et al*. Quantitative objective markers for upper and lower motor neuron dysfunction in ALS. *Neurology* 2007; **68**:1402–10.

51. Block, W, Karitzky, J, Traber, F, *et al*. Proton magnetic resonance spectroscopy of the primary motor cortex in patients with motor neuron disease: subgroup analysis and follow-up measurements. *Arch Neurol* 1998; **55**:931–6.

52. Jones, AP, Gunawardena, WJ, Coutinho, CM, *et al*. Preliminary results of proton magnetic resonance spectroscopy in motor neurone disease (amytrophic lateral sclerosis). *J Neurol Sci* 1995; **129** (Suppl.):85–9.

53. Pioro, EP, Antel, JP, Cashman, NR, Arnold, DL. Detection of cortical neuron loss in motor neuron disease by proton magnetic resonance spectroscopic imaging in vivo. *Neurology* 1994; **44**:1933–8.

54. Rooney, WD, Miller, RG, Gelinas, D, *et al*. Decreased nacetylaspartate in motor cortex and corticospinal tract in ALS. *Neurology* 1998; **50**:1800–5.

55. Pohl, C, Block, W, Karitzky, J, *et al*. Proton magnetic resonance spectroscopy of the motor cortex in 70 patients with amyotrophic lateral sclerosis. *Arch Neurol* 2001; **58**: 729–35.

56. Kalra, S, Vitale, A, Cashman, NR, *et al*. Cerebral degeneration predicts survival in amyotrophic lateral sclerosis. *J Neurol Neurosurg Psychiatry* 2006; **77**:1253–5.

57. Kalra, S, Tai, P, Genge, A, Arnold, DL. Rapid improvement in cortical neuronal integrity in amyotrophic lateral scle-

rosis detected by proton magnetic resonance spectroscopic imaging. *J Neurol* 2006; **253**:1060–3.

58. Nelles, M, Block, W, Traber, F, *et al.* Combined 3T diffusion tensor tractography and 1H-MR spectroscopy in motor neuron disease. *AJNR Am J Neuroradiol* 2008; **29**: 1708–14.

59. Pyra, T, Hui, B, Hanstock, C, *et al.* Combined structural and neurochemical evaluation of the corticospinal tract in amyotrophic lateral sclerosis. *Amyotroph Lateral Scler* 2010; **11**:157–65.

60. Suhy, J, Miller, RG, Rule, R, *et al.* Early detection and longitudinal changes in amyotrophic lateral sclerosis by (1)H MRSI. *Neurology* 2002; **58**:773–9.

61. Wang, S, Poptani, H, Woo, JH, *et al.* Amyotrophic lateral sclerosis: diffusion-tensor and chemical shift MR imaging at 3.0 T. *Radiology* 2006; **239**, 831–8.

62. Cwik, VA, Hanstock, CC, Allen, PS, Martin, WR. Estimation of brainstem neuronal loss in amyotrophic lateral sclerosis with in vivo proton magnetic resonance spectroscopy. *Neurology* 1998; **50**:72–7.

63. Kalra, S, Hanstock, CC, Martin, WR, *et al.* Detection of cerebral degeneration in amyotrophic lateral sclerosis using high-field magnetic resonance spectroscopy. *Arch Neurol* 2006; **63**:1144–8.

64. Ellis, CM, Simmons, A, Andrews, C, *et al.* A proton magnetic resonance spectroscopic study in ALS: correlation with clinical findings. *Neurology* 1998; **51**:1104–9.

65. Abe, K, Takanashi, M, Watanabe, Y, *et al.* Decrease in N-acetylaspartate/creatine ratio in the motor area and the frontal lobe in amyotrophic lateral sclerosis. *Neuroradiology* 2001; **43**:537–41.

66. Kaufmann, P, Pullman, SL, Shungu, DC, *et al.* Objective tests for upper motor neuron involvement in amyotrophic lateral sclerosis (ALS). *Neurology* 2004; **62**:1753–7.

67. Strong, MJ, Grace, GM, Orange, JB, *et al.* A prospective study of cognitive impairment in ALS. *Neurology* 1999; **53**:1665–70.

68. Bowen, BC, Pattany, PM, Bradley, WG, *et al.* MR imaging and localized proton spectroscopy of the precentral gyrus in amyotrophic lateral sclerosis. *AJNR Am J Neuroradiol* 2000; **21**:647–58.

69. Unrath, A, Ludolph, AC, Kassubek, J. Brain metabolites in definite amyotrophic lateral sclerosis. A longitudinal proton magnetic resonance spectroscopy study. *J Neurol* 2007; **254**:1099–106.

70. Rule, RR, Suhy, J, Schuff, N, *et al.* Reduced NAA in motor and non-motor brain regions in amyotrophic lateral sclerosis: a cross-sectional and longitudinal study. *Amyotroph Lateral Scler Other Motor Neuron Disord* 2004; **5**:141–9.

71. Kalra, S, Cashman, NR, Genge, A, Arnold, DL. Recovery of N-acetylaspartate in corticomotor neurons of patients with ALS after riluzole therapy. *Neuroreport* 1998; **9**: 1757–61.

72. Kalra, S, Cashman, NR, Caramanos, Z, *et al.* Gabapentin therapy for amyotrophic lateral sclerosis: lack of improvement in neuronal integrity shown by MR spectroscopy. *AJNR Am J Neuroradiol* 2003; **24**:476–80.

73. Kalra, S, Genge, A, Arnold, DL. A prospective, randomized, placebo-controlled evaluation of corticoneuronal response to intrathecal BDNF therapy in ALS using magnetic resonance spectroscopy: feasibility and results. *Amyotroph Lateral Scler Other Motor Neuron Disord* 2003; **4**:22–6.

74. Cosottini, M, Giannelli, M, Siciliano, G, *et al.* Diffusion-tensor MR imaging of corticospinal tract in amyotrophic lateral sclerosis and progressive muscular atrophy. *Radiology* 2005; **237**:258–64.

75. Ellis, CM, Simmons, A, Jones, DK, *et al.* Diffusion tensor MRI assesses corticospinal tract damage in ALS. *Neurology* 1999; **53**:1051–8.

76. Toosy, AT, Werring, DJ, Orrell, RW, *et al.* Diffusion tensor imaging detects corticospinal tract involvement at multiple levels in amyotrophic lateral sclerosis. *J Neurol Neurosurg Psychiatry* 2003; **74**:1250–7.

77. Abe, O, Yamada, H, Masutani, Y, *et al.* Amyotrophic lateral sclerosis: diffusion tensor tractography and voxel-based analysis. *NMR Biomed* 2004; **17**:411–16.

78. Iwata, NK, Aoki, S, Okabe, S, *et al.* Evaluation of corticospinal tracts in ALS with diffusion tensor MRI and brainstem stimulation. *Neurology* 2008; **70**:528–32.

79. Graham, JM, Papadakis, N, Evans, J, *et al.* Diffusion tensor imaging for the assessment of upper motor neuron integrity in ALS. *Neurology* 2004; **63**:2111–19.

80. Schimrigk, SK, Bellenberg, B, Schluter, M, *et al.* Diffusion tensor imaging-based fractional anisotropy quantification in the corticospinal tract of patients with amyotrophic lateral sclerosis using a probabilistic mixture model. *AJNR Am J Neuroradiol* 2007; **28**:724–30.

81. Senda, J, Ito, M, Watanabe, H, *et al.* Correlation between pyramidal tract degeneration and widespread white matter involvement in amyotrophic lateral sclerosis: a study with tractography and diffusion-tensor imaging. *Amyotroph Lateral Scler* 2009; **10**:288–94.

82. Ciccarelli, O, Behrens, TE, Altmann, DR, *et al.* Probabilistic diffusion tractography: a potential tool to assess the rate of disease progression in amyotrophic lateral sclerosis. *Brain* 2006; **129**:1859–71.

83. Aoki, S, Iwata, NK, Masutani, Y, *et al.* Quantitative evaluation of the pyramidal tract segmented by diffusion tensor tractography: feasibility study in patients with amyotrophic lateral sclerosis. *Radiat Med* 2005; **23**:195–9.

84. Hong, YH, Sung, JJ, Kim, SM, *et al.* Diffusion tensor tractography-based analysis of the pyramidal tract in

patients with amyotrophic lateral sclerosis. *J Neuroimaging* 2008; **18**:282–7.

85. Ciccarelli, O, Behrens, TE, Johansen-Berg, H, *et al.* Investigation of white matter pathology in ALS and PLS using tract-based spatial statistics. *Hum Brain Mapp* 2009; **30**:615–24.

86. Sach, M, Winkler, G, Glauche, V, *et al.* Diffusion tensor MRI of early upper motor neuron involvement in amyotrophic lateral sclerosis. *Brain* 2004; **127**:340–50.

87. Sage, CA, Peeters, RR, Gorner, A, *et al.* Quantitative diffusion tensor imaging in amyotrophic lateral sclerosis. *Neuroimage* 2007; **34**:486–99.

88. Sage, CA, Van Hecke, W, Peeters, R, *et al.* Quantitative diffusion tensor imaging in amyotrophic lateral sclerosis: revisited. *Hum Brain Mapp* 2009; **30**:3657–75.

89. Ince, PG, Evans, J, Knopp, M, *et al.* Corticospinal tract degeneration in the progressive muscular atrophy variant of ALS. *Neurology* 2003; **60**:1252–8.

90. Blain, CR, Williams, VC, Johnston, C, *et al.* A longitudinal study of diffusion tensor MRI in ALS. *Amyotroph Lateral Scler* 2007; **8**:348–55.

91. da Rocha, AJ, Oliveira, AS, Fonseca, RB, *et al.* Detection of corticospinal tract compromise in amyotrophic lateral sclerosis with brain MR imaging: relevance of the T1-weighted spin-echo magnetization transfer contrast sequence. *AJNR Am J Neuroradiol* 2004; **25**:1509–15.

92. Tanabe, JL, Vermathen, M, Miller, R, *et al.* Reduced MTR in the corticospinal tract and normal T2 in amyotrophic lateral sclerosis. *Magn Reson Imaging* 1998; **16**:1163–9.

93. Kato, Y, Matsumura, K, Kinosada, Y, *et al.* Detection of pyramidal tract lesions in amyotrophic lateral sclerosis with magnetization-transfer measurements. *AJNR Am J Neuroradiol* 1997; **18**:1541–7.

94. Dalakas, MC, Hatazawa, J, Brooks, RA, Di Chiro, G. Lowered cerebral glucose utilization in amyotrophic lateral sclerosis. *Ann Neurol* 1987; **22**:580–6.

95. Hatazawa, J, Brooks, RA, Dalakas, MC, *et al.* Cortical motor-sensory hypometabolism in amyotrophic lateral sclerosis: a PET study. *J Comput Assist Tomogr* 1988; **12**:630–6.

96. Kew, JJ, Goldstein, LH, Leigh, PN, *et al.* The relationship between abnormalities of cognitive function and cerebral activation in amyotrophic lateral sclerosis. A neuropsychological and positron emission tomography study. *Brain* 1993; **116**(Pt 6):1399–1423.

97. Kew, JJ, Leigh, PN, Playford, ED, *et al.* Cortical function in amyotrophic lateral sclerosis. A positron emission tomography study. *Brain* 1993; **116**(Pt 3):655–80.

98. Kew, JJ, Brooks, DJ, Passingham, RE, *et al.* Cortical function in progressive lower motor neuron disorders and amyo-

trophic lateral sclerosis: a comparative PET study. *Neurology* 1994; **44**:1101–10.

99. Ludolph, AC, Langen, KJ, Regard, M, *et al.* Frontal lobe function in amyotrophic lateral sclerosis: a neuropsychologic and positron emission tomography study. *Acta Neurol Scand* 1992; **85**:81–9.

100. Abrahams, S, Goldstein, LH, Kew, JJ, *et al.* Frontal lobe dysfunction in amyotrophic lateral sclerosis. A PET study. *Brain* 1996; **119**(Pt 6):2105–20.

101. Abrahams, S, Leigh, PN, Kew, JJ, *et al.* A positron emission tomography study of frontal lobe function (verbal fluency) in amyotrophic lateral sclerosis. *J Neurol Sci* 1995; **129** (Suppl.):44–6.

102. Lloyd, CM, Richardson, MP, Brooks, DJ, *et al.* Extramotor involvement in ALS: PET studies with the GABA(A) ligand [(11)C]flumazenil. *Brain* 2000; **123**(Pt 11):2289–96.

103. Turner, MR, Hammers, A, Al-Chalabi, A, *et al.* Distinct cerebral lesions in sporadic and D90A SOD1 ALS: studies with [11C]flumazenil. *PET. Brain* 2005; **128**:1323–9.

104. Turner, MR, Osei-Lah, AD, Hammers, A, *et al.* Abnormal cortical excitability in sporadic but not homozygous D90A SOD1 ALS. *J Neurol Neurosurg Psychiatry* 2005; **76**: 1279–85.

105. Wicks, P, Turner, MR, Abrahams, S, *et al.* Neuronal loss associated with cognitive performance in amyotrophic lateral sclerosis: an (11C)-flumazenil PET study. *Amyotroph Lateral Scler* 2008; **9**:43–9.

106. Turner, MR, Rabiner, EA, Hammers, A, *et al.* [11C]-WAY100635 PET demonstrates marked 5-HT1A receptor changes in sporadic ALS. *Brain* 2005; **128**:896–905.

107. Bowen, DM, Procter, AW, Mann, DM, *et al.* Imbalance of a serotonergic system in frontotemporal dementia: implication for pharmacotherapy. *Psychopharmacology (Berl)* 2008; **196**:603–10.

108. Sargsyan, SA, Monk, PN, Shaw, PJ. Microglia as potential contributors to motor neuron injury in amyotrophic lateral sclerosis. *Glia* 2005; **51**:241–53.

109. Turner, MR, Cagnin, A, Turkheimer, FE, *et al.* Evidence of widespread cerebral microglial activation in amyotrophic lateral sclerosis: an [11C](R)-PK11195 positron emission tomography study. *Neurobiol Dis* 2004; **15**:601–9.

110. Johansson, A, Engler, H, Blomquist, G, *et al.* Evidence for astrocytosis in ALS demonstrated by [11C](L)-deprenyl-D2 PET. *J Neurol Sci* 2007; **255**:17–22.

111. Lule, D, Ludolph, AC, Kassubek, J. MRI-based functional neuroimaging in ALS: an update. *Amyotroph Lateral Scler* 2009; **10**:258–68.

112. Konrad, C, Henningsen, H, Bremer, J, *et al.* Pattern of cortical reorganization in amyotrophic lateral sclerosis: a functional magnetic resonance imaging study. *Exp Brain Res* 2002; **143**:51–6.

113. Konrad, C, Jansen, A., Henningsen, H. *et al.* Subcortical reorganization in amyotrophic lateral sclerosis. *Exp Brain Res* 2006; **172**:361–9.

114. Schoenfeld, MA, Tempelmann, C, Gaul, C, *et al.* Functional motor compensation in amyotrophic lateral sclerosis. *J Neurol* 2005; **252**:944–52.

115. Stanton, BR, Williams, VC, Leigh, PN, *et al.* Altered cortical activation during a motor task in ALS. Evidence for involvement of central pathways. *J Neurol* 2007; **254**:1260–7.

116. Tessitore, A, Esposito, F, Monsurro, MR, *et al.* Subcortical motor plasticity in patients with sporadic ALS: an fMRI study. *Brain Res Bull* 2006; **69**:489–94.

117. Stanton, BR, Williams, VC, Leigh, PN, *et al.* Cortical activation during motor imagery is reduced in Amyotrophic Lateral Sclerosis. *Brain Res* 2007; **1172**:145–51.

118. Mohammadi, B, Kollewe, K, Samii, A, *et al.* Changes of resting state brain networks in amyotrophic lateral sclerosis. *Exp Neurol* 2009; **217**:147–53.

119. Abrahams, S, Goldstein, LH, Simmons, A, *et al.* Word retrieval in amyotrophic lateral sclerosis: a functional magnetic resonance imaging study. *Brain* 2004; **127**:1507–17.

120. Ng, MC, Ho, JT, Ho, SL, *et al.* Abnormal diffusion tensor in nonsymptomatic familial amyotrophic lateral sclerosis with a causative superoxide dismutase 1 mutation. *J Magn Reson Imaging* 2008; **27**:8–13.

121. Turner, MR, Hammers, A, Allsop, J, *et al.* Volumetric cortical loss in sporadic and familial amyotrophic lateral sclerosis. *Amyotroph Lateral Scler* 2007; **8**:343–7.

122. Stanton, BR, Shinhmar, D, Turner, MR, *et al.* Diffusion tensor imaging in sporadic and familial (D90A SOD1) forms of amyotrophic lateral sclerosis. *Arch Neurol* 2009; **66**:109–15.

123. Turner, MR, Rabiner, EA, Al-Chalabi, A, *et al.* Cortical 5-HT1A receptor binding in patients with homozygous D90A SOD1 vs sporadic ALS. *Neurology* 2007; **68**:1233–5.

124. Riverol, M, Samaranch, L, Pascual, B, *et al.* Forceps minor region signal abnormality 'ears of the lynx': an early MRI finding in spastic paraparesis with thin corpus callosum and mutations in the spatacsin gene (SPG11) on chromosome 15. *J Neuroimaging* 2009; **19**:52–60.

125. Schols, L, Arning, L, Schule, R, *et al.* 'Pseudodominant inheritance' of ataxia with ocular apraxia type 2 (AOA2). *J Neurol* 2008; **255**: 495–501.

CHAPTER 15

Management of low-grade gliomas

R. Soffietti,[1] B. Baumert,[2] L. Bello,[3] A. von Deimling,[4] H. Duffau,[5] M. Frénay,[6] W. Grisold,[7] R. Grant,[8] F. Graus,[9] K. Hoang-Xuan,[10] M. Klein,[11] B. Melin,[12] J. Rees,[13] T. Siegal,[14] A. Smits,[15] R. Stupp[16] and W. Wick[4]

[1]University Hospital San Giovanni Battista, Turin, Italy; [2]Maastricht University Medical Centre, Maastricht, The Netherlands; [3]University of Milan, Milan, Italy; [4]University of Heidelberg, Germany; [5]Hôpital Gui de Chauliac, Montpellier, France; [6]Centre Antoine Lacassagne, Nice, France; [7]Kaiser Franz Josef Hospital, Vienna, Austria; [8]Western General Hospital, Edinburgh, United Kingdom; [9]Hospital Clinic, Barcelona, Spain; [10]Groupe Hospitalier Pitié-Salpêtrière, Paris, France; [11]VU University Medical Centre, Amsterdam, The Netherlands; [12]Umeå University, Umeå, Sweden; [13]National Hospital for Neurology and Neurosurgery, London, United Kingdom; [14]Hadassah Hebrew University Hospital, Jerusalem, Israel; [15]University Hospital, Uppsala, Sweden; [16]University Hospital and University, Lausanne, Switzerland

Background

Low-grade gliomas (LGGs) are a group of tumours with distinct clinical, histological and molecular characteristics. These guidelines focus on the diffuse infiltrative WHO grade II tumours of the cerebral hemispheres in the adult. Brain stem or cerebellar tumours, which are rare and present specific problems of management, are not discussed.

LGGs represent up to 30% of gliomas and affect patients at a younger age than high-grade gliomas. LGGs are commonly located in or close to eloquent areas – those areas of the brain involved in motor, language, visuospatial and memory function [1]. The 5-year overall and progression-free survival rates in randomized studies range from 58% to 72% and 37% to 55% respectively.

Patients with LGGs may survive for up to 20 years [2], but these tumours grow continuously [3, 4] and tend to progress to a higher grade, leading to neurological disa-

bility and ultimately to death. The optimal treatment of patients with LGG is still controversial [5].

Search strategy

We searched the following databases: the Cochrane Library (to date), Medline–Ovid (January 1966 to date), Medline–ProQuest, Medline-EIFL, EMBASE–Ovid (January 1990 to date), CancerNet and Science Citation Index (ISI). We used specific and sensitive keywords, as well as combinations of keywords, and publications in any language of countries represented in the Task Force. The search was completed in June 2009.

Methods for reaching consensus

The panel covered all fields of expertise in neuro-oncology (i.e., neurosurgeons, neurologists, neuropathologists,

European Handbook of Neurological Management: Volume 2, Second Edition. Edited by Nils Erik Gilhus, Michael P. Barnes, Michael Brainin.
© 2012 Blackwell Publishing Ltd. Published 2012 by Blackwell Publishing Ltd.

radiation and medical oncologists and a clinical trial expert). The scientific evidence of papers collected from the literature was evaluated and graded according to EFNS guidelines, and recommendations were given accordingly [6]. Class I evidence was derived from prospective, randomized, well-controlled clinical trials; Class II evidence was derived from prospective studies, including observational studies, cohort studies and case-control studies; Class III evidence was derived from retrospective studies; and Class IV evidence was derived from uncontrolled case series, case reports and expert opinion. As for recommendations, Level A required at least one Class I study or two consistent Class II studies, Level B at least one Class II study or overwhelming Class III evidence and Level C at least two consistent Class III studies. Regarding pathology and genetics, the classification of evidence was limited to the aspects that are mostly strong in terms of prognosis, while clinical features and conventional MRI were reviewed but not graded. When sufficient evidence for Level A–C was not available, we gave a good practice point recommendation if this was agreed by all members of the Task Force. When analysing results and drawing recommendations, differences at any stage were resolved by discussion.

Review of the evidence

Pathology and genetics

The World Health Organization (WHO) classification [7] recognizes grade II astrocytomas, oligodendrogliomas and oligoastrocytomas (Class I). Morphological features distinguish astrocytoma from oligodendroglioma. However, application of the same diagnostic criteria poses difficulties for the separation of oligoastrocytoma from both astrocytoma and oligodendroglioma as the diagnostic features present as a continuum along the histological spectrum and modern surgical approaches and scientific interest in fresh tumour tissue reduce the amount of material seen by the neuropathologists. This aggravates the inherent sampling problem and prevents WHO from providing a recommendation on the proportion of tissues with astrocytic or oligodendroglial differentiation required for the diagnosis of oligoastrocytoma.

Diffuse astrocytomas include fibrillary, gemistocytic and protoplasmic variants. The most common is the fibrillary astrocytoma. It is important to distinguish gemistocytic astrocytoma because it is more prone to malignant progression. Fibrillary astrocytoma is composed of a uniform cell population with only moderate nuclear atypia in a fine fibrillary tumour matrix. The hallmark of the gemistocytic variant are cells with ballooned eosinophilic cytoplasm and eccentric nuclei making up more than 20% of the tumour cells. The mitotic activity in astrocytomas WHO grade II is very low; single mitoses should not result in the diagnosis of anaplastic astrocytoma, while single mitosis in stereotactic biopsy should raise the suspicion of anaplasia. The Ki-67/MIB-1 labelling index in diffuse astrocytoma usually is less than 4%. Tumour necrosis, vascular proliferation, vascular thrombosis and high mitotic activity are not compatible with diffuse astrocytoma WHO grade II. The best immunohistochemical marker is GFAP, which is expressed in both tumour cells and the astrocytic processes. Molecular findings typical for diffuse astrocytoma are *TP53* mutations in 50% of cases; gemistocytic astrocytoma carries *TP53* mutations in more than 80%, while combined 1p/19q deletion is rare [8]. Somatic mutations in the *IDH1* gene have been reported in 75% of astrocytomas [9].

Oligodendrogliomas are moderately cellular and typically exhibit perinuclear halos (the so-called 'fried egg' or 'honeycomb' pattern). Occasionally, tumour cells with a small, strongly eosinophilic cytoplasm are found and are termed 'mini-gemistocytes'. Oligodendrogliomas have a dense network of capillaries and frequently contain calcifications. Occasional mitoses and a Ki-67/MIB-1 labelling index up to 5% are compatible with oligodendroglioma WHO grade II. There is no immunohistochemical marker specific for oligodendroglioma. The molecular hallmark of oligodendrogliomas is a combined loss of 1p/19q occurring in 80% of these tumours [10] (Class II), while TP53 mutations are encountered in only 5%. Somatic *IDH1* mutations are present in 80% of oligodendroglioma [9].

Oligoastrocytomas should be diagnosed on detection of convincing astrocytic and oligodendroglial components, but the inter-observer difference for the diagnosis oligoastrocytoma remains high [11]. Most oligoastrocytomas carry either 1p/19 loss or *TP53* mutations and there is a tendency for these aberrations to be present in both tumour compartments [12]. Up to 80% of oligoastrocytomas carry somatic mutations in *IDH1*. Both genetic (i.e., 1p/19q deletion) and epigenetic (MGMT and RASSF1A promoter methylation) changes seem to be important for gliomagenesis and response/resistance to radiotherapy and chemotherapy [13].

Clinical features

Seizures are the most common presentation and may be partial or generalized. They occur in over 90% of patients and are intractable in 50%. Seizures are more frequently associated with cortically based tumours, particularly in the frontal, temporal and insular/parainsular location, and with oligodendroglial tumours [14]. There is no clear association between severity of epilepsy and behaviour of the tumour. Focal neurological deficits are unusual, developing over many years. Raised intracranial pressure is rare in patients with supratentorial tumours and is typically seen in posterior fossa and intraventricular tumours. Intra-tumoral haemorrhage can occur.

Conventional and advanced neuroimaging

Conventional MRI is useful for differential diagnosis, guiding biopsy or resection, planning radiotherapy and monitoring treatment response [15]. LGGs appear as low-signal mass lesions on T1-weighted MRI and high-signal on T2-weighted and FLAIR sequences. Contrast enhancement is usually absent; when present it may indicate a focal area of high-grade transformation, although some tumours, particularly oligodendrogliomas, have patchy enhancement which remains stable over time.

The use of advanced imaging techniques can increase diagnostic accuracy [16, 17] (Classes II–III). Proton magnetic resonance spectroscopy (MRS) measures major metabolites in tumour tissue. The typical spectrum of a LGG shows elevated choline, reflecting increased membrane turnover, and decreased N-acetyl-aspartate, reflecting neuronal loss, but similar abnormal spectra may be seen in non-neoplastic lesions. Grading of gliomas is not possible by spectroscopy alone, as there is considerable overlap between low-grade and high-grade lesions. The presence of lactate and lipids is associated with higher proliferative activity and more aggressive behaviour [18]. MRS is helpful in guiding a biopsy to an area of high-grade activity, but not in longitudinal monitoring [19].

Dynamic susceptibility contrast MRI (DSC-MRI) allows measurement of relative cerebral blood volume (rCBV) which correlates with vascularity at the histologic level. Increase in rCBV in LGGs predicts high-grade transformation before gadolinium enhancement occurs [20]; however, these observations are limited to astrocytomas, as oligodendrogliomas have significantly higher rCBV [21].

Dynamic contrast enhanced imaging (DCE-MRI) measures the permeability of the blood–brain barrier by means of the transfer coefficient, K^{trans}, which is related to tumour grade, although the correlation is not as strong as for rCBV [22]. Regarding diffusion-weighted imaging (DWI), ADC values are lower and more variable in oligodendrogliomas compared with astrocytomas [23]. There is no correlation between ADC and choline [24].

Quantitative MRI in oligodendrogliomas with loss of heterozygosity of chromosome 1p/19q shows more heterogeneous T1- and T2-dependent signal, less distinct margins and higher rCBV than tumours with intact chromosomes [25, 26].

PET imaging

PET with [18F]-fluorodeoxyglucose (FDG) is of limited value as LGGs show a low FDG-uptake compared to the normal cortex. The usefulness of FDG-PET is limited to the detection of malignant transformation in astrocytomas (Class III) [27] and to the differentiation of radiation necrosis from tumour recurrence (Class II) [28].

PET with 11C-methionine (MET) is most frequently used and the uptake of MET correlates with the proliferative activity of tumour cells. The background uptake with MET-PET in normal brain tissue is lower than with FDG-PET, providing good contrast with tumour uptake and delineation of LGG [29]. LGGs with an oligodendroglial component show a higher MET uptake.

PET with MET is useful in differentiating LGGs from non-tumour lesions (Class II) [30], guiding stereotactic biopsies (Class II) [31], defining pre-operative tumour volume (Class II) [29] and monitoring response to treatment (Class III) [32].

As for novel tracers, 18F-fluoro-L-thymidine is a proliferation marker, but does not enter the brain unless there is a blood–brain barrier defect, and therefore its usefulness seems limited [33].

Prognostic factors

Age over 40 years and the presence of preoperative neurological deficits are adverse prognostic factors (Class I) [34, 35].

Regarding neuroimaging findings, larger tumours and tumours crossing the midline correlate with a short overall and progression-free survival (Class II) [34]. Growth rates are inversely correlated with survival (Class III) [4]. There are conflicting reports as to whether contrast enhancement is associated with a worse prognosis [36, 37].

A low CBV [38] and a low uptake of 11C-MET [39] correlate with longer progression-free and overall survival (Class III).

Oligodendrogliomas have a better prognosis than astrocytomas, whereas oligoastrocytomas have an intermediate outcome (Class I).

1p loss (with or without 19q loss) is a favourable prognostic factor (Class II) [40, 41, 42]. MGMT promoter methylation could predict a shorter time to progression in untreated patients [43], while predicting longer PFS and OS in patients receiving chemotherapy with temozolomide (Class III) [44].

IDH1 codon 132 mutation has been recently suggested as an independent favourable prognostic factor [45].

Antiepileptic treatment

There are no papers dealing with antiepileptic drugs (AEDs) in patients with LGG and seizures. The level of evidence is strong for treatment of seizures in general.

In patients with single seizures, immediate treatment with AEDs increases time to recurrent seizures compared to delayed treatment, without differences with respect to quality of life or serious complications (Class I) [46].

Patients with no history of seizures derive no benefit from prophylactic treatment [47, 48, 49] (Class I). Carbamazepine, phenytoin and valproate have Class I evidence of efficacy [50]. Lamotrigine, gabapentin, oxcarbazepine and topiramate have shown equivalence to carabamazepine, phenytoin and valproate [51]. In the

SANAD study lamotrigine was superior to carbamazepine, gabapentin and topiramate [52]. Valproate may potentiate the hematotoxicity from chemotherapy.

EIAEDs interact with some chemotherapy agents (nitrosoureas, paclitaxel, cyclophosphamide, topotecan, irinotecan, thiotepa, molecular agents), being associated with lower plasma levels and lower bone marrow toxicity (Class II) [47].

Surgery

Surgery is necessary to provide tissue for distinguishing between the histologic types, grading the malignancy and assessing the molecular status of tumours. Moreover, there are scenarios that pose problems of differential diagnosis between LGGs and non-neoplastic lesions (demyelination, inflammation or infection), and thus histological verification is mandatory.

Total resection improves seizure control, particularly in patients with a long epileptic history and insular tumours (Class II) [14].

The use of brain-mapping techniques increases the percentage of patients in whom a total and subtotal resection is achieved and has decreased the percentage of postoperative permanent deficits (Class II) [53, 54, 55].

Awake surgery is a well-tolerated procedure and can 1) increase the indications of resection in eloquent areas; 2) identify the structures crucial for brain functions, especially language, at both cortical and subcortical levels; and 3) optimize the extent of resection, the glioma removal being performed according to functional boundaries (Class III) [55]. Awake surgery has increased the safety of re-operation due to mechanisms of brain plasticity.

The effect of the extent of surgery on overall and progression-free survival is still uncertain as no randomized trials have specifically addressed this question. There is a general trend for most of the recently published articles [56, 57] to support extensive resections based on the surgeon's intraoperative impression (Class II). A critical point is a precise definition of total resection, which for LGGs that do not enhance implies removal of all the hyperintense regions on T2 or FLAIR images, and thus can only be determined by comparing preoperative and postoperative tumour volumes on MRI. This has been done by few studies only, and all have shown that total or near-total resection decreases the incidence of recurrence and the risk of malignant transformation, and improves progression free and overall survival (Class III) [54, 58]. Nonetheless, even with intraoperative MRI-guided surgery, total resection is achieved in no more than 36% of patients [59].

The initial report of RTOG 9802 [60], which performed observation after surgery in patients with age ≤40 years and complete resection, reported a 5-year survival rate of 93%, but 52% of patients progressed within 5 years and received salvage radiotherapy (Class II).

The timing of surgery is controversial in patients who are young, present with an isolated seizure (medically well controlled) and with small tumours. Potential surgical morbidity may compromise the otherwise intact functional status and some authors have advocated deferring surgery in lieu of radiographic control (a 'watch-and-wait policy') [61, 62], especially in oligodendroglial tumours [63]. The risk of deferring surgery includes managing at a later point a larger tumour, which may have undergone anaplastic transformation.

Radiotherapy

Four phase III randomized trials have been performed so far (Table 15.1).

EORTC 22845 [57, 64] investigated the role of radiotherapy (RT) timing. Although improved progression-free survival was demonstrated for patients treated with immediate RT, this did not translate into improved overall survival (Class I). Besides prolonging the time to tumour progression, radiotherapy has several other potential benefits, such as symptom control, particularly epileptic seizures [65].

Two randomized trials investigated different radiation doses. The EORTC 22844 and NCCTG studies showed no advantage for higher versus lower doses (Class I) [66, 67]. If higher doses are used, an increased toxicity is observed, with a 2-year incidence of radiation necrosis of 2.5% [66] or lower levels of functioning, concerning quality of life, especially for fatigue, insomnia and emotional functioning [68].

RTOG 9802 has compared RT alone vs. RT + PCV [69]. As two-thirds of patients in the RT arm who progressed received chemotherapy at progression, this trial might be considered one of early chemotherapy vs. chemotherapy at progression. PFS but not OS were improved (Class I). However, beyond 2 years, the addition of PCV to RT conferred a significant OS and PFS advantage, and reduced the risk of death by 48% and progression by 55%, suggesting a delayed benefit for chemotherapy. Grade 3–4 toxicity was higher among patients receiving RT + PCV (67% vs. 9%) (Class I).

Patients treated with whole-brain radiotherapy have a higher incidence of leuko-encephalopathy and cognitive deficits in comparison with patients treated with focal radiotherapy (Class II) [70]. In studies using modern standards of radiotherapy, less negative impacts on cognition are observed (Class II) [71, 72, 73], although recent data related to patients who had a neuropsychological follow-up at a mean of 12 years and were free of tumour progression suggest that those without radiotherapy maintain their cognitive status, whereas patients receiving radiotherapy do worse on attentional and

Table 15.1 Phase III trials on radiotherapy and chemotherapy for low-grade gliomas.

Study	Treatment Arms/ No. patients	5-year PFS (*P* value)		5-year OS (*P* value)	
EORTC 22845	S (157)	37%		66%	
	S + RT (154)	44%	p = 0.02	63%	NS
EORTC 22844	S + RT 45 Gy (171)	47%		58%	
	S + RT 59.4 Gy (172)	50%	NS	59%	NS
NCCTG	S + RT 50.4 Gy	55%		72%	
	S + RT 64.8 Gy	52%	NS	64%	NS
RTOG 94.02	S + RT (125)	46%		63%	
	S + RT + PCV (126)	63%	p = 0.005	72%	NS

executive functioning, as well as information-processing speed [74].

Chemotherapy

The usefulness of chemotherapy for patients progressing after surgery and radiotherapy is well established (Class II), with more data available for oligodendroglial tumours. PCV (procarbazine, CCNU and vincristine) and temozolomide yield similar objective response rates on CT/MRI (45–62%) and duration of response (10–24 months), with a toxicity profile favouring temozolomide in terms of tolerability (reduced myelotoxicity) and higher dose intensity [75, 76, 77, 78, 79]. The response rate of enhancing tumours, possibly reflecting high-grade pathology, is greater than that of non-enhancing tumours. A clinical benefit (i.e., reduction of seizure frequency and improvement of neurological deficits) is commonly seen in patients responding radiologically and in some patients with stable disease.

Chemotherapy (PCV or TMZ) as initial treatment after surgery has been investigated in high-risk patents (those with incomplete resection, persisting seizures and progression on CT/MRI). All studies have level of evidence of Class II [80, 81, 82, 83]. Complete responses are generally lacking, with a prevalence of minor over partial responses (overall 53%), and maximum tumour shrinkage can be delayed for as long as 24–30 months. Patients more likely to respond have symptomatic/enlarging oligodendroglial tumours, but mixed tumours or astrocytic tumours may respond as well. Most patients with seizures have a clinical benefit, even in the absence of a radiological change. Evaluation of response on conventional MRI (T2-weighted and/or FLAIR images) is difficult in non-enhancing tumours. Chemotherapy with nitrosureas can be an effective initial treatment for unresectable astrocytomas (Class IV) [84].

The response rate after chemotherapy is higher and duration of response is longer in patient with 1p/19q loss than in those with 1p/19q intact [83] (Class III).

Protracted low doses of TMZ could offer potential advantages over standard doses, especially in unmethylated tumours (Class III) [85], but the toxicity could be increased [86]. Preoperative chemotherapy could reduce tumour infiltration/extension and thus improve the surgical resectability (Class IV) [87].

Neurocognitive deficits

Neurocognitive deficits in LGGs can be caused by the tumour itself, tumour-related epilepsy, treatments or psychological distress. The cognitive decline, which might ultimately lead to dementia, negatively affects the patient's quality of life and well-being. Consequently, neurocognitive function is increasingly incorporated as a secondary outcome measure in clinical trials in patients with LGG. In the literature neurocognitive outcome has been assessed systematically in a limited number of studies, with a relatively small number of patients (Class II).

Regarding the effects of the tumour, Tucha *et al.* (2000) [88] found in 91% of patients before surgery neurocognitive deficits such as impairment of executive functions and memory attention. Glioma patients are prone to have more global neurocognitive deficits, unlike patients with stroke, who tend to have site-specific deficits. Patients with tumour in the dominant hemisphere have more memory problems and poorer attention, verbal fluency and verbal learning than those with non-dominant tumours [89], and are less likely to normalize following surgery [90].

Due to the reduction of tumour mass, surgery is more beneficial or at least does not worsen the neurocognitive functioning (Class II). However, surgery can give rise to transient focal neurocognitive deficits [55].

The severity of neurocognitive deficits after radiotherapy ranges from mild attention or memory disturbances to dementia (Class II). A follow-up of the Klein *et al.* (2003) study [74] has demonstrated that there is a relation between neurocognitive status and cerebral atrophy and leukoencephalopathy, and radiological abnormalities increases only in the irradiated group. Neurocognitive side-effects of AEDs can add to previous damage by surgery or radiotherapy (Class II). The older AEDs (phenobarbitone, phenytoin, carbamazepine, valproic acid) can decrease neurocognitive functioning by impairing attention and memory [91]. Among newer AEDs, gabapentin, lamotrigine and levetiracetam have fewer adverse neurocognitive effects, while topiramate is associated with the greatest risk of neurocognitive impairment [92].

A randomized trial has shown that cognitive rehabilitation has a salutary effect on both short- and long-term cognitive complaints and mental fatigue (Class II) [93].

Recommendations

1. Astrocytomas, oligodendrogliomas and oligoastrocytomas are diagnosed using morphological criteria according to WHO classification (Level A).

2. Combined loss of 1p/19q is a marker in favour of the diagnosis of oligodendroglioma or oligoastrocytoma (Level B).

3. MRI with contrast enhancement is the gold standard to monitor LGG after surgery: an MRI examination every 6 months might be sufficient, unless physician thinks otherwise (good practice point).

4. MRS is useful for differentiation of LGG from non-tumorous lesions, preoperative definition of extent and guiding stereotactic biopsies (Level C).

5. DSC-MRI can be employed in the follow-up to predict malignant transformation (Level C).

6. PET with FDG is useful for detecting malignant transformation in astrocytomas (Level C) and for differentiation between radiation necrosis and tumour recurrence (Level B).

7. PET with MET is useful for differentiation of LGG from non-tumorous lesions (Level B), guiding stereotactic biopsies (Level B), pre-treatment evaluation (Level B) and monitoring treatment (Level C).

8. Prophylactic AEDs must not be used before any epileptic seizures have occurred (Level A).

9. AEDs should be started after the first seizure (Level A).

10. AEDs should be individualized according to seizure type, co-medication, comorbidity and patient preferences (good practice point).

11. In patients who need a treatment with chemotherapy, non-EIAEDs are to be preferred (Level B).

12. Surgical resection represents the first treatment option, with the goal to maximally resect the tumour mass whenever possible, while minimizing the postoperative morbidity (Level B). The identification of the eloquent cerebral areas, which have to be preserved during surgery, is performed through preoperative neuroimaging modalities (fMRI, fibre tracking) and intraoperative brain mapping techniques (Level B), and awake surgery could improve the results (Level C).

13. When surgery is not feasible due to tumour location, extension or comorbidities, a biopsy (stereotactic or open) should be performed to obtain a histological diagnosis (good practice point).

14. For patients with unfavourable prognostic factors (older age, incomplete or no resection, existing neurological symptoms) an adjuvant treatment is indicated at any time (Level B), and this is more commonly radiotherapy (good practice point).

15. A total RT dose of 50.4–54 Gy in fractions of 1.8 Gy represents the current standard of care (Level A). Modern radiotherapy techniques (conformal dose delivery or intensity-modulated techniques) should preferably be used (Level B).

16. Younger patients (< 40 years of age) with (near-) complete resection, and tumours with an oligodendroglial component have a more favourable prognosis, and can be observed after surgery (Level B), but close follow-up is needed (good practice point).

17. Chemotherapy is an option for patients with recurrence after surgery and radiation therapy (Level B).

18. Chemotherapy is an option as initial treatment for patients with large residual tumours after surgery or unresectable tumours to delay the risk of late neurotoxicity from large-field radiotherapy, especially when 1p/19q loss is present (Level B).

19. Neuropsychological tests at diagnosis and during the follow-up can be useful, being selected according to the needs of the clinical setting (good practice point). The neuropsychological tests must have standardized materials and administration procedures, published normative data, moderate-to-high test–retest reliability, short administration time (30–40 minutes) and be suitable to monitor changes over time.

20. Cognitive rehabilitation can be helpful (Level B).

References

1. Duffau, L, Capelle, L. Preferential brain locations of low-grade gliomas. *Cancer* 2004; **100**:2622–6.

2. Claus, EB, Black, PM. Survival rates and patterns of care for patients diagnosed with supratentorial low-grade gliomas: data from the SEER program, 1973–2001. *Cancer* 2006; **106**:1358–63.

3. Mandonnet, E, Delattre, JY, Tanguy, ML, *et al.* Continuous growth of mean tumour diameter in a subset of grade II gliomas. *Ann Neurol* 2003; **53**:524–8.

4. Rees, J, Watt, H, Jäger, HR, *et al.* Volumes and growth rates of untreated adult low-grade gliomas indicate risk of early malignant transformation. *Eur J Radiol* 2009; **72**:54–64.

5. Schiff, D, Brown, PD, Giannini, C. Outcome in adult low-grade glioma: the impact of prognostic factors and treatment. *Neurology* 2007; **69**:1366–73.

6. Brainin, M, Barnes, M, Baron, JC, *et al.* Guidance for the preparation of neurological management guidelines by EFNS scientific task forces – revised recommendations 2004. *Eur J Neurol* 2004; **11**:577–81.

7. Louis, D, Ohgaki, H, Wiestler, O, Cavenee, W (eds). *World Health Organization Classification of Tumours of the Central Nervous System*, 4th edn, 2007; IARC, Lyon.

8. Okamoto, Y, Di Patre, PL, Burkhard, C, *et al.* Population-based study on incidence, survival rates, and genetic alterations of low-grade diffuse astrocytomas and oligodendrogliomas. *Acta Neuropathol* 2004; **108**:49–56.

9. Balss, J, Meyer, J, Mueller, W, *et al.* Analysis of the IDH1 codon 132 mutation in brain tumours. *Acta Neuropathol* 2008; **116**:597–602.

10. Kraus, JA, Koopmann, J, Kaskel, P, *et al.* Shared allelic losses on chromosomes 1p and 19q suggest a common origin of oligodendroglioma and oligoastrocytoma. *J Neuropath Exp Neurol* 1995; **54**:91–5.

11. Coons, SW, Johnson, PC, Scheithauer, BW, *et al.* Improving diagnostic accuracy and interobserver concordance in the classification and grading of primary gliomas. *Cancer* 1997; **79**:1381–93.

12. Maintz, D, Fiedler, K, Koopmann, J, *et al.* Molecular genetic evidence for subtypes of oligoastrocytomas. *J Neuropathol Exp Neurol* 1997; **56**:1098–104.

13. Lorente, A, Mueller, W, Urdangarín, E, *et al.* RASSF1A, BLU, NORE1A, PTEN and MGMT expression and promoter methylation in gliomas and glioma cell lines and evidence of deregulated expression of de novo DNMTs. *Brain Pathol* 2009; **19**:279–92.

14. Chang, EF, Potts, MB, Keles, GE, *et al.* Seizure characteristics and control following resection in 332 patients with low-grade gliomas. *J Neurosurg* 2008; **108**:227–35.

15. Sanders, WP, Chistoforidis, GA. Imaging of low-grade primary brain tumours, in *The Practical Management of Low-Grade Primary Brain Tumours* (eds JP Rock, ML Rosenblum, EG Shaw, JG Cairncross), 1999; Lippincott Williams & Wilkins, Philadelphia, pp. 5–32.

16. Law, M, Yang, S, Wang, H, *et al.* Glioma grading: sensitivity, specificity, and predictive values of perfusion MR imaging and proton MR spectroscopic imaging compared with conventional MR imaging. *AJNR Am J Neuroradiol* 2003; **24**:1989–98.

17. Zonari, P, Baraldi, P, Crisi, G. Multimodal MRI in the characterization of glial neoplasms: the combined role of single-voxel MR spectroscopy, diffusion imaging and echo-planar perfusion imaging. *Neuroradiology* 2007; **49**:795–803.

18. Guillevin, R, Menuel, C, Duffau, H, *et al.* Proton magnetic resonance spectroscopy predicts proliferative activity in diffuse low-grade gliomas. *J Neurooncol* 2008; **87**:181–7.

19. Reijneveld, JC, van der Grond, J, Ramos, LM, *et al.* Proton MRS imaging in the follow-up of patients with suspected low-grade gliomas. *Neuroradiology* 2005; **47**:887–91.

20. Danchaivijitr, N, Waldman, AD, Tozer, DJ, *et al.* Low-grade gliomas: do changes in rCBV measurements at longitudinal perfusion-weighted MR imaging predict malignant transformation? *Radiology* 2008; **247**:170–8.

21. Cha, S, Tihan, T, Crawfoed, F, *et al.* Differentiation of low-grade oligodendrogliomas from low-grade astrocytomas by using quantitative blood-volume measurements derived from dynamic susceptibility contrast-enhanced MR imaging. *AJNR Am J Neuroradiol* 2005; **26**:266–73.

22. Law, M, Yang, S, Babb, JS, *et al.* Comparison of cerebral blood volume and vascular permeability from dynamic susceptibility contrast-enhanced perfusion MR imaging with glioma grade. *AJNR Am J Neuroradiol* 2004; **25**: 746–55.

23. Khayal, IS, McKnight, TR, McGue, C, *et al.* Apparent diffusion coefficient and fractional anisotropy of newly diagnosed grade II gliomas. *NMR Biomed* 2009; **22**:449–55.

24. Khayal, IS, Crawford, FW, Saraswathy, S. Relationship between choline and apparent diffusion coefficient in patients with gliomas. *J Magn Reson Imaging* 2008; **27**: 718–25.

25. Jenkinson, MD, du Plessis, DG, Smith, TS, *et al.* Histological growth patterns and genotype in oligodendroglial tumours: correlation with MRI features. *Brain* 2006; **129**:1884–91.

26. Brown, R, Zlatescu, M, Sijben, A, *et al.* The use of magnetic resonance imaging to noninvasively detect genetic signatures in oligodendroglioma. *Clin Cancer Res* 2008; **14**: 2357–62.

27. Di Chiro, G, Brooks, RA. PET-FDG of untreated and treated cerebral gliomas. *J Nucl Med* 1988; **29**:421–3.

28. Minn, H. PET and SPECT in low-grade gliomas. *Eur J Radiol* 2005; **56**:171–8.

29. Kaschten, B, Stevenaert, A, Sadzot, B, *et al.* Preoperative evaluation of 54 gliomas by PET with fluorine-18-fluorodeoxyglucose and/or carbon-11-methionine. *J Nucl Med* 1998; **39**:778–85.

30. Herholz, K, Holzer, T, Bauer, B, *et al.* 11C-methionine PET for differential diagnosis of low-grade gliomas. *Neurology* 1998; **50**:1316–22.

31. Pirotte, B, Goldman, S, Massager, N, *et al.* Comparison of 18F-FDG and 11C-methionine for PET-guided stereotactic brain biopsy of gliomas. *J Nucl Med* 2004; **45**:1293–8.

32. Nuutinen, J, Sonninen, P, Lehikoinen, P. Radiotherapy treatment planning and long-term followup with [(11)C] methionine PET in patients with low-grade astrocytoma. *Int J Radiat Oncol Biol Phys* 2000; **48**:43–52.

33. Jacobs, AH, Thomas, A, Kracht, LW, *et al.* 18F-fluoro-L-thymidine and 11C-methylmethionine as markers of increased transport and proliferation in brain tumours. *J Nucl Med* 2005; **46**:1948–58.

34. Pignatti, F, van den Bent, MJ, Curran, D, *et al.* Prognostic factors for survival in adult patients with cerebral low-grade glioma. *J Clin Oncol* 2002; **20**:2076–84.

35. Lebrun, C, Fontaine, D, Ramaioli, A, *et al.* Long-term outcome of oligodendrogliomas. *Neurology* 2004; **62**: 1783–7.

36. Pallud, J, Capelle, L, Taillandier, L, *et al.* Prognostic significance of imaging contrast enhancement for WHO grade II gliomas. *Neuro Oncol* 2009; **11**:176–82.

37. Chaichana, KL, McGirt, MJ, Niranjan, A. Prognostic significance of contrast-enhancing low-grade gliomas in adults and a review of the literature. *Neurol Res* 2009; **31**:931–9.

38. Law, M, Young, RJ, Babb, JS, *et al.* Gliomas: predicting time to progression or survival with cerebral blood volume measurements at dynamic susceptibility-weighted contrast-enhanced perfusion MR imaging. *Radiology* 2008; **247**: 490–8.

39. Ribom, D, Eriksson, A, Hartman, M, *et al.* Positron emission tomography (11)C-methionine and survival in patients with low-grade gliomas. *Cancer* 2001; **92**:1541–9.

40. Smith, JS, Perry, A, Borell, TJ, *et al.* Alterations of chromosome arms 1p and 19q as predictors of survival in oligodendrogliomas, astrocytomas, and mixed oligoastrocytomas. *J Clin Oncol* 2000; **18**:636–45.

41. Kujas, M, Lejeune, J, Benouaich-Amiel, A, *et al* Chromosome 1p loss: a favorable prognostic factor in low-grade gliomas. *Ann Neurol* 2005; **58**:322–6.

42. Weller, M, Berger, H, Hartmann, C, *et al.* Combined 1p/19q loss in oligodendroglial tumours: predictive or prognostic biomarker? *Clin Cancer Res* 2007; **13**:6933–7.

43. Komine, C, Watanabe, T, Katayama, Y, *et al.* Promoter hypermethylation of the DNA repair gene O6-methylguanine-DNA methyltransferase is an independent predictor of shortened progression free survival in patients with low-grade diffuse astrocytomas. *Brain Pathol* 2003; **13**: 176–84.

44. Everhard, S, Kaloshi, G, Crinière, E, *et al.* MGMT methylation: a marker of response to temozolomide in low-grade gliomas. *Ann Neurol* 2006; **60**:740–3.

45. Sanson, M, Marie, Y, Paris, S, *et al.* Isocitrate dehydrogenase 1 codon 132 mutation is an important prognostic biomarker in gliomas. *J Clin Oncol* 2009; **27**:4150–4.

46. Marson, A, Jacoby, A, Johnson, A, *et al.* Immediate versus deferred antiepileptic drug treatment for early epilepsy and single seizures: a randomised controlled trial. *Lancet* 2005; **365**:2007–13.

47. Glantz, MJ, Cole, BF, Forsyth, PA, *et al.* Practice parameter: anticonvulsant prophylaxis in patients with newly diagnosed brain tumours. Report of the Quality Standards Subcommittee of the American Academy of Neurology. *Neurology* 2000; **54**:1886–93.

48. Perry, J, Zinman, L, Chambers, A, *et al.* The use of prophylactic anticonvulsants in patients with brain tumours – a systematic review. *Curr Oncology* 2006; **13**:222–9.

49. Tremont-Lukas, IW, Ratilal, BO, Armstrong, T, *et al.* Antiepileptic drugs for preventing seizures in patients with brain tumours (Review). *Cochrane Database Syst Rev* 2008; 2, Art No CD004424.

50. ILAE Treatment Guidelines. Evidence-based analysis of antiepileptic drug efficacy and effectiveness as initial monotherapy for epileptic seizures and syndromes. *Epilepsia* 2006; 47:1094–120.

51. Wilby, J, Kainth, A, Hawkins, N, *et al.* Clinical effectiveness, tolerability and cost effectiveness of newer drugs for epilepsy in adults: a systematic review and economic evaluation. *Health Technol Assess* 2005; **9**:1–157.

52. Marson, AG, Appleton, R, Baker, GA, *et al.* A randomised controlled trial examining the longerterm outcomes of standard versus new antiepileptic drugs. The SANAD trial. *Health Technol Assess* 2007; **11**:1–134.

53. Bello, L, Gallucci, M, Fava, M, *et al.* Intraoperative subcortical language tract mapping guides surgical removal of gliomas involving speech areas. *Neurosurgery* 2007; **60**: 67–80.

54. Smith, JS, Chang, EF, Lamborn, KR, *et al.* Role of extent of resection in the long-term outcome of low-grade hemispheric gliomas. *J Clin Oncol* 2008; **26**:1338–45.

55. Duffau, H. Surgery of low-grade gliomas: towards a functional neurooncology. *Curr Opin Oncol* 2009; **21**:543–9.

56. Keles, GE, Lamborn, KR, Berger, MS. Low grade hemispheric gliomas in adults: a critical review of extent of resection as a factor influencing outcome. *J Neurosurg* 2001; 95:735–45.

57. Karim, AB, Afra, D, Cornu, P, *et al.* Randomized trial on the efficacy of radiotherapy for cerebral low-grade glioma in the adult: European Organization for Research and Treatment of Cancer Study 22845 with the Medical Research Council study BRO4: an interim analysis. *Int J Radiat Oncol Biol Phys* 2002; **52**:316–24.

58. Berger, MS, Deliganis, AV, Dobbins, J, Keles, GE. The effect of extent of resection on recurrence in patients with low grade cerebral hemisphere gliomas. *Cancer* 1994; **74**: 1784–91.

59. Claus, EB, Horlacher, A, Hsu, L, *et al.* Survival rates in patients with low-grade glioma after intraoperative magnetic resonance image guidance. *Cancer* 2005; **103**: 1227–33.

60. Shaw, EG, Berkey, B, Coons, SW, *et al.* Recurrence following neurosurgeon-determined grosstotal resection of adult supratentorial low-grade glioma: results of a prospective clinical trial. *J Neurosurg* 2008; **109**:835–41.

61. Recht, LD, Lew, R, Smith, TW. Suspected low-grade glioma: is deferring treatment safe? *Ann Neurol* 1992; **31**:431–6.

62. Reijneveld, JC, Sitskoorn, MM, Klein, M, *et al.* Cognitive status and quality of life in patients with suspected

versus proven low-grade gliomas. *Neurology* 2001; **56**:618–23.

63. Olson, JD, Riedel, E, DeAngelis, LM. Long-term outcome of low-grade oligodendroglioma and mixed glioma. *Neurology* 2000; **54**:1442–8.

64. van den Bent, MJ, Afra, D, de Witte, O, *et al.* EORTC Radiotherapy and Brain Tumour Groups and the UK Medical Research Council. Long-term efficacy of early versus delayed radiotherapy for low-grade astrocytoma and oligodendroglioma in adults: the EORTC 22845 randomised trial. *Lancet* 2005; **366**:985–90.

65. Soffietti, R, Borgognone, M, Ducati, A, *et al.* Efficacy of radiation therapy on seizures in low-grade astrocytomas. *Neuro-Oncol* 2005; **7**:389. (suppl. World Congress of Neuro-Oncology, Ediburgh, 2005).

66. Shaw, E, Arusell, R, Scheithauer, B, *et al.* Prospective randomized trial of low- versus high-dose radiation therapy in adults with supratentorial low-grade glioma: initial report of a North Central Cancer Treatment Group/Radiation Therapy Oncology Group/Eastern Cooperative Oncology Group study. *J Clin Oncol* 2002; **20**:2267–76.

67. Karim, AB, Maat, B, Hatlevoll, R, *et al.* A randomized trial on dose-response in radiation therapy of low-grade cerebral glioma: European Organization for Research and Treatment of Cancer (EORTC) Study 22844. *Int J Radiat Oncol Biol Phys* 1996; **36**:549–56.

68. Kiebert, GM, Curran, D, Aaronson, NK, *et al.* Quality of life after radiation therapy of cerebral low-grade gliomas of the adult: results of a randomised phase III trial on dose response (EORTC trial 22844). *Eur J Cancer* 1998; **34**: 1902–9.

69. Shaw, EG, Wang, M, Coons, SW, *et al.* Final report of Radiation Therapy Oncology Group (RTOG) protocol 9802: radiation therapy (RT) versus RT + procarbazine, CCNU and vincristine (PCV) chemotherapy for adult low-grade gliomas (LGG). *J Clin Oncol* 2008; **26**:90s, 2006.

70. Surma-aho, O, Niemelä, M, Vilkki, J, *et al.* Adverse long-term effects of brain radiotherapy in adult low-grade glioma patients. *Neurology* 2001; **56**:1285–90.

71. Taphoorn, MJ, Schiphorst, AK, Snoek, FJ, *et al.* Cognitive functions and quality of life in patients with low-grade gliomas: the impact of radiotherapy. *Ann Neurol* 1994; **36**: 48–54.

72. Klein, M, Heimans, JJ, Aaronson, NK, *et al.* Effect of radiotherapy and other treatment-related factors on mid-term to long-term cognitive sequelae in low-grade gliomas: a comparative study. *Lancet* 2002; **360**:1361–8.

73. Laack, NN, Brown, PD., Ivnik, RJ, *et al.* Cognitive function after radiotherapy for supratentorial low-grade glioma: a North Central Cancer Treatment Group prospective study. *Int J Radiat Oncol Biol Phys* 2005; **63**:1175–83.

74. Douw, L, Klein, M, Fagel, SS, *et al.* Cognitive and radiological effects of radiotherapy in patients with low-grade glioma: long-term follow-up. *Lancet Neurol* 2009; **8**: 810–18.

75. Soffietti, R, Rudà, R., Bradac, GB, Schiffer, D. PCV chemotherapy for recurrent oligodendrogliomas and oligoastrocytomas. *Neurosurgery* 1998; **43**:1066–73.

76. van den Bent, MJ, Kros, JM, Heimans, JJ, *et al.* Response rate and prognostic factors of recurrent oligodendroglioma treated with procarbazine, CCNU, and vincristine chemotherapy. Dutch Neuro-oncology Group. *Neurology* 1998; **51**:1140–5.

77. van den Bent, MJ, Taphoorn, MJ, Brandes, AA, *et al.* Phase II study of first-line chemotherapy with temozolomide in recurrent oligodendroglial tumours: the European Organization for Research and Treatment of Cancer Brain Tumour Group Study 26971. *J Clin Oncol* 2003; **21**: 2525–8.

78. Pace, A, Vidiri, A, Galiè, E, *et al.* Temozolomide chemotherapy for progressive low-grade glioma: clinical benefits and radiological response. *Ann Oncol* 2003; **14**:1722–6.

79. Quinn, JA, Reardon, DA, Friedman, AH, *et al.* Phase II trial of temozolomide in patients with progressive low-grade glioma. *J Clin Oncol* 2003; **21**:646–51.

80. Brada, M, Viviers, L, Abson, C, *et al.* Phase II study of primary temozolomide chemotherapy in patients with WHO grade II gliomas. *Ann Oncol* 2003; **14**:1715–21.

81. Buckner, JC, Gesme, D, Jr, O'Fallon, JR, *et al.* Phase II trial of procarbazine, lomustine, and vincristine as initial therapy for patients with low-grade oligodendroglioma or oligoastrocytoma: efficacy and associations with chromosomal abnormalities. *J Clin Oncol* 2003; **21**:251–5.

82. Hoang-Xuan, K, Capelle, L, Kujas, M, *et al.* Temozolomide as initial treatment for adults with low-grade oligodendrogliomas or oligoastrocytomas and correlation with chromosome 1p deletions. *J Clin Oncol* 2004; **22**:3133–8.

83. Kaloshi, G, Benouaich-Amiel, A, Diakite, F, *et al.* Temozolomide for low-grade gliomas: predictive impact of 1p/19q loss on response and outcome. *Neurology* 2007; **68**: 1831–6.

84. Frenay, MP, Fontaine, D, Vandenbos, F, *et al.* First-line nitrosourea-based chemotherapy in symptomatic non-resectable supratentorial pure low-grade astrocytomas. *Eur J Neurol* 2005; **12**:685–90.

85. Kesari, S, Schiff, D, Drappatz, J, *et al.* Phase II study of protracted daily temozolomide for lowgrade gliomas in adults. *Clin Cancer Res* 2009; **15**:330–7.

86. Tosoni, A, Franceschi, E, Ermani, M, *et al.* Temozolomide three weeks on and one week off as first-line therapy for patients with recurrent or progressive low-grade gliomas. *J Neurooncol* 2008; **89**:179–85.

87. Duffau, H, Taillandier, L, Capelle, L. Radical surgery after chemotherapy: a new therapeutic strategy to envision in grade II glioma. *J Neurooncol* 2006; **80**:171–6.

88. Tucha, O, Smely, C, Preier, M, Lange, KW. Cognitive deficits before treatment among patients with brain tumours. *Neurosurgery* 2000; **47**:324–33.

89. Hahn, CA, Dunn, RH, Logue, PE, *et al.* Prospective study of neuropsychologic testing and quality-of-life assessment of adults with primary malignant brain tumours. *Int J Radiat Oncol Biol Phys* 2003; **55**:992–9.

90. Yoshii, Y, Tominaga, D, Sugimoto, K, *et al.* Cognitive function of patients with brain tumour in pre- and postoperative stage. *Surgical Neurol* 2008; **69**:51–61.

91. Meador, KJ. Cognitive outcomes and predictive factors in epilepsy. *Neurology* 2002; **58**:21–6.

92. Meador, KJ. Cognitive and memory effects of the new antiepileptic drugs. *Epilepsy Res* 2006; **68**:63–7.

93. Gehring, K, Sitskoorn, MM, Gundy, CM, *et al.* Cognitive rehabilitation in patients with gliomas: a randomized, controlled trial. *J Clin Oncol* 2009; **27**: 3712–22.

CHAPTER 16

Treatment of tension-type headache

L. Bendtsen,[1] S. Evers,[2] M. Linde,[3] D. D. Mitsikostas,[4] G. Sandrini[5] and J. Schoenen[6]

[1]Glostrup Hospital, University of Copenhagen, Denmark; [2]University of Münster, Münster, Germany; [3]University of Gothenburg and St Olav's Hospital, Trondheim Norway and Norwegian University of Science and Technology, Trondheim, Norway; [4]Athens Naval Hospital, Athens, Greece; [5]IRCCS Catholic University of Pavia, Pavia, Italy; [6]University of Liège, Liège, Belgium

Objectives

These guidelines aim to give evidence-based recommendations for the acute and prophylactic drug treatment of tension-type headache (TTH). In addition, the guidelines aim to provide a short overview on non-drug treatment of TTH based on the best-performed controlled trials, reviews and meta-analyses, whereas the vast amount of uncontrolled reports of non-drug treatment will not be considered. A brief clinical description of the headache disorders is included. The definitions follow the diagnostic criteria of the International Headache Society (IHS) [1].

Background

Tension-type headache is classified into three subtypes according to headache frequency: infrequent episodic TTH (less than one day of headache per month), frequent episodic TTH (1–14 days of headache per month) and chronic TTH (≥15 days per month) [1] (Table 16.1). This division may seem artificial but has proved to be highly relevant for several reasons. First, impact on quality of life differs considerably between the subtypes. A person having a headache every day from the time of waking, persisting until bedtime, month in and month out, is disabled. At the other extreme, a mild headache once every other month has very little impact on health or functional ability and needs little if any medical atten-

tion. Second, the pathophysiological mechanisms may differ significantly between the subtypes; peripheral mechanisms are probably more important in episodic TTH, whereas central pain mechanisms are pivotal in chronic TTH [2]. Third, treatment differs between the subtypes, with symptomatic and prophylactic treatments being more appropriate for episodic and chronic TTH respectively. Therefore, a precise diagnosis is mandatory and should be established by means of a headache diary [3] completed for at least 4 weeks.

The recommendations in this paper are based on the scientific evidence from clinical trials and on the expert consensus by the respective task force of the European Federation of Neurological Societies (EFNS). The legal aspects of drug prescription and drug availability in the different European countries will not be considered. The definitions of the recommendation levels follow the EFNS criteria [4]. Briefly, a level A rating (established as effective, ineffective or harmful) requires at least one convincing class I study or at least two consistent, convincing class II studies. A level B rating (probably effective, ineffective or harmful) requires at least one convincing class II study or overwhelming class III evidence, whereas a level C rating (possibly effective, ineffective or harmful) requires at least two convincing class III studies [4].

In general, non-pharmacological management should always be considered in TTH [5]. When it comes to pharmacological management, the general rule is that patients

European Handbook of Neurological Management: Volume 2, Second Edition. Edited by Nils Erik Gilhus, Michael P. Barnes, Michael Brainin.
© 2012 Blackwell Publishing Ltd. Published 2012 by Blackwell Publishing Ltd.

Table 16.1 Diagnostic criteria of tension-type headache of the IHS classification [1].

2.1 Infrequent episodic tension-type headache
  A. At least 10 episodes occurring on <1 day per month on average (<12 days per year) and fulfilling criteria B–D
  B. Headache lasting from 30 min to 7 days
  C. Headache has at least two of the following characteristics:
    (1) bilateral location
    (2) pressing/tightening (non-pulsating) quality
    (3) mild or moderate pain intensity
    (4) not aggravated by routine physical activity such as walking or climbing stairs
  D. Both of the following:
    (1) no nausea or vomiting (anorexia may occur)
    (2) no more than one of photophobia or phonophobia
  E. Not attributed to another disorder
2.2 Frequent episodic tension-type headache
As 2.1 except for:
A. At least 10 episodes occurring on ≥1 but <15 days per month for at least 3 months (≥12 and <180 days per year) and fulfilling
    criteria B–D
2.3 Chronic tension-type headache
As 2.1 except for:
Headache occurring on ≥15 days per month on average for >3 months (≥180 days per year) and fulfilling criteria B–D
  B. Headache lasts hours or may be continuous
  D. Both of the following:
    (1) no more than one of photophobia, phonophobia or mild nausea
    (2) neither moderate nor severe nausea or vomiting

with episodic TTH [1] are treated with symptomatic (acute) drugs, whereas prophylactic drugs should be considered in patients with very frequent episodic TTH and chronic TTH [1]. Analgesics are often ineffective in patients with chronic TTH. Furthermore, their frequent use produces risk of toxicity (e.g. kidney and liver problems) as well as of medication-overuse headache [6].

Search strategy

A literature search was performed using the reference databases MedLine, Science Citation Index and the Cochrane Library; the keywords used were 'tension-type headache' (last search October 2009). In addition, a review book [7] and treatment recommendations from the British Association for the Study of Headache [8] were considered. Trials published in English and conducted among adult patients (aged 18 years and older) with reasonable criteria designed to distinguish TTH from migraine were considered. For drug treatments, randomized placebo-controlled trials and trials comparing different treatments were considered. For non-drug treatments controlled trials were considered.

Method for reaching consensus

All authors performed an independent literature search. The first draft of the manuscript was written by the chairman of the task force. All other members of the task force read the first draft and discussed changes by email. Three more drafts were then written by the chairman and each time discussed by email. All recommendations had to be agreed to by all members of the task force unanimously. The background of the research strategy and reaching consensus and the definitions of the recommendation levels used in this paper have been described in the EFNS recommendations [4].

Epidemiology

The lifetime prevalence of TTH was as high as 78% in a population-based study in Denmark, but the majority had episodic infrequent TTH (1 day a month or less) without specific need of medical attention [9]. Nevertheless, 24–37% had TTH several times a month, 10% had it weekly and 2–3% of the population had chronic TTH usually lasting for the greater part of a lifetime [9, 10].

The female:male ratio of TTH is 5:4, indicating that, unlike migraine, women are only slightly more affected than men [11, 12]. The average age of onset of TTH is higher than in migraine, namely 25–30 years in cross-sectional epidemiological studies [10]. The prevalence peaks between the age of 30 and 39 years and decreases slightly with age. Poor self-rated health, inability to relax after work and sleeping few hours per night have been reported as risk factors for developing TTH [13].

A recent review of the global prevalence and burden of headaches [11] showed that the disability of TTH as a burden of society was greater than that of migraine, which indicates that the overall cost of TTH is greater than that of migraine. Two Danish studies have shown that the number of work days missed in the population was three times higher for TTH than for migraine [10, 14] and a US study has also found that absenteeism due to TTH is considerable [15]. The burden is particularly high for the minority who have substantial and complicating co-morbidities [16].

Clinical aspects

TTH is characterized by a bilateral, pressing, tightening pain of mild-to-moderate intensity, occurring either in short episodes of variable duration (episodic forms) or continuously (chronic form). The headache is not associated with the typical migraine features such as vomiting, severe photophobia and phonophobia. In the chronic form, only one of the last two accompanying symptoms or mild nausea is accepted [1] (see Table 16.1). Due to a lack of accompanying symptoms and the relatively milder pain intensity, patients are rarely severely incapacitated by their pain. TTH is the most featureless of the primary headaches and, as many secondary headaches may mimic TTH, a diagnosis of TTH requires exclusion of other organic disorders.

Diagnosis

The diagnosis of TTH is based on the typical patient's history and a normal neurological examination. A correct diagnosis should be assured by means of a headache diary [3] recorded over at least 4 weeks. The diagnostic problem most often encountered is to discriminate between TTH and mild migraine. If the headache is strictly unilateral the debated entity cervicogenic headache should be considered [17]. The diary may also reveal triggers and medication overuse, and it will establish the baseline against which to measure the efficacy of treatments. Identification of a high intake of analgesics is essential because medication overuse requires specific treatment [6].

Paraclinical investigations, in particular brain imaging, is necessary if secondary headache is suspected (e.g. the headache characteristics are atypical), if the course of headache attacks changes or if persistent neurological or psychopathological abnormalities are present. Significant co-morbidity, e.g. anxiety or depression, should be identified and treated concomitantly. Poor compliance with prophylactic treatment may be a problem in chronic TTH as it is in migraine [18]. It should be explained to the patient that frequent TTH can only seldom be cured, but that a meaningful improvement can often be obtained with the combination of drug and non-drug treatments.

Acute drug treatment of TTH

Acute drug therapy refers to the treatment of individual attacks of headache in patients with episodic and chronic TTH. Most headaches in patients with episodic TTH are mild to moderate and the patients often can self-manage by using simple analgesics (paracetamol or aspirin) or non-steroidal anti-inflammatory drugs (NSAIDs). The efficacy of the simple analgesics tends to decrease with increasing frequency of the headaches. In patients with chronic TTH, the headaches are often associated with stress, anxiety and depression, and simple analgesics are usually ineffective and should be used with caution because of the risk of medication-overuse headache at a regular intake of simple analgesics for more than 14 days a month or triptans or combination analgesics for more than 9 days a month [19]. Other interventions such as non-drug treatments and prophylactic pharmacotherapy should be considered.

The effect of acute drugs in TTH has been examined in many studies, and these have used many different methods for measurement of efficacy. The guidelines for drug trials in TTH from the International Headache Society recommends being pain free after 2 hours as the primary efficacy measure [20]. This has been used in some studies whereas many studies have used other efficacy measures such as pain intensity difference, time to meaningful relief. This makes comparison of results between studies difficult.

Simple analgesics and NSAIDs

Paracetamol 1000 mg was significantly more effective than placebo in most [21–27] but not all [28, 29] trials, whereas three trials found no significant effect of paracetamol 500–650 mg compared with placebo [21, 28, 30].

Aspirin has consistently been reported to be more effective than placebo in doses of 1000 mg [21, 31, 32], 500–650 mg [21, 32–34] and 250 mg [32]. One study found no difference in efficacy between solid and effervescent aspirin [34].

Ibuprofen 800 mg [33], 400 mg [24, 25, 33, 35, 36] and 200 mg [37] are more effective than placebo, as are ketoprofen 50 mg [28, 37], 25 mg [27, 29, 37] and 12.5 mg [29]. One study could not demonstrate a significant effect of ketoprofen 25 mg possibly due to a low number of patients [28]. Diclofenac 25 mg and 12.5 mg have been reported as effective [35], whereas there are no trials of the higher doses of 50–100 mg that proved effective in migraine. Naproxen 375 mg [26] and 550 mg [30, 38] and metamizole 500 mg and 1000 mg [31] have also been demonstrated to be effective. The latter drug is not available in many countries, because it carries a minimal (if at all) risk of causing agranulocytosis. Treatment with intramuscular injection of ketorolac 60 mg in an emergency department has been reported as effective [39].

Optimal dose

There are only a few studies investigating the ideal dose for drugs used for the acute treatment of TTH. One study demonstrated a significant dose–response relationship of aspirin, with 1000 mg being superior to 500 mg and 500 mg being superior to 250 mg [32]. Ketoprofen 25 mg tended to be more effective than 12.5 mg [29], whereas another study found very similar effects of ketoprofen 25 mg and 50 mg [37]. Paracetamol 1000 mg seems to be superior to 500 mg, because only the former dose has been demonstrated to be effective. In case of lack of evidence, the most effective dose of a drug well tolerated by a patient should be chosen. Suggested doses are presented in Table 16.2.

Comparison of simple analgesics

Five studies reported NSAIDs to be significantly more effective than paracetamol [24, 25, 28–30], whereas three studies could not demonstrate a difference [21, 26, 27]. Five studies have compared efficacy of different NSAIDs, and it has not be possible to clearly demonstrate superiority of any particular drug [31, 33, 35, 37, 44].

Adverse events

A thorough review of the acute drug treatment of TTH could not detect any difference in adverse events between paracetamol and NSAIDs or between these drugs and placebo [45]. However, it is well known that NSAIDs have more gastrointestinal side effects than paracetamol, whereas the use of large amounts of paracetamol may cause liver injury. Among the NSAIDs, ibuprofen seem to have the most favourable side-effect profile [45].

Table 16.2 Recommended drugs for acute therapy of tension-type headache.

Substance	Dose (mg)	Level of recommendation	Comment
Ibuprofen	200–800	A	Gastrointestinal side effects, risk of bleeding
Ketoprofen	25	A	Side effects as for ibuprofen
Aspirin	500–1000	A	Side effects as for ibuprofen
Naproxen	375–550	A	Side effects as for ibuprofen
Diclofenac	12.5–100	A	Side effects as for ibuprofen, only doses of 12.5–25 mg tested in tension-type headache
Paracetamol	1000 (oral)	A	Less risk of gastrointestinal side effects compared with NSAIDs
Caffeine combination	65–200	B	[a]

The level of recommendation considers side effects and consistency of the studies. There is sparse evidence for optimal doses. The most effective dose of a drug well tolerated by a patient should be chosen.
[a]Combination with caffeine 65–200 mg increases the efficacy of ibuprofen [40] and paracetamol [23, 41], but possibly also the risk for developing medication-overuse headache [42, 43]. Level of recommendation of combination drugs containing caffeine is therefore level B.

Combination analgesics

The efficacy of simple analgesics and NSAIDs is increased by combination with caffeine 64–200 mg [22, 23, 40, 41, 46, 47]. There are no comparative studies examining the efficacy of combination with codeine. It is clinically well known that caffeine withdrawal can cause headache, and chronic daily headache has been reported associated with use of over-the-counter caffeine combination products [42]. Therefore it is probable that combinations of simple analgesics or NSAIDs with caffeine are more likely to induce MOH than simple analgesics or NSAIDs alone. Until otherwise proven, we therefore recommend that simple analgesics or NSAIDs are the drugs of first choice, and that combinations of one of these drugs with caffeine should be drugs of second choice for the acute treatment of TTH. Combinations of simple analgesics with codeine or barbiturates should not be used, because use of the latter drugs increases the risk of developing medication-overuse headache [42].

Triptans, muscle relaxants and opioids

Triptans have been reported to be effective for the treatment of interval headaches [48], which were most likely mild migraines [49], in patients with migraine. Triptans most probably do not have a clinically relevant effect in patients with TTH [50, 51] and cannot be recommended. Muscle relaxants have not been demonstrated effective in episodic TTH [52]. Use of opioids increases the risk of developing medication-overuse headache [42]. Opioids are not recommended for the treatment of TTH.

Conclusions

Simple analgesics and NSAIDs are the mainstays in the acute therapy of TTH (see Table 16.2). Paracetamol 1000 mg is probably less effective than the NSAIDs, but has a better gastric side-effect profile [53]. Ibuprofen 400 mg may be recommended as drug of choice among the NSAIDs because of a favourable gastrointestinal side-effect profile compared with other NSAIDs [53]. Combination analgesics containing caffeine are more effective than simple analgesics or NSAIDs alone, but are regarded by some experts [43] as more likely to induce medication-overuse headache. Physicians should be aware of the risk of developing medication-overuse headache as a result of frequent and excessive use of all types of analgesics in acute therapy [6]. Triptans, muscle relax-

ants and opioids do not play a role in the treatment of TTH.

Although simple analgesics and NSAIDs are effective in episodic TTH, the degree of efficacy has to be put in perspective. For example, the proportion of patients that were pain free 2 hours after treatment with paracetamol 1000 mg, naproxen 375 mg and placebo were 37%, 32% and 26%, respectively [26]. The corresponding rates for paracetamol 1000 mg, ketoprofen 25 mg and placebo were 22%, 28% and 16% in another study, with 61%, 70% and 36% of participants reporting worthwhile effect [27]. Thus, efficacy is modest and there is clearly room for better acute treatment of episodic TTH.

> ### Recommendations
>
> Simple analgesics and NSAIDs are recommended for treatment of episodic TTH. Combination analgesics containing caffeine are drugs of second choice. It is crucial to avoid frequent and excessive use of analgesics to prevent the development of medication-overuse headache.

Prophylactic drug treatment of TTH

Prophylactic pharmacotherapy should be considered in patients with chronic TTH, and it can be considered in patients with very frequent episodic TTH. Co-morbid disorders, e.g. being overweight or depression, should be taken into account. For many years the tricyclic antidepressant amitriptyline has been used. More lately other antidepressants, NSAIDs, muscle relaxants, anticonvulsants and botulinum toxin have been tested in chronic TTH. The effect of prophylactic drugs in TTH has been examined in surprisingly few placebo-controlled studies, which have used different methods for measurement of efficacy. The guidelines for drug trials in TTH from the IHS recommends days with TTH or area-under-the-headache curve (AUC) to be used as primary efficacy measure [20]. These parameters have been used in some studies, whereas other studies have used other efficacy measures such as pain reduction from baseline, headache intensity. This makes comparison of results between studies difficult.

Amitriptyline

Lance and Curran [54] reported amitriptyline 10–25 mg three times daily to be effective, whereas Diamond and

Baltes [55] found amitriptyline 10 mg/day, but not 60 mg/day, to be effective. Amitriptyline 75 mg/day was reported to reduce headache duration in the last week of a 6-week study [56], whereas no difference in effect size between amitriptyline 50–75 mg/day or amitriptylinoxide 60–90 mg/day and placebo was found in one study [57]. However, in addition the frequencies of side effects were similar on amitriptyline and placebo in the latter study. The inability to detect the well-known side effects of amitriptyline suggests insensitivity of the trial for reasons that remain obscure. Bendtsen *et al.* [58] found that amitriptyline 75 mg daily reduced the AUC (calculated as headache duration times headache intensity) by 30% compared with placebo, which was highly significant. Holroyd and colleagues [59] treated patients with antidepressants (83% took amitriptyline median dose 75 mg daily and 17% took nortriptyline median dose 50 mg daily) and compared this with stress management therapy and a combination of stress management and antidepressant treatment. After 6 months, all three treatments reduced headache index, with approximately 30% more than placebo, which was highly significant.

Other antidepressants.

The tricyclic antidepressant clomipramine 75–150 mg daily [60] and the tetracyclic antidepressants maprotiline 75 mg daily [61] and mianserin 30–60 mg daily [60] have been reported to be more effective than placebo. Interestingly, some of the newer more selective antidepressants, with action on serotonin and noradrenaline, seem to be as effective as amitriptyline, with the advantage that they are tolerated in doses needed for the treatment of concomitant depression. Thus, the noradrenergic and specific serotoninergic antidepressant mirtazapine 30 mg/day reduced headache index by 34% more than placebo in difficult-to-treat patients without depression including patients who had not responded to amitriptyline [62]. The efficacy of mirtazapine was comparable to that of amitriptyline reported by the same group [58]. A systematic review concluded that the two treatments may be equally effective for the treatment of chronic TTH [63]. The serotonin and noradrenaline reuptake inhibitor venlafaxine 150 mg/day [64] reduced headache days from 15 per month to 12 per month in a mixed group of patients with either frequent episodic or chronic TTH. Low-dose mirtazapine 4.5 mg/day alone or in combination with ibuprofen 400 mg/day was not effective in chronic TTH. The selective serotonin reuptake inhibitors (SSRIs) citalopram [58] and sertraline [65] have not been found to be more effective than placebo. SSRIs have been compared with other antidepressants in six studies, which were reviewed in a Cochrane analysis that concluded that SSRIs are less efficacious than tricyclic antidepressants for the treatment of chronic TTH [66].

Miscellaneous agents.

There have been conflicting results for treatment with the muscle relaxant tizanidine [61, 67], whereas the NMDA (*N*-methyl-D-aspartic acid) antagonist memantine was not effective [68]. Botulinum toxin has been extensively studied [69–79]. It was concluded in a systematic review that it is likely to be ineffective or harmful for the treatment of chronic TTH [63]. The prophylactic effect of daily intake of simple analgesics has not been studied in trials that had this as the primary efficacy parameter, but explanatory analyses indicated that ibuprofen 400 mg/day was not effective in one study [80]. On the contrary, ibuprofen increased headache compared with placebo, indicating a possible early onset of medication-overuse headache [80]. Topiramate [81] and buspirone [82] have been reported as effective in open-label studies.

Conclusions

Amitriptyline has a clinically relevant prophylactic effect in patients with chronic TTH and should be drug of first choice (Table 16.3). Mirtazapine or venlafaxine is prob-

Table 16.3 Recommended drugs for prophylactic therapy of tension-type headache. The level of recommendation considers side effects and number and quality of the studies.

Substance	Daily dose (mg)	Level of recommendation
Drug of first choice		
Amitriptyline	30–75	A
Drugs of second choice		
Mirtazapine	30	B
Venlafaxine	150	B
Drugs of third choice		
Clomipramine	75–150	B
Maprotiline	75	B
Mianserin	30–60	B

ably effective, whereas the older tricyclic and tetracyclic antidepressants clomipramine, maprotiline and mianserin may be effective. A recent systematic review [63] concluded that amitriptyline and mirtazapine are the only forms of treatment that can be considered to have been proved beneficial for the treatment of chronic TTH. However, the last search was performed in 2007 before publication of the study on venlafaxine [64].

Amitriptyline should be started at low dosages (10–25 mg/day) and titrated by 10–25 mg weekly until either the patient has good therapeutic effect or side effects are encountered. It is important that patients be informed that this is an antidepressant agent but that it has an independent action on pain. The maintenance dose is usually 30–75 mg daily administered 1–2 hours before bedtime to help to circumvent any sedative adverse effects. The effect is not related to the presence of depression [58]. A significant effect of amitriptyline may be observed already in the first week on the therapeutic dose [58]. It is therefore advisable to change to other prophylactic therapy if the patient does not respond after 4 weeks on the maintenance dose. The side effects of amitriptyline include dry mouth, drowsiness, dizziness, obstipation and weight gain. Mirtazapine, of which the major side effects are drowsiness and weight gain, or venlafaxine, of which the major side effects are vomiting, nausea, dizziness and loss of libido, should be considered if amitriptyline is not effective or not tolerated. Discontinuation should be attempted every 6–12 months. The physician should bear in mind that the efficacy of preventive drug therapy in TTH is often modest, and that the efficacy should outweigh the side effects.

Recommendations

Amitriptyline is drug of first choice for the prophylactic treatment of chronic TTH. Mirtazapine and venlafaxine are drugs of second choice.

Non-pharmacological treatment of TTH

Information, reassurance and identification of trigger factors

Non-drug management should be considered for all patients with TTH and is widely used (Table 16.4).

Table 16.4 Non-pharmacological treatments for tension of tension-type headache.

Treatment	Level of recommendation
Psychobehavioural treatments	
EMG biofeedback	A
Cognitive–behavioural therapy	C
Relaxation training	C
Physical therapy	C
Acupuncture	C

The level of recommendation considers number and quality of the studies.

However, the scientific evidence for efficacy of most treatment modalities is sparse [83–86]. The very fact that the physician takes the problem seriously may have a therapeutic effect, particularly if the patient is concerned about serious disease, e.g. brain tumour, and can be reassured by thorough examination. Identification of trigger factors should be performed, because coping with triggers may be of value [87]. The most frequently reported triggers for TTH are stress (mental or physical), irregular or inappropriate meals, high intake or withdrawal of coffee and other caffeine-containing drinks, dehydration, sleep disorders, too much or too little sleep, reduced or inappropriate physical exercise and psychobehavioural problems, as well as variations during the female menstrual cycle and hormonal substitution [88–90]. It has been demonstrated that stress induces more headache in patients with chronic TTH than in healthy controls probably through hyperalgesic effects on already sensitized pain pathways [91].

Information about the nature of the disease is important. It can be explained that muscle pain can lead to a disturbance of the brain's pain-modulating mechanisms [2, 92, 93], so that normally innocuous stimuli are perceived as painful, with secondary perpetuation of muscle pain and risk of anxiety and depression. The prognosis in the longer run was found to be favourable in a population-based 12-year epidemiological follow-up study, because approximately half of all individuals with frequent or chronic TTH had remission of their headaches [13]. It is not known whether the same is true for individuals who seek medical consultation.

Psychobehavioural treatments

A large number of psychobehavioural treatment strategies have been used to treat chronic TTH. Electromyographic (EMG) biofeedback, cognitive–behavioural therapy and relaxation training have been investigated the most. However, only a few trials have been performed controlled with sufficient power and clear outcome measures [85]. Hypnotherapy has been reported as effective [94] but there is no convincing evidence for its effect in TTH [85, 95].

EMG biofeedback

The aim of EMG biofeedback is to help the patient to recognize and control muscle tension by providing continuous feedback about muscle activity. Sessions typically include an adaptation phase, baseline phase, training phase where feedback is provided and self-control phase where the patient practises controlling muscle tension without the aid of feedback [96]. A recent review including 11 studies concluded that, because of low power, there is conflicting evidence to support or refute the effectiveness of EMG biofeedback compared with placebo or any other treatments [85]. However, a recent extensive and thorough meta-analysis, including 53 studies, concluded that biofeedback has a medium-to-large effect. The effect was found to be long lasting and enhanced by combination with relaxation therapy [97]. Most of the studies included employed EMG biofeedback. It was not possible to draw reliable conclusions as to whether the effect differed between patients with episodic and chronic TTH.

Cognitive–behavioural therapy

The aim of cognitive–behavioural therapy is to teach the patient to identify thoughts and beliefs that generate stress and aggravate headaches. These thoughts are then challenged, and alternative adaptive coping self-instructions are considered. A variety of exercises may be used to challenge thoughts and beliefs, including experimenting with adoption of another person's view of the situation, actively generating other possible views of a situation, and devising a behavioural experiment to test the validity of a particular belief [96]. One study found cognitive–behavioural therapy, treatment with tricyclic antidepressants and a combination of the two treatments

better than placebo, with no significant difference between treatments [59], although another study reported no difference between cognitive–behavioural therapy and amitriptyline [98]. Cognitive–behavioural therapy may be effective but there is no convincing evidence [63, 85].

Relaxation training

The goal of relaxation training is to help the patient to recognize and control tension as it arises in the course of daily activities. Relaxation training involves a range of affective, cognitive and behavioural techniques, such as breathing exercises and meditation. Relaxation training has been compared with no treatment or waiting list control [99–103] and with other interventions [104–107]. A recent review concluded that there is conflicting evidence that relaxation is better than no treatment, waiting list or placebo [85].

Conclusions

EMG biofeedback has an effect in TTH, whereas cognitive–behavioural therapy and relaxation training may have an effect in TTH, but at this moment in time there is no convincing evidence to support this [63, 85]. These treatments are relatively time-consuming, but unfortunately there are no documented guidelines for which psychobehavioural treatment(s) to choose for the individual patient. Therefore until scientific evidence is provided common sense must be used. Thus, it is, for example, likely that cognitive–behavioural therapy will be most beneficial for the patient in whom psychobehavioural problems or affective distress plays a major role [96], whereas biofeedback or relaxation training may be preferable for the tense patient.

Non-invasive physical therapy

Physical therapy is widely used for the treatment of TTH and includes the improvement of posture, massage, spinal manipulation, oromandibular treatment, exercise programmes, hot and cold packs, ultrasound and electrical stimulation, but most of these modalities have not been properly evaluated [108]. Active treatment strategies are generally recommended [108]. A recent review concluded that exercise may have a value for TTH [109]. Carlson et al. [110] reported better effect of physiotherapy than acupuncture. A controlled study [111] combined various techniques such as massage, relaxation and home-based exercises, and found a modest effect. It was reported that adding craniocervical training to classic physiotherapy was better than physiotherapy alone [112]. A recent study found no significant long-lasting differences in efficacy among relaxation training, physical training and acupuncture [113]. Spinal manipulation has no effect in episodic TTH [114] and no convincing effect in chronic TTH [115, 116]. Oromandibular treatment with occlusal splints is often recommended but has not yet been tested in trials of reasonable quality and cannot be recommended in general [117]. There is no firm evidence for efficacy of therapeutic touch, cranial electrotherapy or transcutaneous electrical nerve stimulation [84].

It can be concluded that there is a huge contrast between the widespread use of physical therapies and the lack of robust scientific evidence for the efficacy of these therapies, and that further studies of improved quality are necessary to either support or refute the effectiveness of physical modalities in TTH [84, 108, 118, 119].

Acupuncture and nerve block

The prophylactic effect of acupuncture has been investigated in several trials in patients with frequent episodic or chronic TTH. A review [63] and a meta-analysis [120] concluded that there is no evidence for efficacy of acupuncture in TTH. Two trials reported better effect of acupuncture than basic care or waiting list but no better effect of Chinese acupuncture compared with sham acupuncture [121, 122], whereas a recent Cochrane analysis [86] concluded that there was overall a slightly better effect from acupuncture than from sham acupuncture, based on the results from five trials [122–126]. Four trials compared acupuncture with physiotherapy [110, 113, 127], relaxation [113] and a combination of massage and relaxation [128]. Collectively these trials suggest slightly better results for some outcomes with the latter therapies according to the recent Cochrane analysis [86]. Together, the available evidence suggests that acupuncture could be a valuable option for patients with frequent TTH, but more research is needed before final conclusions can be made.

A recent study reported no effect of greater occipital nerve block in patients with chronic TTH [129].

Recommendations

Non-drug management should always be considered although the scientific basis is limited. Information, reassurance and identification of trigger factors may be rewarding. EMG biofeedback has a documented effect in TTH, whereas cognitive–behavioural therapy and relaxation training are most likely effective, but there is no convincing evidence. Physical therapy and acupuncture may be valuable options for patients with frequent TTH, but there is no robust scientific evidence for efficacy.

Need of update

These recommendations should be updated within 5 years.

Conflicts of interest

The present guidelines were developed without external financial support. The authors report the following financial supports:

Lars Bendtsen: salary by Glostrup University Hospital. Honoraria in 2009 from MSD and Pfizer.

Stefan Evers: salary by the University of Münster. Honoraria or grants by Addex Pharma, AGA Medical Corporation, Allergan, AstraZeneca, Berlin Chemie, Boehringer Ingelheim, CoLucid, Desitin, Eisai, GlaxoSmithKline, Ipsen, Janssen-Cilag, Merz, MSD, Novartis, Pfizer, Reckitt-Benckiser and UCB.

Mattias Linde: salary from the Cephalea Headache Centre and Gothenburg University, Sweden. Honoraria or grants in 2009 from Allergan, AstraZeneca, MSD and the Swedish Migraine Association.

Dimos D. Mitsikostas: salary by Athens Naval Hospital. Honoraria or grants for 2009 by Bayer-Schering, Janssen-Cilag, Lilly, Merk-Serono, Novartis, MSD and UCB.

Giorgio Sandrini: salary from University of Pavia. Honoraria in 2009 from Allergan, Solvay Pharma and Newrons Alpha.

Jean Schoenen: salary from the University of Liège. Honoraria or grants in 2009 from Janssen-Cilag, GSK, Coherex, Medtronic and STX-Med.

References

1. Headache Classification Subcommittee of the International Headache Society. *The International Classification of Headache Disorders*, 2nd edn. *Cephalalgia* 2004; **24**(suppl 1):1–160.

2. Bendtsen, L. Central sensitization in tension-type headache – possible pathophysiological mechanisms. *Cephalalgia* 2000; **20**:486–508.

3. Russell, MB, Rasmussen, BK, Brennum, J, Iversen, HK, Jensen, R, Olesen, J. Presentation of a new instrument: the diagnostic headache diary. *Cephalalgia* 1992; **12**: 369–74.

4. Brainin, M, Barnes, M, Baron, JC. *et al.* Guidance for the preparation of neurological management guidelines by EFNS scientific task forces – revised recommendations 2004. *Eur J Neurol* 2004; **11**:577–81.

5. Bendtsen, L. Tension-type headache. In: MacGregor, A, Jensen, R. (eds), *Migraine and Other Headaches*. Oxford: Oxford University Press, 2008; pp. 103–12.

6. Katsarava, Z, Jensen, R. Medication-overuse headache: where are we now? *Curr Opin Neurol* 2007; **20**: 326–30.

7. Olesen, J, Goadsby, PJ, Ramadan, N, Tfelt-Hansen, P, Welch, KM. *The Headaches*, 3rd edn. Philadelphia: Lippincott Williams & Wilkins, 2006; pp. 1–1169.

8. Steiner, TJ, MacGregor, EA, Davies, PTG. *Guidelines for All Healthcare Professionals in the Diagnosis and Management of Migraine, Tension-Type, Cluster and Medication-overuse Headache*, 3rd edn. British Association for the Study of Headache, 2007; pp. 1–52.

9. Lyngberg, AC, Rasmussen, BK, Jorgensen, T, Jensen, R. Has the prevalence of migraine and tension-type headache changed over a 12-year period? A Danish population survey. *Eur J Epidemiol* 2005; **20**:243–9.

10. Rasmussen, BK. Epidemiology of headache. *Cephalalgia* 1995; **15**:45–68.

11. Stovner, L, Hagen, K, Jensen, R. *et al.* The global burden of headache: a documentation of headache prevalence and disability worldwide. *Cephalalgia* 2007; **27**: 193–210.

12. Andlin-Sobocki, P, Jonsson, B, Wittchen, HU, Olesen, J. Cost of disorders of the brain in Europe. *Eur J Neurol* 2005; **12**(suppl 1):1–27.

13. Lyngberg, AC, Rasmussen, BK, Jorgensen, T, Jensen, R. Prognosis of migraine and tension-type headache: a population-based follow-up study. *Neurology* 2005; **65**: 580–5.

14. Lyngberg, AC, Rasmussen, BK, Jorgensen, T, Jensen, R. Secular changes in health care utilization and work absence for migraine and tension-type headache: a population based study. *Eur J Epidemiol* 2005; **20**:1007–14.

15. Schwartz, BS, Stewart, WF, Lipton, RB. Lost workdays and decreased work effectiveness associated with headache in the workplace. *J Occup Environ Med* 1997; **39**:320–7.

16. Jensen, R, Stovner, LJ. Epidemiology and comorbidity of headache. *Lancet Neurol* 2008; **7**:354–61.

17. Haldeman, S, Dagenais, S. Cervicogenic headaches: a critical review. *Spine J* 2001; **1**:31–46.

18. Mulleners, WM, Whitmarsh, TE, Steiner, TJ. Noncompliance may render migraine prophylaxis useless, but once-daily regimens are better. *Cephalalgia* 1998; **18**:52–6.

19. Olesen, J, Bousser, MG, Diener, HC. *et al.* New appendix criteria open for a broader concept of chronic migraine. *Cephalalgia* 2006; **26**:742–6.

20. Bendtsen, L, Bigal, ME, Cerbo, R. *et al.* Guidelines for controlled trials of drugs in tension-type headache: second edition. *Cephalalgia* 2010; **30**:1–16.

21. Steiner, TJ, Lange, R, Voelker, M. Aspirin in episodic tension-type headache: placebo-controlled dose-ranging comparison with paracetamol. *Cephalalgia* 2003; **23**: 59–66.

22. Schachtel, BP, Thoden, WR, Konerman, JP, Brown, A, Chaing, DS. Headache pain model for assessing and comparing the efficacy of over-the-counter analgesic agents. *Clin Pharmacol Ther* 1991; **50**:322–9.

23. Migliardi, JR, Armellino, JJ, Friedman, M, Gillings, DB, Beaver, WT. Caffeine as an analgesic adjuvant in tension headache. *Clin Pharmacol Ther* 1994; **56**:576–86.

24. Schachtel, BP, Furey, SA, Thoden, WR. Nonprescription ibuprofen and acetaminophen in the treatment of tension-type headache. *J Clin Pharmacol* 1996; **36**:1120–5.

25. Packman, B, Packman, E, Doyle, G. *et al.* Solubilized ibuprofen: evaluation of onset, relief, and safety of a novel formulation in the treatment of episodic tension-type headache. *Headache* 2000; **40**:561–7.

26. Prior, MJ, Cooper, KM, May, LG, Bowen, DL. Efficacy and safety of acetaminophen and naproxen in the treatment of tension-type headache. A randomized, double-blind, placebo-controlled trial. *Cephalalgia* 2002; **22**: 740–8.

27. Steiner, TJ, Lange, R. Ketoprofen (25 mg) in the symptomatic treatment of episodic tension-type headache: double-blind placebo-controlled comparison with acetaminophen (1000 mg). *Cephalalgia* 1998; **18**:38–43.

28. Dahlöf, CGH, Jacobs, LD. Ketoprofen, paracetamol and placebo in the treatment of episodic tension-type headache. *Cephalalgia* 1996; **16**:117–23.

29. Mehlisch, DR, Weaver, M, Fladung, B. Ketoprofen, acetaminophen, and placebo in the treatment of tension headache. *Headache* 1998; **38**:579–89.

30. Miller, DS, Talbot, CA, Simpson, W, Korey, A. A comparison of naproxen sodium, acetaminophen and placebo in

the treatment of muscle contraction headache. *Headache* 1987; **27**:392–6.

31. Martinez-Martin, P, Raffaelli, E. Jr, Titus, F, *et al.* Efficacy and safety of metamizol vs. acetylsalicylic acid in patients with moderate episodic tension-type headache: a randomized, double-blind, placebo- and active-controlled, multicentre study. *Cephalalgia* 2001; **21**:604–10.

32. Von Graffenried, B, Nuesch, E. Non-migrainous headache for the evaluation of oral analgesics. *Br J Clin Pharmacol* 1980; **10**(suppl 2):225S–31S.

33. Diamond, S. Ibuprofen versus aspirin and placebo in the treatment of muscle contraction headache. *Headache* 1983; **23**:206–10.

34. Langemark, M, Olesen, J. Effervescent ASA versus solid ASA in the treatment of tension headache. A double-blind, placebo controlled study. *Headache* 1987; **27**:90–5.

35. Kubitzek, F, Ziegler, G, Gold, MS, Liu, JM, Ionescu, E. Low-dose diclofenac potassium in the treatment of episodic tension-type headache. *Eur J Pain* 2003; **7**:155–62.

36. Schachtel, BP, Thoden, WR. Onset of action of ibuprofen in the treatment of muscle-contraction headache. *Headache* 1988; **28**:471–4.

37. van Gerven, JM, Schoemaker, RC, Jacobs, LD. *et al.* Self-medication of a single headache episode with ketoprofen, ibuprofen or placebo, home-monitored with an electronic patient diary. *Br J Clin Pharmacol* 1996; **42**:475–81.

38. Pini, LA, Del, BE, Zanchin, G, *et al.* Tolerability and efficacy of a combination of paracetamol and caffeine in the treatment of tension-type headache: a randomised, double-blind, double-dummy, cross-over study versus placebo and naproxen sodium. *J Headache Pain* 2008; **9**: 367–73.

39. Harden, RN, Rogers, D, Fink, K, Gracely, RH. Controlled trial of ketorolac in tension-type headache. *Neurology* 1998; **50**:507–9.

40. Diamond, S, Balm, TK, Freitag, FG. Ibuprofen plus caffeine in the treatment of tension-type headache. *Clin Pharmacol Ther* 2000; **68**:312–19.

41. Ward, N, Whitney, C, Avery, D, Dunner, D. The analgesic effects of caffeine in headache. *Pain* 1991; **44**:151–5.

42. Scher, AI, Lipton, RB, Stewart, WF, Bigal, M. Patterns of medication use by chronic and episodic headache sufferers in the general population: results from the frequent headache epidemiology study. *Cephalalgia* 2009; **13**: 59–63.

43. Bigal, ME, Lipton, RB. Overuse of acute migraine medications and migraine chronification. *Curr Pain Headache Rep* 2009; **13**:301–7.

44. Lange, R, Lentz, R. Comparison ketoprofen, ibuprofen and naproxen sodium in the treatment of tension-type headache. *Drugs Exp Clin Res* 1995; **21**:89–96.

45. Verhagen, AP, Damen, L, Berger, MY, Passchier, J, Merlijn, V, Koes, BW. Is any one analgesic superior for episodic tension-type headache? *J Fam Pract* 2006; **55**:1064–72.

46. Diener, HC, Pfaffenrath, V, Pageler, L, Peil, H, Aicher, B. The fixed combination of acetylsalicylic acid, paracetamol and caffeine is more effective than single substances and dual combination for the treatment of headache: a multicentre, randomized, double-blind, single-dose, placebo-controlled parallel group study. *Cephalalgia* 2005; **25**:776–87.

47. Cerbo, R, Centonze, V, Grazioli, I, *et al.* Efficacy of a fixed combination of indomethacin, prochlorperazine, and caffeine in the treatment of episodic tension-type headache: a double-blind, randomized, nimesulide-controlled, parallel group, multicentre trial. *Eur J Neurol* 2005; **12**:759–67.

48. Cady, RK, Gutterman, D, Saiers, JA, Beach, ME. Responsiveness of non-IHS migraine and tension-type headache to sumatriptan. *Cephalalgia* 1997; **17**:588–90.

49. Lipton, RB, Cady, RK, Stewart, WF, Wilks, K, Hall, C. Diagnostic lessons from the spectrum study. *Neurology* 2002; **58**:S27–31.

50. Brennum, J, Brinck, T, Schriver, L, *et al.* Sumatriptan has no clinically relevant effect in the treatment of episodic tension-type headache. *Eur J Neurol* 1996; **3**:23–8.

51. Brennum, J, Kjeldsen, M, Olesen, J. The 5-HT1-like agonist sumatriptan has a significant effect in chronic tension-type headache. *Cephalalgia* 1992; **12**:375–9.

52. Mathew, N, Ashina, M. Acute pharmacotherapy of tension-type headaches. In: Olesen, J, Goadsby, PJ, Ramadan, N, Tfelt-Hansen, P, Welch, KM. (eds), *The Headaches*, 3rd edn. Philadelphia: Lippincott Williams & Wilkins, 2005; pp. 727–33.

53. Langman, MJ, Weil, J, Wainwright, P, *et al.* Risks of bleeding peptic ulcer associated with individual non-steroidal anti-inflammatory drugs. *Lancet* 1994; **343**:1075–8.

54. Lance, JW, Curran, DA. Treatment of chronic tension headache. *Lancet* 1964; **i**:1236–9.

55. Diamond, S, Baltes, BJ. Chronic tension headache – treated with amitriptyline – a double-blind study. *Headache* 1971; **11**:110–16.

56. Göbel, H, Hamouz, V, Hansen, C, *et al.* Chronic tension-type headache: amitriptyline reduces clinical headache-duration and experimental pain sensitivity but does not alter pericranial muscle activity readings. *Pain* 1994; **59**: 241–9.

57. Pfaffenrath, V, Diener, HC, Isler, H, *et al.* Efficacy and tolerability of amitriptylinoxide in the treatment of chronic tension-type headache: a multi-centre controlled study. *Cephalalgia* 1994; **14**:149–55.

58. Bendtsen, L, Jensen, R, Olesen, J. A non-selective (amitriptyline), but not a selective (citalopram), serotonin reuptake inhibitor is effective in the prophylactic treatment

of chronic tension-type headache. *J Neurol Neurosurg Psychiatry* 1996; **61**: 285–90.

59. Holroyd, KA, O'Donnell, FJ, Stensland, M, Lipchik, GL, Cordingley, GE, Carlson, BW. Management of chronic tension-type headache with tricyclic antidepressant medication, stress management therapy, and their combination: a randomized controlled trial. *JAMA* 2001; **285**:2208–15.

60. Langemark, M, Loldrup, D, Bech, P, Olesen, J. Clomipramine and mianserin in the treatment of chronic tension headache. A double-blind, controlled study. *Headache* 1990; **30**:118–21.

61. Fogelholm, R, Murros, K. Tizanidine in chronic tension-type headache: a placebo controlled double-blind crossover study. *Headache* 1992; **32**:509–13.

62. Bendtsen, L, Jensen, R. Mirtazapine is effective in the prophylactic treatment of chronic tension-type headache. *Neurology* 2004; **62**:1706–11.

63. Silver, N. Headache (chronic tension-type). *Clinical Evidence* 2007; 1–21.

64. Zissis, N, Harmoussi, S, Vlaikidis, N, *et al.* A randomized, double-blind, placebo-controlled study of venlafaxine XR in out-patients with tension-type headache. *Cephalalgia* 2007; **27**:315–24.

65. Singh, NN, Misra, S. Sertraline in chronic tension-type headache. *J Assoc Physicians India* 2002; **50**:873–8.

66. Moja, PL, Cusi, C, Sterzi, RR, Canepari, C. Selective serotonin re-uptake inhibitors (SSRIs) for preventing migraine and tension-type headaches. *Cochrane Database Syst Rev* 2005; (3):CD002919.

67. Murros, K, Kataja, M, Hedman, C, *et al.* Modified-release formulation of tizanidine in chronic tension-type headache. *Headache* 2000; **40**:633–7.

68. Lindelof, K, Bendtsen, L. Memantine for prophylaxis of chronic tension-type headache – a double-blind, randomized, crossover clinical trial. *Cephalalgia* 2009; **29**:314–21.

69. Padberg, M, de Bruijn, SF, de Haan, RJ, Tavy, DL. Treatment of chronic tension-type headache with botulinum toxin: a double-blind, placebo-controlled clinical trial. *Cephalalgia* 2004; **24**:675–80.

70. Relja, M, Telarovic, S. Botulinum toxin in tension-type headache. *J Neurol* 2004; **251**(suppl 1):12–14.

71. Rollnik, JD, Tanneberger, O, Schubert, M, Schneider, U, Dengler, R. Treatment of tension-type headache with botulinum toxin type A: a double-blind, placebo-controlled study. *Headache* 2000; **40**:300–5.

72. Schmitt, WJ, Slowey, E, Fravi, N, Weber, S, Burgunder, JM. Effect of botulinum toxin A injections in the treatment of chronic tension-type headache: a double-blind, placebo-controlled trial. *Headache* 2001; **41**:658–64.

73. Schulte-Mattler, WJ, Krack, P, BoNTTH Study Group. Treatment of chronic tension-type headache with botulinum toxin A: a randomized, double-blind, placebo-controlled multicenter study. *Pain* 2004; **109**:110–14.

74. Smuts, JA, Baker, MK, Smuts, HM. Prophylactic treatment of chronic tension-type headache using botulinum toxin type A. *Eur J Neurol* 1999; **6**(suppl 4):S99–102.

75. Göbel, H, Lindner, V, Krack, PK. Treatment of chronic tension-type headache with botulinum toxin, a double blind, placebo-controlled clinical trial. *Cephalalgia* 1999; **19**:455.

76. Silberstein, SD, Gobel, H, Jensen, R, *et al.* Botulinum toxin type A in the prophylactic treatment of chronic tension-type headache: a multicentre, double-blind, randomized, placebo-controlled, parallel-group study. *Cephalalgia* 2006; **26**:790–800.

77. Kokoska, MS, Glaser, DA, Burch, CM, Hollenbeak, CS. Botulinum toxin injections for the treatment of frontal tension headache. *J Headache Pain* 2004; **5**:103–9.

78. Harden, RN, Cottrill, J, Gagnon, CM, *et al.* Botulinum toxin a in the treatment of chronic tension-type headache with cervical myofascial trigger points: a randomized, double-blind, placebo-controlled pilot study. *Headache* 2009; **49**:732–43.

79. Straube, A, Empl, M, Ceballos-Baumann, A, Tolle, T, Stefenelli, U, Pfaffenrath, V. Pericranial injection of botulinum toxin type A (Dysport) for tension-type headache – a multicentre, double-blind, randomized, placebo-controlled study. *Eur J Neurol* 2008; **15**:205–13.

80. Bendtsen, L, Buchgreitz, L, Ashina, S, Jensen, R. Combination of low-dose mirtazapine and ibuprofen for prophylaxis of chronic tension-type headache. *Eur J Neurol* 2007; **14**:187–93.

81. Lampl, C, Marecek, S, May, A, Bendtsen, L. A prospective, open-label, long-term study of the efficacy and tolerability of topiramate in the prophylaxis of chronic tension-type headache. *Cephalalgia* 2006; **26**:1203–8.

82. Mitsikostas, DD, Gatzonis, S, Thomas, A, Ilias, A. Buspirone vs amitriptyline in the treatment of chronic tension-type headache. *Acta Neurol Scand* 1997; **96**:247–51.

83. Vernon, H, McDermaid, CS, Hagino, C. Systematic review of randomized clinical trials of complementary/alternative therapies in the treatment of tension-type and cervicogenic headache. *Complement Ther Med* 1999; **7**:142–55.

84. Bronfort, G, Nilsson, N, Haas, M, *et al.* Non-invasive physical treatments for chronic/recurrent headache. *Cochrane Database Syst Rev* 2004; (3):CD001878.

85. Verhagen, AP, Damen, L, Berger, MY, Passchier, J, Koes, BW. Behavioral treatments of chronic tension-type headache in adults: are they beneficial? *CNS Neurosci Ther* 2009; **15**:183–205.

86. Linde, K, Allais, G, Brinkhaus, B, Manheimer, E, Vickers, A, White, AR. Acupuncture for tension-type headache. *Cochrane Database Syst Rev* 2009; (1):CD007587.

87. Martin, PR, MacLeod, C. Behavioral management of headache triggers: avoidance of triggers is an inadequate strategy. *Clin Psychol Rev* 2009; **29**:483–95.

88. Nash, JM, Thebarge, RW. Understanding psychological stress, its biological processes, and impact on primary headache. *Headache* 2006; **46**:1377–86.

89. Ulrich, V, Russell, MB, Jensen, R, Olesen, J. A comparison of tension-type headache in migraineurs and in non-migraineurs: a population-based study. *Pain* 1996; **67**: 501–6.

90. Rasmussen, BK, Jensen, R, Schroll, M, Olesen, J. Interrelations between migraine and tension-type headache in the general population. *Arch Neurol* 1992; **49**:914–18.

91. Cathcart, S, Petkov, J, Winefield, AH, Lushington, K, Rolan, P. Central mechanisms of stress-induced headache. *Cephalalgia* 2009; **9**:411–27.

92. Fumal, A, Schoenen, J. Tension-type headache: current research and clinical management. *Lancet Neurol* 2008; **7**:70–83.

93. Bendtsen, L, Jensen, R. Tension-type headache. *Neurol Clin* 2009; **27**:525–535.

94. Hammond, DC. Review of the efficacy of clinical hypnosis with headaches and migraines. *Int J Clin Exp Hypn* 2007; **55**:207–19.

95. Kroner-Herwig, B. Chronic pain syndromes and their treatment by psychological interventions. *Curr Opin Psychiatry* 2009; **22**:200–4.

96. Holroyd, KA, Martin, PR, Nash, JM. Psychological treatments of tension-type headache. In: Olesen, J, Goadsby, PJ, Ramadan, N, Tfelt-Hansen, P, Welch, KM. (eds), *The Headaches*, 3rd edn. Philadelphia: Lippincott Williams & Wilkins, 2005; pp. 711–19.

97. Nestoriuc, Y, Rief, W, Martin, A. Meta-analysis of biofeedback for tension-type headache: efficacy, specificity, and treatment moderators. *J Consult Clin Psychol* 2008; **76**: 379–96.

98. Holroyd, KA, Nash, JM, Pingel, JD, Cordingley, GE, Jerome, A. A comparison of pharmacological (amitriptyline HCL) and nonpharmacological (cognitive-behavioral) therapies for chronic tension headaches. *J Consult Clin Psychol* 1991; **59**:387–93.

99. Wojciechowski, FL. Behavioural treatment of tension headache: a contribution to controlled outcome research methodology. *Tijdschr Psychol* 1984; **12**:16–30.

100. Chesney, MA, Shelton, JL. A comparison of muscle relaxation and electromyogram biofeedback treatments for muscle contraction headache. *J Behav Ther Exp Psychiatry* 1976; **7**:221–5.

101. Schlutter, LC, Golden, CJ, Blume, HG. A comparison of treatments for prefrontal muscle contraction headache. *Br J Med Psychol* 1980; **53**:47–52.

102. Janssen, K. Differential effectiveness of EMG-feedback versus combined EMG-feedback and relaxation instructions in the treatment of tension headache. *J Psychosom Res* 1983; **27**:243–53.

103. Hutchings, DF, Reinking, RH. Tension headaches: what form of therapy is most effective? *Biofeedback Self Regul* 1976; **1**:183–90.

104. Arena, JG, Bruno, GM, Hannah, SL, Meador, KJ. A comparison of frontal electromyographic biofeedback training, trapezius electromyographic biofeedback training, and progressive muscle relaxation therapy in the treatment of tension headache. *Headache* 1995; **35**:411–19.

105. Gada, MT. A comparative study of efficacy on EMG biofeedback and progressive muscular relaxation in tension headache. *Indian J Psychiatry* 1984; **26**:121–7.

106. Murphy, AI, Lehrer, PM, Jurish, S. Cognitive coping skills training and relaxation training as treatments for tension headaches. *Behavioral Therapy* 1990; **21**:89–98.

107. Finn, T, DiGiuseppe, R, Culver, C. The effectiveness of rational-emotive therapy in the reduction of muscle contraction headaches. *J Cogn Psychother* 1991; **5**: 93–103.

108. Jensen, R, Roth, JM. Physiotherapy of tension-type headaches. In: Olesen, J, Goadsby, PJ, Ramadan, N, Tfelt-Hansen, P, Welch, KM. (eds), *The Headaches*, 3rd edn. Philadelphia: Lippincott Williams & Wilkins, 2005; pp. 721–6.

109. Fricton, J, Velly, A, Ouyang, W, Look, JO. Does exercise therapy improve headache? A systematic review with meta-analysis. *Curr Pain Headache Rep* 2009; **13**:413–19.

110. Carlsson, J, Fahlcrantz, A, Augustinsson, LE. Muscle tenderness in tension headache treated with acupuncture or physiotherapy. *Cephalalgia* 1990; **10**:131–41.

111. Torelli, P, Jensen, R, Olesen, J. Physiotherapy for tension-type headache: a controlled study. *Cephalalgia* 2004; **24**:29–36.

112. van Ettekoven, H, Lucas, C. Efficacy of physiotherapy including a craniocervical training programme for tension-type headache; a randomized clinical trial. *Cephalalgia* 2006; **26**:983–91.

113. Soderberg, E, Carlsson, J, Stener-Victorin, E. Chronic tension-type headache treated with acupuncture, physical training and relaxation training. Between-group differences. *Cephalalgia* 2006; **26**:1320–9.

114. Bove, G, Nilsson, N. Spinal manipulation in the treatment of episodic tension-type headache: a randomized controlled trial. *JAMA* 1998; **280**:1576–9.

115. Boline, PD, Kassak, K, Bronfort, G, Nelson, C, Anderson, AV. Spinal manipulation vs. amitriptyline for the treatment

of chronic tension-type headaches: a randomized clinical trial. *J Manipulative Physiol Ther* 1995; **18**:148–54.

116. Hoyt, WH, Shaffer, F, Bard, DA, *et al.* Osteopathic manipulation in the treatment of muscle-contraction headache. *J Am Osteopath Assoc* 1979; **78**:322–5.

117. Graff-Radford, SB, Canavan, DW. Headache attributed to orofacial/temporomandibular pathology. In: Olesen, J, Goadsby, PJ, Ramadan, N, Tfelt-Hansen, P, Welch, KM. (eds), *The Headaches*, 3rd edn. Philadelphia: Lippincott Williams & Wilkins, 2005; pp. 1029–35.

118. Biondi, DM. Physical treatments for headache: a structured review. *Headache* 2005; **45**:738–46.

119. Lenssinck, ML, Damen, L, Verhagen, AP, Berger, MY, Passchier, J, Koes, BW. The effectiveness of physiotherapy and manipulation in patients with tension-type headache: a systematic review. *Pain* 2004; **112**:381–8.

120. Davis, MA, Kononowech, RW, Rolin, SA, Spierings, EL. Acupuncture for tension-type headache: a meta-analysis of randomized, controlled trials. *J Pain* 2008; **9**:667–77.

121. Jena, S, Witt, CM, Brinkhaus, B, Wegscheider, K, Willich, SN. Acupuncture in patients with headache. *Cephalalgia* 2008; **28**:969–79.

122. Melchart, D, Streng, A, Hoppe, A, *et al.* Acupuncture in patients with tension-type headache: randomised controlled trial. *BMJ* 2005**331**:376–82.

123. Tavola, T, Gala, C, Conte, G, Invernizzi, G. Traditional Chinese acupuncture in tension-type headache: a controlled study. *Pain* 1992; **48**:325–9.

124. Endres, HG, Bowing, G, Diener, HC, *et al.* Acupuncture for tension-type headache: a multicentre, sham-controlled, patient-and observer-blinded, randomised trial. *J Headache Pain* 2007; **8**:306–14.

125. Karst, M, Reinhard, M, Thum, P, Wiese, B, Rollnik, J, Fink, M. Needle acupuncture in tension-type headache: a randomized, placebo-controlled study. *Cephalalgia* 2001; **21**:637–642.

126. White, AR, Resch, KL, Chan, JC, *et al.* Acupuncture for episodic tension-type headache: a multicentre randomized controlled trial. *Cephalalgia* 2000; **20**:632–7.

127. Ahonen, E, Hakumaki, M, Mahlamaki, S, Partanen, J, Riekkinen, P, Sivenius, J. Effectiveness of acupuncture and physiotherapy on myogenic headache: a comparative study. *Acupunct Electrother Res* 1984; **9**:141–50.

128. Wylie, KR, Jackson, C, Crawford, PM. Does psychological testing help to predict the response to acupuncture or massage/relaxation therapy in patients presenting to a general neurology clinic with headache? *J Tradit Chin Med* 1997; **17**:130–9.

129. Leinisch-Dahlke, E, Jurgens, T, Bogdahn, U, Jakob, W, May, A. Greater occipital nerve block is ineffective in chronic tension type headache. *Cephalalgia* 2005; **25**:704–8.

CHAPTER 17

Diagnosis, therapy and prevention of Wernicke's encephalopathy

R. Galvin,[1] G. Brathen,[2] A. Ivashynka,[3] M. Hillbom,[4] R. Tanasescu[5] and M.A. Leone[6]

[1]Cork University Hospital, Wilton, Cork, Ireland; [2]Trondheim University Hospital, Trondheim, Norway; [3]National Neurology and Neurosurgery Research Centre, Minsk, Belarus; [4]Oulu University Hospital, Oulu, Finland; [5]Colentina Hospital, University of Medicine and Pharmacy, Carol Davila, Bucharest, Romania.; [6]Azienda Ospedaliero-Universitaria Maggiore della Carita, Novara, Italy

Introduction

Wernicke's encephalopathy (WE) is a devastating acute or subacute neurological disorder resulting from thiamine (vitamin B_1) deficiency. Although vitamins were discovered at the beginning of the twentieth century, and we learned to treat thiamine deficiency some decades later, WE remains the most important encephalopathy due to a single vitamin deficiency. The disease that we now recognize as wet beri-beri, caused by thiamine deficiency from eating polished rice, was probably recognized 1000 years ago in China [1], but WE and the associated Korsakoff's amnestic syndrome were not described until the late nineteenth century [2–4]. The classic clinical triad of signs of WE comprises ocular signs, cerebellar dysfunction and confusion.

The reported prevalence of WE in postmortem studies ranges from 0.4% to 2.8%, accounting on average for 1.3% of all postmortem examinations (Table 17.1), and seems to be much higher in people with than those without alcohol problems. WE is traditionally regarded as a condition related to alcohol abuse. Interestingly, one of Carl Wernicke's index cases was a young woman with repeated vomiting after the ingestion of sulphuric acid,

and we now increasingly recognize that WE can arise in many situations other than alcohol abuse.

The disease is rare, catastrophic in onset, clinically complex and often delayed in diagnosis. We lack controlled studies on its management, although the literature abounds with small series and individual case reports. As a result of ethical problems in conducting controlled trials in a disease with a high mortality and an established therapy, new controlled data are also unlikely to be published in the future. Evidence is scarce for many aspects concerning the diagnosis and treatment of WE, but we consider guidelines to be important because it is potentially preventable and treatable and frequently remains undiagnosed particularly in situations where alcohol is not involved.

Search strategy

We searched MEDLINE with the following string: (1) *Wernicke Encephalopathy/ OR (2) ('Thiamine Deficiency/complications'[Mesh] OR 'Thiamine Deficiency/diagnosis'[Mesh] OR 'Thiamine Deficiency/drug therapy'[Mesh] OR 'Thiamine Deficiency/

European Handbook of Neurological Management: Volume 2, Second Edition. Edited by Nils Erik Gilhus, Michael P. Barnes, Michael Brainin.
© 2012 Blackwell Publishing Ltd. Published 2012 by Blackwell Publishing Ltd.

Table 17.1 Frequency of Wernicke's encephalopathy in series of consecutive postmortem examinations.

Author (reference)	Years of survey	Area	Source	Alcohol-dependent and non-alcohol-dependent individuals			Alcohol-dependent individuals			Non-alcohol-dependent individuals		
				N	WE	Percentage	N	WE	Percentage	N	WE	Percentage
Cravioto 1961 [5]	1957–60	USA, New York	H	1600	28	1.7						
Jellinger 1976 [6]	NS	Austria	H	1009	11	1.1						
Victor 1971 [7]	1963–66	USA	H	1539	29	1.9						
Torvik 1982 [8]	1975–9	Norway	H	8735	75	0.9	713	70	9.8			
Harper 1979, 1983 [9, 10]	1973–81	Australia, Perth	H + CO	4677	131	2.8						
Hauw 1988 [11]	1952–83	France	H	8200	111	1.4						
Harper 1989 [12]	NS	Australia, Sydney	H + CO	285	6	2.1						
Lindboe 1989 [13]	1983–7	Norway	H	6964	52	0.7	604	40	6.6	6360	12	0.2
Pollak 1989 [14]	NS	Germany	H				154	13	8.4			
Skullerud 1991 [15]	1984–7	Norway	CO				127	18	14.2			
Naidoo 1991 [16]	1988–9	South Africa	H				29	17	58.6			
Riethdorf 1991 [17]	1983–86	Germany	H	2372	14	0.6	223	14	6.3			
Vege 1991 [18]	1988	Norway	H	279	4	1.4						
Lana-Peixoto 1992 [19]	1978–90	Brazil	H	1655	36	2.2						
Boldorini 1992 [20]	NS	Italy	H									
Harper 1995 [21]	1989–94	France	H + CO	256	1	0.4				380	65	17.1
Sheedy 1999 [22], Harper 1998 [23]	1996–7	Australia, Sydney	CO	2212	25	1.1						
Bleggi-Torres 2000 [24]	1987–98	Brazil	H							180	10	5.6
Bertrand, 2009 [25]	2001–6	France	CJD national register							657	19	2.9
Total				**39783**	**523**	**1.3**	**1850**	**172**	**9.3**	**6920**	**87**	**1.3**

CJD, Creutzfeldt–Jakob disease; NS, not specified; H, hospital series; CO, coroner series.

epidemiology'[Mesh] OR 'Thiamine Deficiency/etiology' [Mesh] OR 'Thiamine Deficiency/prevention and control'[Mesh]) OR (3) Korsakoff Syndrome/ NOT Wernicke Encephalopathy/). We also searched EMBASE, LILACS (Wernicke Encephalopathy OR Thiamine) and the Cochrane Library. All searches were done from database inception up to 31 May 2009. All papers published in European languages were considered. Titles and abstracts were double-checked by two panel members who were blinded to the other details and relevant papers were fully read. Secondary searching was carried out using the bibliography of relevant articles. Congress abstracts were not searched.

Methods for reaching consensus

Articles were graded for evidence according to the revised European Federation of Neurological Societies (EFNS) scientific task force guidance for guidelines [26] by two members of the panel; in case of disagreement, grading was discussed in a panel meeting. Each successive guideline draft was circulated among panellists and modified after their comments. All members of the task force agreed to all recommendations unanimously; where there was lack of evidence, but consensus was clear, we have stated our opinion as a good practice point (GPP).

Findings

How often is WE diagnosed in life?

Postmortem studies indicate that WE is frequently undiagnosed during life. Table 17.2 lists the postmortem studies reporting the percentage of patients with or without alcohol problems and WE diagnosed *ante mortem*. All were class IV studies. WE was suspected during life in only about a third of patients with and 6% of patients without alcohol problems. These series are likely to be biased towards more severe cases and the number of patients remaining undiagnosed before death is probably higher. These observations would suggest that thiamine deficiency and its consequences are likely to remain undiagnosed during life in significant numbers of cases. We are probably underestimating the real incidence of the disease, and it seems reasonable to recommend that a postmortem examination has to be performed when patients die in situations with a suspicion of thiamine deficiency.

> **Recommendation**
>
> Patients dying from symptoms suggesting WE should have a postmortem examination (GPP).

When should we suspect WE in patients with no alcohol problems?

We found more than 600 cases of WE reported in clinical settings other than alcohol use (Table 17.3). Among the most frequent settings were malignant disease, gastrointestinal disease and surgery, and vomiting due to hyperemesis gravidarum. Other causes included fasting, starvation, malnutrition and the use of unbalanced diets. Systematic reviews have been published for bariatric surgery [29, 30] and hyperemesis gravidarum [31]. After bariatric surgery, i.e. the surgical procedures for obesity (gastric banding, gastric bypass, biliopancreatic diversion, etc.), the risk for WE is long lasting. According to one report, 94% of WE cases were seen within 6 months of surgery [29]. Whenever a pregnant woman with persistent vomiting develops neurological signs or symptoms, WE should be considered [31]. Prevalence studies of WE among patients with no alcohol problems have not been done and we can only speculate about the real prevalence of the disease in at-risk situations. Some conditions, such as bariatric surgery, may increase in the future, whereas others may disappear.

> **Recommendation**
>
> The level of suspicion for WE should be high in all clinical conditions that could lead to thiamine deficiency in the absence of alcoholism (GPP). After bariatric surgery we recommend follow-up of the thiamine status for at least 6 months (recommendation level B).

Which clinical features accurately identify WE?

Table 17.4 lists the studies comparing postmortem series (including three or more cases) with clinical features of patients with acute WE. Most patients had alcohol

Table 17.2 Number of cases of Wernicke's encephalopathy diagnosed *ante mortem* in postmortem series.

Author (reference)	Years of the survey	Area	Evidence class	Source	Alcohol-dependent patients			Non-alcohol-dependent patients		
					No. of postmortem examinations	No. diagnosed *ante mortem*	Percentage	No. of postmortem examinations	No. diagnosed *ante mortem*	Percentage
Victor 1971 [7]	1950–61	USA	IV	H	53	45	84.9			
Torvik 1982 [8]	1975–9	Norway	IV	H	19	1	5.3			
Harper 1979, 1983 [9, 10]	1973–81	Australia, Perth^a	IV	H + CO	131	26	19.8			
Harper 1989 [12]	NS	Australia, Sydney	IV	H + CO	6	2	33.3			
Lindboe 1989 [13]	1983–7	Norway	IV	H	11	4	36.4	7	0	0
Naidoo 1991 [16]	1988–9	South Africa	IV	H	17	0	0			
Riethdorf 1991 [17]	1983–86	Germany	IV	H	14	3	21.4			
Vege 1991 [18]	1988	Norway	IV	H	3	1	33.3	1	0	0
Sheedy 1999 [22] Harper 1998 [23]	1996–7	Australia, Sydney	IV	CO	18	4	22.2			
Ogershok 2002 [27]	1984–99	USA	IV	H	1	1	100	3	1	33
Kuo 2009 [28]	NS	USA	IV	H				5	1	20
Bertrand, 2009 [25]	2001–6	France	IV	CJD national register				19	0	0
Total					**273**	**87**	**31.9**	**35**	**2**	**5.7**

CJD, Creutzfeldt–Jakob disease; NS, not specified; H, hospital series; CO, coroner series.
^a>90% alcohol-dependent patients.

Table 17.3 List of cases of Wernicke's encephalopathy reported in non-alcohol-dependent patients.[a]

Clinical condition	No.	Percentage
Cancer	113	18.1
Gastrointestinal surgery	105	16.8
Hyperemesis gravidarum	76	12.2
Starvation/Fasting	64	10.2
Gastrointestinal tract diseases	48	7.7
AIDS	31	5.0
Malnutrition	26	4.2
Dialysis and renal diseases	24	3.8
Parenteral nutrition	24	3.8
Vomiting	15	2.4
Psychiatric diseases	15	2.4
Stem cell/marrow transplantation	14	2.2
Infections	9	1.4
Intoxication	9	1.4
Thyroid diseases	8	1.3
Unbalanced diet	6	1.0
Iatrogenic	5	0.8
Hypoxic encephalopathy	2	0.3
Others	12	1.9
Unknown etiology	19	3.0
Total	**625**	**100.0**

[a]Search performed in MEDLINE, EMBASE, LILACS from database inception until 31 May 2009.

reviewed by three researchers: sensitivity of each domain (recalculated from the paper) ranged from 20% (seizures) to 75% (cerebellar signs). Sensitivity of the classic triad was 23%, but rose to 85% if the patients had at least two of the four following features: dietary deficiencies, eye signs, cerebellar signs, and either mild memory impairment or an altered mental state.

Thiamine deficiency may also result in other manifestations such as dry beri-beri (neuropathy), wet beri-beri (neuropathy with high-output congestive heart failure), gastrointestinal beri-beri (abdominal pain, vomiting and lactic acidosis) and coma followed by Marchiafava–Bignami syndrome [36, 37]. Heart failure with lactic acidosis is an important syndrome to be noted, because several papers have reported favourable outcome after thiamine treatment [38, 39].

Recommendation

The clinical diagnosis of WE in alcohol-dependent patients requires two of the following four signs: (1) dietary deficiencies, (2) eye signs, (3) cerebellar dysfunction and (4) either an altered mental state or mild memory impairment (level B). It is reasonable to apply the same criteria to non-alcohol-dependent patients (GPP).

---

problems. Consecutive postmortem examinations were collected without knowledge of clinical data. However, it is unknown whether the clinical data evaluation was blinded to postmortem results, so all these studies are considered class IV. The classic diagnostic triad (eye signs, cerebellar signs and confusion) was reported in only 8% of patients with clinical details. Although it should be considered as a minimum estimate due to a possible reporting bias, this figure prompts the need to reconsider diagnostic criteria for in-life diagnosis of WE. Caine *et al.* [35] (class II) studied clinical features of 28 postmortem-proven alcohol-dependent patients with WE who were well evaluated during life. They divided signs and symptoms into eight clinical domains (see Table 17.4 for definitions): dietary deficiencies, eye signs, cerebellar signs, seizures, frontal lobe dysfunction, amnesia, mild memory impairment and altered mental state. Reproducibility and validity of the criteria were then tested on 106 alcohol-dependent patients who had postmortem examinations. Clinical records of the patients were blindly

Are clinical features of alcohol-dependent WE different from non-alcohol-dependent WE?

Table 17.5 lists case series (including three or more cases) published after Caine's criteria and compares clinical features of alcohol-dependent and non-alcohol-dependent patients with WE. All but two were class IV studies. In most studies, the MRI investigations were not performed blind to clinical evaluation and vice versa. Although these studies cannot give reliable information on the frequency of clinical features, they allow a comparison of the clinical features in alcohol-dependent and non-alcohol-dependent patients. There is evidence that clinical features were unevenly distributed: dietary deficiency and vomiting were more frequent among non-alcohol-dependent patients ($p < 0.0001$), whereas eye and cerebellar signs were more frequent among alcohol-dependent ones ($p < 0.0001$). The classic triad was significantly more frequent in alcohol-dependent than in the

Table 17.4 Clinical features of patients with an autopsy proved diagnosis of Wernicke's encephalopathy.

Author (reference)	Evidence class	Total no. patients	Dietary deficiencies	Nausea and vomiting	Any eye sign	Cerebellar signs	Seizures	Amnesia, mild memory impairment	Altered mental state	Triad
Cravioto 1961 [5]	IV	28	14		9	5			26	4
Grunnet 1969 [32]	IV	24	1		9	3	4	4	17	0
Torvik 1982 [8]	IV	19			4	0			18	0
Harper 1986 [33]	IV	97			28	36		29	41	16
Lindboe 1989 [13]	IV	18	1		3	0			11	0
Naidoo 1991 [16]	IV	17		8	0	2			9	0
Vege 1991 [18]	IV	4	2	1	0	0		2	3	0
Ogershok 2002 [27]	IV	4	3		4	1	1		4	1
Bleggi-Torres 1997 [34]	IV	8			3	0			6	0
Harper 1998 [23]	IV	18			0	3	3	6		0
Bertrand 2009 [25]	IV	19			2	15		19	1	0
Total no. (%)		256	21 (8.2)	9 (3.5)	62 (24.2)	65 (25.4)	8 (3.1)	60 (23.4)	136 (53.1)	21 (8.2)

Empty cell means that not mentioned; 0 = specified as absent

Definition of domains [35] Domain 6 and 7 are combined in the table. Domain 5 was sporadically mentioned in the papers and it is not included here.

1. Dietary deficiencies (a body mass index lower than 2 SD below normal as evidence of undernutrition, a history of grossly impaired dietary intake, or an abnormal thiamine status); the column including nausea and vomiting is added here, but they were not considered by Caine *et al.*

2. Eye signs (oculomotor abnormalities such as ophthalmoplegia, nystagmus or gaze palsy).

3. Cerebellar signs (ataxia, unsteadiness, abnormalities of past pointing, dysdiadokokinesia, impaired heel-shin testing).

4. Seizures (either as part of a withdrawal syndrome or in isolation or a longstanding history of anticonvulsant medication).

5. Frontal lobe dysfunction (abnormalities in planning, insight, or abstraction with formal neuropsychological testing or when neurological examination elicited these characteristics).

6. Amnesia (a stable and persisting inability to form new memories).

7. Mild memory impairment (failure to remember two or more words in the four item memory test, or impairment on more elaborate neuropsychological tests of memory function).

8. Altered mental state (disorientation in two of three fields, confused, an abnormal digit span or comatose).

non-alcohol-dependent patients ($p < 0.005$). Reasons for the difference are unclear, but may be due to the fact that WE in non-alcohol-dependent patients usually presents as a dramatic acute syndrome, whereas WE in alcohol-dependent patients may more frequently present as a subclinical syndrome. Furthermore, alcohol-dependent patients may develop thiamine deficiency several times during their lifespan, whereas non-alcohol-dependent patients are not likely to do so. Magnesium deficiency could also contribute to the poor recovery from WE in alcohol-dependent patients [56].

Recommendation

The clinical diagnosis of WE should take into account the different presentations of clinical signs between alcohol-dependent and non-alcohol-dependent patients and the higher prevalence of the disease in the former (level C).

Is there any laboratory test that accurately identifies patients with thiamine deficiency?

The erythrocyte transketolase activity assay, including thiamine pyrophosphate effect, has been replaced by direct measurement of thiamine and its phosphate esters in human blood by high-performance liquid chromatography (HPLC) [57, 58]. This thiamine assay is now commercially available in many countries. Adult normal range (60–220 nmol/l) and the lowest detectable level (3–35 nmol/l) are given. The sample (2–ml EDTA blood) should be taken before administration of thiamine and should be protected from light. However, normal thiamine levels do not necessarily exclude WE in exceptional cases, i.e. in the presence of thiamine transporter gene mutations [59].

The concentration of thiamine and thiamine monophosphate and diphosphate in plasma and whole blood samples were assessed in six healthy individuals for 12 h and in urine for 24 h after either an intravenous or oral bolus dose of 50 mg thiamine-HCl. Unphosphorylated thiamine increased rapidly in plasma after intravenous administration and then decreased to its initial value within 12 h. The half-life was 96 min. Thiamine mono- and diphosphate increased moderately (56%), and

decreased slowly; the half-life of diphosphate was 664 min. Within 24 h, 53% of the administered dose was recovered in the urine, indicating a restricted distribution [60].

Recommendation

Whenever WE is suspected a blood sample for measurement of total thiamine should be drawn immediately before administration of thiamine and sent for HPLC analysis (GPP).

Does radiology accurately identify patients with WE?

Computed tomography (CT) is not a reliable test for WE [41] (class II). Table 17.6 lists MRI series including three or more cases of WE. Seven compare alcohol-dependent with non-alcohol-dependent patients and one additional paper alcohol-dependent patients with acute WE with controls and asymptomatic alcohol-dependent patients without WE. In this class II retrospective study alcohol-dependent patients with and without WE were compared and MR images were randomly and blindly assessed by two neuroradiologists [41]. The sensitivity and specificity of MRI were 53% and 93%. Positive predictive value was 89%.

Pooled data in Table 17.6 showed that among alcohol-dependent patients with a clinically verified acute WE, conventional MRI revealed lesions in almost two-thirds of the subjects. Little additional information was obtained by using fluid-attenuated inversion recovery (FLAIR) images and diffusion-weighted imaging (DWI). In non-alcohol-dependent patients, the available data showed a higher yield of lesions, varying from 97% (DWI) to 99% (conventional) and 100% (FLAIR). Location of lesions was more frequently atypical among non-alcohol-dependent than alcohol-dependent patients, whereas contrast enhancement of the thalamus and mammillary bodies was observed to associate more frequently with alcohol abuse [63]. Typically, the lesions were symmetrical and seen in the thalami, mammillary bodies, tectal plate and periaqueductal area. Atypical lesions were located in the cerebellum, vermis, cranial nerve nuclei, red nuclei, dentate nuclei, caudate nuclei, splenium and cerebral cortex. Reversible cytotoxic oedema was

Table 17.5 Clinical features of alcohol-dependent and non-alcohol-dependent patients with Wernicke's encephalopathy.

Author (reference)	Evidence class	Total no. patients	Dietary deficiencies	Nausea and vomiting	Any eye sign	Cerebellar signs	Seizures	Amnesia, mild memory impairment	Altered mental state	Triad
Alcohol-dependent patients										
Gallucci 1990 [40]	IV	5		5	5	4			3	3
Antunez 1998 [41]	II	15			14	12			10	9
Park 2001 [42]	III	12			11	10		1	5	4
Varnet 2002 [43]	IV	25	1		20	22			19	11
Ogershok 2002 [27]	IV	6			6	3			6	3
Weidauer 2003 [44]	IV	11			11	10		5	10	9
Chung SP 2003 [45]	IV	1	1		0	1			1	0
Halavaara 2003 [46]	IV	2	1	1	2	2		2	2	2
White 2005 [47]	IV	1	1	1	1	1		1	1	1
Zuccoli 2009 [48]	IV	24			22	17			20	13
Total no. (%)		**102**	**4 (3.9)**	**7 (6.9)**	**92 (90.2)**	**82 (80.4)**	**0 (–)**	**9 (8.8)**	**77 (75.5)**	**55 (53.9)**
Non-alcohol-dependent patients										
Shikata 2000 [49]	IV	3	3		3	1		3		1
Merkin-Zaborsky 2001 [50]	IV	3	1	2	3	3				0
Park 2001 [42]	III	3	2	2	2	2		1	3	2
Ogershok 2002 [27]	IV	6	6	3	5	2			6	2
Weidauer 2003 [44]	IV	1		1	1	1		1	1	1
Chung SP 2003 [45]	IV	3	1	0	1	3			3	1
Halavaara 2003 [46]	IV	3	3	2	3	3		1	2	2
Zhong 2005 [51]	IV	6	6		2	2		2	6	
White 2005 [47]	IV	2	2	2	2	2		1	1	1
Sun 2006 [52]	IV	4	1	3	3	0		1	4	0
Unlu 2006 [53]	IV	6	6		6	6			6	6
Fei 2008 [54]	IV	12	12		9	3				2
Kirbas 2008 [55]	IV	25	25	7	14	10		3	9	4
Francini-Pesenti 2009 [62]	IV	7	7	3	6	7			7	6
Zuccoli 2009 [48]	IV	32	21	11	22	13			30	11
Total		**116**	**96 (82.8)**	**36 (31.0)**	**82 (70.7)**	**58 (50.0)**	**0 (–)**	**13 (11.2)**	**78 (67.2)**	**39 (33.6)**

Empty cell means that not mentioned; 0. specified as absent.

See Table 17.4 for the definition of domains.

Table 17.6 MRI features of alcohol-dependent and non-alcohol-dependent patients with Wernicke's encephalopathy.

Author (reference)	Evidence class	Type of MRI	Conventional MRI		MRI gadolinium enhancement		FLAIR MRI		DWR MRI	
			Total no.	Positive no. (%)	Total no.	Positive no. (%)	Total no.	Positive no. (%)	Total no.	Positive no. (%)
Alcohol-dependent patients										
Gallucci 1990 [40]	IV	0.5 T	5	5						
Antunez 1998 [41]	II	1.5 T	15	8	2	0				
Park 2001 [42]	III	2.0 T	8	8						
Varnet 2002 [43]	III	1–1.5 T	25	16	25	3				
Ogershok 2002 [27]	IV	?	2	0						
Chung SP 2003 [45]	IV	1.5 T	11	2	11	4	11	3	1	1
Weidauer 2003 [44]	IV	1.5 T	2	2	2	0	2	2	2	2
Halavaara 2003 [46]	IV	1.5 T	1	1	2	0			1	1
White 2005 [47]	IV	?					1	1		
Zuccoli 2009 [48]	IV	1.0/1.5 T	24	17	18	17	24	17		
TOTAL			93	59 (63.4)	58	24 (41.4)	38	23 (60.5)	4	4 (100)
Non-alcohol-dependent patients										
Mascalchi 1999 [61]	IV	?	3	3	2	1				
Park 2001 [42]	III	2.0 T	3	3						
Ogershok 2002 [27]	IV	?	1	1						
Chung SP 2003 [45]	IV	1.5T	1	0	1	1	1	1	1	1
Weidauer 2003 [44]	IV	1.5 T	3	3	1	1	1	1		
Halavaara 2003 [46]	IV	1.5 T	2	2	3	0	3	3	3	3
White 2005 [47]	IV	?	6	6			2	2	2	2
Zhong 2005 [51]	IV	1.5 T	6	6			6	6	6	6
Unlu 2006 [53]	IV	1.0 T	12	12	6	5	6	6	4	3
Fei 2008 [54]	IV	1.5 T	7	7	3	3	10	10	7	7
Francini-Pesenti 2009 [62]	IV	?					7	7		
Zuccoli 2009 [48]	IV	1.0/1.5 T	32	32	23	9	32	32	6	6
Total			77	76 (98.7)	43	22 (51.0)	72	72 (100)	29	28 (97.0)

DWI, diffusion-weighted imaging; FLAIR, fluid-attenuated inversion recovery; MRI, magnetic resonance imaging.

considered the most distinctive lesion of WE [63]. The heterogeneity of MRI lesions may result from disease severity, acuteness of the disease and timing of imaging. We cannot say which of the MRI techniques used is most useful.

What is the efficacy of thiamine treatment in WE?

The efficacy of thiamine for WE has been assessed in only one double-blind randomized clinical trial [64]. Due to several methodological shortcomings it is, in our opinion, a class III study. Thiamine hydrochloride was given to 107 patients in doses of 5, 20, 50, 100 and 200 mg daily for 2 days, with assessment of effect on the third day by a single neuropsychological test, suggested to be sensitive to cognitive impairment. The authors concluded that the 200 mg dose was superior to the mean result of all the other dosages. This study was evaluated in a Cochrane review concluding that, in comparison to the 5 mg dose, 200 mg was significantly more effective [65]. In another randomized double-blind study 10 mg thiamine or placebo was given to elderly people with subclinical thiamine deficiency [66]. These people did not have WE. Quality of life was enhanced by providing thiamine supplements.

There is no consensus on the optimal dose of thiamine, its preparation form, duration of treatment or the number of daily doses. Pharmacokinetic studies show a blood half-life of free thiamine of only 96 min [60] so it can be speculated that giving thiamine in two or three daily doses might achieve better penetrance to the brain and other tissues than a single daily dose [67].

According to many case reports, treatment with either 100 or 200 mg thiamine given intravenously has cured the disease in non-alcohol-dependent patients. On the other hand, this has not always been the case in alcohol-dependent patients. Alcohol-dependent patients with

WE may need higher daily doses and 500 mg three times daily has been recommended [68, 69]. The reason for the discrepancy is unclear. Alcohol-dependent patients may have had previous subclinical episodes of the disease, leading to permanent damage in the brain before admission to hospital with WE, or the often coexistent severe alcohol withdrawal syndrome may have resulted in permanent damage of the brain tissue due to excess glutamate liberated in the brain [70].

Experimental [60] and clinical data [71–73] indicate that orally administered thiamine hydrochloride is ineffective in increasing blood thiamine or curing WE. The critical blood concentrations of thiamine for treating WE have not been determined. It could be speculated that patients in a catabolic state and alcohol-dependent patients have reduced ability to store thiamine because the enzymes depending on thiamine are downregulated or protein binding is altered by the influence of alcohol. In such patients even high doses of thiamine might not cause a sufficient increase of thiamine stores unless a balanced diet has been instituted at the same time. Thus, normalization of diet might be an important factor in the acute treatment of suspected or manifest WE.

As the unwanted side effects to B vitamins are most commonly seen after multiple administrations, and the necessary dose of thiamine amounts to a rather painful volume when given intramuscularly, we suggest an intravenous infusion of thiamine diluted with 100 ml physiological saline or 5% glucose, given over 30 min. It is also important to give thiamine before any carbohydrate, because it is well known that glucose infusion precipitates WE in thiamine deficiency [69].

Is thiamine therapy safe?

The overall safety of intravenous thiamine is very good. In a prospective study of 989 patients receiving 100 mg thiamine hydrochloride as a single intravenous injection over 10 s or less, one patient reacted with generalized pruritus and 11 had transient local irritation [74] (class II). In a retrospective survey Wrenn and Slovis identified no cases of significant adverse reactions to thiamine in more than 300 000 treatments [74]. Sporadic anaphylactic reactions have been reported, but it is not documented that thiamine was the cause in all cases. However, it has been suggested that thiamine should be given in circumstances where facilities for resuscitation are available [68]. This is preferable, but because a delay in treatment may cause irreversible brain damage and is life threatening, we recommend starting treatment immediately, even in the absence of facilities for resuscitation.

Recommendation

The overall safety of thiamine is very good, regardless of route of administration (level B). Thiamine should be given without delay in all circumstances irrespective of whether or not facilities for resuscitation are immediately available (GPP).

Is there a place for prophylactic thiamine therapy?

Studies from several countries show a thiamine deficiency in the elderly population [75] and thiamine has been added to foods in many countries [76]. Some observational studies from Australia [76, 77] suggest that this preventive effort has resulted in a decrease of the occurrence of the disease, although no controlled studies have been performed on this matter and are unlikely to be done in the future. Supplementation of thiamine to alcoholic beverages has also been suggested [75]. However, the mechanisms via which alcohol ingestion predisposes to thiamine deficiency suggest that adding thiamine into alcoholic beverages is a useless strategy. First, alcohol inhibits the absorption of thiamine from the intestine; second, during alcohol metabolism thiamine will be neither phosphorylated nor incorporated into enzymes in body tissues [78]. Thiamine ingested together with alcohol will therefore be excreted in urine as free thiamine.

Thiamine deficiency is frequently not clinically apparent and WE can easily be worsened or precipitated if the treating physician gives glucose to a patient unaware that there is a thiamine deficiency. In many countries emergency ward guidelines include recommendations to administer parenteral thiamine, e.g. to patients who are in status epilepticus [79], before any infusion of carbohydrates is started.

There are also other conditions (see Table 17.3) in which administration of thiamine in food or oral preparation is inefficient (e.g. vomiting). Such conditions require parenteral administration of thiamine. In hunger strikers there is evidence from one cohort study (class IV) [80] that up to 600 mg thiamine orally, together with one tablespoon of sugar daily, did not prevent the development of WE. We did not find any other studies evaluating the prophylactic administration of thiamine in other risk conditions in alcohol-dependent or non-alcohol-dependent patients. Administration of multivitamin pills has been recommended after bariatric surgery. However, parenteral administration of vitamins may be a better strategy to prevent vitamin deficiency, because these patients frequently vomit [30].

Recommendation

Supplementation of thiamine into food may prevent the development of WE (GPP). There is no evidence that supplementation into beverages may be useful. We recommend prophylactic parenteral administration of 200 mg thiamine before carbohydrates are started in all individuals with a risk condition managed in accident and emergency (GPP). After bariatric surgery we recommend parenteral thiamine supplementation (GPP). We think that hunger strikers should be carefully informed of the risk of WE and persuaded to accept a parenteral administration of thiamine followed by glucose (GPP). However, in both these situations we do not have any evidence of an effective dosage.

Conflict of interest

The present guidelines were developed without external financial support. None of the authors reports any conflict of interest.

References

1. Fan, KW. Jiao Qi disease in medieval China. *Am J Chin Med* 2004; **32**:999–1011.

2. Thomson, AD, Cook, CC, Guerrini, I, Sheedy, D, Harper, C, Marshall, EJ. Wernicke's encephalopathy revisited. Translation of the case history section of the original manuscript by Carl Wernicke 'Lehrbuch der Gehirnkrankheiten fur Aerzte and Studirende' 1881;with a commentary. *Alcohol Alcoholism* 2008; **43**:174–9.

3. Wernicke, C. *Lehrbuch der Gehirnkrankheiten fur Aerzte und Studirende*, vol 2. 1881; pp. 229–42.

4. Korsakow, SS. Über eine besondere form psychischer Störung combiniert mit multipler neurotis. *Arch Psychiatr Nervenkr* 1890; **21**:669–704.

5. Cravioto, H, Korein, J, Silberman, J. Wernicke's encephalopathy. A clinical and pathological study of 28 autopsied cases. *Arch Neurol* 1961; **4**:510–19.

6. Jellinger, K. Neuropathological aspects of dementias resulting from abnormal blood and cerebrospinal fluid dynamics. *Acta Neurol Belg* 1976; **76**:83–102.

7. Victor, M, Adams, RD, Collins, GH. The Wernicke–Korsakoff syndrome. A clinical and pathological study of 245 patients, 82 with post-mortem examinations. *Contemp Neurol Ser* 1971; **7**:1–206.

8. Torvik, A, Lindboe, CF, Rogde, S. Brain lesions in alcoholics. A neuropathological study with clinical correlations. *J Neurol Sci* 1982; **56**:233–48.

9. Harper, C. Wernicke's encephalopathy: a more common disease than realised. A neuropathological study of 51 cases. *J Neurol Neurosurg Psychiatry* 1979; **42**:226–31.

10. Harper, C. The incidence of Wernicke's encephalopathy in Australia – a neuropathological study of 131 cases. *J Neurol Neurosurg Psychiatry* 1983; **46**:593–8.

11. Hauw, JJ, De Baecque, C, Hausser-Hauw, C, Serdaru, M. Chromatolysis in alcoholic encephalopathies. Pellagra-like changes in 22 cases. *Brain* 1988; **111**:843–57.

12. Harper, C, Gold, J, Rodriguez, M, Perdices, M. The prevalence of the Wernicke–Korsakoff syndrome in Sydney, Australia: a prospective necropsy study. *J Neurol Neurosurg Psychiatry* 1989; **52**:282–5.

13. Lindboe, CF, Loberg, EM. Wernicke's encephalopathy in non-alcoholics. An autopsy study. *J Neurol Sci* 1989; **90**:125–9.

14. Pollak, KH. Alcoholism and morphologic findings of the nervous system in autopsy cases. *Psychiatr Neurol Med Psychol (Leipz)* 1989; **41**:664–79.

15. Skullerud, K, Andersen, SN, Lundevall, J. Cerebral lesions and causes of death in male alcoholics. A forensic autopsy study. *Int J Legal Med* 1991; **104**:209–13.

16. Naidoo, DP, Bramdev, A, Cooper, K. Wernicke's encephalopathy and alcohol-related disease. *Postgrad Med J* 1991; **67**:978–81.

17. Riethdorf, L, Warzok, R, Schwesinger, G. Die Alkoholenzephalopathien im Obduktionsgut. *Zentralbl Pathol* 1991; **137**:48–56.

18. Vege, A, Sund, S, Lindboe, CF. Wernicke's encephalopathy in an autopsy material obtained over a one-year period. *APMIS* 1991; **99**:755–8.

19. Lana-Peixoto, MA, Dos Santos, EC, Pittella, JE. Coma and death in unrecognized Wernicke's encephalopathy. An autopsy study. *Arq Neuropsiquiatr* 1992; **50**:329–33.

20. Boldorini, R, Vago, L, Lechi, A, Tedeschi, F, Trabattoni, GR. Wernicke's encephalopathy: occurrence and pathological aspects in a series of 400 AIDS patients. *Acta Biomed Ateneo Parmense* 1992; **63**:43–9.

21. Harper, C, Fornes, P, Duyckaerts, C, Lecomte, D, Hauw, JJ. An international perspective on the prevalence of the Wernicke–Korsakoff syndrome. *Metab Brain Dis* 1995; **10**:17–24.

22. Sheedy, D, Lara, A, Garrick, T, Harper, C. Size of mammillary bodies in health and disease: useful measurements in neuroradiological diagnosis of Wernicke's encephalopathy. *Alcohol Clin Exp Res* 1999; **23**:1624–8.

23. Harper, CG, Sheedy, DL, Lara, AI, Garrick, TM, Hilton, JM, Raisanen, J. Prevalence of Wernicke–Korsakoff syndrome in Australia: has thiamine fortification made a difference? *Med J Aust* 1998; **168**:542–545.

24. Bleggi-Torres, LF, de Medeiros, BC, Werner, B. *et al.* Neuropathological findings after bone marrow transplantation: an autopsy study of 180 cases. *Bone Marrow Transplant* 2000; **25**:301–7.

25. Bertrand, A, Brandel, JP, Grignon, Y. *et al.* Wernicke encephalopathy and Creutzfeldt-Jakob disease. *J Neurol* 2009; **256**:904–9.

26. Brainin, M, Barnes, M, Baron, J-C. *et al.* Guidance for the preparation of neurological management guidelines by EFNS scientific task forces – revised recommendations 2004. *Eur J Neurol* 2004; **11**:577–81.

27. Ogershok, PR, Rahman, A, Nestor, S, Brick, J. Wernicke encephalopathy in nonalcoholic patients. *Am J Med Sci* 2002; **323**:107–11.

28. Kuo, SH, Debnam, JM, Fuller, GN, de Groot, J. Wernicke's encephalopathy: an underrecognized and reversible cause of confusional state in cancer patients. *Oncology* 2009; **76**:10–18.

29. Aasheim, ET. Wernicke encephalopathy after bariatric surgery: a systematic review. *Ann Surg* 2008; **248**:714–20.

30. Singh, S, Kumar, A. Wernicke encephalopathy after obesity surgery: a systematic review. *Neurology* 2007; **68**:807–11.

31. Chiossi, G, Neri, I, Cavazzuti, M, Basso, G, Facchinetti, F. Hyperemesis gravidarum complicated by Wernicke encephalopathy: background, case report, and review of the literature. *Obstet Gynecol Surv* 2006; **61**:255–68.

32. Grunnet, ML. Changing incidence, distribution and histopathology of Wernicke's polioencephalopathy. *Neurology* 1969; **19**:1135–9.

33. Harper, CG, Giles, M, Finlay-Jones, R. Clinical signs in the Wernicke-Korsakoff complex: a retrospective analysis of 131 cases diagnosed at necropsy. *J Neurol Neurosurg Psychiatry* 1986; **49**:341–5.

34. Bleggi-Torres, LF, de Medeiros, BC, Ogasawara, VS. *et al.* Iatrogenic Wernicke's encephalopathy in allogeneic bone marrow transplantation: a study of eight cases. *Bone Marrow Transplant* 1997; **20**:391–5.

35. Caine, D, Halliday, GM, Kril, JJ, Harper, CG. Operational criteria for the classification of chronic alcoholics: identification of Wernicke's encephalopathy. *J Neurol Neurosurg Psychiatry* 1997; **62**:51–60.

36. Campbell, CH. The severe lactic acidosis of thiamine deficiency: acute pernicious or fulminating beriberi. *Lancet* 1984; **ii**:446–9.

37. Hillbom, M, Pyhtinen, J, Pylvanen, V, Sotaniemi, K. Pregnant, vomiting, and coma. *Lancet* 1999; **353**:1584.

38. Brady, JA, Rock, CL, Horneffer, MR. Thiamin status, diuretic medications, and the management of congestive heart failure. *J Am Diet Assoc* 1995; **95**:541–4.

39. Shimon, I, Almog, S, Vered, Z. *et al.* Improved left ventricular function after thiamine supplementation in patients with congestive heart failure receiving long-term furosemide therapy. *Am J Med* 1995; **98**:485–90.

40. Gallucci, M, Bozzao, A, Splendiani, A, Masciocchi, C, Passariello, R. Wernicke encephalopathy: MR findings in five patients. *AJR Am J Roentgenol* 1990; **155**:1309–14.

41. Antunez, E, Estruch, R, Cardenal, C, Nicolas, JM, Fernandez-Sola, J, Urbano-Marquez, A. Usefulness of CT and MR imaging in the diagnosis of acute Wernicke's encephalopathy. *AJR Am J Roentgenol* 1998; **171**:1131–7.

42. Park, SH, Kim, M, Na, DL, Jeon, BS. Magnetic resonance reflects the pathological evolution of Wernicke encephalopathy. *J Neuroimaging* 2001; **11**:406–11.

43. Varnet, O, de Seze, J, Soto-Ares, G. *et al.* Wernicke–Korsakoff syndrome: diagnostic contribution of magnetic resonance imaging. *Rev Neurol (Paris)* 2002; **158**:1181–5.

44. Weidauer, S, Nichtweiss, M, Lanfermann, H, Zanella, FE. Wernicke encephalopathy: MR findings and clinical presentation. *Eur Radiol* 2003; **13**:1001–9.

45. Chung, SP, Kim, SW, Yoo, IS, Lim, YS, Lee, G. Magnetic resonance imaging as a diagnostic adjunct to Wernicke encephalopathy in the ED. *Am J Emerg Med* 2003; **21**:497–502.

46. Halavaara, J, Brander, A, Lyytinen, J, Setala, K, Kallela, M. Wernicke's encephalopathy: is diffusion-weighted MRI useful? *Neuroradiology* 2003; **45**:519–23.

47. White, ML, Zhang, Y, Andrew, LG, Hadley, WL. MR imaging with diffusion-weighted imaging in acute and chronic Wernicke encephalopathy. *AJNR Am J Neuroradiol* 2005; **26**:2306–10.

48. Zuccoli, G, Santa Cruz, D, Bertolini, M. *et al.* MR imaging findings in 56 patients with Wernicke encephalopathy: nonalcoholics may differ from alcoholics. *AJNR Am J Neuroradiol* 2009; **30**:171–6.

49. Shikata, E, Mizutani, T, Kokubun, Y, Takasu, T. 'Iatrogenic' Wernicke's encephalopathy in Japan. *Eur Neurol* 2000; **44**:156–61.

50. Merkin-Zaborsky, H, Ifergane, G, Frisher, S, Valdman, S, Herishanu, Y, Wirguin, I. Thiamine-responsive acute neurological disorders in nonalcoholic patients. *Eur Neurol* 2001; **45**:34–7.

51. Zhong, C, Jin, L, Fei, G. MR Imaging of nonalcoholic Wernicke encephalopathy: a follow-up study. *AJNR Am J Neuroradiol* 2005; **26**:2301–5.

52. Sun, GH, Yang, YS, Liu, QS, Cheng, LF, Huang, XS. Pancreatic encephalopathy and Wernicke encephalopathy in association with acute pancreatitis: a clinical study. *World J Gastroenterol* 2006; **12**:4224–7.

53. Unlu, E, Cakir, B, Asil, T. MRI findings of Wernicke encephalopathy revisited due to hunger strike. *Eur J Radiol* 2006; **57**:43–53.

54. Fei, GQ, Zhong, C, Jin, L. *et al.* Clinical characteristics and MR imaging features of non-alcoholic Wernicke encephalopathy. *AJNR Am J Neuroradiol* 2008; **29**:164–9.

55. Kirbas, D, Sutlas, N, Kuscu, DY, Karagoz, N, Tecer, O, Altun, U. The impact of prolonged hunger strike: clinical and laboratory aspects of twenty-five hunger strikers. *Ideggyogy Sz* 2008; **61**:317–24.

56. Traviesa, DC. Magnesium deficiency: a possible cause of thiamine refractoriness in Wernicke-Korsakoff encephalopathy. *J Neurol Neurosurg Psychiatry* 1974; **37**:959–62.

57. Tallaksen, CM, Bohmer, T, Bell, H, Karlsen, J. Concomitant determination of thiamin and its phosphate esters in human blood and serum by high-performance liquid chromatography. *J Chromatogr* 1991; **564**:127–36.

58. Lu, J, Frank, EL. Rapid HPLC measurement of thiamine and its phosphate esters in whole blood. *Clin Chem* 2008; **54**:901–6.

59. Kono, S, Miyajima, H, Yoshida, K, Togawa, A, Shirakawa, K, Suzuki, H. Mutations in a thiamine transporter gene and Wernicke's-like encephalopathy. *N Engl J Med* 2009; **360**:1792–4.

60. Tallaksen, C, Sande, A, Bøhmer, T, Bell, H, Karlsen, J. Kinetics of thiamin and thiamin phosphate esters in human blood,

plasma and urine after 50 mg intravenously or orally. *Eur J Clin Pharmacol* 1993; **44**:73–8.

61. Mascalchi, M, Simonelli, P, Tessa, C. *et al.* Do acute lesions of Wernicke's encephalopathy show contrast enhancement? Report of three cases and review of the literature. *Neuroradiology* 1999; **41**:249–54.

62. Francini-Pesenti, F, Brocadello, F, Manara, R, Santelli, L, Laroni, A, Caregaro, L. Wernicke's syndrome during parenteral feeding: not an unusual complication. *Nutrition* 2009; **25**:142–6.

63. Zuccoli, G, Pipitone, N. Neuroimaging findings in acute Wernicke's encephalopathy: review of the literature. *AJR Am J Roentgenol* 2009; **192**:501–8.

64. Ambrose, ML, Bowden, SC, Whelan, G. Thiamin treatment and working memory function of alcohol-dependent people: preliminary findings. *Alcohol Clin Exp* 2001; *Res* **25**:112–16.

65. Day, E, Bentham, P, Callaghan, R, Kuruvilla, T, George, S. Thiamine for Wernicke-Korsakoff Syndrome in people at risk from alcohol abuse. *Cochrane Database Syst Rev* 2004; (4):1–20.

66. Wilkinson, TJ, Hanger, HC, Elmslie, J, George, PM, Sainsbury, R. The response to treatment of subclinical thiamine deficiency in the elderly. *Am J Clin Nutr* 1997; **66**: 925–8.

67. Donnino, MW, Vega, J, Miller, J, Walsh, M. Myths and misconceptions of Wernicke's encephalopathy: what every emergency physician should know. *Ann Emerg Med* 2007; **50**:715–21.

68. Thomson, AD, Cook, CC, Touquet, R, Henry, JA, Royal College of Physicians L. The Royal College of Physicians report on alcohol: guidelines for managing Wernicke's encephalopathy in the accident and Emergency Department. *Alcohol Alcoholism* 2002; **37**:513–21.

69. Sechi, G, Serra, A. Wernicke's encephalopathy: new clinical settings and recent advances in diagnosis and management. *Lancet Neurol* 2007; **6**:442–55.

70. Thomson, AD, Marshall, EJ. The natural history and pathophysiology of Wernicke's encephalopathy and Korsakoff's psychosis. *Alcohol Alcoholism* 2006; **41**:151–8.

71. Baker, H, Frank, O. Absorption, utilization and clinical effectiveness of allithiamines compared to water-soluble thiamines. *J Nutr Sci Vitaminol (Tokyo)* 1976; **22**(suppl):63–8.

72. Thomson, AD, Ryle, PR, Shaw, GK. Ethanol, thiamine and brain damage. *Alcohol Alcoholism* 1983; **18**:27–43.

73. Brown, LM, Rowe, AE, Ryle, PRMSK, Jones, D, Thomson, AD, Shaw, GK. Efficacy of vitamin supplementation in chronic alcoholics undergoing detoxification. *Alcohol Alcoholism* 1983; **18**:157–66.

74. Wrenn, KD, Murphy, F, Slovis, CM. A toxicity study of parenteral thiamine hydrochloride. *Ann Emerg Med* 1989; **18**:867–70.

75. Thomson, AD, Marshall, EJ. The treatment of patients at risk of developing Wernicke's encephalopathy in the community. *Alcohol Alcoholism* 2006; **41**:159–67.

76. Harper, C. Thiamine (vitamin B1) deficiency and associated brain damage is still common throughout the world and prevention is simple and safe! *Eur J Neurol* 2006; **13**: 1078–82.

77. Rolland, S, Truswell, AS. Wernicke-Korsakoff syndrome in Sydney hospitals after 6 years of thiamine enrichment of bread. *Public Health Nutr* 1998; **1**:117–22.

78. Hoyumpa, AM, Jr. Mechanisms of thiamin deficiency in chronic alcoholism. *Am J Clin Nutr* 1980; **33**:2750–61.

79. Meierkord, H, Boon, P, Engelsen, B. *et al.* EFNS guideline on the management of status epilepticus in adults. *Eur J Neurol* 2010; **17**:348–55.

80. Basoglu, M, Yetimalar, Y, Gurgor, N. *et al.* Neurological complications of prolonged hunger strike. *Eur J Neurol* 2006; **13**:1089–97.

CHAPTER 18

Recommendations for the diagnosis and management of spontaneous intracerebral haemorrhage

T. Steiner,[1] M. Kaste,[2] M. Forsting,[3] D. Mendelow,[4] H. Kwiecinski,[5] I. Szikora,[6] S. Juvela,[2] A. Marchel,[5] R. Chapot,[7] C. Cognard,[8] A. Unterberg[1] and W. Hacke[1,9]

The European Stroke Initiative (EUSI) Writing Committee Writing Committee for the EUSI Executive Committee
[1]Heidelberg University Hospital, Heidleberg, Germany; [2]Helsinki, Finland; [3]Essen University Hospital ; [4]University Hospital, Newcastle Upon Tyne, UK; [5]formerly Medical University of Warsaw, Warsaw, Poland; [6]National Institute of Neurosciences, Budapest, Hungary; [7]Klinik für Radiologie und Neuroradiologie, Alfried Krupp Krankenhaus, Rüttenscheid, Essen, Germany; [8]Le Centre Régional de Radiochirurgie Stéréotaxique, Centra Hopitalier Universitaire de Toulouse, Toulouse, France; [9]For the ESO (European Stroke Organization) writing committee

Introduction

Intracerebral haemorrhage (ICH) and subarachnoid haemorrhage (SAH) are responsible for about 20% of all strokes [1–6]. Within the last 15 years knowledge in this field based on prospective and randomized controlled trials (RCTs) has accumulated. The concept of rebleeding or growth of haematoma in spontaneous ICH has been prospectively described [7–9], coiling has been shown to become an important therapeutic option in SAH [10] and the molecular mechanisms of consecutive damage after haemorrhage were further identified. Several RCTs for treatment of ICH or SAH are available [11–13].

After the second edition of the European Stroke Initiative (EUSI) Recommendations for acute ischaemic stroke in 2003 [14], the Executive Committee of the EUSI felt that there were enough data to address recommendations for the treatment of spontaneous ICH including spontaneous and subarachnoid haemorrhage.

In December 2004 members of the executive committee and writing committee met for 2 days in Heidelberg, Germany and prepared these recommendations: on the management of ICH.

The levels of evidence in this chapter correspond to those published by the European Federation of Neurological Societies (EFNS) and are listed in Table 18.1 [15]. In the recommendations we give levels A–C and, if the data represents good clinical practice or are unknown, we refer to class IV.

Incidence, mortality and prognosis

ICH is responsible for 10–17% of all strokes [6, 16–18]. The incidence of ICH is influenced by racial factors and was found to be higher in black, Hispanic and Asian individuals compared with the white population [16, 19, 20].

The 30-day mortality rate correlates with the size and location of the initial bleeding [7, 21]. In patients with an initial volume of >60 cm^3 the mortality rate was 93%

European Handbook of Neurological Management: Volume 2, Second Edition. Edited by Nils Erik Gilhus, Michael P. Barnes, Michael Brainin.
© 2012 Blackwell Publishing Ltd. Published 2012 by Blackwell Publishing Ltd.

Table 18.1 Evidence classification scheme.

	For therapeutic intervention	For diagnostic procedures
Class I	An adequately powered prospective, randomized controlled, clinical trial with masked outcome assessment in a representative population OR an adequately powered systematic review of prospective, randomized controlled, clinical trials with masked outcome assessment in representative populations. The following are required: (a) Randomization concealment (b) Primary outcome(s) is/are clearly defined (c) Exclusion/inclusion criteria are clearly defined (d) Adequate accounting for dropouts and crossovers with numbers sufficiently low to have minimal potential for bias (e) Relevant baseline characteristics are presented and substantially equivalent among treatment groups or there is appropriate statistical adjustment for differences	A prospective study in a broad spectrum of people with the suspected condition, using a 'gold standard' for case definition, where the test is applied in a blinded evaluation, and enabling the assessment of appropriate tests of diagnostic accuracy
Class II	Prospective matched group cohort study in a representative population with masked outcome assessment that meets a–e above or a randomized controlled trial in a representative population that lacks one criteria of a–e	A prospective study of a narrow spectrum of people with the suspected condition, or a well-designed retrospective study of a broad spectrum of persons with an established condition (by 'gold standard') compared with a broad spectrum of controls, where test is applied in a blinded evaluation, and enabling the assessment of appropriate tests of diagnostic accuracy
Class III	All other controlled trials (including well-defined natural history controls or patients serving as own controls) in a representative population, where outcome assessment is independent of patient treatment	Evidence provided by a retrospective study where either people with the established condition or controls are of a narrow spectrum, and where the test is applied in a blinded evaluation
Class IV	Evidence from uncontrolled studies, case series, case reports or expert opinion	Any design where test is not applied in blinded evaluation OR evidence provided by expert opinion alone or in descriptive case series (without controls)
Rating of recommendations		
Level A	Effective, ineffective or harmful – requires at least one convincing class I study or at least two consistent, convincing class II studies	established as useful/ predictive or not useful/ predictive – requires at least one convincing class I study or at least two consistent, convincing class II studies
Level B	Probably effective, ineffective, or harmful) requires at least one convincing class II study or overwhelming class III evidence	Probably useful/ predictive or not useful/ predictive – requires at least one convincing class II study or overwhelming class III evidence
Level C	Possibly effective, ineffective or harmful – rating requires at least two convincing class III studies	Possibly useful/ predictive or not useful/ predictive – requires at least two convincing class III studies

According to Brainin et al. 2004 [15].

for deep haemorrhage and 71% for lobar bleeding. In patients with a volume between 30 and 60 cm³ the mortality rate was 64% for deep haemorrhage, 60% for lobar bleeding and 75% for cerebellar haemorrhages. If initial volumes were <30 cm³ the mortality rate decreased to 23% for deep haemorrhage, 7% for lobar location and 57% for cerebellar haemorrhages [22].

In retrospective studies between 35 and 52% of patients were found to have died within 1 month of ICH onset and only 20% of patients regain functional independence by 6 months [22–24]. Treatment within specialized neurological/neuro surgical (neurosurgical) intensive care units (NICUs) can decrease the mortality rate to 28–38% compared with treatment on general intensive care units (ICUs) of 25–83% [25]. Besides volume of ICH and Glasgow Coma Scale (GCS) score on admission, age >80 years, infratentorial origin of ICH and the presence of intraventricular blood were found to be independent predictors of the 30-day mortality rate [26]. However, this should be applied with caution, because the single most important factor predicting survival after ICH was the implementation of do-not-resuscitate orders [27]. This may be responsible for a pessimistic overestimation of prognosis in ICH.

Complications of ICH

Subsequent increase of the bleeding is an early complication after ICH. The frequency of increasing bleeding is high, although it is not clear whether growth of volume is due to rebleeding or continuous bleeding. Brott et al. [7] showed that 'growth', defined as a 33% increase of haematoma volume on cerebral computed tomography (CCT), occurred in 26% of 103 patients within 4 hours of first symptoms. Another 12% had growth within the following 20 hours. Haemorrhage growth was significantly associated with clinical deterioration [7]. These findings are supported by three retrospective studies [8, 9, 28]. Enlargements of ICH are also seen when observation periods are extended up to 48 hours, although the frequency diminishes with time from onset of symptoms [9]. Predictors of haemorrhage expansion include initial haematoma volume, early presentation, irregular shape, liver disease, hypertension, hyperglycaemia, alcohol use and hypofibrinogenaemia [8, 21].

Of patients with spontaneous ICH 36–50% have additional IVH [29]. Tuhrim reported that the 30-day mortality rate was 43% for patients with ICH compared with

9% in patients with only intraparenchymal blood. Intraventricular blood volume was significantly associated with the probability of mortality at day 30 [29]. Location of parenchymal origin of the ICH, distribution of ventricular blood and total volumes have been reported to be predictors of outcome in patients with spontaneous ICH and intraventricular extension [30, 31]. Furthermore hydrocephalus was found to be an independent predictor of early mortality [32].

Brain oedema after ICH is observed in the acute and subacute phase and may increase for up to 14 days [33, 34]. Shrinking of the haematoma due to clot retraction leads to an accumulation of serum in the early phase [35]. Thrombin and several serum proteins were found to be involved in the inflammatory reaction of the perihaematomal zone [36–39]. Factors released from activated platelets at the site of bleeding, such as vascular endothelial growth factor, may interact with thrombin to increase vascular permeability and contribute to the development of oedema [40]. Several studies in spontaneous ICH suggest that the role of perihaematomal ischaemia is small at most. Magnetic resonance imaging (MRI) found decreased perfusion but no ischaemia in the perilesional zone [41, 42], whereas positron emission tomography (PET) found intact autoregulation in the perihaematomal area [43] and only a reactive reduction of cerebral blood flow (CBF) consistent with oligaemia and diaschisis [43, 44].

Causes

ICH should be classified into spontaneous ICH, where no cause for ICH are found or secondary (15–20%) causes were found. About 30% of ICHs are found in association with cerebral amyloid angiopathy (CAA) [45]. Other causes may be aneurysms, arteriovenous malformations (AVMs), coagulopathies, liver cirrhosis, neoplasms, trauma, vasculitis, moyamoya disease, sinus venous thrombosis, eclampsia and cerebral endometriosis.

ICHs preferentially occur at certain locations, which are associated with specific underlying diseases. Thus, lobar bleeding is often seen in elderly patients with CAA [46, 47]. Amyloid angiopathy is a common cause of ICH in occipital and parietal regions, particularly in elderly people (>70 years) [48, 49]. In a recent study of genotype and haplotype association, apolipoprotein E$_4$ was found to be independently associated with lobar ICH but not with non-lobar ICH [50].

Risk factors

Arterial hypertension is the most common risk factor for spontaneous ICH and the frequency has been estimated to be between 70 and 80% [5]. The role of hypertension is supported by the high frequency of left ventricular hypertrophy at postmortem examination of patients with ICH, although there are clinical series where the history of hypertension, EEG and chest X-ray evidence suggested hypertension in only 56% of patients with ICH [51]. The role of hypertension and the beneficial effect of antihypertensive treatment with regard to risk of ICH were verified in the PROGRESS trial [52]. The relative risk of ICH was reduced by 50% in comparison with the placebo-treated group after 4 years of follow-up.

Other risk factors for ICH, in addition to age, hypertension and ethnicity, include cigarettes, oral anticoagulants, antiplateletes, smoking, alcohol consumption and low serum cholesterol levels [53]:

In a population-based case–control study hypercholesterolaemia was associated with a lower risk of ICH. On the other hand, treatment with statins did not increase the risk of ICH [54]. This may be in contrast to the findings from a recently presented secondary prevention trail (STARCL).

The risk of haemorrhagic stroke including ICH was 2.5 times higher in smokers [55]. Both the Physicians' Health Study [56] and the Women's Health Study [57] confirmed the role of smoking as a risk factor for ICH. For men smoking 20 cigarettes or more the relative risk of ICH was 2.06 (95% confidence interval [CI] 1.08–3.96) and for women smoking 15 cigarettes or more the relative risk was 2.67 (95% CI 1.04–6.90) [56, 57].

An increasing body mass index (BMI) was found to be correlated with an increasing size of IVH volume [58].

Several studies document an increased risk of ICH in relation to alcohol consumption [59, 60]. Spontaneous ICH can probably also be triggered by binge drinking [60].

A variety of coagulopathies can lead to cerebral haemorrhage and anticoagulation accounts from 4% up to 20% of ICH in different series. Anticoagulation increases the risk of ICH 8–11 times to that in patients with similar age who are not on anticoagulation [48, 61, 62]. In a meta-analysis of 16 RCTs ($n = 55462$), aspirin therapy was shown to increase the risk of ICH (12 events per 10 000). However, this effect did not outweigh the net benefit of reducing the risk in myocardial infarction (reduction of 137 per 10 000) or ischaemic stroke (reduc-

tion of 39 per 10 000) [63]. The risk of ICH was significantly increased by the combination of aspirin and clopidogrel when compared with aspirin alone, given for secondary prevention in high-risk patients with recent ischaemic stroke or transient ischaemic attack (TIA) [64]. Moreover, Toyoda and colleagues published a retrospective study in which they found prior antiplatelet to be an independent predictor of haematoma enlargement, measured on the second day in the hospital [65].

A variety of illicit drugs is known to cause ICH. The best known of these are amphetamines and cocaine and this possibility should be kept in mind in young patients in whom other causes such as AVMs or traumas have been excluded [49, 61]. Also, thrombolysis of cerebral ischaemic infarction may increase the risk of ICH [66]. Brain tumours, vasculitis and various vasculopathies including sinus thrombosis are important causes of ICH [49, 61].

Location and clinical symptoms

The clinical presentation of ICH depends on its site, size and speed of development. About 80% of ICHs occur in the cerebral hemispheres, with about 40% in the basal ganglia, 30% in the thalamus, 20% lobar, and about 10% in the cerebellum and pons [7, 11, 13, 67].

The striatum (caudate nucleus and putamen) is the most common site of ICH. The most common type of spontaneous onset is a gradual smooth progression of symptoms over minutes and sometimes over hours, usually beginning with hemiparesis [49]. Gradual development is due to bleeding from small penetrating vessels under arteriolar or capillary pressure. Another type of onset is an abrupt development of symptoms with a reduced level of consciousness over a few moments.

Bleeding directly in the brain parenchyma rather than the cerebrospinal fluid (CSF) space is painless due to the fact that the brain is devoid of pain fibres, so that the initial bleed causes no headache but neurological symptoms based in the region. If the haematoma starts in the putamen, it causes contralateral limb weakness and hemisensory symptoms, whereas bleeding in the thalamus causes greater hemisensory loss and hemiparesis. As the bleeding area grows, the weakness becomes more severe and sensory symptoms, loss of speech depending on the side of the bleed and conjugate eye deviation to the side of ICH might ensue, together with reduced level of consciousness. If the haematoma continues to grow, it may lead to coma and death as a result of increased intracranial pressure (ICP) and compression of brain-stem centres. Oculomotor signs such as forced downward gaze, convergence paralysis and unreactive miotic pupils suggest thalamic haemorrhage. The clinical presentation also involves slight contralateral motor hemiparesis and greater hemisensory loss.

Vomiting is a typical sign of ICH caused by increased intracranial pressure and distortion of the brain structures. Nearly half of patients with hemispheric ICH and more than half of those with posterior circulation haemorrhages vomit, whereas patients with cerebellar haemorrhages almost always vomit early in the clinical course.

Headache is not an invariable symptom of ICH. Patients with small deep haematomas often have no headache any time during their illness, whereas headache is much more common in large haematomas and those rupturing in the CSF with meningeal irritation. Headache is often accompanied by vomiting and decreased level of consciousness when the haematoma enlarges, but it may be the sole manifestation of caudate haemorrhage, which is usually accompanied by ventricular extension of the haemorrhage.

Several attempts were made to clinically differentiate supratentorial haemorrhagic from ischaemic stroke [68, 69]. Weir and co-workers showed that the sensitivity and specificity of scoring systems is not reliable in predicting haemorrhagic stroke [70]. In conclusion, symptoms of haemorrhagic stroke cannot be differentiated from those caused by an ischaemic stroke. Imaging is always needed to confirm the diagnosis of ICH.

Imaging intracerebral haemorrhage

The sensitivity of CT in intracerebral haemorrhage has been proven in several studies [71–73]. Acute haemorrhage is hyperdense, with Hounsfield units between 40 and 60 HU. The only clinical exceptions are patients with a low haematocrit, due to the low haemoglobin concentration when even the acute haematoma can be isodense [74]. Over time – with a decrease of 2 HU/day – the haematoma becomes isodense and then hypodense.

The appearance of ICH on MRI depends on a variety of technical and biological variables, such as field strength, sequences and age of the haematoma [75]. As a rule of thumb for 1.5 tesla: a hyperacute haematoma is isointense on T1-weighted and hyperintense on T2-weighted images. During the hyperacute stage, the MRI protocol should always include T2*- and/or proton density (PD)-weighted images. Later on (beyond 7 days) the methaemoglobin appears bright on T1- and T2-weighted images. In the chronic stage a dark rim of haemosiderin is typical on MR images and best seen on T2- or T2*-weighted images.

When analysing the images, an attempt should be made to differentiate between hypertensive and non-hypertensive ICH in order to optimize the subsequent diagnostic work-up. Haemorrhages that originate in the putamen, globus pallidus, thalamus, internal capsule, periventricular white matter, pons and cerebellum, particularly in a patient with known hypertension, are often attributed to hypertensive small-vessel disease [76]. In these patients further imaging studies investigating the underlying vascular pathology are not necessary. Follow-up with CT or MRI might be necessary, particularly for patients with intraventricular haemorrhages and those with clinical deterioration.

There is an ongoing discussion about whether further work-up is needed for patients with deep basal ganglia location of the ICH, who have chronic hypertension. This goes back to the old concept that ICH in association with chronic hypertension is a 'disease entity' in itself. This concept can no longer be regarded as sufficient: first, because hypertension can be found in as many patients with deep as with lobar location of the ICH [77]; and second, because there should be an underlying cerebrovascular disease as a consequence of chronic hypertension that caused the bleeding. This might be arteriosclerotic micro- or macroangiopathy which increases with age. Thus, particularly in younger patents with ICH and chronic hypertension, it seems not sufficient to stop searching for a cause of the ICH by just performing one initial CT. Further diagnostic work-up should include MR angiography (MRA), CT angiography (CTA) and/or digital subtraction angiography (DSA). The same is true for patients with lobar haemorrhages. T2*-weighted MRI is suspicious of an underlying amyloid angiopathy if it reveals multiple cortical and subcortical old haemorrhages [78].

For patients requiring emergency surgical evacuation, the fastest and most effective technique revealing the underlying vascular pathology is CTA [79]. Alternatively, MRA can be performed [80]. Under such emergency conditions, DSA is also acceptable, but generally not required. Aneurysms larger than 3 mm and larger AVMs – not requiring a specific technique – can be recognized with cross-sectional angiographic methods [79–81].

MRI is the optimal technique to demonstrate low-flow vascular malformations (cavernomas), haemorrhagic tumours and other vascular pathologies. CTA or MRA is the method of choice to demonstrate dural sinus thrombosis as the underlying cause of ICH.

DSA is the optimal technique to demonstrate underlying high-flow vascular malformations. As larger ICHs may change the haemodynamics of AVMs to an extent that the malformation cannot be seen on CTA or MRA, DSA can be electively performed in a delayed fashion.

Recommendations

1. The sensitivity for acute ICH – including SAH – is almost equal between CT and MRI, if the MRI protocol includes T2*- and/or PD-weighted images. However, patient monitoring is still easier in CT (level A recommendation).

2. If urgent surgical evacuation of a non-hypertensive ICH is indicated, the underlying vascular pathology should be studied preferably by CTA, or alternatively by MRA or DSA (class IV evidence).

3. If urgent surgical evacuation of a supposedly non-hypertensive ICH is not indicated, the underlying vascular pathology should be investigated by:

   (a) MRI if the suspected lesion is a cavernoma, or cerebral amyloid angiopathy

   (b) CTA or MRA if the suspected lesion is dural sinus thrombosis

   (c) DSA if the suspected lesion is a ruptured aneurysm or a pial or dural AVM. These studies may be done as elective procedure except if aneurysm rupture is assumed (class IV evidence).

Emergency management and general treatment

There are five main areas in the treatment of acute intracerebral haemorrhage:

1. General treatment does not substantially differ from the treatment of ischaemic stroke. The neurological status and vital functions (blood pressure, pulse rate, oxygenation, temperature) should be continuously or regularly monitored.

2. Specific therapy directed against the growth of the haematoma is currently subject to surgery and ongoing RCTs.

3. Prevention and treatment of complications, which may be either neurological (such as space-occupying oedema or seizures) or medical (such as aspiration, infections, decubital ulcers, DVT or PE).

4. Early secondary prevention to reduce the incidence of early recurrence of ICH. Apart from treatment of increased blood pressure and withholding the use of antithrombotic drugs, early secondary prevention does not substantially differ from secondary prevention in stroke in general, which was detailed in the 2003 EUSI recommendations [14].

5. Early rehabilitation is also essential for ICH patients. Again, there are no substantial differences to the 2003 EUSI recommendations for acute ischaemic stroke [14].

General stroke treatment and monitoring

The term 'general treatment' refers to clinical and instrumental monitoring as well as treatment strategies aimed at stabilizing the acutely ill patient. This not only provides an optimum physiological basis upon which specific therapeutic strategies can be applied [14, 82], but also represents a cornerstone of stroke treatment by treating other medical problems that may significantly influence stroke outcome. All patients with ICH should be treated in stroke units if such a unit exists in the hospital or on an ICU if the patient's condition requires this. Stroke unit care reduces mortality and increases the likelihood of good functional outcome of stroke in general [25]. There is a consensus that the management of general medical problems is the basis for stroke treatment [14, 82]. It is generally believed that ICH survivors have better neurological and functional prognoses than the survivors of ischaemic stroke [83].

General treatment of patients with stroke and ICH needs monitoring of clinical development and physiological functions. Neurological status is best monitored using validated neurological scales. The National Institutes of Heath (NIH) Stroke Scale [84] and the GCS [85] are the most frequently used. Other scales such as Scandinavian Stroke Scale [86] or the Unified Neurological Stroke Scale may also used. However, it is essential that a centre concentrate on the use of one scale only. The ICH score is an instrument that may allow risk stratification of ICH patients on admission [26].

General management of all stroke patients including those with ICH comprises respiratory and cardiac care, fluid and metabolic management and blood pressure control. In addition prophylactic measures concerning deep venous thrombosis (DVT), pulmonary embolism (PE), aspiration pneumonia, other infections and decubital ulcer are part of the general treatment of the patients.

Vital functions, pulmonary function, airway protection, glucose, body temperature, fluid balance, electrolytes and decubital ulcers are mostly comparable with the ESO recommendations for ischaemic stroke [87]. In the next sections we describe only those management procedures in ICH patients that are different from ischaemic stroke.

Blood pressure management

Blood pressure monitoring and treatment are a critical issue in acute ICH general treatment, although it remains controversial due to the fact that there are no randomized trials to guide the management. Reducing blood pressure in acute ICH may prevent or retard the growth of the haematoma and also decrease the risk of rebleeding, but reduced cerebral perfusion pressure (CPP) could compromise adequate CBF due to increased intracranial pressure. Qureshi and co-workers kept the blood pressure of 27 patients with acute ICH <160 mmHg (systolic) and 90 mmHg (diastolic) in a prospective trial [88]. They found a haematoma growth in 9%. This is remarkably lower than the number found by Brott et al. in a prospective study that did not primarily target blood pressure measurement. In Brott et al.'s study the growth was observed in 38% within 24 hours of symptom onset [7]. Stroke patients are frequently chronically hypertensive and their brain hydraulic autoregulatory curve is shifted to the right. This means that, although in normal individuals CBF is constant at a mean arterial pressure (MAP) of approximately 50–150 mmHg, hypertensive stroke patients can tolerate higher MAP levels better, whereas they are at risk of critical hypoperfusion at MAP levels usually well tolerated by normotensive individuals. MAP should be gradually reduced to <130 mmHg in people with a history of chronic hypertension, but a reduction of more than 20% should be avoided and MAP should not be reduced to <84 mmHg [89].

The INTERACT study randomized 200 patients to either intensive blood pressure-lowering therapy below a systolic pressure of 140 mmHg or to a group that was treated according to the American Heart Association [AHA] guidelines (blood pressure <180 mmHg) [90]. It was found that there was a significant difference in the mean proportional difference of blood volume increase in favour of patient who did receive intensive blood pressure-lowering therapy.

The ATACH looked at safety and feasibility of blood pressure-lowering therapy in three target groups (systolic pressure within a range of 170–200 mmHg [group 1], 140–170 mmHg [group 2] and 110–140 mmHg [group 3]). None of the predefined stopping thresholds needed to be activated [91].

Currently INTERACT-2 and ATACH-2 are running to confirm their results on a clinical endpoint.

Based on these data, and until results are available from ongoing trials, an upper limit of systolic blood pressure of 180 mmHg and a diastolic blood pressure of 105 mmHg is recommended for patients with known prior hypertension or signs (ECG, retina) of chronic hypertension. If treatment is necessary, target blood pressure should be 170/100 (or MAP 125 mmHg). In patients without known hypertension, upper recommended limits are 160/95 mmHg). If treatment is necessary, the target blood pressure should be 150/90 (or MAP 110 mmHg).

These limits and targets should be adapted (increased) to higher values in patients with monitoring of increased intracranial pressure (ICP) to guarantee a sufficient cerebral perfusion pressure (CCP = MAP − ICP) of at least 60 to 70 mmHg, however these are data derived from traumatic brain injury.

Treatment may be appropriate in the setting of concomitant acute myocardial ischaemia (although extreme lowering of blood pressure is deleterious for myocardial infarction patients as well), cardiac insufficiency, acute renal failure, acute hypertensive encephalopathy or aortic arch dissection.

In patients with ischaemic stroke, sublingual calcium antagonists should be avoided because of the risk of abrupt reduction of blood pressure [92], possible ischaemic steal [82, 93–96] and overshoot hypertension. However, these concepts may possibly not apply to spontaneous ICH, because there is no evidence of an ischaemic penumbra [41, 42, 44]. Nevertheless, oral and intravenous administration of calcium antagonists should be used carefully, because of their rapid and excessive effect. The same may be true for subcutaneous clonidine. In both cases, the duration of action is hard to predict. Oral captopril (6.25–12.5 mg) has been recommended as an oral first-line drug [97], but has a short duration of action and can have an abrupt effect. In USA and Canada, intravenous labetalol 10 mg, which is not available everywhere in Europe, or enalapril is frequently recommended. Intravenous urapidil is also increasingly used. Finally, sodium nitroprusside is sometimes necessary despite some major side effects, such as reflex tachycardia coronary artery ischaemia, antiplatelet action and increasing ICP [98]. Intravenous treatment of hypertension should always be accompanied by continuous regular blood pressure monitoring. In an ICU, blood pressure monitoring with an intra-arterial line is advisable [99]. Intravenous antihypertensive drugs that may be used in acute ICH are listed in the Table 18.2.

Treatment of complications
Management of increased ICP

Increased ICP, brain oedema and mass effect are associated with high morbidity and mortality after ICH. Some patients with suspected intracranial hypertension and decreasing level of consciousness might require invasive ICP monitoring, although its added value beyond clinical or radiological monitoring has not been proven yet. The aim of treating elevated ICP is to maintain the CPP above 60–70 mmHg, knowing that CPP = MAP − ICP.

The main methods of medical decompression for increased ICP include: controlled hyperventilation, osmotic diuretics and intravenous barbiturates (Table 18.3). They are most useful to bridge the time to surgery, if the latter is planned. Corticosteroids are not recommended and they should be avoided in the treatment of the acute phase of ICH [5, 100].

The aim of therapeutic hyperventilation is to achieve arterial PCO_2 levels of 4.0–4.7 kPa (30–35 mmHg). The beneficial effects of controlled hyperventilation are transient and this method is usually most useful in the first hours after its institution. Lack of reduction of increased ICP with hyperventilation means is a poor prognostic sign for ICH patients. Mannitol produces a rapid lowering of ICP and the effect is observed already within 20 min from the intravenous bolus, which suggests that this effect may be independent of subsequent diuresis.

Mannitol (20%) in a dose of 0.75–1.0 g/kg is given as intravenous bolus that is followed by 0.25–0.5 g/kg every 3–6 hours depending on the neurological status, fluid balance and serum osmolality, which should be kept at ≤310 mosmol/l. Mannitol can be safely used for periods of not more than 5 days, after which it can cause renal failure and electrolyte disturbances. Prolonged use leads to mannitol accumulation within the tissue, producing an osmotic effect that exacerbates oedema. If intracranial hypertension cannot be controlled with osmotic therapy and hyperventilation, induced barbiturate coma may be considered [101]. Barbiturates have been shown to reduce CBF and metabolism, which result in a decline in ICP. Pentobarbital is the most commonly used agent in a loading dose 3–10 mg/kg, by infusing at a rate of 1 mg/kg per min. The experience with high doses of barbiturates in ICH patients is still limited and further clinical studies are needed.

Seizure

In a prospective study, the incidence of post-haemorrhagic seizures – as proven by continuous EEG – was found to be higher than for ischaemic stroke. Eighteen of 63 (28%) patients with ICH showed electrographic evidence of seizure compared with 3 of 46 (6%) patients who had had an ischaemic stroke [102]. Seizures occurred in 21% of subcortical haemorrhages. They were more common in lobar haemorrhages. Seizures were associated with neurological worsening and an increase in midline shift. The rate of increase on NIHSS was significantly higher in patients with seizures. Age and initial NIHSS were independent predictors of outcome [105].

In another prospective, study, 4.2% (32/761) had their clinically detected initial seizure at the onset of the haemorrhage or within 24 hours [103]. Twenty-five patients (3.8%) had their first seizures within 29 days. One of the 32 patients with immediate (within 24 hours) seizure had a recurrent seizure within the next 29 days though it is not clear whether this patient did receive prophylactic treament. The occurrence of seizures was elevated in patients with lobar location and small-sized ICH. Early seizures were associated with lobar location and neurological complications, mainly rebleeding. In this study the prophylactic use of antiepileptic treatment in patients with lobar location did lead to a reduction in seizures.

Table 18.2 Intravenous antihypertensive drugs that may be used in acute ICH.

Drug	Dose	Onset of action (min)	Duration of action	Comments
Adrenergic inhibitors				
Labetalol	20–80 mg bolus every 10 min, up to 300 mg; 0.5–2.0 mg/min infusion	5–10	3–6 h	Indicated in ischaemic and haemorrhagic stroke; contraindicated in acute heart failure
Esmolol	250–500 µg/kg per min bolus, then 50–100 µg/kg per min infusion	1–2	10–30 min	Indicated in stroke and aortic dissection; contraindicated in bradycardia, atrioventricular block, heart failure and bronchospasm
Urapidil	12.5–25 mg bolus; 5–40 mg/h infusion	3–5	4–6 h	Indicated in most hypertensive emergencies including stroke; avoid in coronary ischaemia
Vasodilators				
Nitroprusside[a]	0.25–10 µg/kg per min as infusion	Within seconds	2–5 min	Indicated in most hypertensive emergencies including stroke, when diastolic BP >140 mmHg; contraindicated in high ICP
Nicardipine	5–15 mg/h infusion	5–10	0.5–4 h	Indicated in stroke; contra-indicated in acute heart failure, coronary ischemia and aortic stenosis
Enalaprilat	1.25–5 mg every 6 h	15–30	6–12 h	Indicated in acute left ventricular failure; avoid in acute MI and hypotension
Hydralazine	10–20 mg bolus	10–20	1–4 h	Indicated in eclampsia; avoid in tachycardia and coronary ischaemia
Fenoldopam	0.1–0.3 µg/kg per min infusion	<5	30 min	Indicated in most hypertensive emergencies including stroke; avoid in glaucoma, tachycardia and portal hypertension
Diuretics				
Furosemide	20–40 mg bolus	2–5	2–3 h	Avoid in hypokalaemia, eclampsia and phaeochromocytoma

[a] Nitroprusside is contraindicated in patients with high ICP;

AV, atrioventricular; ICH, intracerebral haemorrhage; ICP, intracranial pressure; MI, myocardial infarction.
Modified from Ringleb *et al.* [97]).

Table 18.3 Escalation scheme for treatment of intracranial pressure.

Measurement	Comment
Avoid situations that may lead to an elevation or aggravation of intracerebral pressure: pain, fever, psychological stress, physical stress (e.g. body positioning), hyponatraemia, hypertension	
Elevation of body positioning up to 30°	CCP >60 mmHg[a]
Mannitol (20%), intravenous, 100 ml (bolus), up to six times a day	Serum osmolarity <320 mmol/l
HyperHAES (NaCl 7.5%; HES 6%), intravenous, 150 ml bolus	Serum sodium <155 mmol/l
Paralytics, (e.g. vercuronium), titrate to effect	
Tris buffer, intravenous (central line), 1 mmol/kg bolus; 0.25 mmol/kg as permanent infusion	pH <7.5–7.55
	Caution: tissue necrosis (central line needed)
Consider haematoma evacuation with or without decompressive hemicraniectomy	
Barbiturates (thiopental), intravenous, 250–500 mg bolus	Caution: tissue necrosis, central line needed
	Caution: liver function disturbances
	Caution: usually marked decrease in MAP
Hyperventilation, increasing respiratory rate and tidal volume	PaO$_2$ 30–35 mmHg

[a]In case monitoring probe is in place, cerebral perfusion pressure should be kept >70 mmHg.
Tris, 2-amino-2-hydroxymethyl-propane-1,3-diol.

In an older study all epileptic seizures (17%; 19/112) occurred at ICH onset [104]. In this study there was no association between seizure and the size of the haemorrhage, but there was an association if the blood had extended into the cerebral cortex.

Furthermore, non-convulsive seizure or status epilepticus have been detected in 28% of stuporous or comatose patients [105, 106].

Prevention of DVT and PE

Prevention of DVT/PE is of major importance in the care of every stroke patient [107] and patients with ICH are no exception. Although graded compression stockings are effective in surgical patients, their efficacy in haemorrhagic stroke patients has not been verified [108–110]. The randomized controlled CLOTS study (routine care plus graduated compression stockings, thigh-length compression stocking versus routine care without stockings) in stroke patients did not find a benefit for stockings. Although subcutaneous heparin and low-molecular-weight heparin (LMWH) reduce venous thromboembolism, their effect is counterbalanced by an increase in haemorrhagic complications [111]. In patients with ICH they are usually withheld during the first days and administered only in patients at high risk of DVT or PE with half of the ordinary dose [112]. Depending on the choice of the drug, either activated prothrombin time (APTT) or anti-factor Xa tests should be used to monitor the level of anticoagulation. The initial use of intermittent pneumatic compression devices for DVT/PE prophylaxis in patients with acute ICH has been recently recommended by experts of the Seventh ACCP Conference on Antithrombotic and Thrombolytic Therapy [112]. Only in one small trial was low-dose heparin (5000 U) given subcutaneously to patients with ICH on day 2. They were compared with patients who had received their first dose of heparin either on day 4 or 10. There was a significantly smaller number of PE in patients who had received early heparin on day 2, whereas the number of patients with intracranial rebleeding was not increased [113]. The Seventh ACCP Conference on Antithrombotic and Thrombolytic Therapy panel of experts recommends that, in neurologically stable patients, a low dose of subcutaneous heparin (or LMWH) can be started on the second day after the onset of acute ICH [112].

Recommendations

1. All patients with ICH should preferably be treated in stroke units or on ICUs if the patient's condition requires this. Stroke unit care reduces mortality and increases the likelihood of good functional outcome of stroke in general [25]. Continuous cardiac monitoring is recommended in the first 48–72 hours of stroke onset, particularly in patients with: previously known cardiopathies, history of arrhythmias, unstable blood pressure, clinical signs/symptoms of heart failure, abnormal baseline ECG, haemorrhage involving the insular cortex (level C recommendation).

2. Immediate antihypertensive therapy is recommended in cases of ICH and heart failure, aortic dissection, acute myocardial infarction and acute renal failure, but it should be applied cautiously (class IV evidence).

3. Treatment is recommended if blood pressure is elevated above the following levels, confirmed by repeated measurements (class IV evidence):

    (a) Patients with known history of hypertension or signs (ECG, retina) of chronic hypertension: systolic blood pressure >180 mmHg and/or diastolic blood pressure >105 mmHg. If treated, target blood pressure should be 170/100 (or MAP 125 mmHg).

    (b) Patients without known hypertension: systolic blood pressure >160 mmHg and/or diastolic blood pressure >95 mmHg. If treated, target blood pressure should be 150/90 (or MAP 110 mmHg).

    (c) Reduction of MAP by more than 20% should be avoided.

    (d) These limits and targets should be adapted to higher values in patients with monitoring of increased ICP to guarantee a sufficient CPP >70 mmHg Recommended drugs for blood pressure treatment: intravenous labetalol or urapidil, intravenous sodium nitroprusside or nitroglycerin, and captopril (p.o.). Avoid oral nifedipine and any drastic blood pressure decrease (see Table 18.3).

4. Continuous ICP monitoring should be considered in patients who need mechanical ventilation for further therapeutic options (class IV evidence).

5. Medical treatment of elevated ICP should be started if deterioration can be related to increasing oedema (on CCT or MRI) (class IV evidence).

6. Medical treatment of elevated ICP includes glycerol, mannitol, HyperHAES and short-term hyperventilation (class IV evidence).

7. Compression stockings and intermittent pneumatic compression are not recommended for prevention of thromboembolism in patients with disabling limb weakness from the start of treatment (class Ia, level B). Low-dose subcutaneous heparin or LMWH should be considered after 24 h, especially in patients who are at high risk of thromboembolism (class IV evidence).

8. Early prophylactic treatment of seizures is not recommended for all patients, but may be considered for selected patients with lobar ICH. In all other cases seizures should be treated only if they occur (level C recommendation). If seizures occur, a step-wise administration of antiepileptic drugs is generally recommended (Table 18.4). Antiepileptic treatment should be continued for 30 days. After this time, treatment should be reduced and eventually discontinued. If seizures recur, patients should receive chronic treatment with anticonvulsants.

9. Other general measures (control of hyperglycaemia, hyperthermia, fluid management, nutrition, and prevention of aspiration pneumonia and bed sores) are the same as for patients with ischaemic stroke [14].

10. Early mobilization is recommended unless intracranial hypertension is present.

11. Early rehabilitation is recommended in patients with neurological deficits and should follow the same principles as in patients with ischaemic stroke (class IV evidence).

Specific treatment

Surgery

ICH represents a heterogeneous group of pathological conditions that deserve differentiation in order to clarify the different surgical treatment options. Surgical treatments should be considered separately according to whether the haemorrhage is supratentorial or infratentorial, and the presence or absence of aneurysms or other causes of spontaneous ICH.

Supratentorial non-aneurysmal ICH

Ten trials with 2059 participants were included in the latest Cochrane review on surgery in ICH. Surgery was associated with statistically significant reduction in the odds of being dead or dependent at final follow-up (odds ratio [OR] 0.71, 95% CI 0.58–0.88; $2P = 0.001$) with no significant heterogeneity among the study results. Surgery was also associated with significant reduction in the odds of death at final follow-up (OR 0.74, 95% CI 0.61–0.90; $2P = 0.003$). Although the quality of most of the trials

Table 18.4 Recommendation for the treatment of seizure/status epilepticus.

Step 1	
Lorazepam *or*	0.1 mg/kg body weight intravenously; 2 mg/min., if necessary repeated, max. 10 mg
Diazepam[a] *or*	0.25 mg/kg body weight intravenously; 5 mg/min, if necessary repeated, max. 30 mg
Clonazepam[a] *or*	1–2 mg intravenously; 0.5 mg/min., if necessary repeated, max. about 6 mg
Step 2	
Phenytoin[b]	15-20 mg/kg body weight intravenously at 50 mg/min over 5 min, remainder over 20–30 min, max. 30 mg/kg body weight
Step 3	
Phenobarbital	20 mg/kg body weight intravenously; 100 mg/min, higher doses possible if continuous EEG monitoring is available
Step 4	
Thiopental *or*	4–7 mg/kg body weight bolus, then 500 mg/h. EEG monitoring and burst-suppression pattern over 24 h
Propofol *or*	1–2 mg/kg body weight intravenous bolus, then 2–10 mg/kg per h
Midazolam *or*	0.2 mg/kg body weight intravenous bolus, then 0.8–1 µg/kg per min
Valproic acid	10–20 mg/kg body weight bolus or 1200 mg within the first hour, then 6 mg/kg per h (possibly significant elevation of phenytoin level)

[a]Diazepam or clonazepam, but not lorazepam, may be started within 10 min of the administration of phenytoin – through a separate intravenous line.
[b]If there is no effect and phenytoin was already used initially: benzodiazepine (as step 1), otherwise phenobarbital.
Modified following the recommendations of the German Neurological Society [194] and Mayer and Rincon [195].

was acceptable but not high, there was significant heterogeneity for death as the outcome (see Figure 18.1) [114].

There is thus some tendency towards support for early surgery. The adverse effect of ventricular blood [29] has not been considered in any of these trials, so that the effect of surgery on pure parenchymal ICH, without ventricular haemorrhage, has yet to be determined.

The largest of these trials was the Surgical Trial in Spontaneous Intracerebral Haemorrhage (STICH) and this showed, in 1033 patients, that early surgery (within 24 hours) was no different from initial conservative treatment (OR 0.89 with 95% CI 0.66–1.19) [11]. Clinical observation (with or without ICP/CPP monitoring) is therefore a reasonable management policy initially.

Prespecified post-hoc analysis in the STICH trial showed that two subgroups – deterioration in consciousness (from a GCS of between 9 and 12) and location (deep versus superficial) – approached significant benefit with early surgery and these permit the following considerations: consider craniotomy if there is deterioration from a GCS score of between 9 and 12 and/or if the clot is superficial (≤1 cm from surface). Deep-seated haematomas do not benefit from craniotomy. Stereotaxic aspiration may be considered. Both these procedures certainly call for more trials [115].

Cerebellar non-aneurysmal ICH

Cerebellar haemorrhage causes damage in two ways: it may produce direct compression of the cerebellum and brain stem with relevant symptoms and signs or hydrocephalus. Clot evacuation should be considered if there is neurological dysfunction or radiological evidence of obliteration of CSF spaces infratentorially [116]. Surprisingly good results have been reported with surgical evacuation of cerebellar haematomas, but the optimal timing has not been established and there are no prospective RCTs of surgery in cerebellar haemorrhage. By contrast there is universal clinical agreement on ventricular drainage for hydrocephalus at any time after ictus [117]. For this reason ventricular drainage and evacuation of the cerebellar haematoma should be considered if hydrocephalus occurs or if haematomas are larger than 2–3 cm in diameter, although advanced age and coma militate against favourable outcomes. All these data are derived from personal experience or retrospective studies.

Intraventricular haemorrhage

The outcome from ICH is much worse with intraventricular haemorrhage (IVH) [118]. This has not been taken into account in any of the surgical trials in ICH to date [119]. With intraventricular haemorrhage (IVH), hydrocephalus is common but blood clots will often block the drainage catheters. For this reason methods to maintain their patency have been evaluated. Intraventricular thrombolysis with urokinase or recombinant tissue plasminogen activator (rt-PA) via external ventricular drainage seems to

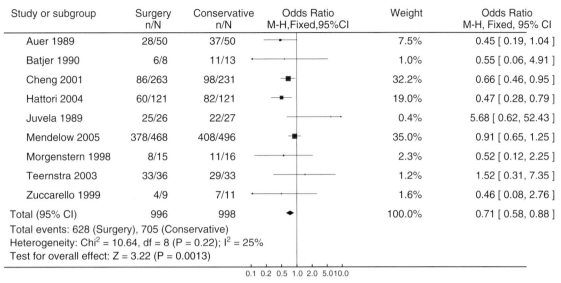

Study or subgroup	Surgery n/N	Conservative n/N	Odds Ratio M-H,Fixed,95%CI	Weight	Odds Ratio M-H, Fixed, 95% CI
Auer 1989	28/50	37/50		7.5%	0.45 [0.19, 1.04]
Batjer 1990	6/8	11/13		1.0%	0.55 [0.06, 4.91]
Cheng 2001	86/263	98/231		32.2%	0.66 [0.46, 0.95]
Hattori 2004	60/121	82/121		19.0%	0.47 [0.28, 0.79]
Juvela 1989	25/26	22/27		0.4%	5.68 [0.62, 52.43]
Mendelow 2005	378/468	408/496		35.0%	0.91 [0.65, 1.25]
Morgenstern 1998	8/15	11/16		2.3%	0.52 [0.12, 2.25]
Teernstra 2003	33/36	29/33		1.2%	1.52 [0.31, 7.35]
Zuccarello 1999	4/9	7/11		1.6%	0.46 [0.08, 2.76]
Total (95% CI)	996	998		100.0%	0.71 [0.58, 0.88]

Total events: 628 (Surgery), 705 (Conservative)
Heterogeneity: Chi^2 = 10.64, df = 8 (P = 0.22); I^2 = 25%
Test for overall effect: Z = 3.22 (P = 0.0013)

0.1 0.2 0.5 1.0 2.0 5.0 10.0
Favours surgery Favours conservative

Figure 18.1 Meta-analysis of the 9 prospective randomized controlled trials in spontaneous supratentorial intracerebral haemorrhage for death or dependency [114]).

be effective [120, 121]. More trials are needed and several are being conducted.

Treatment of hydrocephalus

Hydrocephalus may occur with any type of ICH. With SAH it is often the non-obstructive or 'communicating' type of hydrocephalus, whereas with intraventricular or parenchymal haemorrhage it is more likely to be of the obstructive or 'non-communicating' type, and with cerebellar haemorrhage it is always obstructive.

The methods of treatment depend on the type of hydrocephalus, although all types can be treated with ventricular access. The communicating type of hydrocephalus can be treated via the lumbar route, which is less invasive (no risk of epilepsy or brain haemorrhage).

Methods of treatment include observation if it is mild and does not cause any disturbance of consciousness. External drainage can be ventricular or via the lumbar route if it is a communicating type of hydrocephalus. Lumbar drainage is definitely contraindicated with all types of obstructive hydrocephalus or if the aetiology is in doubt. Intraventricular thrombolysis trials have been encouraging [121] but not in infants [122].

Internal drainage is achieved with a ventricular peritoneal shunt, or a lumbar peritoneal shunt if the hydrocephalus is of the communicating type. Endoscopic third ventriculostomy is seldom successful with hydrocephalus associated with acute haemorrhage [123] except perhaps in neonates [124]. Favourable results have been described in case series with intraoperative opening of the lamina terminalis and Lilliequist's membrane [125, 126]. There are no efficacy trials comparing any type of drainage with non-intervention or different routes of CSF access. There are a few trials comparing different shunt types but these have failed to show any difference. Antibiotic prophylaxis has been shown to be effective in CSF shunt operations [127].

ICH caused by AVMs

AVMs that cause haemorrhage are also a particular problem because of the risk of rebleeding. Management options include observation, embolization, surgical excision and stereotactic radiotherapy. Combinations of these treatments afford the best results and have to be considered at the time of the haemorrhage [128]. No prospective RCTs have been conducted but surgeons agree that surgical treatment of the AVM may be facilitated by the clot's, presence so timing of the surgery for the AVM should take place within about 2–3 months of the ictus if the surgeon is to take advantage of the dissection created by the haematoma. With unruptured AVMs a trial of surgery compared with conservative treatment has been initiated [129].

In general, endovascular embolization is an optional treatment modality for the treatment of the underlying vascular pathology including aneurysm, AVMs and developmental arteriovenous malformations (DAVMs), but excluding cavernomas [130, 131].

The goal of the endovascular embolization of an AVM or DAVM is to eliminate or reduce the size of and blood flow through the AVM nidus either as a sole treatment or as a preoperative method [130, 131].

Cavernous angiomas

Cavernous angiomas are structural vascular lesions of the brain and spinal cord that occasionally bleed. The estimated annual bleeding rate is 0.7% per year and per lesion [132–134]. Patients with one previous haemorrhage had an annual 4.5% risk of rebleeding. Usually, the consecutive haematoma is not life threatening, because cavernomas are part of the low-pressure system. The latter is the reason for the often negative DSA findings. In less than 10% of patients angiography reveals the vascular malformation. The highest diagnostic sensitivity is given by T2*-weighted MR sequences [132, 133]. In up to 30% cavernomas are associated with developmental venous anomalies (DVAs) and vice versa. All patients with a cavernoma should, therefore, have a contrast-enhanced MR scan in order to rule out an accompanying DVA. This is specifically important if the cavernoma is a candidate for surgical removal.

Therapy

Treatment options in cavernomas depend mainly on the natural course of the lesion, as well as its location and surgical accessibility. The last depends on the skill of the surgeon and the position of the lesion relative to eloquent areas of the brain [135].

In general, therapeutic strategies include:
• Observation of patients with asymptomatic or inaccessible lesions (class IV evidence)

• Surgical excision of symptomatic and accessible lesions (class IV evidence)
• Radiosurgery for progressively symptomatic but surgically inaccessible lesions [136] (class IV evidence).

The main indication for surgical removal of a cavernoma is prevention of haemorrhage. Therefore, many surgical groups recommend surgical removal of a cavernoma if it is located in a non-eloquent brain area and easily accessible [137]. However, it is quite difficult to predict the natural course of an individual cavernoma and, therefore, it is impossible to balance the individual bleeding risk of the individual patient against the morbidity and mortality of a surgical procedure (class IV evidence).

Haemostatic therapy

The use of haemostatic agents to control bleeding has been tried in ICH and SAH with various agents (tranexamic acid, ε-aminocaproic acid, aprotinin) [138–140]. These trials could not demonstrate safety or efficacy. Recombinant activated factor VIIa (rFVIIa) was developed for the treatment of patients with haemophilia and is thus also used to stop intracerebral bleeding in these patients [141, 142]. Factor VIIa initiates coagulation at the site of vessel disruption, so it may lead to thrombotic side effects.

Two prospective, randomized, placebo-controlled, dose-escalating, phase IIa trials demonstrated safety and feasibility for the use of (rFVIIa in 88 patients with spontaneous ICH within 4 hours of first symptoms [12, 143].

In a prospective, randomized, placebo-controlled trial, 400 patients with spontaneous ICH were treated with rFVIIa (40, 80, 160 μg/kg) within 4 h of ictus. Diagnosis had to be confirmed within 3 h. Patients with any history of ischaemic events were excluded. Treatment of ICH with rFVIIa within 4 h of onset limited haematoma expansion, decreased mortality and improved the 3-month clinical outcome, despite a significant 5% increase of arterial thromboembolic events within the highest dose rate (160 μg/kg) [13]. These included seven myocardial ischaemic events and nine cases of cerebral infarction; all but four of these occurred within 3 days of dosing. Two of the cases of cerebral infarction were massive and fatal, five were moderate in severity and disabling (two of these occurred 26 and 54 days after treatment and were not felt to be treatment related), and two were asymptomatic. With the exception of one patient with an anterior wall myocardial infarction who recovered with sequelae, the cardiac events that occurred in the rFVIIa-treated patients were characterized by small troponin I elevations, non-ST elevation ECG abnormalities and good recovery. Possibly or probably (as opposed to unlikely) treatment-related thromboembolic subarachnoid events that were fatal or disabling occurred in 2.0% of rFVIIa-treated patients compared with 2.1% in the placebo group.

Finally, the phase III trial, which included 816 patients, compared placebo and 20 and 80 µg/kg rFVIIa. That trial confirmed a significant reduction of haematoma expansion, but it failed to find a clinical effect of the treatment. Thromboembolic events were clearly increased in patients who had received rFVIIa [144].

Recommendations

- Consider craniotomy if there is deterioration in consciousness (from GCS level of between 12 and 9 to 8 or lower), if the ICH is superficial (the clot is subcortical ≤1 cm from the surface and does not reach deep basal ganglia) or if it is located in the cerebellum (level C recommendation).

- Deep-seated haematomas do not benefit from craniotomy. Stereotaxic aspiration may be considered (class IV evidence), especially if mass effect is present.

- Management options of AVMs include observation, embolization, surgical excision and focused radiotherapy. Combinations of these treatments afford the best results and have to be considered at the time of the haemorrhage. Surgical treatment takes place within about 2–3 months of the ictus if surgical excision is to be undertaken (class IV evidence).

- If patients have impaired level of consciousness and a haematoma at least 3 cm in diameter, consider emergency evacuation of the clot with excision of the AVM in the same operation if possible (class IV evidence).

- Use of rFVIIa leads to a reduction in haematoma expansion, but was not proved to be clinically effective. Furthermore the number of thromboembolic events was higher in patients treated with rFVIIa. Treatment of ICH with rFVIIa should is not recommended (class Ia, level A).

- External drainage (EVD) for hydrocephalus can be ventricular or via the lumbar route if it is a communicating type of hydrocephalus (class IV evidence). Lumbar drainage is definitely contraindicated with all types of obstructive hydrocephalus or if the aetiology is in doubt.

- Intraventricular thrombolysis trials may be considered if an EVD becomes necessary (class IV evidence) but not in infants.

Special aspects in the management of ICH

Treatment of ICH related to oral anticoagulants

The annual risk of ICH in patients who are on oral anticoagulation treatment (OAT) is between 0.3 and 3.7% when the international normalized ratio (INR) is in a range between 2.0 and 4.5 [145]. The annual risk in the placebo groups was about 0.1% [146–148]. Every elevation of 0.5 unit of the INR increases the risk for major bleedings (intracranial or fatal) by 1.4 [149].

A rather high annual risk of a thromboembolic complication of 5–10% without OAT, a figure representative for high–risk patients with mechanical valves, can be translated as a 2–week risk of 0.2–0.4%, i.e. a rather low risk. This risk should be compared with the very high risk of early rebleeding, especially in patients with OAT-related ICH.

A few studies actually support this view and have indicated that the rate of embolic events is low, even in high-risk patients, if OATs are interrupted for up to 10–14 days [150–152]. Studies have indicated that ICH in patients on OAT has a more severe prognosis with larger bleedings and higher case fatality than ICH in patients not receiving OAT [153, 154]. Furthermore, the use of warfarin is associated with worse outcome in patients with ICH [145]. Flibotte et al. found that the use of warfarin significantly increases the likelihood of death when controlling for baseline ICH and intraventricular haemorrhage volumes [153]. In addition, the use of warfarin and increased intensity of anticoagulation are independent predictors of 3-month mortality [155].

Based on these experiences it has been suggested that the INR should be normalized as an emergency in all patients who have an OAT-associated ICH. Principally, this can be achieved by administration of prothrombin complex (PCC), fresh frozen plasma (FFP) or vitamin K, but there are no randomized trials comparing the different methods. Goldstein and co-workers demonstrated that time to treatment is an important determinant of 24-hour anticoagulation reversal, when using FFP and vitamin K [156]. Fredricksson and co-workers retrospectively studied 17 patients with OAT-associated ICH [157]. Ten of these patients were treated with PCC and 7 with FFP. Both agents led to a significant decrease of the INR. However, in PCC-treated patients the effect was stronger in both the speed and the quantity of decrease of the INR. Clinical deterioration was less common in those patients who had received PCC. A disadvantage of FFP was the larger infusion volumes that had to be used, because the concentration of coagulation factors in FFP is significantly lower than in PCC.

In a Swedish multicentre study of 151 patients who had had OAT-associated ICH the use of FFP, PCC and vitamin K was studied. The management strategies varied considerably between the 10 hospitals involved. In some cases no special treatment was given. Early clinical deterioration, most probably due to haematoma enlargement, was seen in 48% of the patients. None of the three active interventions seemed to have a significant influence on mortality, although the non-randomized observational design of the study has to be admitted [158].

It is necessary to combine PCC or FFP treatment with vitamin K, because the half-life time (HLT) of warfarin and phenprocoumon (2 and up to 7 days, respectively) is much longer than the HLT of the vitamin K-dependent factors. The dosage of PCC and FFP is specified in Table 18.5. Further details about dosages should be obtained from the manufacturers. Repeat measurement of coagulation status and haematology consultation should be obtained in the acute phase.

Recombinant factor VIIa was used to lower the INR in volunteers who had received acecoumarol and in patients treated with warfarin, which excessively elevated INRs [159, 160]. The substances have been used singly or in combination with FFP in two small retrospective series of patients with spontaneous ICH [161, 162]. In patients who received rFVIIa or the combination the authors observed a faster normalization of INR and smaller volumes of FFP respectively. However, it must be borne in mind that the INR might not reflect the actual status of all vitamin K-dependent coagulation factors [163].

Table 18.5 Recommendation for the treatment of anticoagulation-associated intracerebral haemorrhage (ICH).

Normalization of INR (INR <1.2)	
PCC	10 U/kg will reduce an increased INR with about 50%. If INR >1.8, give 1000 U. Measure INR after 10 min. If INR still >1.8, give 500 U Beriplex P/N. Further details should be obtained from the manufacturer
FFP	10 ml/kg will reduce an INR of 4.2 to 2.4, an INR of 3.0–2.1, or an INR of 2.4 to 1.8. To reduce an INR of 4.2–1.4 would require 40 ml/kg
Vitamin K	Once or twice 5–10 mg p.o or i.v.[a]
Normalization of PTT after heparin	
Protamine sulphate	1–1.5 ml protamine sulphate inactivates 1000 IU heparin of the total amount applied within the last 4 h
Prevention of deep vein thrombosis	
Low-dose heparin/heparinoids	

[a]Anaphylactic reactions with intravenous application.
FFP, fresh frozen plasma; INR, international normalized ratio; PCC, prothrombin complex; PTT, prothrombin time.

As there are no RCTs available, there are some guidelines on treatment of OAT-associated ICH: UK guidelines issued by the British Committee for Standards in Haematology recommend 5 mg intravenous or oral vitamin K, and 50 U/kg of PCC or 15 ml/kg of FFP [164]. Another UK guideline, issued by the Northern Region Haematologists' Group, reduces the recommended dose of PCC to 30 U/kg [165]. The American Thoracic Society recommend 10 mg intravenous vitamin K and PCC, without specifying the dose of PCC [166]. The Australasian Society of Thrombosis and Haemostasis recommends 5–10 mg intravenous vitamin K, 25–50 IU/kg of PCC, and 150–300 ml FFP [167]. The recommendation for the concomitant use of PCC and FFP is because the PCC preparation licensed in Australia and New Zealand at the time the guidelines were published (in 2004) did not contain factor VII. These considerations call for prospective trials that will test the effectiveness of FFP and/or PCC in OAT-associated ICH and the hypothesis to see whether rFVIIa may be an alternative treatment in this indication [145].

Considerations concerning whether and when to resume therapeutic anticoagulation in patients who have had OAT-associated ICH include whether intracranial bleeding has been fully arrested, the estimated existing risk of thromboembolism and the presumed pathophysiology of the ICH, which will determine the risk of haemorrhage recurrence [150–152, 168–171]. The indication for secondary prophylactic treatment with OAT should be carefully re-evaluated after an ICH before restarting it. Currently, the EUSI recommends the preventive use of anticoagulation for patients who had embolic stroke associated with atrial fibrillation, prosthetic heart valves or other proven cardioembolic source [14]. In the state transition decision model stratified by location of haemorrhage, it turned out that patients with atrial fibrillation and lobar location of their bleedings restarting anticoagulation would not lead to a benefit in terms of quality-adjusted life-years (QUALYs), because the risk of rebleeding and a higher chance of death would outweigh the risk of occurrence of cerebral ischaemia. This was different for patients with deep location ICH [170].

Previously, the AHA has recommended the use of dabigatran for secondary prophylaxis in patients with atrial fibrillation [172]. There may be other alternative oral anticoagulants that become available in the future [173].

Recommendations

In patients with an OAT-associated ICH and an INR >1.4:

1. OAT should be discontinued, the INR should be normalized with prothrombin complex or FFP. Intravenous vitamin K should be added (class IV evidence).

2. After having re-checked the indication for anticoagulation following ESO recommendations on ischaemic stroke, OAT may be continued after 14–21 days, depending on the perceived risk of thromboembolic occlusion and the perceived risk of ICH recurrence (class IV evidence).

Prevention of recurrence: modification of risk factors

Antihypertensive treatment

Earlier studies suggested that hypertensive ICH rarely rebleeds [174, 175] but in recent reports the rate of recur-

rent hypertensive ICH is from 4.% to 5.4% [176, 177], and in one report it is 2.9% per year [178]. About 70% of recurrent haemorrhagic strokes can be fatal.

There is good evidence that blood pressure is a determinant of the risk of stroke among both normotensive and hypertensive individuals [179]. However, there was no strong evidence until recently that reducing blood pressure after stroke reduces the rate of new vascular events or death. A meta-analysis from nine RCTs on antihypertensive drugs, in which a small number of stroke survivors had been included, led to an estimated relative risk reduction (RRR) for stroke of 29% (95% CI: 5–47%) [180], but these trials suffered severe limitations. In most trials, ICH patients were either not included or not prospectively studied (e.g. PATS, HOPE) [181–183].

The Perindopril PROtection aGainst REcurrent Stroke Study (PROGRESS) was a double-blind, randomized trial comparing perindopril (4 mg daily), with or without indapamide (2–2.5 mg daily), with placebo for the prevention of recurrent ischaemic stroke in individuals with a history of non-disabling cerebrovascular disease (minor stroke or TIA) irrespective of blood pressure [52]. Antihypertensive treatment was initialized at least 2 weeks after stroke. The PROGRESS study included 6105 patients and showed that lowering blood pressure by an average of 9/4 mmHg with perindopril-based therapy decreased the risk of recurrent stroke by 28% versus placebo. Patients receiving both perindopril and indapamide had a mean drop in blood pressure of 12/5 mmHg and a 43% reduction in the risk of stroke. Interestingly, the observed benefit was achieved regardless of blood pressure at entry and type of stroke. These beneficial effects were present in all stroke subtypes, but greater in haemorrhagic strokes (RRR: 50%; 95% CI: 33–74%) and in Asian individuals. The combination therapy prevented 1 recurrent stroke for 14 patients treated over a 5-year period. A recent systematic review of blood pressure reduction in prevention of stroke recurrences including ICHs revealed a positive association between the magnitude of blood pressure reduction and the risk of vascular events [184].

Alcohol consumption

The association between alcohol consumption and stroke is complex and may differ between white and other populations, e.g. Japanese. In the Honolulu Heart Program, heavy drinkers had a three times higher risk of haemorrhagic stroke (SAH or ICH) than non-drinkers [185]. A case–control study in a multiethnic population suggested that moderate consumption (up to two drinks of spirits, two cans of beer or two glasses of wine, equivalent to 20–30 g ethyl alcohol, per day) was associated with a decreased risk of ischaemic stroke, whereas heavy alcohol consumption was associated with an increased risk of ischaemic and haemorrhagic stroke [186]. A recent meta-analysis has given similar results by showing that heavy alcohol drinking (>60 g/day) increases the relative risk of stroke, whereas light or moderate alcohol consumption may protect against total and ischaemic stroke [187]: a consumption of <12 g alcohol/day was associated with a reduced risk of total stroke (RR = 0.83) and ischaemic stroke (RR = 0.80) and a moderate consumption of alcohol (12–24 g/day) was associated with an RRR for ischaemic stroke of 0.72 [187], but there is no evidence to support any alcohol consumption in the prevention of ICH.

Antiplatelet agents

Patients with ICH who have preceding or ensuing ischaemic disease (coronary artery syndrome, ischaemic stroke, peripheral arterial disease) or are at risk for ischaemia (symptomatic carotid stenosis, cerebral microangiopathy) may need secondary prophylaxis with antiplatelet drugs. There are no studies that have looked into the risk of rebleeding in patients who receive antiplatelet drugs for secondary prophylaxis after an ICH. However, it is known that small vessel disease is a risk factor for both ischaemic stroke and intracerebral haemorrhage, cerebral amyloid angiopathy in particular is a risk factor of ICH, and there are some studies that have looked into the risk of secondary ICH in patients with pre-existing small vessel disease or cerebral ischaemia. Thus it was suspected that cerebral small vessel disease and the intake of aspirin are associated with an increased risk of ICH in patients with ischaemic infarct of arterial origin [188]. However, an analysis of nine randomized clinical trials did not confirm this association [189]. Hypertension additionally increases the risk of ICH [190], but no increase in risk of ICH was found among aspirin users. Other antiplatelet drugs – such as clopidogrel or the combination of dipyridamole and aspirin – have also been shown to be effective in secondary prophylaxis of vascular events. The risk of rebleeding was not increased by either of these substances. Adding aspirin to clopidogrel

in high-risk patients is associated with increased risk of life-threatening major bleedings (MATCH study 2004). [191, 192]. Furthermore, pretreatment with aspirin before thrombolysis with rt-PA did not increase the risk of ICH, if selection criteria for thrombolysis were applied properly [193]. In conclusion, all these studies are only *indirect* information. The risk of ICH in patients who are on secondary prophylaxis with aspirin after ICH is not known. No definitive answer can be given to this problem, because there is insufficient evidence.

Recommendations

1. Diagnosis and control of hypertension after ICH are strongly recommended as the most effective means to decrease morbidity, mortality and recurrence due to spontaneous ICH (level A recommendation).

2. After ICH blood pressure should be lowered, irrespective of its level, with a diuretic and an angiotensin-converting enzyme (ACE) inhibitor, subject to toleration of the treatment (level A recommendation). The effectiveness of other classes of blood pressure-lowering drugs has not yet been established by controlled trials.

3. Despite lack of evidence, people with elevated BMI should take a weight-reducing diet, those with hypertension should reduce their salt intake and smokers should quit smoking (class IV evidence).

4. Excessive use of alcohol must be discouraged (class IV evidence).

5. After ICH, antiplatelet treatment has to be individualized depending on the presence of ischaemic vascular diseases or anticipated risk, on the one hand, and the perceived risk of ICH recurrence (class IV evidence), on the other.

Conclusion

These recommendations were set up in a period of transition: knowledge of pathophysiology, diagnosis and possible therapies in patients with intracerebral haemorrhage has drastically increased within the last few years. Still, most of the recommendations cannot be based on level A evidence. At this point it is possible though to identify more clearly those areas of research priority. For example, surgical treatment of patients with spontaneous ICH cannot be recommended on the basis of current trials, but these trials enable us to define target populations more clearly in the future. Acute hematoma expansion has been identified as the acute problem of ICH in the first few hours. Further studies are needed to identify the role of treatments that prevent or limit hematoma expansion, to the precise timing of various treatments and the role of hypertension.

References

1. Flaherty, ML, Woo, D, Haverbusch, M, *et al.* Racial variations in location and risk of intracerebral hemorrhage. *Stroke* 2005; **36**:934–7.

2. Zhang, LF, Yang, J, Hong, Z, *et al.* Proportion of different subtypes of stroke in China. *Stroke* 2003; **34**:2091–6.

3. Ayala, C, Croft, JB, Greenlund, KJ, *et al.* Sex differences in US mortality rates for stroke and stroke subtypes by race/ethnicity and age, 1995–1998. *Stroke* 2002; **33**:1197–201.

4. Skidmore, CT, Andrefsky, J. Spontaneous intracerebral hemorrhage: epidemiology, pathophysiology, and medical management. *Neurosurg Clin N Am* 2002; **13**:281–8, v.

5. Qureshi, AI, Tuhrim, S, Broderick, JP, *et al.* Spontaneous intracerebral hemorrhage. *N Engl J Med* 2001; **344**:1450–60.

6. Broderick, JP, Brott, T, Tomsick, T, Miller, R, Huster, G. Intracerebral hemorrhage more than twice as common as subarachnoid hemorrhage. *J Neurosurg* 1993; **78**:188–91.

7. Brott, T, Broderick, J, Kothari, R, *et al.* Early hemorrhage growth in patients with intracerebral hemorrhage. *Stroke* 1997; **28**:1–5.

8. Kazui, S, Naritomi, H, Yamamoto, H, Sawada, T, Yamaguchi, T. Enlargement of spontaneous intracerebral hemorrhage. Incidence and time course. *Stroke* 1996; **27**:1783–7.

9. Fujii, Y, Tanaka, R, Takeuchi, S, *et al.* Hematoma enlargement in spontaneous intracerebral hemorrhage. *J Neurosurg* 1994; **80**:51–7.

10. International Subarachnoid Aneurysm Trial (ISAT) Collaborative Group. International Subarachnoid Aneurysm Trial (ISAT) of neurosurgical clipping versus endovascular coiling in 2143 patients with ruptured intracranial aneurysms: a randomised trial. *Lancet* 2002; **360**:1267–74.

11. Mendelow, AD, Gregson, BA, Fernandes, HM, *et al.* Early surgery versus initial conservative treatment in patients with spontaneous supratentorial intracerebral haematomas in the International Surgical Trial in Intracerebral Haemorrhage (STICH): a randomised trial. *Lancet* 2005; **365**:387–97.

12. Mayer, S, Brun, N, Broderick, J, *et al.* Safety and feasibility of recombinant factor VIIa for acute intracerebral hemorrhage. *Stroke* 2005; **36**:74–9.

13. Mayer, S, Brun, N, Broderick, J, *et al.* Recombinant activated factor VII for acute intracerebral hemorrhage. *N Engl J Med* 2005; **352**:777–85.

14. European Stroke Initiative (EUSI) Executive Committee and the EUSI Writing Committee. European stroke initiative recommendations for stroke management – update 2003. *Cerebrovasc Dis* 2003; **16**:311–37.

15. Brainin, M, Barnes, M, Baron, JC, *et al.* Guidance for the preparation of neurological management guidelines by EFNS scientific task forces – revised recommendations 2004. *Eur J Neurol* 2004; **11**:577–81.

16. Sacco, RL, Boden-Albala, B, Gan, R, *et al.* Stroke incidence among white, black, and Hispanic residents of an urban community: the Northern Manhattan Stroke Study. *Am J Epidemiol* 1998; **147**:259–68.

17. Kolominsky-Rabas, PL, Sarti, C, Heuschmann, PU, *et al.* A prospective community-based study of stroke in Germany – the Erlangen Stroke Project (ESPro): incidence and case fatality at 1, 3, and 12 months. *Stroke* 1998; **29**:2501–6.

18. Weimar, C, Weber, C, Wagner, M, *et al.* Management patterns and health care use after intracerebral hemorrhage. A cost-of-illness study from a societal perspective in Germany. *Cerebrovasc Dis* 2003; **15**:29–36.

19. Bruno, A, Carter, S. Possible reason for the higher incidence of spontaneous intracerebral hemorrhage among Hispanics than non-Hispanic whites in New Mexico. *Neuroepidemiology* 2000; **19**:51–2.

20. Ayala, C, Greenlund, KJ, Croft, JB, *et al.* Racial/ethnic disparities in mortality by stroke subtype in the United States, 1995–1998. *Am J Epidemiol* 2001; **154**:1057–63.

21. Fujii, Y, Takeuchi, S, Sasaki, O, Minakawa, T, Tanaka, R. Multivariate analysis of predictors of hematoma enlargement in spontaneous intracerebral hemorrhage. *Stroke* 1998; **29**:1160–6.

22. Broderick, J, Brott, T, Duldner, JE, Tomsick, T, Huster, G. Volume of intracerebral hemorrhage: a powerful and easy-to-use predictor of 30-day mortality. *Stroke* 1993; **24**:987–93.

23. Counsell, C, Boonyakarnkul, S, Dennis, M, *et al.* Primary intracerebral haemorrhage in the Oxfordshire community stroke project, 2: prognosis. *Cerebrovasc Dis* 1995; **5**:26–34.

24. Anderson, CS, Chakera, TM, Stewart-Wynne, EG, Jamrozik, KD. Spectrum of primary intracerebral haemorrhage in Perth, Western Australia, 1989–90: incidence and outcome. *J Neurol Neurosurg Psychiatry* 1994; **57**:936–40.

25. Diringer, MN, Edwards, DF. Admission to a neurologic/neurosurgical intensive care unit is associated with reduced mortality rate after intracerebral hemorrhage. *Crit Care Med* 2001; **29**:635–40.

26. Hemphill, JC. 3rd, Bonovich, DC, Besmertis, L, Manley, GT, Johnston, SC. The ICH score: a simple, reliable grading

scale for intracerebral hemorrhage. *Stroke* 2001; **32**: 891–7.

27. Becker, KJ, Baxter, AB, Cohen, WA, *et al.* Withdrawal of support in intracerebral hemorrhage may lead to self-fulfilling prophecies. *Neurology* 2001; **56**:766–72.

28. Fujitsu, K, Muramoto, M, Ikeda, Y, *et al.* Indications for surgical treatment of putaminal hemorrhage. Comparative study based on serial CT and time-course analysis. *J Neurosurg* 1990; **73**:518–25.

29. Tuhrim, S, Horowitz, DR, Sacher, M, Godbold, JH. Volume of ventricular blood is an important determinant of outcome in supratentorial intracerebral hemorrhage. *Crit Care Med* 1999; **27**:617–21.

30. Young, WB, Lee, KP, Pessin, MS, *et al.* Prognostic significance of ventricular blood in supratentorial hemorrhage: a volumetric study. *Neurology* 1990; **40**:616–19.

31. Juvela, S. Risk factors for impaired outcome after spontaneous intracerebral hemorrhage. *Arch Neurol* 1995; **52**: 1193–200.

32. Diringer, MN, Edwards, DF, Zazulia, AR. Hydrocephalus: a previously unrecognized predictor of poor outcome from supratentorial intracerebral hemorrhage. *Stroke* 1998; **29**:1352–7.

33. Zazulia, AR, Diringer, MN, Derdeyn, SP, Powers, WJ. Progression of mass effect after intracerebral hemorrhage. *Stroke* 1999; **30**:1167–73.

34. Gebel, JM. Jr, Jauch, EC, Brott, TG, *et al.* Relative edema volume is a predictor of outcome in patients with hyperacute spontaneous intracerebral hemorrhage. *Stroke* 2002; **33**:2636–41.

35. Xi, G. Intracerebral hemorrhage: pathophysiology and therapy. *Neurocrit Care* 2004; **1**:5–18.

36. Lee, KR, Colon, GP, Betz, AL, *et al.* Edema from intracerebral hemorrhage: the role of thrombin. *J Neurosurg* 1996; **84**:91–6.

37. Castillo, J, Davalos, A, Alvarez-Sabin, J, *et al.* Molecular signatures of brain injury after intracerebral hemorrhage. *Neurology* 2002; **58**:624–9.

38. Abilleira, S, Montaner, J, Molina, CA, *et al.* Matrix metalloproteinase-9 concentration after spontaneous intracerebral hemorrhage. *J Neurosurg* 2003; **99**:65–70.

39. Xi, G, Wagner, KR, Keep, RF, *et al.* Role of blood clot formation on early edema development after experimental intracerebral hemorrhage. *Stroke* 1998; **29**:2580–6.

40. Sansing, LH, Kaznatcheeva, EA, Perkins, CJ, *et al.* Edema after intracerebral hemorrhage: correlations with coagulation parameters and treatment. *J Neurosurg* 2003; **98**: 985–92.

41. Schellinger, PD, Fiebach, JB, Hoffmann, K, *et al.* Stroke MRI in intracerebral hemorrhage: is there a perihemorrhagic penumbra? *Stroke* 2003; **34**:1674–9.

42. Butcher, KS, Baird, T, MacGregor, L, *et al.* Perihematomal edema in primary intracerebral hemorrhage is plasma derived. *Stroke* 2004; **35**:1879–85.

43. Powers, WJ, Zazulia, AR, Videen, TO, *et al.* Autoregulation of cerebral blood flow surrounding acute (6 to 22 hours) intracerebral hemorrhage. *Neurology* 2001; **57**:18–24.

44. Zazulia, AR, Diringer, MN, Videen, TO, *et al.* Hypoperfusion without ischemia surrounding acute intracerebral hemorrhage. *J Cereb Blood Flow Metab* 2001; **21**:804–10.

45. Greenberg, SM, Briggs, ME, Hyman, BT, *et al.* Apolipoprotein E epsilon 4 is associated with the presence and earlier onset of hemorrhage in cerebral amyloid angiopathy. *Stroke* 1996; **27**:1333–7.

46. Lang, EW, Ren Ya, Z, Preul, C, *et al.* Stroke pattern interpretation: the variability of hypertensive versus amyloid angiopathy hemorrhage. *Cerebrovasc Dis* 2001; **12**: 121–30.

47. Knudsen, KA, Rosand, J, Karluk, D, Greenberg, SM. Clinical diagnosis of cerebral amyloid angiopathy: validation of the Boston criteria. *Neurology* 2001; **56**:537–9.

48. Rosand, J, Hylek, EM, O'Donnell, HC, Greenberg, SM. Warfarin-associated hemorrhage and cerebral amyloid angiopathy: a genetic and pathologic study. *Neurology* 2000; **55**:947–51.

49. Caplan, LR. Intracerebral hemorrhage. In Caplan, L.R. (ed.), *Caplan's Stroke: A clinical approach*. Boston: Butterworth-Heinemann, 2000: 383–418.

50. Woo, D, Kaushal, R, Chakraborty, R, *et al.* Association of apolipoprotein E4 and haplotypes of the apolipoprotein E gene with lobar intracerebral hemorrhage. *Stroke* 2005; **36**:1874–9.

51. Brott, T, Thalinger, K, Hertzberg, V. Hypertension as a risk factor for spontaneous intracerebral hemorrhage. *Stroke* 1986; **17**:1078–83.

52. PROGRESS Collaborative Group. Randomised trial of a perindopril-based blood-pressure-lowering regimen among 6105 individuals with previous stroke or transient ischaemic attack. *Lancet* 2001; **358**:1033–41.

53. Segal, AZ, Chiu, RI, Eggleston-Sexton, PM, Beiser, A, Greenberg, SM. Low cholesterol as a risk factor for primary intracerebral hemorrhage: A case-control study. *Neuroepidemiology* 1999; **18**:185–93.

54. Woo, D, Kissela, BM, Khoury, JC, *et al.* Hypercholesterolemia, HMG-CoA reductase inhibitors, and risk of intracerebral hemorrhage: a case–control study. *Stroke* 2004; **35**: 1360–4.

55. Abbott, RD, Yin, Y, Reed, DM, Yano, K. Risk of stroke in male cigarette smokers. *N Engl J Med* 1986; **315**:717–20.

56. Kurth, T, Kase, CS, Berger, K, *et al.* Smoking and the risk of hemorrhagic stroke in men. *Stroke* 2003; **34**:1151–5.

57. Kurth, T, Kase, CS, Berger, K, *et al.* Smoking and risk of hemorrhagic stroke in women. *Stroke* 2003; **34**:2792–5.

58. Zhou, JF, Wang, JY, Luo, YE, Chen, HH. Influence of hypertension, lipometabolism disorders, obesity and other lifestyles on spontaneous intracerebral hemorrhage. *Biomed Environ Sci* 2003; **16**:295–303.

59. Donahue, RP, Abbott, RD, Reed, DM, Yano, K. Alcohol and hemorrhagic stroke. The Honolulu Heart Program. *JAMA* 1986; **255**:2311–14.

60. Juvela, S, Hillbom, M, Palomaki, H. Risk factors for spontaneous intracerebral hemorrhage. *Stroke* 1995; **26**:1558–64.

61. Kase, CS, Mohr, JP, Caplan, LR. Intracerebral hemorrhage. In: Mohr, J.P., Choi, D.C., Grotta, J.C., Weir, B., Wolf, P.A. (eds), *Stroke: Pathophysiology, diagnosis, and management*, Philadelphia: Churchill Livingstone, 2004: 327–76.

62. Hart, RG, Boop, BS, Anderson, DC. Oral anticoagulants and intracranial hemorrhage. Facts and hypotheses. *Stroke* 1995; **26**:1471–7.

63. He, J, Whelton, PK, Vu, B, Klag, MJ. Aspirin and risk of hemorrhagic stroke: a meta-analysis of randomized controlled trials. *JAMA* 1998; **280**:1930–5.

64. Diener, HC, Bogousslavsky, J, Brass, LM, *et al.* Aspirin and clopidogrel compared with clopidogrel alone after recent ischaemic stroke or transient ischaemic attack in high-risk patients (MATCH): randomised, double-blind, placebo-controlled trial. *Lancet* 2004; **364**:331–7.

65. Toyoda, K, Okada, Y, Minematsu, K, *et al.* Antiplatelet therapy contributes to acute deterioration of intracerebral hemorrhage. *Neurology* 2005; **65**:1000–4.

66. Hacke, W, Donnan, G, Fieschi, C, *et al.* Association of outcome with early stroke treatment: pooled analysis of ATLANTIS, ECASS, and NINDS rt-PA stroke trials. *Lancet* 2004; **363**:768–74.

67. McCormick, WF, Rosenfield, DB. Massive brain hemorrhage: a review of 144 cases and an examination of their causes. *Stroke* 1973; **4**:946–54.

68. Allen, CM. Clinical diagnosis of the acute stroke syndrome. *Q J Med* 1983; **52**:515–23.

69. Poungvarin, N, Viriyavejakul, A, Komontri, C. Siriraj stroke score and validation study to distinguish supratentorial intracerebral haemorrhage from infarction. *BMJ* 1991; **302**:1565–7.

70. Weir, CJ, Murray, GD, Adams, FG, *et al.* Poor accuracy of stroke scoring systems for differential clinical diagnosis of intracranial haemorrhage and infarction. *Lancet* 1994; **344**:999–1002.

71. Smith, EE, Rosand, J, Greenberg, SM. Hemorrhagic stroke. *Neuroimaging Clin N Am* 2005; **15**:259–72.

72. Broderick, JP, Brott, TG, Tomsick, T, Barsan, W, Spilker, J. Ultra-early evaluation of intracerebral hemorrhage. *J Neurosurg* 1990; **72**:195–9.

73. Weisberg, LA. Computerized tomography in intracranial hemorrhage. *Arch Neurol* 1979; **36**:422–6.

74. Boyko, OB, Cooper, DF, Grossman, CB. Contrast-enhanced CT of acute isodense subdural hematoma. *AJNR Am J Neuroradiol* 1991; **12**:341–3.

75. Gomori, JM, Grossmann, RI. Mechanisms responsible for the MR appearance and evolution of intracranial hemorrhage. *Radiographics* 1988; **8**:427–40.

76. Laissy, JP, Normand, G, Monroc, M, *et al.* Spontaneous intracerebral hematomas from vascular causes. *Neuroradiology* 1991; **33**:291–5.

77. Sacco, S, Marini, C, Toni, D, Olivieri, L, Carolei, A. Incidence and 10-year survival of intracerebral hemorrhage in a population-based registry. *Stroke* 2009; **40**:394–9.

78. van Straaten, EC, Scheltens, P, Barkhof, F. MRI and CT in the diagnosis of vascular dementia. *J Neurol Sci* 2004; **226**(1–2):9–12.

79. Uysal, E, Yanbuloglu, B, Erturk, M, Kilinc, BM, Basak, M. Spiral CT angiography in diagnosis of cerebral aneurysms of cases with acute subarachnoid hemorrhage. *Diagn Interv Radiol* 2005; **11**:77–82.

80. Kouskouras, C, Charitanti, A, Giavroglou, C, *et al.* Intracranial aneurysms: evaluation using CTA and MRA. Correlation with DSA and intraoperative findings. *Neuroradiology* 2004; **46**:842–50.

81. Dammert, S, Krings, T, Moller-Hartmann, W, *et al.* Detection of intracranial aneurysms with multislice CT: comparison with conventional angiography. *Neuroradiology* 2004; **36**:427–34.

82. Adams, H, Brott, T, Crowell, R, *et al.* Guidelines for the management of patients with acute ischemic stroke. A statement for healthcare professionals from a special writing group of the Stroke Council of the American Heart Association. *Circulation* 1994; **90**:1588–601.

83. Paolucci, S, Antonucci, G, Grasso, MG, *et al.* Functional outcome of ischemic and hemorrhagic stroke patients after inpatient rehabilitation: a matched comparison. *Stroke* 2003; **34**:2861–5.

84. Lyden, P, Brott, T, Tilley, B, *et al.* Improved reliability of the NIH Stroke Scale using video training. NINDS TPA Stroke Study Group. *Stroke* 1994; **25**:2220–6.

85. Teasdale, G, Jennett, B. Assessment of coma and impaired consciousness. A practical scale. *Lancet* 1974; **2**:81–4.

86. Lindstrom, E, Boysen, G, Christiansen, LW, Nansen, BR, Nielsen, PW. Reliability of Scandinavian neurological stroke scale. *Cerebrovasc Dis* 1991; **1**:103–7.

87. ESO. ESO Guideline Update – January 2009: Guidelines for management of ischaemic stroke and transient ischaemic attack 2008. 2009. http://www.eso-stroke.org/recommendations (accessed 9.5.2011).

88. Qureshi, AI, Mohammad, YM, Yahia, AM, et al. A prospective multicenter study to evaluate the feasibility and safety of aggressive antihypertensive treatment in patients with acute intracerebral hemorrhage. J Intens Care Med 2005; 20:34–42.

89. Morgenstern, LB. Medical therapy of intracerebral and intraventricular hemorrhage. In: Mohr, J.P., Choi, D.C., Grotta, J.C., Weir, B., Wolf, P.A. (eds), Stroke: Pathophysiology, Diagnosis, and Management, Philadelphia: Churchill Livingstone, 2004; 1079–87.

90. Anderson, CS, Huang, Y, Wang, JG, et al. Intensive blood pressure reduction in acute cerebral haemorrhage trial (INTERACT): a randomised pilot trial. Lancet Neurol 2008; 7:391–9.

91. Qureshi, AI, ATACH investigators. Antihypertensive treatment of acute cerebral hemorrhage. Crit Care Med 2010; 38:637–48.

92. Grossman, E, Messerli, FH, Grodzicki, T, Kowey, P. Should a moratorium be placed on sublingual nifedipine capsules given for hypertensive emergencies and pseudoemergencies? JAMA 1996; 276:1328–31.

93. Ahmed, N, Nasman, P, Wahlgren, NG. Effect of intravenous nimodipine on blood pressure and outcome after acute stroke. Stroke 2000; 31:1250–5.

94. Graham, DI, McGeorge, A, Fitch, W, Jones, JV, MacKenzie, ET. Ischaemic brain damage induced by rapid lowering of arterial pressure in hypertension. J Hypertens 1984; 2:297–304.

95. Powers, WJ. Acute hypertension after stroke: the scientific basis for treatment decisions. Neurology 1993; 43:461–7.

96. Jorgensen, H, Nakayama, H, Rasschou, H, Olsen, T. Effects of blood pressure and diabetes on stroke progression. Lancet 1994; 334:156–9.

97. Ringleb, PA, Bertram, M, Keller, E, Hacke, W. Hypertension in patients with cerebrovascular accident. To treat or not to treat? Nephrol Dial Transplant 1998; 13:2179–81.

98. Bath, P, Chalmers, J, Powers, W, et al. International Society of Hypertension (ISH): statement on the management of blood pressure in acute stroke. J Hypertens 2003; 21: 665–72.

99. Steiner, T. Stroke Unit design: intensive monitoring should be routine. Stroke 2003; 35:1018–19.

100. Poungvarin, N, Bhoopat, W, Viriyavejakul, A, et al. Effects of dexamethasone in primary supratentorial intracerebral hemorrhage. N Engl J Med 1987; 316:1229–33.

101. Broderick, JP, Adams, HP. Jr, Barsan, W, et al. Guidelines for the management of spontaneous intracerebral hemorrhage: a statement for healthcare professionals from a special writing group of the Stroke Council, American Heart Association. Stroke 1999; 30:905–15.

102. Vespa, PM, O'Phelan, K, Shah, M, et al. Acute seizures after intracerebral hemorrhage: a factor in progressive midline shift and outcome. Neurology 2003; 60:1441–6.

103. Passero, S, Rocchi, R, Rossi, S, Ulivelli, M, Vatti, G. Seizures after spontaneous supratentorial intracerebral hemorrhage. Epilepsia 2002; 43:1175–80.

104. Berger, AR, Lipton, RB, Lesser, ML, Lantos, G, Portenoy, RK. Early seizures following intracerebral hemorrhage: implications for therapy. Neurology 1988; 38:1363–5.

105. Vespa, P. Continuous EEG monitoring for the detection of seizures in traumatic brain injury, infarction, and intracerebral hemorrhage: 'to detect and protect'. J Clin Neurophysiol 2005; 22:99–106.

106. Varelas, PN, Mirski, MA. Management of seizures in critically ill patients. Curr Neurol Neurosci Rep 2004; 4: 489–96.

107. Silver, F, Norris, JW, Lewis, AJ, Hachinski, VC. Early mortality following stroke: a prospective review. Stroke 1984; 15:492–6.

108. Adams, HP. Jr. Effective prophylaxis for deep vein thrombosis after stroke. low-dose anticoagulation rather than stockings alone. Stroke 2004; 35:2911.

109. Davis, SM, Donnan, GA. Effective prophylaxis for deep venous thrombosis after stroke. both low-dose anticoagulation and stockings for most cases. Stroke 2004; 35:2910.

110. Dennis, MS. Effective prophylaxis for deep vein thrombosis after stroke. low-dose anticoagulation rather than stockings alone: against. Stroke 2004; 35:2912–13.

111. Gubitz, G, Counsel, C, Sandercock, P, Signorini, D. Anticoagulants for acute ischaemic stroke. Oxford: Update Software, 2000, issue 2, page CD000024.

112. Albers, GW, Amarenco, P, Easton, JD, Sacco, RL, Teal, P. Antithrombotic and thrombolytic therapy for ischemic stroke: the Seventh ACCP Conference on Antithrombotic and Thrombolytic Therapy. Chest 2004; 126:483S–512S.

113. Boeer, A, Voth, E, Henze, T, Prange, HW. Early heparin therapy in patients with spontaneous intracerebral haemorrhage. J Neurol Neurosurg Psychiatry 1991; 54:466–7.

114. Prasad, K, Mendelow, AD, Gregson, B. Surgery for primary supratentorial intracerebral haemorrhage. Cochrane Database Syst Rev 2008; (4):CD000200.

115. Teernstra, OP, Evers, SM, Lodder, J, et al. Stereotactic treatment of intracerebral hematoma by means of a plasminogen activator: a multicenter randomized controlled trial (SICHPA). Stroke 2003; 34:968–74.

116. Dunne, JW, Chakera, T, Kermode, S. Cerebellar haemorrhage – diagnosis and treatment: a study of 75 consecutive cases. Q J Med 1987; 64:739–54.

117. Salazar, J, Vaquero, J, Martinez, P, et al. Clinical and CT scan assessment of benign versus fatal spontaneous cerebellar haematomas. Acta Neurochir (Wien) 1986; 79:80–6.

118. Bhattathiri P, Gregson B, Prasad K, Mendelow AD. Intraventricular Haemorrhage (IVH) and hydrocephalus after spontaneous intracerebral haematoma: results from the STICH trial. In: Hoff JT, Keep RF, Xi G, Hua Y eds, *Brain Edema XIII – Acta Neurochirurgica.* Wien: Springer Verlag; 2006:65–68

119. Mathew, P, Teasdale, G, Bannan, A, *et al.* Neurosurgical management of cerebellar haematoma and infarct. *J Neurol Neurosurg Psychiatry* 1995; **59**:287–92.

120. Naff, NJ, Carhuapoma, JR, Williams, MA, *et al.* Treatment of intraventricular hemorrhage with urokinase: effects on 30-day survival. *Stroke* 2000; **31**:841–7.

121. Naff, NJ, Hanley, DF, Keyl, PM, *et al.* Intraventricular thrombolysis speeds blood clot resolution: results of a pilot, prospective, randomized, double-blind, controlled trial. *Neurosurgery* 2004; **54**:577–83, discussion 583–574.

122. Haines, S, Lapointe, M. Fibrinolytic agents in the management of posthemorrhagic hydrocephalus in preterm infants: the evidence. *Child's Nerv Syst* 1999;**15**:226–34.

123. Siomin V, Cinalli G, Grotenhuis A, *et al.* Endoscopic third ventriculostomy in patients with cerebrospinal fluid infection and/or hemorrhage. *J Neurosurg* 2002; **97**:519–24

124. Pikus, H, Levy , ML, Gans, W, *et al.* Outcome, cost analysis, and long-term follow-up in preterm infants with massive grade IV germinal matrix hemorrhage and progressive hydrocephalus. *Neurosurgery* 1997; **40**:983–8.

125. Andaluz, N, Zuccarello, M. Fenestration of the lamina terminalis as a valuable adjunct in aneurysm surgery. *Neurosurgery* 2004; **55**:1050–9.

126. Sindou, M. Favourable influence of opening the lamina terminalis and Lilliequist's membrane on the outcome of ruptured intracranial aneurysms. A study of 197 consecutive cases. *Acta Neurochir* 1994; **127**:15–16.

127. Haines, S, Walters, B. Antibiotic prophylaxis for cerebrospinal fluid shunts: a metanalysis. *Neurosurgery* 1994; **34**:87–92.

128. Pan, HC, Sun, MH, Yang, DY, *et al.* Multidisciplinary treatment of cavernous sinus dural arteriovenous fistulae with radiosurgery and embolization. *J Clin Neurosci* 2005; **12**:744–9.

129. Choi, J, Mohr, J. Brain arteriovenous malformations in adults. *Lancet Neurol* 2005; **4**:299–308.

130. Castel, JP, Kantor, G. Postoperative morbidity and mortality after microsurgical exclusion of cerebral arteriovenous malformations. Current data and analysis of recent literature. *Neurochirurgie* 2000; **47**:369–83.

131. Ogivy, CS, Stieg, PE, Awad, I, *et al.* Recommendation for the management of intracranial arteriovenous malformations: a statement for health-care professional from a special writing group of the Stroke Council, American Stroke Association. *Stroke* 2010; **32**:1457–71.

132. Porter, RW, Detwiler, PW, Spetzler, RF, *et al.* Cavernous malformations of the brainstem: experience with 100 patients. *J Neurosurg* 1999; **90**:50–8.

133. Kupersmith, MJ, Kalish, H, Epstein, F, *et al.* Natural history of brainstem cavernous malformations. *Neurosurgery* 2001; **48**:47–53.

134. Aiba, T, Tanaka, R, Koike, T, *et al.* Natural history of intracranial cavernous malformations. *J Neurosurg* 1995; **83**: 56–9.

135. Maraire, JN, Awad, IA. Intracranial cavernous malformations: lesions behavior and management strategies. *Neurosurgery* 1995; **37**:591–605.

136. Hasegawa, T, McInerney, J, Kondziolka, D, *et al.* Long-term results after stereotactic radiosurgery for patients with cavernous malformations. *Neurosurgery* 2002; **50**:1190–8.

137. Purdy, PD, Batjer, HH, Samson, D. Management of hemorrhagic complications from preoperative embolization of arteriovenous malformations. *J Neurosurg* 1991; **74**: 205–11.

138. Piriyawat, P, Morgenstern, LB, Yawn, D, Hall, CE, Grotta, JC. Treatment of acute intracerebral hemorrhage with e-aminocaproic acid – a pilot study. *Neurocrit Care* 2004; **1**:47–51.

139. Kassell, NF, Haley, EC, Torner, JC. Antifibrinolytic therapy in the treatment of aneurysmal subarachnoid hemorrhage. *Clin Neurosurg* 1986; **33**:137–45.

140. Roos, YB, Rinkel, GJ, Vermeulen, M, Algra, A, van Gijn, J. Antifibrinolytic therapy for aneurysmal subarachnoid haemorrhage. *Cochrane Database Syst Rev* 2003; (2): CD001245.

141. Hedner, U. NovoSeven as a universal haemostatic agent. *Blood Coag Fibrinolysis* 2000; **11**(suppl 1):S107–11.

142. Hedner, U, Erhardtsen, E. Potential role for rFVIIa in transfusion medicine. *Transfusion* 2002; **42**:114–24.

143. Mayer, S, Brun, N, Broderick, J, *et al.* Recombinant activated factor VII for acute intracerebral hemorrhage: US phase IIA trial. *Neurocrit Care* 2005; **4**:206–14.

144. Mayer, S, Brun, N, Broderick, J, *et al.* Efficacy and safety of recombinant activated factor VII for acute intracerebral hemorrhage. *N Engl J Med* 2008; **358**:2127–37.

145. Steiner, T, Diringer, M, Rosand, J. Intracerebral hemorrhage associated with oral anticoagulant therapy: current practices and open questions. *Stroke* 2005; **37**: 256–62.

146. Stroke Prevention in Atrial Fibrillation Investigators. Bleeding during antithrombotic therapy in patients with atrial fibrillation. *Arch Intern Med* 1996; **156**:409–16.

147. Stroke Prevention in Atrial Fibrillation Investigators. Warfarin versus aspirin for prevention of thromboembolism in atrial fibrillation. Stroke Prevention in Atrial Fibrillation II Study. *Lancet* 1994; **343**:687–91.

148. Stroke Prevention in Atrial Fibrillation Investigators. Adjusted-dose warfarin versus low-intensity, fixed-dose warfarin plus aspirin for high-risk patients with atrial fibrillation: Stroke Prevention in Atrial Fibrillation III randomised clinical trial. *Lancet* 1996; **348**:633–8.

149. The Stroke Prevention in Reversible Ischemia Trial (SPIRIT) Study Group. A randomized trial of anticoagulants versus aspirin after cerebral ischemia of presumed arterial origin. *Ann Neurol* 1997; **42**:857–65.

150. Phan, TG, Koh, M, Wijdicks, EF. Safety of discontinuation of anticoagulation in patients with intracranial hemorrhage at high thromboembolic risk. *Arch Neurol* 2000; **57**:1710–13.

151. Ananthasubramaniam, K, Beattie, JN, Rosman, HS, Jayam, V, Borzak, S. How safely and for how long can warfarin therapy be withheld in prosthetic heart valve patients hospitalized with a major hemorrhage? *Chest* 2001; **119**: 478–84.

152. Bertram, M, Bonsanto, M, Hacke, W, Schwab, S. Managing the therapeutic dilemma: patients with spontaneous intracerebral hemorrhage and urgent need for anticoagulation. *J Neurol* 2000; **247**:209–14.

153. Flibotte, JJ, Hagan, N, O'Donnell, J, Greenberg, SM, Rosand, J. Warfarin, hematoma expansion, and outcome of intracerebral hemorrhage. *Neurology* 2004; **63**:1059–64.

154. Neau, JP, Couderq, C, Ingrand, P, Blanchon, P, Gil, R. Intracranial hemorrhage and oral anticoagulant treatment. *Cerebrovasc Dis* 2001; **11**:195–200.

155. Rosand, J, Eckman, MH, Knudsen, KA, Singer, DE, Greenberg, SM. The effect of warfarin and intensity of anticoagulation on outcome of intracerebral hemorrhage. *Arch Intern Med* 2004; **164**:880–4.

156. Goldstein, JN, Thomas, SH, Frontiero, V, *et al.* Timing of fresh frozen plasma administration and rapid correction of coagulopathy in warfarin-related intracerebral hemorrhage. *Stroke* 2006; **37**:151–5.

157. Fredriksson, K, Norrving, B, Stromblad, LG. Emergency reversal of anticoagulation after intracerebral hemorrhage. *Stroke* 1992; **23**:972–7.

158. Sjöblom, L, Hardemark, HG, Lindgren, A, *et al.* Management and prognostic features of intracerebral hemorrhage during anticoagulant therapy: a Swedish multicenter study. *Stroke* 2001; **32**:2567–74.

159. Erhardtsen, E, Nony, P, Dechavanne, M, *et al.* The effect of recombinant factor VIIa (NovoSeven) in healthy volunteers receiving acenocoumarol to an International Normalized Ration above 2.0. *Blood Coagul Fibrinolysis* 1998; **9**:741–8.

160. Deveras, RA, Kessler, CM. Reversal of warfarin-induced excessive anticoagulation with recombinant human factor VIIa concentrate. *Ann Intern Med* 2002; **137**:884–8.

161. Freeman, WD, Brott, TG, Barrett, KM, *et al.* Recombinant factor VIIa for rapid reversal of warfarin anticoagulation in acute intracranial hemorrhage. *Mayo Clin Proc* 2004; **79**:1495–500.

162. Brody, DL, Aiyagari, V, Shakleford, AM, Diringer, MN. Use of recombinant factor VIIa in patients with warfarin-associated intracranial hemorrhage. *Neurocritical Care* 2005; **2**:263–7.

163. O'Shaughnessy, DF, Atterbury, C, Bolton Maggs, P, *et al.* Guidelines for the use of fresh-frozen plasma, cryoprecipitate and cryosupernatant. *Br J Haematol* 2004; **126**: 11–28.

164. British Committee for Standards in Haematology. Guidelines on oral anticoagulation: third edition. *Br J Haematol* 1998; **101**:374–87.

165. Hanley, JP. Warfarin reversal. *J Clin Pathol* 2004; **57**: 1132–9.

166. Ansell, J, Hirsh, J, Dalen, J, *et al.* Managing oral anticoagulant therapy. *Chest* 2001; **119**:22S–38S.

167. Baker, RI, Coughlin, PB, Gallus, AS, *et al.* Warfarin reversal: consensus guidelines, on behalf of the Australasian Society of Thrombosis and Haemostasis. *Med J Aust* 2004; **181**: 492–7.

168. Butler, AC, Tait, RC. Management of oral anticoagulant-induced intracranial haemorrhage. *Blood Rev* 1998; **12**:35–44.

169. Hacke, W. The dilemma of anticoagulation for patients with intracranial hemorrhage or how wide is the strait between Skylla and Karybdis? Editorial. *Neurology* 2000; **57**:1682–4.

170. Eckman, MH, Rosand, J, Knudsen, KA, Singer, DE, Greenberg, SM. Can patients be anticoagulated after intracerebral hemorrhage? A decision analysis. *Stroke* 2003; **34**:1710–16.

171. Wijdicks, EF, Diringer, MN. Middle cerebral artery territory infarction and early brain swelling: progression and effect of age on outcome. *Mayo Clin Proc* 1998; **73**: 829–36.

172. Wann, LS, Curtis, AB, Ellenbogen, KA, *et al.* 2011 ACCF/AHA/HRS focused update on the management of patients with atrial fibrillation (update on dabigatran): a report of the American College of Cardiology Foundation/American Heart Association task force on practice guidelines. *Circulation* 2011; in press.

173. Cleland, JG, Coletta, AP, Buga, L, *et al.* Clinical trials update from the American Heart Association Meeting 2010: EMPHASIS-HF, RAFT, TIM-HF, Tele-HF, ASCEND-HF, ROCKET-AF, and PROTECT. *Eur J Heart Fail* 2011; **13**:460–5.

174. Douglas, MA, Haerer, AF. Long-term prognosis of hypertensive intracerebral hemorrhage. *Stroke* 1982; **13**:488–91.

175. Kunitz, SC, Gross, CR, Heyman, A, *et al.* The pilot Stroke Data Bank: definition, design, and data. *Stroke* 1984; **15**:740–6.

176. Chen, CH, Huang, CW, Chen, HH, Lai, ML. Recurrent hypertensive intracerebral hemorrhage among Taiwanese. *Kaohsiung J Med Sci* 2001; **17**:556–63.

177. Bae, H, Jeong, D, Doh, J, *et al.* Recurrence of bleeding in patients with hypertensive intracerebral hemorrhage. *Cerebrovasc Dis* 1999; **9**:102–8.

178. Hasimoto, Y, Moriyasu, H, Miyashita, T, *et al.* Recurrence of hypertensive intracerebral hemorrhage. *Jpn J Stroke* 1992; **14**:172–8.

179. Rodgers, A, MacMahon, S, Gamble, G, *et al.* Blood pressure and risk of stroke in patients with cerebrovascular disease. The United Kingdom Transient Ischaemic Attack Collaborative Group. *BMJ* 1996; **313**:147.

180. The INDANA (INdividual Data ANalysis of Antihypertensive intervention trials) Project Collaborators. Effect of antihypertensive treatment in patients having already suffered from stroke. Gathering the evidence. The INDANA (INdividual Data ANalysis of Antihypertensive intervention trials) Project Collaborators. *Stroke* 1997; **28**: 2557–62.

181. PATS Collaborating Group. Post-stroke antihypertensive treatment study. A preliminary result. *Chin Med J (Engl)* 1995; **108**:710–17.

182. Yusuf, S, Gerstein, H, Hoogwerf, B, *et al.* Ramipril and the development of diabetes. *JAMA* 2001; **286**:1882–5.

183. Bosch, J, Yusuf, S, Pogue, J, *et al.* Use of ramipril in preventing stroke: double blind randomised trial. *BMJ* 2002; **324**:699–702.

184. Rashid, P, Leonardi-Bee, J, Bath, P. Blood pressure reduction and secondary prevention of stroke and other vascular events: a systematic review. *Stroke* 2003; **34**:2741–8.

185. Donahue, RP, Abbott, RD. Alcohol and haemorrhagic stroke. *Lancet* 1986; **2**:515–16.

186. Goldstein, LB, Adams, R, Becker, K, *et al.* Primary prevention of ischemic stroke : a statement for healthcare professionals from the stroke council of the American Heart Association. *Stroke* 2001; **32**:280–99.

187. Reynolds, K, Lewis, B, Nolen, JD, *et al.* Alcohol consumption and risk of stroke: a meta-analysis. *JAMA* 2003; **289**: 579–88.

188. Gorter, JW. Major bleeding during anticoagulation after cerebral ischemia: patterns and risk factors. Stroke Prevention In Reversible Ischemia Trial (SPIRIT). European Atrial Fibrillation Trial (EAFT) study groups. *Neurology* 1999; **53**:1319–27.

189. Ariesen, MJ, Algra, A, Koudstaal, PJ, Rothwell, PM, van Walraven, C. Risk of intracerebral hemorrhage in patients with arterial versus cardiac origin of cerebral ischemia on aspirin or placebo: analysis of individual patient data from 9 trials. *Stroke* 2004; **35**:710–14.

190. Thrift, AG, McNeil, JJ, Forbes, A, Donnan, GA. Three important subgroups of hypertensive persons at greater risk of intracerebral hemorrhage: Melbourne risk factor group. *Hypertension* 1998; **31**:1223–9.

191. Diener, HC, Cunha, L, Forbes, C, *et al.* European Stroke Prevention Study 2. Dipyridamol and acetylsalicylic acid in the secondary prevention of stroke. *J Neurol Sci* 1996; **143**:1–13.

192. CAPRIE Steering Committee. A randomised, blinded, trial of clopidogrel versus aspirin in patients at risk if ischaemic events (CAPRIE). *Lancet* 1996; **348**:1329–39.

193. Schmulling, S, Rudolf, J, Strotmann-Tack, T, *et al.* Acetylsalicylic acid pretreatment, concomitant heparin therapy and the risk of early intracranial hemorrhage following systemic thrombolysis for acute ischemic stroke. *Cerebrovasc Dis* 2003; **16**:183–90.

194. Deutsche Gesellschaft für Neurologie (DGN). Leitlinien: Status epilepticus im Erwachsenenalter. 2003 http://www. dgn.org/, Access: 8.7.2003.

195. Mayer, SA, Rincon, F. Treatment of intracerebral haemorrhage. *Lancet Neurol* 2005; **4**:662–72.

CHAPTER 19

Diagnostic approach to pauci- or asymptomatic hyperCKemia

T. Kyriakides,[1] C. Angelini,[2] J. Schaefer,[3] S. Sacconi,[4] G. Siciliano,[5] J. J. Vilchez,[6] and D. Hilton-Jones[7]

[1]The Cyprus Institute of Neurology and Genetics, Nicosia, Cyprus; [2]University of Padova, Padova, Italy; [3]Uniklinikum C. G.Carus, University of Dresden, Dresden, Germany; [4]Nice University Hospital, Nice, France; [5]Section of Neurology, University of Pisa, Pisa, Italy; [6]Hospital Universitari La Fe, Valencia, Spain; [7]John Radcliffe Hospital, Oxford, UK

Background

The normal values quoted for serum creatine kinase (sCK) are usually supplied by the manufacturer of the assay and have been derived from population samples that do not accurately reflect the entire population and do not take into account a number of extremely important variables which can affect sCK activity, notably gender, ethnic origin and the effects of exercise [1]. As a consequence, many normal individuals will wrongly be considered to have hyperCKemia and may be investigated unnecessarily or be denied treatment with statins because of unfounded concerns about the presence of subclinical muscle disease [2].

A practical definition of hyperCKemia

In the present context, we aim to define an upper reference value of CK above which further investigation for a possible subclinical myopathy may be appropriate.

Consideration has to be given to the sensitivity and specificity of measuring sCK. Sensitivity means the likelihood of there being an abnormal result in somebody with a muscle disease; thus an elevated sCK is a true-positive result. Specificity relates to a normal individual being classified as having a normal CK – a true-negative result. A low upper limit of normal will increase sensitivity at the cost of reduced specificity so that in practice more normal individuals will be investigated inappropriately. On the other hand, if the upper limit is set higher it will reduce the sensitivity of the test but increase the specificity – fewer normal individuals will be investigated inappropriately, but some patients with muscle disease may be missed. Recent evidence suggests that adopting newly proposed upper reference limits has little practical clinical impact with respect to reducing sensitivity [3].

The first priority is therefore to establish appropriate 97.5 percentile values for each sex and ethnic group. Table 19.1 show the 97.5 percentile values by gender and ethnicity, published in a recent Dutch study. This is the largest study to date looking at the distribution of CK in a large random population sample with standardization of exercise and we propose using these figures as a basis for defining practical upper reference limits for CK activity. Limited evidence suggests that these figures can be applied to patient populations in other countries [3]. Manufacturer quoted upper limits for serum CK activity should be replaced by these figures from Brewster *et al.* [4].

European Handbook of Neurological Management: Volume 2, Second Edition. Edited by Nils Erik Gilhus, Michael P. Barnes, Michael Brainin.
© 2012 Blackwell Publishing Ltd. Published 2012 by Blackwell Publishing Ltd.

Table 19.1 97.5 percentile for serum CK activity (iu/l).

	Non-black	Non-black	Black	Black
	Female	*Male*	*Female*	*Male*
CK iu/l	217	336	414	801

Derived from Brewster *et al.*, 2007.

Table 19.2 Percentage of normal individuals with CK activity above the upper limit of normal.

	Non-black	Non-black	Black	Black
	Female	*Male*	*Female*	*Male*
1.0 ULN	2.5	2.5	2.5	2.5
1.5 ULN	1.5(325)	1.0(504)	1.3(621)	0.5(1201)
2.0 ULN	0.2	0.8	0.5	0

Brewster *et al.*, 2007, pers. comm.
ULN = upper limit of normal. The value in bracket represents
1.5 × ULN.

Table 19.3 Causes of hyperCKemia unrelated to a recognized neuromuscular disease.

Medications
Strenuous muscle exercise (especially eccentric)
Trauma (EMG studies, IM injections)
Surgery
Toxins (alcohol, heroin, cocaine)
Endocrine (hypothyroidism, hypoparathyroidism)
Viral illness
Metabolic (hypokalaemia, hyponatraemia)
'Idiopathic' (sporadic and familial)
Race (black > non-black)
Sex (male > female)
Chronic cardiac disease (CK-MB)
Obstructive sleep apnoea
Neuroacanthocytosis syndromes
Macro-CK
Malignant hyperthermia syndrome

Table 19.4 Drugs frequently associated with chronic hyperCKemia.

Statins (HMG-CoA reductase inhibitors)
Fibrates
Colchicine
Anti-psychotic drugs (including neuroleptic malignant
   syndrome)
Zidovudine
Certain beta blockers
Isoretinoin

In routine clinical practice laboratory results slightly above the defined upper limit (97.5 percentile) are often safely ignored, presumably reflecting the fact that by definition 2.5% of normal individuals will fall in this category and experience indicates that ignoring such values has little clinical impact. It may thus be reasonable, in a population of asymptomatic individuals, to set the level above which investigation is appropriate to a level higher than the 97.5 percentile. Brewster *et al.* (2007) [4], following personal contact, calculated the figures shown in Table 19.2.

If a figure of 1.5 times ULN is taken as the cut-off value for further investigation, as opposed to the 97.5 percentile, then it would approximately half the number of people being investigated, with probably only a small reduction in sensitivity.

Non-myopathic hyperCKemia

Serum CK activity is commonly, but not always, elevated in patients with skeletal muscle disease. It also important to recognize that hyperCKemia can occur in those without a primary muscle disorder. There may be secondary involvement as in neurogenic disorders such as amyotrophic lateral sclerosis, hereditary spinal muscular atrophy type III and IV, post-polio syndrome, bulbospinal muscular atrophy and some neuropathies. In these conditions there are usually no diagnostic difficulties as additional features on examination and the history point to the correct interpretation. sCK may also be elevated in patients without primary neuromuscular disease (Tables 19.3 and 19.4).

These guidelines consider the diagnostic approach in patients with paucior asymptomatic hyperCKemia who otherwise do not have an apparent medical explanation for their hyperCKemia. One of the aims is to provide guidelines to identify in which patients it is appropriate to perform a muscle biopsy.

Search strategy

The Task Force members met in 2009 and decided on a search policy. This included a search for existing guidelines and articles dealing with series of patients investigated for asymptomatic/pauci-symptomatic hyperCKemia, as well as articles dealing with myopathies that can present with asymptomatic hyperCKemia.

Medline 1966–2009 was searched and key terms included: creatine kinase, creatine kinase AND high, creatine kinase AND increase, hyperCKaemia/hyperCKemia AND idiopathic, hyperCKaemia/hyperCKemia AND asymptomatic, hyperCKaemia/hyperCKemia AND biopsy, hyperCKaemia or hyperCKemia AND investigation, CK elevation or elevated AND idiopathic, CK elevation or elevated AND asymptomatic, creatine kinase elevation or elevated AND asymptomatic, creatine kinase elevation or elevated AND idiopathic rhabdomyolysis AND asymptomatic.

The Cochrane Library and the American Academy of Neurology were accessed for any guidelines on the investigation of HyperCKemia and none was found. The only guidelines found were those approved by the Italian Association of Myology Committee [5].

Abstracts were reviewed and relevant articles identified and circulated among members of the Task Force. To evaluate articles we followed the critical review of guidelines as recommended by the EFNS [6]. Only Class IV studies were identified. A first draft was prepared and circulated to all members of the Task Force for a consensus position. Several revisions to the first draft were made and the Task Force met again to finalize the guidelines.

Patients and definitions

Once non-myopathic hyperCKemia has been excluded, pauci-symptomatic patients are those patients without any objective signs of muscle disease such as muscle weakness, atrophy, hypertrophy or myotonia but who have nonspecific and vague neuromuscular symptoms such as myalgias, unexplained fatigue, exercise intolerance, cramps and stiffness. Patients with asymptomatic hyperCKemia are those who do not have any neuromuscular symptoms or signs. Patients with pauci- or asymptomatic hyperCKemia form a heterogeneous group

including among others 'normal' individuals (see above), patients with subclinical myopathy and patients with 'idiopathic hyperCKemia'. The latter term was initially coined by Rowland *et al.* and can be defined as those individuals who have persistent hyperCKemia but no clinical, neurophysiological or histopathological evidence of neuromuscular disease using current laboratory methodologies [7]. There is some evidence that 'idiopathic hyperCKemia' is sometimes familial and may be genetically determined [8].

Results

Muscle biopsy diagnoses in patients with pauci- or asymptomatic hyperCKemia

Several genetically well-defined myopathies can rarely present with isolated hyperCKemia as shown in Table 19.5.

However an indication of the relative frequencies of various myopathies diagnosed in patients with pauci- or asymptomatic hyperCKemia can be gleaned from some retrospective studies [9, 17, 26, 27, 28, 29, 30, 31]. Patients with non-neuromuscular causes of hyperCKemia and/or with a family history of documented neuromuscular disorder were excluded in these studies. Although none was prospective, patient inclusion was probably representative of everyday practice. The frequency of definitive or probable diagnoses provided by muscle biopsy varied from 8% to 63%.

The frequency of a normal biopsy result after all laboratory tests had been performed varied between 8% and

Table 19.5 Genetic myopathies that can present as isolated hyperCKemia.

Adult onset glycogenosis type II	[9]
Caveolinopathy (Caveolin-3)	[10–12]
Calpainopathy (Calpain-3)	[13, 14]
Desminopathy	[15, 16]
Dysferlinopathy (LGMD & Miyoshi)	[14, 17–19]
Fukutin-related protein (FKRP) LGMD 2I	[19]
Dystrophinopathy(also female carriers)	[20–23]
Sarcoglycanopathy	[24]
Myotonic dystrophy type 2	[25]

55%. What is perhaps distressing to both patient and physician is the frequency of nonspecific myopathic abnormalities which prevented a diagnosis to be made in 16–83% of patients.

There are several reasons for the discrepancy in reaching a final diagnosis between series, including differences in the age of patients, the level of hyperCKemia and the range of testing performed on muscle biopsies. Three large studies (>100 patients each) have included comprehensive testing beyond routine histology and histochemistry, such as immunocytochemistry, respiratory chain and glycolytic enzyme assays [9, 17, 28]. Of a total of 323 patients in these three studies a specific diagnosis was made in 92 (28%), an abnormal, nonspecific myopathic biopsy was found in 138 (43%) and a normal biopsy in 93 (29%). The specific diagnoses made in 460 patients with pauci- or asymptomatic hyperCKemia are shown in Table 19.6. Of the 121 specific diagnoses the most common were metabolic myopathies (42%) and subclinical muscular dystrophies (21%). The former were presumably asymptomatic or only minimally symptomatic, while the latter were mostly diagnosed in the first two decades, presumably prior to the appearance of the typical phenotypes. As can be seen from Table 19.6, although only a small minority of the myopathies have specific treatments, an accurate diagnosis of an untreatable condition is often enormously beneficial to the patient and the family in terms of discussing prognosis, potential complications which may be treatable (e.g., cardiomyopathy and ventilatory muscle involvement) and genetic counselling.

Variables that increase the likelihood of a diagnostic muscle biopsy

The patient is best served if a muscle biopsy results in a specific diagnosis. A few studies have looked for clinical and laboratory indicators, which, if present, indicate that muscle biopsy is more likely to give a specific diagnosis.

Level of hyperCKemia

Fernandez et al. identified that a CK > 10 × normal was statistically associated with an increased probability of arriving at a specific diagnosis following biopsy [9]. Similarly Prelle et al. [17] found a CK > 5 × normal, combined with an age of <24 years, to be predictive of arriving at a specific diagnosis. In Filosto et al., seven out

of 105 had a metabolic myopathy; five myophosphorylase deficiency (glycogenosis type V), one phosphofructokinase deficiency; and one mitochondrial myopathy [28]. All six patients with a glycogenosis had a CK > 7 × normal.

The role of electromyography

With rare exceptions (e.g., myotonic dystrophy) an electromyogram (EMG) is not expected to provide any specific diagnosis other than to give information about motor unit physiology. There are several studies on the sensitivity and specificity of EMG in the literature but what is relevant in the context of paucior asymptomatic hyperCKemia can only be gleaned from the studies in this particular group of patients. The key questions that need to be answered are: does an abnormal EMG increase the likelihood of an abnormal biopsy and, conversely, does a normal EMG decrease the likelihood of an abnormal biopsy?

In Prelle et al. 100 patients had both EMG and biopsy [17]. The sensitivity of EMG (the proportion of patients with an abnormal biopsy who also had an abnormal EMG) biopsy was 73%. Thus an abnormal EMG increases the chances of obtaining an abnormal biopsy. The specificity of EMG (proportion of patients with normal biopsy who also have a normal EMG) was only 53%. Thus an abnormal EMG may be associated with a normal biopsy. If one uses the data in Prelle et al., the positive predictive value of an abnormal EMG (i.e., the likelihood that an abnormal EMG will predict an abnormal biopsy in a group of pauci- or asymptomatic hyperCKemia patients) is 51%. Similarly, the negative predictive value of a normal EMG (i.e., the likelihood that a normal EMG will predict a normal biopsy) is 74%.

In the study by Joy and Oh the sensitivity of an abnormal EMG was 92% and its specificity 100% [29]. The positive predictive value of an abnormal EMG in predicting an abnormal biopsy was 100%, while the negative predictive value of a normal EMG in predicting a normal biopsy was 80%. On the basis of our extensive personal experience the figures from this much smaller study (19 patients) are far too optimistic. However, it is noteworthy that both studies agree on the high negative predictive value of a normal EMG (74–80%).

As far as can be ascertained, in none of the above studies was quantitative EMG employed and therefore its contribution in helping to select patients for biopsy is unknown.

Table 19.6 Diagnoses in patients with pauci- or asymptomatic hyperCKemia.

Diagnoses	Joy et al, 1989	Reijneveld et al, 2001	Prelle et al, 2002	Simmons et al, 2003	Fernandez et al, 2006	Dabby et al, 2006	Filosto et al, 2007	Malan-drini et al 2008	Total
Specific myopathies	12/19	6/37	21/114	6/20	55/104	3/40	15/105	3/37	121/460
Muscular Dystrophies									25
Dystrophinopathy		2	5		9	3		1	17
Dysferlinopathy			1		1				2
Caveolinopathy					1				1
Calpainopathy					1				1
Sarcoglycanopathy		1							1
LGMD-unspecified			1						1
Fukutin related protein					2				2
Metabolic myopathies									50
CPT 2 def.									6
Myophosphorylase	1	1	4	2	15		5		22
Phosphofructokinase def.							1		1
1 α, glucosidase def.					9				9
glycogenoses (unspecified)					1				1
Phosphorylase-b Kinase				3					3
Adenylate Deaminase			1	1					2
Mitochondrial	2		2		1		1		6
Inflammatory myopathy									20
Polymyositis	5				6			1	12
Inclusion body myositis	1				2				3
Macrophagic myositis					5				5
Congenital myopathy									8
Central core	1	1	1				2	1	6
Centronuclear							1		1
Multicore	1								1
Miscellaneous									14
Malignant Hyperthermia myopathy			3						3
Tubular aggregates		1					3		5
Myofibrillar myopathy			1						2
Lobulated fiber myopathy					2		2		2
Desminopathy			1						1
Sarcoid myopathy	1								1
Myotonia fluctuans			1						1
Non-specific myopathic	3/19	24/37	18/114	3/20	26/104	19/40	68/105	29/37	190/460
Neurogenic			13/114		2/104		8/105	2/37	25/460
Normal	4/19	7/37	62/114	11/20	15/104	18/40	14/105	3/37	134/460

283

Clinical parameters

Fernandez *et al.* (2006) found age < 15 years to be statistically associated with a higher probability of reaching a specific diagnosis. Other variables associated with increased probability, but which did not reach statistical significance, were female vs. male (63 vs. 51%) and pauci-symptomatic vs. asymptomatic (59 vs. 50%) [9]. Among pauci-symptomatic patients with hyperCKemia investigated by Filosto *et al.*, all six patients with glycogenoses had exercise-induced myalgias and no patients with isolated rest pain had a metabolic myopathy [28].

Prognosis in patients with pauci- or asymptomatic hyperCKemia

Prelle *et al.* reported a 6-year follow-up study of 55 of the 93 undiagnosed asymptomatic hyperCKemic patients of their original cohort (38 were lost to follow-up) [32]. Most patients (43/55 or 78%) still had persistent hyperCKemia but at a lower level. CK had normalized in 12/55 (22%). Statistical analysis revealed a correlation between CK normalization and a normal biopsy. One patient was diagnosed to have limb girdle muscular dystrophy and one to be a dystrophinopathy carrier. Thus long-term prognosis for the whole group was favourable.

An earlier, long-term follow-up study (mean 7.2 years) of 23 out of the original 31 idiopathic hyperCKemia patients also provided a benign prognosis, with none of the patients developing neurological abnormalities except for one who developed an axonal neuropathy [33]. The mean values of CK did not differ significantly at follow-up.

Risk for malignant hyperthermia

Malignant hyperthermia (MH) susceptibility may be seen in association with central core disease, in which case additional features of myopathy may be present, but can also occur in isolation. In the latter group of asymptomatic patients some may have hyperCKemia. The question therefore arises as to the possibility of MH susceptibility in an individual with asymptomatic hyperCKemia in whom all other investigations have failed to reveal a cause. There are practical problems in that confirmation of MH susceptibility involves what will usually be a second muscle biopsy, few centres offer such testing and even then there are limits to sensitivity and specificity.

There have been few large studies. Weglinski *et al.* (1997) [34] reported that 24 out of 49 (49%) patients with asymptomatic hyperCKemia had positive contracture tests. More recently Malandrini *et al.* (2008) found one susceptible and one equivocal subject in 37 patients with asymptomatic hyperCKemia [31]. The facility for MH testing varies widely between neuromuscular centres and countries. We advise that local guidelines be followed, but that a pragmatic approach is to advise patients with otherwise unexplained hyperCKemia that they may be MH-susceptible and that appropriate anaesthetic guidelines should be followed. Consideration also has to be given to assessing and advising other family members.

Recommendations

The recommendations are based on the limited number of Class IV studies available and the expert opinion of the panel and as a result can be viewed as Level C recommendations. They outline the sequential steps in a diagnostic approach to pauci- or asymptomatic hyperCKemia.

1. HyperCKemia is defined as sCK > 1.5 × the ULN (see revised values in Table 19.2).
2. Consider all non-neuromuscular causes in Tables 19.3 and 19.4 and other non-myopathic causes of hyperCKemia that might explain their high sCK.
3. Inquire about any family history of neuromuscular disease, hyperCKemia or malignant hyperthermia.
4. Before embarking on long and expensive investigations it is advised that hyperCKemia is confirmed by repeat assay, and that the possibility of normal, exercise-induced elevation is excluded. The patient should therefore be advised to avoid strenuous exercise for 7 days prior to sampling and at least two samples one month apart should be taken.
5. If hyperCKemia is confirmed, perform a nerve conduction study and electromyogram (EMG).
6. A biopsy may be performed in a patient with hyperCKemia if one or more of the following applies:
   a. the EMG is abnormal (myopathic);
   b. sCK is ≥ 3 × normal;
   c. the patient is aged < 25 years;
   d. Presence of exercised-induced pain or exercise intolerance;

    e. women with hyperCKemia but sCK< 3 × normal (because of the possibility of Duchenne/Becker mutation carrier status). However, prior to biopsy DNA analysis on blood lymphocytes should be undertaken. Currently, MLPA analysis will identify ~70% of carriers. Developing technology is likely to improve that and all such cases should be discussed with local genetic services.

    f. Men with hyperCKemia and a sCK < 3 times normal may be offered a biopsy if they are seriously concerned about neuromuscular disease or alternatively they may be followed up in the neurology clinic.

7. The extent of diagnostic work-up to be performed on a muscle biopsy will vary, but must include histology, histochemistry and immunohistochemistry (Table 19.7). Further investigations may be needed, directed by the biopsy appearance, including western blotting, enzymolog and mitochondrial DNA analysis. A frozen sample should be stored at the time of biopsy to be available for such studies.

Table 19.7 Minimal muscle biopsy investigations.

Histology & histochemistry

Haematoxylin &eosin, modified Gomori trichrome, Oil red O, periodic acid-schiff, adenosine triphosphatase (9.4, 4.2, and 4.6), succinate dehydrogenase (SDH), Nicotinamide Adenine Dinucleotide Hydrogenase (NADH), cytochrome c oxidase, myophosphorylase, acid phosphatase.

Immunohistochemistry

Dystrophin, α, β, γ and δ sarcoglycans, dysferlin, caveolin-3, MHC-1, α-dystroglycan.

References

1. Sewright, KA, Hubal, MJ, Kearns, A, *et al.* Sex differences in response to maximal eccentric exercise. *Med Sci Sports Exerc* 2008; **40**:242–51.

2. Glueck, CJ, Rawal, B, Khan, NA, *et al.*Should high creatine kinase discourage the initiation or continuance of statins for the treatment of hypercholesterolemia? *Metabolism* 2009; **58**:233–8.

3. Nardin, RA, Zarrin, AR, Horowitz, GL, Tarulli, AW. Effect of newly proposed CK reference limits on neuromuscular diagnosis. *Muscle Nerve* 2009; **39**:494–7.

4. Brewster, LM, Mairuhu, G, Sturk, A, van Montfrans, GA. Distribution of creatine kinase in the general population: implications for statin therapy. *Am Heart J* 2007; **154**: 655–61.

5. Morandi, ., Angelini, C, Prelle, A, *et al.* High plasma creatine kinase: review of the literature and proposal for a diagnostic algorithm. *Neurol Sci* 2006; **2**:303–11.

6. Brainin, M, Barnes, M, Baron, JC, *et al.* Guidance for the preparation of neurological management guidelines by EFNS scientific task forces – revised recommendations. *Eur J Neurol* 2004; **11**:577–81.

7. Rowland, LP, Willner, J, Cerri, C, *et al.* Approaches to the membrane theory of Duchenne muscular dystrophy, in *Muscular Dystrophy Research: Advances and New Trends* (eds C Angelini, GA Danielli, D Fontanari) 1980; Excerpta Medica, Amsterdam, pp. 3–13.

8. Capasso, M, De Angelis, MV, Di Muzio, A, *et al.* Familial idiopathic hyper-CK-emia: an underrecognized condition. *Muscle Nerve* 2006; **33**:760–5.

9. Fernandez, C, de Paula, AM, Figarella-Branger, D, *et al.* Diagnostic evaluation of clinically normal subjects with chronic hyperCKemia. *Neurology* 2006; **66**:1585–7.

10. Carbone, I, Bruno, C, Sotgia, F, *et al.* Mutation in the CAV3 gene causes partial caveolin-3 deficiency and hyperCKemia. *Neurology* 2000; **54**:1373–6.

11. Woodman, SE, Sotgia, F, Galbiati, F, *et al.* Caveolinopathies: mutations in caveolin-3 cause four distinct autosomal dominant muscle diseases. *Neurology* 2004; **62**:538–43.

12. Merlini, L, Carbone, I, Capanni, C, *et al.* Familial isolated hyperCKaemia associated with a new mutation in the caveolin-3 (CAV-3) gene. *J Neurol Neurosurg Psychiatry* 2002; **73**:65–7.

13. Hanisch, F, Muller, CR, Grimm, D, *et al.* Frequency of calpain-3 c.550delA mutation in limb girdle muscular dystrophy type 2 and isolated hyperCKemia in German patients. *Clin Neuropathol* 2007; **26**:157–63.

14. Fanin, M, Nascimbeni, AC, Aurino, S, *et al.* Frequency of LGMD gene mutations in Italian patients with distinct clinical phenotypes. *Neurology* 2009; **72**:1432–5.

15. Prelle, A, Rigoletto, C, Moggio, M, *et al.* Asymptomatic familial hyperCKemia associated with desmin accumulation in skeletal muscle. *J Neurol Sci* 1996; **140**:132–6.

16. Strach, K, Sommer, T, Grohe, C, *et al.* Clinical, genetic, and cardiac magnetic resonance imaging findings in primary desminopathies. *Neuromuscul Disord* 2008; **18**:475–82.

17. Prelle, A, Tancredi, L, Sciacco, M, *et al.* Retrospective study of a large population of patients with asymptomatic or minimally symptomatic raised serum creatine kinase levels. *J Neurol* 2002; **249**:305–11.

18. Nguyen, K, Bassez, G, Krahn, M, *et al.* Phenotypic study in 40 patients with dysferlin gene mutations: high frequency of atypical phenotypes. *Arch Neurol* 2007; **64**:1176–82.

19. Boito, CA, Melacini, P, Vianello, A, *et al.* Clinical and molecular characterization of patients with limb-girdle muscular dystrophy type 2I. *Arch Neurol*, 2005; **62**:1894–9.

20. Ferreiro, V, Giliberto, F, Muniz, GM, *et al.* Asymptomatic Becker muscular dystrophy in a family with a multiexon deletion. *Muscle Nerve* 2009; **39**:239–43.

21. Ramelli, GP, Joncourt, F, Luetschg, J, *et al.* Becker muscular dystrophy with marked divergence between clinical and molecular genetic findings: case series. *Swiss Med Wkly* 2006; **136**:189–93.

22. Hoffman, EP, Arahata, K, Minetti, C, *et al.* Dystrophinopathy in isolated cases of myopathy in females. *Neurology* 1992; **42**:967–75.

23. Doriguzzi, C, Palmucci, L, Mongini, T, *et al.* Systematic use of dystrophin testing in muscle biopsies: results in 201 cases. *Eur J Clin Invest* 1997; **27**:352–8.

24. Angelini, C, Fanin, M, Menegazzo, E, *et al.* Homozygous alpha-sarcoglycan mutation in two siblings: one asymptomatic and one steroid-responsive mild limb-girdle muscular dystrophy patient. *Muscle Nerve* 1998; **21**:769–75.

25. Merlini, L, Sabatelli, P, Columbaro, M, *et al.* Hyper-CK-emia as the sole manifestation of myotonic dystrophy type 2. *Muscle Nerve* 2005; **31**:764–7.

26. Simmons, Z, Peterlin, BL, Boyer, PJ, Towfighi, J. Muscle biopsy in the evaluation of patients with modestly elevated creatine kinase levels. *Muscle Nerve* 2003; **27**:242–4.

27. Reijneveld, JC, Notermans, NC, Linssen, WH, *et al.* Hyper-CK-aemia revisited. *Neuromuscul Disord* 2001; **11**:163–4.

28. Filosto, M, Tonin, P, Vattemi, G, *et al.* The role of muscle biopsy in investigating isolated muscle pain. *Neurology* 2007; **68**:181–6.

29. Joy, JL, Oh, SJ. Asymptomatic hyper-CK-emia: an electrophysiologic and histopathologic study. *Muscle Nerve* 1989; **12**:206–9.

30. Dabby, R, Sadeh, M, Herman, O, *et al.* Asymptomatic or minimally symptomatic hyperCKemia: histopathologic correlates. *Isr Med Assoc J* 2006; **8**,:110–13.

31. Malandrini, A, Orrico, A, Gaudiano, C, *et al.* Muscle biopsy and in vitro contracture test in subjects with idiopathic HyperCKemia. *Anesthesiology* 2008; **109**:625–8.

32. D'Adda, E, Sciacco, M, Fruguglietti, ME, *et al.* Follow-up of a large population of asymptomatic/oligosymptomatic hyperckemic subjects. *J Neurol*, 2006; **253**:1399–1403.

33. Reijneveld, JC, Notermans, NC, Linssen, WH, Wokke, JH. Benign prognosis in idiopathic hyper-CK-emia. *Muscle Nerve* 2000; **23**:575–9.

34. Weglinski, MR, Wedel, DJ, Engel, AG. Malignant hyperthermia testing in patients with persistently increased serum creatine kinase levels. *Anesth Analg* 1997; **84**:1038–41.

CHAPTER 20

Diagnosis and management of neuromyelitis optica

J. Sellner,[1] M. Boggild,[2] M. Clanet,[3] R. Q. Hintzen,[4] Z. Illes,[5] X. Montalban,[6] R. A. Du Pasquier,[7] C. H. Polman,[8] P. Soelberg Sørensen[9] and B. Hemmer[1]

[1]Klinikum rechts der Isar, Technische Universität München, Munich, Germany; [2]The Walton Centre for Neurology and Neurosurgery, Liverpool, United Kingdom; [3]Purpan University Hospital, Toulouse, France; [4]Erasmus MC, University Medical Centre, Rotterdam, The Netherlands; [5]University of Pecs, Pecs, Hungary; [6]Hospital Universitari Vall d' Hebron (HUVH), Barcelona, Spain; [7]Centre Hospitalier Universitaire Vaudois and University of Lausanne, Lausanne, Switzerland; [8]VU University Medical Centre, MS Center, Amsterdam, The Netherlands; [9]Copenhagen University and Rigshospitalet, Copenhagen, Denmark

Objectives

To provide guidelines for best practice diagnosis and management of adult neuromyelitis optica based on the current state of clinical and scientific knowledge.

Introduction

Neuromyelitis optica (NMO, also known as Devic's disease) is a severe idiopathic immune-mediated demyelinating and necrotizing disease that predominantly involves optic nerves and the spinal cord. Cases of NMO have been reported in all continents and races, but ethnic variations suggest that genetic factors are relevant [1, 2, 3, 4, 5, 6, 7, 8, 9, 10]. In Europe, the prevalence of NMO among autoimmune disorders of the central nervous system (CNS) is relatively low compared with multiple sclerosis (MS). However, NMO makes up a substantial proportion of inflammatory demyelinating disorders of the CNS in non-Caucasian populations, such as Afro-Brazilians (15%), East Asians (up to 48%) and Indians (9%), most likely due to the divergent prevalence of MS [9, 11, 12, 13].

The association between optic neuritis (ON) and spinal cord impairment was first described by Sir Clifford Albutt in 1870 [14]. In 1894, Eugene Devic and his student Fernand Gault evaluated further cases and proposed the nature of the pathological process, named the syndrome 'neuro-myélite optique' or 'neuroptico-myélite', and discussed a relationship with MS [15, 16]. However, it was not until the 1990s that further clinical and histopathological studies changed the concept and place of NMO within the expanding range of autoimmune disorders of the CNS.

Historically, the diagnosis of NMO was restricted to a monophasic course of bilateral ON and myelitis as well as cases with short intervals between the index events. More recently, NMO has been recognized as a recurrent autoimmune CNS disorder with clinical, neuroimaging and laboratory findings that are distinct from MS. Accordingly, NMO immunoglobulin G (NMO-IgG, referred to as aquaporin 4 antibody when using antigen-specific detection techniques), an autoantibody that binds to the water channel aquaporin 4 (AQP4), in combination with diagnostic criteria support distinction of NMO from other autoimmune disorders of the CNS [17]. NMO-IgG/AQP4 antibodies are also detected in

European Handbook of Neurological Management: Volume 2, Second Edition. Edited by Nils Erik Gilhus, Michael P. Barnes, Michael Brainin.

NMO spectrum disorders, which include: 1) spatially limited forms, such as longitudinally extensive transverse myelitis (LETM) and recurrent isolated optic neuritis (RION)/bilateral optic neuritis (BON) [18, 19]; 2) NMO in the context of organ- and non-organ-specific autoimmune diseases [20, 21]; 3) atypical cases with clinically manifest or subclinical brain lesions; and 4) Asian opticospinal MS (OSMS) [22].

The natural history of untreated NMO is significantly worse than that of MS, with acquisition of residual disability from initial relapses in the majority of patients. Hence, NMO requires early recognition and concepts for treatment of acute attacks and long-term disease modification. However, studies on diagnosis and evaluation of treatments are scarce and most diagnostic and therapeutic recommendations reflect consensus opinion of individual experts in the field.

Search strategy and grading of recommendations

Evidence for this guideline was collected by searches for original articles, case reports and meta-analyses in the Medline and Cochrane databases by employing relevant keywords, combinations and abbreviations. The period for eligible articles was 1965–September 2009, and following suggestions from the reviewers some individual articles beyond this period were included. Clinical practice guidelines were searched for within databases of the European Federation of Neurological Societies (EFNS, www.efns.org/EFNS-Guideline-Papers.270.0.html), the American Academy of Neurology (AAN, www.aan.com/go/practice/guidelines), the American College of Rheumatology (ACR, www.rheumatology.org/index.org) and the British Society for Rheumatology (www.rheumatology.org.uk).

Scientific evidence for diagnostic investigations and treatments were evaluated according to pre-specified levels of certainty (Classes I, II, III and IV) [23]. The recommendations were graded according to the strength of evidence (Level A, B or C), using definitions given in the EFNS guidance. When sufficient evidence for recommendations A–C were not available, we gave a good practice point recommendation if agreed by all members of the Task Force.

The Task Force was initiated by the EFNS Scientific Panel on Multiple Sclerosis/Demyelinating Disorders and commissioned by the Scientific Committee of the EFNS. JS and BH wrote the first draft. Consensus was reached after three rounds of circulating questionnaires and drafts to the Task Force members.

Results

Diagnostic strategies
Demographics and disease-specific features
Ethnic variations in the condition suggest that genetic factors are important and rare familial cases have been reported (Class IV) [24, 25]. NMO primarily affects non-whites and populations with a minor European contribution to their genetic composition (Class IV) [13, 26, 27, 28, 29]. Among a cohort of 850 patients with demyelinating disorders in north-east Tuscany, the prevalence of NMO spectrum disorders was 1.5% ($n = 13$), the MS:NMO ratio was 42.7:1 (Class IV) [30]. Similar neuroimaging, autoantibody and immunopathological characteristics of NMO and Asian opticospinal MS support the hypothesis that the latter, or a subset, is identical to Western NMO (Class IV) [9, 29, 31]. Yet, Japanese opticospinal MS was associated with the human leukocyte antigen (HLA) Class II DPB1*0501 allele, which could not be confirmed in a European NMO cohort (Class III) [1, 10, 32]. Moreover, different diagnostic criteria for Japanese and Western forms impede a detailed comparison (Class IV) [22].

In monophasic NMO (no recurrence, simultaneous or closely related ON and LETM [<30 days]), men and women are affected equally but in the more frequent recurrent disease course, women are overrepresented (ratio 5–10:1) (Class IV) [2, 4, 7, 8, 29, 33, 34]. The age of onset in NMO ranges from childhood to late adulthood, the median onset age is in the late 30s, with the incidence tapering off after the fifth decade [35, 36, 37, 38] (Class IV). In MS, 70% of first manifestations occur between the age of 20 and 40 (median onset at ~30 years) [39].

The majority of patients suffer from a recurrent course (80–90%), while monophasic (10–20%) and primary or secondary progressive courses are rare (Class IV) [2, 8, 40, 41]. Relapses usually occur early, in clusters and at unpredictable intervals (Class IV) [8, 40]. In the Mayo Clinic series, the second relapse occurred within 1 year in 60%, within 3 years in 90%, but also decades after the index events (Class IV) [8]. Likewise, in a Cuban NMO study the next relapse developed after a mean time of 15 months (range 1–158 months) from the index events (Class IV) [33]. In contrast, among Mexican NMO patients who were followed for more than 3 years, 82% (14/17 patients) still had a monophasic course (Class IV) [7]. Predictors of a recurrent course were a longer inter-attack interval between the first two clinical episodes, older age at onset, female sex and less severe motor impairment at the sentinel myelitis event (Class IV) [40].

There are no disease-specific clinical features. Clinical manifestations include involvement of the optic nerve, spinal cord, or both, but also many other symptoms and signs. Resulting from a cumulative attack-related injury of the CNS, the natural history of NMO is characterized by a stepwise deterioration of motor, sensory, visual and bowel/bladder function (Class IV) [8, 33, 40]. Severe attacks of myelitis or ON should raise suspicion of NMO. Most relapses worsen over several days and then slowly improve in the weeks or months after the maximum clinical deficit is reached (Class IV) [8]. An antecedent viral illness was reported in 30% of patients with monophasic and 23% of patients with recurrent NMO (Class IV) [8].

Conclusions

NMO is a different clinical entity from MS, characterized by a worldwide occurrence with ethnic variations, and (compared to MS) is a relatively rare disorder in Europe. Most frequently, NMO develops as a recurrent disorder, which predominantly affects women.

Recommendations

In the diagnosis of NMO it is recommended to take the following disease characteristics into consideration: the predominant course is characterized by recurrent severe attacks of myelitis and/or uni- or bilateral ON with incomplete recovery, and is up to 10 times more prevalent in women than in men. Age of onset (the late 30s) is approximately 10 years later than age of onset in MS, but NMO may also occur in children and elderly people.

Clinical features
Optic neuritis

Visual loss is generally more severe in NMO than in MS (Class IV) [42]. The occurrence of bilateral simultaneous ON or sequential ON in rapid succession is more sugges-tive for NMO (Class IV) [40]. Other clinical features of ON, including pain, pattern of visual loss, occurrence of positive visual phenomena such as movement-induced phosphenes and findings on examination, do not differ from MS-related ON attacks (Class IV) [8]. Blindness in at least one eye developed in 60% of recurrent (mean follow-up 16.9 years) and 22% of monophasic NMO patients (mean follow-up 7.7 years) (Class IV) [8]. Ophthalmoscopic examination may be normal or exhibit signs of ON, and optic atrophy with disc pallor is typi-cally more pronounced than in MS. In addition, demy-elination and necrosis is predominantly seen at the centre of the nerve and may form cavitation (Class IV) [43, 44].

Visual field testing typically reveals central scotoma, although other visual field changes, such as colour blind-ness, bitemporal hemianopsia, paracentral scotoma and altitudinal deficits, are possible. Optic coherence tomog-raphy studies in NMO reported a thinner retinal fibre layer than in MS, indicating more widespread axonal injury (Class IV) [45, 46].

Myelitis

Spinal cord involvement usually presents in the form of complete transverse myelitis with para- or tetraparesis, an almost symmetrical sensory level and sphincter dys-function (Class IV) [2, 8, 34, 47]. In contrast, spinal cord symptoms in MS are milder and asymmetric, and caused by acute partial transverse myelitis (Class IV) [48, 49]. Radicular pain, paroxysmal tonic spasms and Lhermitte's signs develop in a third of the recurrent cases, but are rare or absent in patients with monophasic NMO (Class IV) [8]. Nausea and intractable hiccups were found in 8 of 47 (17%) patients with recurrent NMO due to expansion of the lesion to the medulla (Class IV) [50]. Other brain-stem symptoms include vomiting, vertigo, hearing loss, facial weakness, trigeminal neuralgia, diplopia, ptosis and nystagmus (Class IV) [8, 51, 52]. Due to involvement of the medullary centres of neuromuscular respiration control, neurogenic respiratory failure and subsequent death can occur (Class IV) [8].

Other manifestations

CNS involvement beyond the optic nerve and spinal cord/brainstem is observed in about 15% of NMO patients and includes encephalopathy, hypothalamic dysfunction and cognitive impairment (Class IV) [8, 53, 54]. The latter is present in NMO with a similar frequency as that reported in MS (Class IV) [55]. Magana *et al.* reported five NMO-IgG seropositive women ($n = 3$ NMO, $n = 2$ recurrent LETM), who developed confusion and depressed consciousness consistent with posterior reversible encephalopathy syndrome (PRES) (Class IV) [53]. The immune-mediated disruption of the AQP4 water channel function may play a central role in the pathogenesis of PRES in these patients. Endocrinopathies associated with NMO include amenorrhea, galactorrhea, diabetes insipidus, hypothyroidism and hyperphagia (Class IV) [56].

Outcome

The index events (visual acuity, motor, sensory and sphincter dysfunction) are more severe in monophasic than recurrent NMO (Class IV) [40]. Repeated NMO attacks are the main cause of accumulation of neurological impairment, whereas permanent disability in MS is primarily a feature of secondary progression. In a Brazilian cohort, incomplete recovery from the index event predicted future disability (Class IV) [4].

A history of other autoimmune diseases, higher attack frequency during the first 2 years of disease and better motor recovery following the index myelitis event was associated with increased risk for fatality in recurrent NMO (Class IV) [40]. In this study (published in 2003), which may have been biased towards more severe and complicated cases, 32% of patients with recurrent NMO died (median follow-up 60.2 months) while no death occurred in patients with monophasic NMO [40]. Twenty four out of 96 (25%) patients of a cohort from the French West indies died; predictors of mortality were higher attack frequency during the first year of disease, blindness and sphincter signs at onset (Class IV) [57]. Mortality in a cohort of recurrent NMO from Brazil (published in 2002) was even higher (50%) (Class IV) [12], but recent progress in understanding the disease and its management are likely to have decreased mortality rates.

Conclusions

A recurrent course with rapid development of further events is frequent. Individual episodes of ON/LETM are severe and permanent disability is more attack-related in NMO than in MS. CNS involvement beyond optic nerve and spinal cord/brainstem need to be taken into account. NMO is associated with a more detrimental short- and long-term outcome than MS, and neurogenic respiratory failure is the most frequent cause of death. Prognostic factors need to be confirmed in independent prospective studies.

Recommendations

ON with severe visual loss and in rapid succession may be indicative for NMO. Optic atrophy is more pronounced than in MS and may form cavitation. Complete transverse myelitis is typical for NMO and partial transverse myelitis syndromes are more indicative of MS. Expansion of the spinal cord lesion may lead to brainstem symptoms and life-threatening complications.

Imaging
Optic nerve

There are no studies evaluating differences in MRI presentation of ON in the setting of NMO and MS. Short-tau inversion recovery (STIR) sequences provide fat suppression, which is advantageous for evaluation of the optic nerve. Using STIR sequences, increased signal intensity on T2-weighted scans of the optic nerve is reported in acute ON in 84% and during remission in 20% (Class IV) [58]. Disruption of the blood–nerve barrier leads to gadolinium enhancement on T1-weighted spin echo sequences. Gadolinium-enhancement is a sensitive finding in acute ON (94%) (Class IV) [59], is of variable extent and can occasionally extend into the optic chiasm. In a Cuban study of patients with long-duration NMO, gadolinium-enhancement of the optic nerve was found in 32.5% (Class III) [60].

Spinal cord

Spinal cord lesions extending over three or more vertebral segments are the most reliable finding for the diagnosis of NMO (Class IV) [52]. However, normal appearances or shorter lesions can be found very early during relapse or in residual atrophic stage [52]. Lesions are predominantly located in the cervical and thoracic cord with a central grey matter pattern, reflected by hyperintensities on T2-weighted axial scans and corresponding T1 hypointensities (Class IV) [47, 61]. Cervical lesions may extend to the lower medulla. Cavity-like longitudinally extensive lesions are seen in cases of severe disease. Acute spinal cord lesions tend to occupy most of the cross-sectional area of an affected segment and are associated with swelling and gadolinium-enhancement (detectable days to months following relapse) (Class IV) [2, 62, 63]. In a study on LETM relapses in NMO ($n = 11$), gadolinium-enhancement disappeared in all patients following treatment with high-dose methyl-prednisolone, and lesions may almost entirely disappear during remission (Class IV) [61].

Conversely, spinal cord lesions over two or more vertebral segments are rarely found in MS [48]. Lesions in MS usually appear as short-segment, asymmetric and often posterior cord lesions (Class IV) [49, 64]. A 'snake-eye' or 'owl-eye' sign is a common feature of spinal artery ischemia and may be a transient finding at an early stage of NMO (Class IV) [61].

Brain

Normal brain MRI is initially present in 55–84% of NMO patients, though a development of cerebral white matter lesions can be expected over the course of the disease (Class IV) [2, 8, 34]. Indeed, brain MRI lesions can be detected with serial scans in up to 84.8% of NMO patients (Class IV) [4, 51, 65, 66, 67]. Distribution of NMO-typical brain lesions (8/120 patients) corresponded to structures with high AQP4 expression, such as ependymal cells, hypothalamus and brainstem (Class IV) [51, 65]. The presence of brain lesions may be more common in childhood NMO. A cross-sectional study reported that brain lesions were found in 68% and predominantly involved the periventricular region (Class IV) [68].

Most lesions are nonspecific and asymptomatic; Pittock *et al.* reported the presence of brain MRI lesions in 60% of patients, of which 10% were rated MS-like and fulfilled the Barkhof criteria for dissemination in space (Class III) [51]. Two or more brain MRI lesions were found in 66% of a Cuban NMO cohort, but presence of lesions did not correlate with disease severity (Class IV) [60]. In a Chinese study most supratentorial lesions were rated as nonspecific punctate or small round dot, and located in juxtacortical, subcortical and deep white matter regions (Class IV) [67]. Callosal lesions were described in 18.2% (4/22) of AQP4 antibody-positive Japanese patients with NMO spectrum disorders (Class III) [69]. These callosal lesions were classified as acute, large and oedematous in 3 of 4 patients and appeared with a heterogeneous lesion intensity ('marbled pattern'), whereas callosal lesions in MS (36/56, 64.3%) were reported to be small, isolated and non-oedematous. Another study described a cloud-like enhancement of brain lesions in terms of multiple patchy enhancement with blurred margin as typical for NMO (Class IV) [70].

Symptomatic brain lesions are not an exclusion criterion for NMO [54, 56]. Brain MRI of NMO spectrum disorder patients experiencing a PRES episode revealed bilateral T2-hyperintensities primarily in frontal, parieto-occipital and cerebellar regions (Class IV) [53].

Conclusions

The most characteristic MRI finding is a spinal cord lesion expanding over 3 or more vertebral segments on T2-weighted images, occupying most of the cross-sectional area, frequently hypointense on T1-weighted images and displaying gadolinium-enhancement. Brain MRI can be normal, disclose NMO-typical lesions, show nonspecific white matter lesions or rarely exhibit MS-like lesions fulfilling the Barkhof criteria for dissemination in space. NMO-typical brain lesions are present in areas with high AQP4 expression such as peri-ependymal in the hypothalamus and the brainstem. Gadolinium-enhancement within the optic nerve is a frequent finding on MRI in the setting of ON but may also be present during remission. Typical MRI characteristics of brain lesions need to be confirmed in larger studies.

Recommendations

The MRI appearance of spinal cord lesions plays a central role in the diagnosis of NMO. Brain MRI is a mainstay in the work-up and may display Gadolinium-enhancement of the optic nerve and both symptomatic and asymptomatic brain lesions.

Cerebrospinal fluid analysis

CSF abnormalities are detected in most NMO patients and concern cell count, protein level and oligoclonal bands (OCB). Pleocytosis, usually consisting of monocytes and lymphocytes, is present in 14–79% of patients

(Class IV) [8, 34]. CSF pleocytosis can include or be dominated by neutrophils; eosinophils may also be found (Class IV) [8, 71]. CSF cell count is greater than 50 cells/μL in 13–35% of patients and in a few cases up to 1,000 cells/μL (Class IV) [8, 34, 72]. Patients with LETM are more likely to exhibit a pleocytosis than patients with ON (Class IV) [73]. Increased protein levels are present in 46–75% of cases (Class IV) [2, 34]. The frequency of OCB in NMO ranges from 0 to 37% and presence of OCB can be transient in NMO (Class IV) [2, 4, 8, 34, 74]. CSF analysis in MS rarely reveals a pleocytosis exceeding 50 cells/μL, and OCB are present in over 90% in established MS (Class III) [74]. One study found a positive MRZ (measles, rubella and zoster) reaction, as defined by a combination of at least two positive antibody indices, in MS in 37 of 42, but in NMO in only 1 of 20 (Class III) [75].

Neurofilaments are released into CSF following axonal injury. Neurofilament heavy chain (NfH) levels are significantly higher in the CSF of NMO than MS patients (Class III) [76]. Also, glial fibrillary acidic protein (GFAP) is significantly higher in CSF of NMO patients compared to MS, spinal cord infarction and ADEM (Class III) [77].

Conclusions

Analysis of CSF provides supportive data for the diagnosis of NMO, and CSF should be obtained during or shortly after an acute attack. The findings are useful but not highly sensitive or specific. The value of NfH and GFAP determination need to be evaluated in further studies.

Recommendations

CSF findings with a lymphomononuclear pleocytosis >50 cells/μL, occasional presence of neutrophils/eosinophils and lack of OCB may be indicative but is not specific for NMO and NMO spectrum disorders.

Electrophysiological evaluation

There are only a few studies reporting electrophysiological examinations in NMO. An Australian study revealed abnormal visual evoked potentials (VEP) more frequently in opticospinal demyelinating disease than in conventional MS (85% and 71.4%, respectively) (Class IV) [27]. In a multi-ethnic Cuban NMO study, somatosensory-evoked potentials (SEP) were abnormal in 86% (42/49), VEP in 83% (44/53) and brain stem acoustic-evoked potentials (BAEP) in 37% (19/51) (Class IV) [33]. BAEP abnormalities were more frequent in blacks than in other patients (78% vs. 29%, $P = 0.003$). Peripheral motor and sensory nerve conduction was normal in all patients of a Japanese study with 9 opticospinal MS patients (Class IV) [78].

Conclusions

VEP, SEP and BAEP examination in NMO patients frequently reveal abnormalities while peripheral nerve conduction studies are expected to be normal.

Aquaporin 4
Expression of AQP4 within the CNS

AQP4 is an osmosis-driven, bidirectional water channel that belongs to the subfamily of mammalian aquaporins. In the CNS, AQP4 is expressed at the astrocytic foot processes in close vicinity to the basement membranes, in the optic nerve, in a subpopulation of ependymal cells, in hypothalamic nuclei and in the subfornical organ [79, 80]. In NMO, the third extracellular loop of AQP4 is considered as the major epitope for AQP4 antibodies [81]. Astrocytes were shown to undergo necrosis in a complement-dependent manner when exposed to AQP4 antibody containing sera, and disease was induced by passive transfer of antibodies to rats, suggesting a primary pathogenic role of AQP4 antibodies in NMO [82, 83]. A recent study evaluated the plasma cell population taken from an early NMO patient at the molecular level and reported that AQP4-specific IgG is synthesized intrathecally at disease onset, and contributes directly to CNS pathology [84].

NMO-IgG/AQP4 antibody assay

The diagnosis of NMO and its distinction from MS has been facilitated by the discovery of NMO-IgG/AQP4 antibodies. The initial assay was based on an indirect immunofluorescence method using mouse cerebellum (IIF) (Class II) [17]. With this assay, testing for NMO-IgG had a reported sensitivity of 58–76% and a specificity of

85–99% for NMO. There are four other assay techniques allowing detection of AQP4 antibodies including cell-based assays (CBA), radioimmunoprecipitation assays (RIPA), fluoroimmunoprecipitation assays (FIPA) and enzyme-linked immunosorbent assays (ELISA) [85, 86]. Sensitivities and specificities of the assays differ and the gold standard remains to be elucidated [85, 86, 87, 88, 89, 90, 91]. Cell-based techniques such as CBA may show the best results (Class IV) [86].

NMO-IgG/AQP4 antibody and disease characteristics

NMO-IgG/AQP4 antibodies can be detected years before the onset of NMO [92]. A French study using IIF did not report differences with regard to age and onset of disease, annualized relapse rate, brain MRI findings and CSF abnormalities when comparing NMO-IgG positive and negative patients (Class II) [87]. A Cuban study evaluating 48 recurrent NMO patients (diagnostic criteria of 1999) reported a relatively low prevalence of NMO-IgG (33.3%, method: IIF); however presence of NMO-IgG was associated with a worse course defined by more frequent relapses, occurrence of myelitis and greater attack-related disability (Class II) [87]. Detection of NMO-IgG was also associated with a higher probability for > 3 periventricular lesions and localization within the deep white matter, and a more extensive lesion on spinal cord images during remission. A European study reported that AQP4 antibody levels in serum correlated with disease activity and were reduced by treatments such as rituximab, azathioprine, cyclophosphamide (method: FIPA) (Class IV) [93]. Antibody titres were attenuated by methyl-prednisolone and remained low during remission, while high titres were associated with complete blindness and more extensive brain lesions (methods: CBA) (Class II) [88]. The study also revealed that AQP4 antibody titres positively correlated with the length of spinal cord lesions at the lowest point of exacerbations. In another study measures of complement-mediated cell injury but not AQP4 antibody titres were indicative of disease severity [94]. A recent Japanese study evaluated the frequency of AQP4 antibodies in idiopathic demyelinating diseases [10] and found that the HLA-DPB1*0501 allele was associated with seropositive opticospinal MS but not with classical MS or seronegative opticospinal MS (Class II). A French NMO study reported that the presence of NMO-IgG was linked to HLA-DRB1*01*03 (majority DR3) [1]. In a cohort of 130 patients with relapsing-remitting MS none tested positive for NMO-IgG [95].

AQP4 antibodies in spatially limited syndromes

NMO-IgG is also found in patients with LETM (37.9–50%) or RION (14.3–20%) and importantly appear to predict outcome in terms of conversion to NMO (Class II) [18, 19]. Detection of NMO-IgG in serum of patients with RION (5 of 25) was associated with a more severe initial ON episode, poor visual outcome and development of NMO (Class II) [18]. Of 9 NMO-IgG-positive LETM patients, 5 (65%) experienced either another episode of myelitis ($n = 4$) or ON ($n = 1$) within 1 year (Class II) [19]. The probability of detecting NMO-IgG in the serum of patients with acute partial transverse myelitis (lesion < 3 vertebral segments) is low; NMO-IgG was found in 1 of 22 patients (4.5%) (Class III) [96]; this patient subsequently developed recurrent LETM. Recently, four cases of AQP4 antibody-negative recurrent LETM which did not seem to be related to NMO were reported (Class IV) [97]. Of note, some NMO or spectrum disorder cases can be NMO-IgG-positive and AQP4 antibody-negative, or vice versa (Class IV) [85]. In a series of three rapidly recurring LETM patients, AQP4 antibodies could not be detected in serum but in CSF (Class IV), confirming the diagnosis of a spatially limited NMO spectrum disorder and mandating initiation of immunosuppressive treatment [98].

Conclusions

The presence of NMO-IgG/AQP4 antibodies supports the diagnosis of NMO (Level A) and is a prognostic marker for high-risk syndromes (Level A). NMO-IgG/AQP4 antibodies are routinely evaluated in serum. Whether determination of NMO-IgG/AQP4 antibodies in CSF of seronegative patients is helpful is currently unclear. NMO-IgG/AQP4 antibodies can be present in patients years before and after clinical disease activity. The ideal method for determination of the antibodies has not yet been established and testing with different methods may be reasonable in cases with a high suspicion for AQP4 CNS autoimmunity. It also remains to be determined whether NMO-IgG/AQP4 antibodies are a reliable marker of disease activity and treatment response.

Diagnostic criteria

Criteria for diagnosis of NMO

The following two diagnostic criteria were developed on the basis of the most recent clinical, MRI and laboratory findings and have incorporated the determination of the NMO-IgG/AQP4 antibody. Of note, the Wingerchuk criteria refer to NMO-IgG and were set up when antigen-specific assays were not available.

Revised diagnostic criteria by Wingerchuk *et al.* (2006) (Class IV) [52]

Two absolute criteria:
• optic neuritis; and
• myelitis.

At least two of three supportive criteria:
• the presence of a contiguous spinal cord MRI lesion extending over three or more vertebral segments;
• MRI criteria not satisfying the revised McDonald diagnostic criteria for MS; and
• NMO-IgG in serum.

These revised diagnostic criteria and the criteria set up in 1999 (excluding patients with brain lesions and without considering NMO-IgG) were applied in a series of Spanish and Italian patients with suspected NMO ($n = 28$) and NMO spectrum disorders (LETM and RION, $n = 18$); 115 MS patients served as controls (Class IV) [91]. IIF was used to determine NMO-IgG. Compared to the 1999 criteria, the revised criteria were found to be associated with a higher specificity (83.3% vs. 25%), but slightly lower sensitivity (87.5% vs. 93.7%).

NMSS task force on differential diagnosis of MS, Miller *et al.* (2008) (Class IV) [99]

Major criteria
• ON in one or both eyes;
• transverse myelitis, clinically complete or incomplete, but associated with radiological evidence of spinal cord

lesion extending over three or more spinal segments on T2-weighted MRI images and hypointensities on T1-weighted images when obtained during acute episode of myelitis; and
• no evidence for sarcoidosis, vasculitis, clinically manifest systemic lupus erythematosus (SLE) or Sjögren's syndrome (SS), or other explanation for the syndrome.

All major criteria are required but may be separated by an unspecified interval.

Minor criteria, of which at least one must be fulfilled:
• most recent brain MRI scan of the head must be normal or may show abnormalities not fulfilling the Barkhof criteria used for McDonald diagnostic criteria, including: a) nonspecific brain T2-signal abnormalities not satisfying the Barkhof criteria for dissemination in space used in the revised McDonald criteria, b) lesions in the dorsal medulla, either contiguity or not in contiguity with a spinal cord lesion, c) hypothalamic and/or brainstem lesions, d) 'linear' periventricular/corpus callosum signal abnormality, but not ovoid, not extending into the parenchyma of the cerebral hemispheres in Dawson finger configuration; or
• positive test in serum or CSF for NMO-IgG/AQP4 antibodies.

NMO spectrum disorders

NMO spectrum disorders comprise the spatially limited syndromes, presentations with atypical features, including brain lesions and comorbidities, and OSMS. Among 13 patients NMO spectrum disorders from north-east Tuscany, seven had clinically definite NMO after a follow-up of at least 2 years, the other six (46%) remained NMO spectrum disorders (Class IV) [30].

Spatially limited NMO spectrum disorders: NMO-IgG/AQP4 positive LETM and RION/BON

NMO-IgG/AQP4 antibody-positive LETM or RION/BON are limited or inaugural syndromes of NMO. (For details on the risk of such patients for converting to NMO refer to 'AQP4 antibodies in spatially limited syndromes', above.) The NMSS Task Force concluded that these limited syndromes should not qualify as NMO, even in the presence of NMO-IgG/AQP4 antibody (Class IV) [99]. Currently, there are no diagnostic criteria

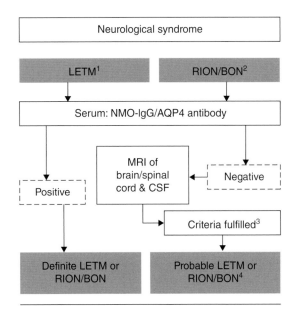

Neurological syndrome

LETM[1]   RION/BON[2]

Serum: NMO-IgG/AQP4 antibody

MRI of brain/spinal cord & CSF ← Negative

Positive

Criteria fulfilled[3]

Definite LETM or RION/BON   Probable LETM or RION/BON[4]

[1] Diagnosis of LETM is based on a spinal cord syndrome in combination with a spinal cord lesion expanding over 3 or more vertebral segments
[2] Diagnosis of ON is based on clincal, ophthalmologic and VEP examination
[3] Criteria: brain MRI negative OR NMO-typical brain lesions AND negative OCB/no intrathecal IgG-synthesis
[4] Pathological VEP (for LETM) or SEP (for RION/BON) is further supportive of probable NMO spectrum disorder if criteria[3] are fulfilled

Figure 20.1 Flow-chart of panel recommendations for the work-up and diagnosis of suspected spatially limited NMO spectrum disorders LETM and RION/BON.

for spatially limited NMO syndromes, so the panel proposed potential guidelines for work-up and diagnosis (Figure 20.1).

NMO and spatially limited NMO spectrum disorders: association with comorbidities

NMO and spatially limited manifestations can occur in association with organ- and non-organ-specific autoimmune disorders. Hypothyroidism, pernicious anaemia, ulcerative colitis, primary sclerosing cholangitis and idiopathic thrombocytopenic purpura are organ-specific autoimmune disorders associated with NMO. Also NMO patients can be seropositive for acetylcholine receptor (AChR) antibodies and 1–2% have clinical and electrophysiological findings compatible with myasthenia gravis (MG) (Class IV) [21, 100, 101]. Moreover, NMO and

NMO spectrum disorders can occur with endocrinopathies (Class IV) [56, 102, 103, 104, 105].

Among the non-organ-specific autoimmune diseases are SLE, SS, antiphospholipid syndrome and sarcoidosis (Class IV) [20, 106,107, 108, 109, 110, 111, 112]. Autoantibodies against nuclear antigens can be detected in NMO without clinical evidence of systemic autoimmune diseases. Some authors consider this as an epiphenomenon in the context of disordered humoral autoimmunity (Class IV) [2, 20, 113]. Pittock and colleagues evaluated the presence of autoantibodies in North-American patients with NMO ($n = 78$) and LETM ($n = 75$) and most frequently detect antinuclear antibodies (43.8%) followed by antibodies for SS (15.7%) (Class IV) [20]. Both antibodies were found more frequently in NMO-IgG-positive than in NMO-IgG-negative patients ($P = 0.001$). No patient was positive for NMO-IgG among the 49 control patients with SS/SLE; none of these patients had a presentation involving the optic nerve or spinal cord. The frequency for detection of autoantibodies was even higher in paediatric NMO, where autoantibodies were found in 57 of 75 (76%) patients (Class IV) [68]. In these patients a coexisting autoimmune disease was diagnosed in 16 of 58 patients (28%). Occurrence of ON and LETM in these syndromes can either be considered as a vasculitic neurological complication or the currently more favoured coexistence of two autoimmune disorders (Class IV) [20]. In addition, in a cohort of NMO patients ($n = 78$) 3% met the international criteria for SLE or SS (Class IV) [20]. Stating that it was a conservative decision, the NMSS Task Force concluded that, pending further studies, clinical evidence of SLE or SS should exclude a diagnosis of NMO [99]. Conversely, the panel commented that in the lack of clinical evidence for SLE or SS, seropositivity for anti-nuclear antibodies (ANA) or SSA/SSB would not exclude the diagnosis of NMO.

Atypical cases

Patients with clinically manifest or subclinical brain MRI lesions (hypothalamic, periventricular, brainstem) are referred to as atypical cases when other clinical characteristics are typical of NMO and when they are seropositive for NMO-IgG/AQP4 antibodies [114]. Brain lesions in some NMO spectrum disorder patients are accompanied by vasogenic oedema and may manifest as PRES (Class IV) [53].

Asian opticospinal MS (OSMS)

OSMS shares some clinical, immunological and MRI features with recurrent NMO and it has been suggested that OSMS may be the same entity as NMO (Class IV) [31]. However, differences of nomenclature in Asia and Western countries hamper comparative analyses. While the diagnosis of NMO requires ON and LETM in Western countries, in Asia, regardless of the length of their spinal cord lesion, associations of ON and myelitis are classified as OSMS [99]. NMO-IgG/AQP4 antibody seropositivity has been reported in OSMS in about 60% of the patients (Class IV) [17, 31]. NMO-IgG/AQP4 antibody-negative OSMS is associated with significantly fewer brain lesions and some authors suggest that the immunopathogenesis of OSMS is more heterogeneous (Class IV) [22].

Differential diagnosis

Despite the availability of diagnostic criteria there is an overlap between MS and NMO, and MS remains the most important differential diagnosis. In a cohort of 320 patients with CIS suggestive of MS, 23 patients (7.2%) fulfilled the revised absolute NMO criteria of 2006 at some time (Class III) [115]. In paediatric NMO particularly, ADEM has to be considered (Class IV) [68]. Other differential diagnoses include spinal cord and/or optic nerve manifestations of viral, bacterial and fungal infections. Toxic exposures, nutritional and metabolic disorders, ischemia, neoplasia and neurodegenerative diseases may mimic inflammation within the spinal cord and the optic nerve. Also hereditary optic neuropathies and retinal disorders have to be considered. Furthermore, spinal cord compression, arteriovenous malformations and non-cord mimics such as Guillain-Barré syndrome and MG have to be taken into account.

Conclusions

NMO and NMO spectrum disorders need to be distinguished from MS due to divergent course, treatment strategies and outcome. 'High-risk' syndromes among NMO spectrum disorders include NMO-IgG/AQP4 antibody-positive LETM and RION/BON. Overlap with organ- and non-organ-specific autoimmune disorders and a broad range of other differential diagnoses have to be taken into account.

Recommendations

Diagnostic criteria are the cornerstone of NMO diagnosis and inception cohort studies in patients with first episodes are needed to refine the diagnostic criteria. A diagnostic guideline for spatially limited NMO spectrum disorders was assembled by the European Task Force (Figure 20.1).

Management

Treatment of acute exacerbations
Steroids

Initial or recurrent episodes are usually treated with high-dose intravenous methyl-prednisolone (1 g daily for 3–5 consecutive days). This recommendation is taken from studies of MS and idiopathic ON since there are no controlled therapeutic trials which investigated the effectiveness of steroids specifically in NMO. Acute NMO symptoms respond to short courses of high-dose intravenous corticosteroids in up to 80% of patients within 1–5 days and treatment is generally well tolerated (Class IV) [8]. In many EU countries intravenous therapy with methyl-prednisolone for MS-related relapses is followed by an oral taper, which lacks controlled trials and needs to be performed slowly.

Plasma exchange

Therapeutic plasmapheresis was effective in patients with severe symptoms that fail to improve or progress despite treatment with corticosteroids. Plasma exchange (1–1.5 plasma volume per exchange) for the treatment of steroid-unresponsive severe mostly MS-related attacks was compared in a double-blind, sham-controlled protocol (a total of 7 treatments every other day) in a North American study (Class II only for MS, rating not possible for NMO since only two NMO patients were included) [116]. Patients who did not achieve moderate or greater improvement after the first treatment phase crossed over to the opposite treatment. Improvement was found in 8 of 19 (42.1%) patients receiving plasma exchange and only in 1 of 17 (5.9%) receiving sham exchange. In an extension of this study, moderate or marked improvement was detected in 6 of 10 NMO patients after switching to plasma exchange (Class III) [117]. However, in three patients no improvement could be achieved. Predictive factors for better prognosis were male gender, preserved reflexes and early initiation of plasma exchange. Llufriu *et al.* performed plasma exchange in four NMO patients with severe episodes of CNS demyelination unresponsive to steroids; one patient had improved at discharge (25%) and three when reassessed after 6 months (75%) (Class IV) [118]. Watanabe *et al.* reported the therapeutic efficacy of plasma exchange (median 4 exchanges over a period of 1–2 weeks) in six NMO-IgG seropositive patients who were unresponsive to high-dose intravenous methyl-prednisolone treatment (Class IV) [119]. Following plasma exchange, three patients experienced significant functional improvement, while one had mild and two no improvement. Clinical response commenced quickly after one or two exchanges. Benefits were also seen in patients with severe isolated optic neuritis who were unresponsive to high-dose corticosteroids (Class IV) [120]. Efficacy of plasma exchange for severe spinal cord attacks in patients with NMO spectrum disorders was shown to be independent of NMO-IgG seropositivity (Class IV) [121]. Miyamoto *et al.* reported 4 AQP4 antibody-positive NMO patients with steroid-refractory relapses in which plasmapheresis was effective (Class IV) [122]. Lymphocyte apheresis, a procedure that removes only lymphocytes but not plasma from the blood, was effectively applied in a single NMO-IgG-negative NMO patient who did not respond to methyl-prednisolone or IVIG (Class IV) [123].

Intravenous Immunoglobulins (IVIG)

IVIG has not been specifically evaluated for ON/LETM relapses of NMO/NMO spectrum disorders and is rarely used for corticosteroid-refractory attacks [124].

Conclusions

Disability in NMO is attack-related and relapses require a rapid treatment approach with high-dose i.v. corticosteroids, followed by a slow tailoring; however, they may have limited or no effect in a subgroup of patients. A repeated course of corticosteroids may be considered prior to further treatment escalation. Corticosteroid tapering is standard for treatment of MS relapses in many countries of the EU. However, it needs to be acknowledged that there is no evidence based on RCT for corticosteroid tapering. In case of unresponsiveness to steroids early initiation of a rescue therapy with plasmapheresis is indicated (up to seven treatments every other day). There is currently no evidence for the effectiveness of

other pharmacological approaches in the treatment of NMO relapses. Whether NMO spectrum disorders associated with other autoimmune disorders require a different approach for treatment of acute relapses has yet to be determined.

Recommendations

We suggest the following approach for treatment of relapses: high-dose steroids (methyl-prednisolone; 1 g for 3–5 consecutive days) as first-line therapy, followed by an oral prednisolone taper. Early initiation of an escalation therapy with plasma exchange is recommended in steroid-unresponsive relapses. Prior to escalation therapy, a repeated course of high dose corticosteroids may be considered.

Attack prevention (alphabetical order)
Immunomodulatory treatment

Some patients with recurrent NMO receive the initial diagnosis of MS and are treated with approved immunomodulatory therapies such as interferon-β and glatiramer acetate. A randomized-controlled trial for interferon-β 1b in Japan revealed effectiveness in relapsing-remitting MS but was not powered for evaluation of treatment effects in opticospinal MS (Class I for MS) [125]. However, exacerbations of severe ON and myelitis were reported from a Japanese OSMS trial with interferon-β 1b and treatment was discontinued in 5 of 6 patients (Class IV) [126]. A retrospective Japanese study of 104 consecutive patients revealed that interferon-β 1b significantly reduced the relapse rate in the first year in MS ($n = 69$; $P < 0.00001$), whereas the annualized relapse rate was not altered in NMO patients ($n = 35$, $P = 0.56$) (Class III) [127]. The development of extensive brain lesions after treatment with interferon-β was observed in two Japanese patients (Class IV) [128]. In a French study, 26 patients with recurrent NMO receiving either immunosuppressive (cyclophosphamide, mitoxantrone, or azathioprine) or immunomodulatory treatment (interferon-β) were followed for a mean of 32 months (Class III) [129]. The retrospective analysis revealed that the probability of further relapses was significantly lower in patients receiving immunosuppressive treatment ($P = 0.0007$). A 48-year-old patient with NMO who was unresponsive to cyclophosphamide but was effectively treated with glatiramer-acetate was reported (Class IV) [130].

Intravenous Immunoglobulins (IVIG)

IVIG might be effective in NMO given the potential humoral immunopathogenesis. However, there are only very few supportive data in the literature, including the case of two recurrent NMO patients who responded to IVIG while prior azathioprine and prednisone therapies were not effective (Class IV) [131]. An open-label study, including five patients with NMO and three with recurrent LETM treated with bi-monthly IVIG (0.7 g per kg bodyweight per day for 3 consecutive days), reported an effect on the annualized relapse rate (from 1.6 in the previous year to 0.0006 in the follow-up, $P = 0.01$) and the EDSS (from 3.3 to 2.6, $P = 0.04$) (Class IV) [132]. A total of 83 infusions during a mean follow-up of 19.3 months (range 4–21) was well tolerated, minor adverse events included headache in three patients and a mild cutaneous rash in one patient.

Immunosuppressive treatment

Azathioprine and steroids

Azathioprine is a purine synthesis inhibitor and interferes with the proliferation of cells, especially leukocytes. Azathioprine (75–100 mg daily) in combination with oral prednisolone (1 mg/kg/daily) was evaluated in a prospective open-label case-series of seven patients with newly diagnosed NMO (Class IV) [133]. The combination was effective over a treatment period of 19 months by means of sustained improvement in the EDSS scores and absence of relapses. Treatment with azathioprine may be carried out in analogy to the recommendations for myasthenia gravis. Haematological evaluations are required every 2–4 weeks, the dosage may be reduced in the course and treatment duration of up to 5 years may be considered. The evaluation of long-term side-effects of azathioprine treatment in MS revealed that gastrointestinal complaints and leukopenia were very common adverse events (>10%), while infections, allergy and haematological disturbances were common (1–10%) [134]. Corticosteroids are used for rapid immunosuppression until azathioprine exerts its full effect. Some patients experience clinical worsening when prednisone is reduced below 5–15 mg/d (Class IV) [135]. Long-term treatment with corticosteroids requires osteoporosis prophylaxis.

Cyclophosphamide

Cyclophosphamide, an alkylating chemotherapeutic drug related to nitrogen mustards, is a nonspecific immunosuppressant that affects both T- and B-cell function. Immunosuppression is transient when cyclophosphamide is given in standard pulse doses, and the immune function recovers within a few months to a year after cessation [136]. Published treatment regimens for i.v. cyclophosphamide vary and range from 7 to 25 mg/kg every month over a period of 6 months. Uromitexan administration with every dose needs to be included for prevention of haemorrhagic cystitis.

A few case reports suggest that cyclophosphamide is partially effective in NMO syndromes associated with other autoimmune disorders including SLE and SS (Class IV) [137, 138, 139, 140]. In neuropsychiatric SLE, low-dose i.v. cyclophosphamide (200–400 mg per month, $n = 37$) and oral prednisone was superior to oral prednisone alone ($n = 23$, average daily dose of prednisone 20.5 mg in both groups) [141]. In MS, cyclophosphamide is considered a treatment option in aggressive courses refractory to immunomodulatory treatment. However, a recent Cochrane systematic review found only four randomized-controlled MS trials with sufficient data and concluded cyclophosphamide does not prevent worsening of the EDSS [142]. Side effects including the occurence of amenorrhea and sepsis has to be taken into account.

Methotrexate

Methotrexate exerts its immunosuppressive activity via inhibition of dihydrofolate reductase and has anti-inflammatory and immunomodulatory effects. Among 8 patients with NMO, 4 treated with a combination of methotrexate (i.v. 50 mg weekly) and prednisolone (1 mg/kg/daily) were stabilized (Class IV) [143]. Among the four patients who were treated with cyclophosphamide only, 1 stabilized and the remaining 3 responded positively after switching to the combination of methotrexate and prednisolone.

Mitoxantrone

Mitoxantrone is an anthracenedione antineoplastic agent that intercalates with DNA and inhibits both DNA and RNA synthesis, suppressing T- and B-cell immunity. A prospective 2-year case-series ($12 \, mg/m^2$ monthly for 6 months, followed by three more treatments, each 3 months apart) reported that 4 of 5 patients with recurrent NMO experienced disease stabilisation and improvement of MRI measures (Class IV) [144]. Mitoxantrone is a toxic agent that must be administered with care to reduce the likelihood of bone marrow suppression, opportunistic infection and cardiomyopathy. Amenorrhoea is a major concern in the treatment of young women. Therapy-related acute leukaemia (TRAL) was studied in 5,472 MS patients treated with a mean dose of $74.2 \, mg/m^2$ (range: $12–120 \, mg/m^2$) [145]. TRAL occurred in 0.3%, median onset was at 18.5 months (range 40–60 months) after start of mitoxantrone treatment and among the 25 patients for which the outcome was reported, six died (24%). A relationship with the total dose is suggested since over 80% of the patients in which acute leukaemia occurred had received $>60 \, mg/m^2$.

Mycophenolate mofetil

Mycophenolate (p.o. 1–3 g per day) is suggested in several conditions requiring immunosuppression and is mostly used when a rapid onset of treatment effects is not required and azathioprine is not tolerated. The occurrence of treatment effect is more rapid for mycophenolate than for azathioprine. Jacob and colleagues reported a retrospective study of 24 patients suffering from NMO ($n = 15$) and NMO spectrum disorders (relapsing LETM $n = 7$, RION and LETM $n = 1$ each) with a median treatment duration of 27 months (Class IV) [146]. At a median follow-up of 28 months (range 18–89 months), 19 patients (79%) were continuing treatment and 1 had died. The median annualized post-treatment relapse rate was lower than the pre-treatment rate ($P < 0.001$). A 9-year-old girl with NMO was treated with mycophenolate and achieved sustained improvement over a 2-year follow-up (Class IV) [147]. Some panel members have had very good experience with mycophenolate as long-term treatment of NMO and would also consider this therapy as first-line treatment (expert opinion).

Prednisolone

Low-dose oral prednisolone (5–20 mg daily) was shown to reduce relapse frequency in a retrospective study of 9 Japanese NMO patients (Class IV) [148]. However, relapses occurred significantly more frequently when steroids were tapered to 10 mg/day or less (odds ratio 8.75).

Rituximab

Rituximab, a chimeric anti-CD20 monoclonal antibody capable of depleting mature and precursor B cells, was shown to reduce disease activity and prevent disability in two studies. The first study, a retrospective analysis of 25 NMO patients treated with rituximab as escalation therapy, was performed in patients from the US and UK (Class IV) [149]. Two rituximab regimens were used: 1) $375 \, mg/m^2$ infused once per week for 4 weeks ($n = 18$); and 2) 1,000 mg infused twice, with a 2-week interval between the infusions ($n = 4$). The median annualized pre-treatment relapse rate was 1.7 (range 0–3.2) and dropped to 0 relapses (range 0–3.2) at a median follow-up of 19 months. The EDSS improved in 11 patients, did not change in nine and worsened in five, of whom two died. The second study is an open-label study which evaluated eight NMO patients who had failed other therapeutic regimens and were treated with rituximab (four infusions $375 \, mg/m^2$, once per week) (Class IV) [150]. Mean follow-up time was 12 months and 6/8 patients remained relapse-free. B-cell counts were evaluated bi-monthly and patients were given the option to be retreated with rituximab when B-cell counts became detectable (re-treatment of two 1,000 mg infusions, 2 weeks apart).

A 2005 report on the safety of rituximab in patients with cancer and rheumatoid arthritis concluded that overall usage is safe [151]. Infusion-related reactions were reported in 84% and included nausea, headache, fatigue, rash and flu-like symptoms. The incidence of these symptoms is highest after the first infusion and decreases in the course. Thus, the use of acetaminophen, antihistamines and corticosteroids is recommended as pretreatment. Infections are reported in 30% of rituximab-treated patients, but only 1–2% acquire severe infections. Of note, concomitant immunosuppressive therapies enhance the susceptibility to infection.

Other treatment options

There are no studies of fingolimod (FTY-720) or natalizumab in NMO.

Plasmapheresis

The potential therapeutic efficacy of plasmapheresis for relapse prevention is derived from a study by Miyamoto et al. in which two NMO patients received intermittent plasma exchange in combination with immunosuppressants (Class

IV) [122]. One patient received prednisolone and cyclophosphamide and additional double filtration plasmapheresis; the other patient additional azathioprine and cyclophosphamide.

Conclusions

Long-term treatment options should be initiated as soon as the diagnosis of NMO is made since prevention of attacks is the key issue for reducing permanent disability (Table 20.1). Seronegative NMO is treated in the same way as seropositive NMO. However, there are no randomized controlled trials and currently only Class IV evidence for the effect of any medication for relapse prevention. Hence, data favouring specific therapies are weak. Immunosuppression is the preferred treatment but optimal drug regimen and treatment duration have yet to be determined; the decision on treatment options has to consider the time until the treatment effect is reached and potential long-term side-effects. Intermittent plasmapheresis might be considered in case of insufficient relapse prevention with immunosuppressants. Whether NMO-IgG/AQP4 antibody titres may serve as a marker of treatment response remains to be elucidated.

Spatially limited NMO spectrum disorders such as LETM and RION/BON should be considered as inaugural manifestations of NMO and treatment should be started in accordance with the clinical course (Table 20.2). Currently it is not clear whether NMO syndromes associated with other autoimmune disorders have a divergent course and require different or additional treatment strategies. However, by analogy to NMO, there is a lack of large randomized trials for the treatment CNS manifestations of systemic autoimmune disorders [152].

Recommendations

First- and second-line therapy schemes for NMO and spatially limited NMO spectrum disorders are suggested by the Task Force (Table 20.1 and 20.2, respectively). The categorization in first- and second-line therapies is based on expert preference.

First-line therapy: As first-line therapy oral treatment with azathioprine (2.5–3 mg/kg daily), in combination with oral prednisolone (1 mg/kg daily or equivalent given every other day) until azathioprine has taken full effect, is recommended. Slow tapering of prednisolone should be considered after 2–3 months. Optimal treatment duration has yet to be determined; considering the experience in MG, a treatment duration of up

Table 20.1 Panel recommendations for immunosuppressive treatment of NMO.

	Drug name	Regimen
First-line therapy		
	Azathioprine	Oral 2.5–3 mg/kg/day
plus	Prednisolone	Oral 1 mg/kg/day, tapered when azathioprine becomes effective (after 2–3 months)
OR		
	Rituximab	Option 1: i.v. 375 mg/m² weekly for 4 weeks (lymphoma protocol)
		Option 2: 1000 mg infused twice, with a 2-week interval between the infusions (rheumatoid arthritis protocol)
		Options 1and 2: re-infusion after 6–12 months; however, optimal treatment duration unknown
Second-line therapy		
	Cyclophophosphamide	i.v. 7–25 mg/kg every month over a period of 6 months, especially considered in case of association with SLE/SS
OR		
	Mitoxantrone	i.v. 12 mg/m² monthly for 6 months, followed by 12 mg/m² every 3 months for 9 months
OR		
	Mycophenolate mofetil	p.o. 1–3 g per day
Other therapies	IVIG, Methotrexate	
Escalation therapy		
AND	Intermittent plasma exchange	

Table 20.2 Panel recommendation for starting immunosuppressive treatment in spatially limited NMO spectrum disorders RION/BON and LETM.

	NMO-IgG/AQP4 antibody	Severity/recovery of acute attacks	Immunosuppressive treatment
RION/BON	+	severe/poor	+
	+	acceptable/good	+/−*
	−	severe/poor	+/−*
	−	acceptable/good	−
LETM	+	severe/poor	+
	+	acceptable/good	+/−*
	−	severe/poor	+/−*
	−	acceptable/good	−

*Depending on follow-up and number of episodes.

to 5 years should be expected for azathioprine. A further first-line therapy is rituximab. However, the optimal surrogate measures, treatment intervals and duration remain unclear.

Second-line therapy: If first-line treatment is ineffective or the patient develops steroid dependence for clinical remission, alternative immunosuppressive therapies need to be considered. We suggest cyclophosphamide (7–25 mg/kg every month over a period of 6 months), mitoxantrone (12 mg/m^2 every 3 months for 9 months) or mycophenolate mofetil (1–3 g/day) as second-line therapy (alphabetical order). Other potentially effective drugs include IVIG and methotrexate. Additional intermittent plasma exchange may be an option for treatment escalation.

Spatially limited NMO spectrum disorders

Whether spatially limited NMO spectrum disorders should be handled as if they are NMO or if long-term treatment should be deferred until the relationship with NMO is better established by the occurrence of corresponding symptoms (LETM or ON, respectively) is unclear. The panel has set up a treatment scheme adapted from classical NMO which considers initiation of immunosuppressive treatment depending on the clinical course (Table 20.2). Of note, the likelihood for NMO-IgG/AQP4-negative ON to be associated with MS or other disorders is higher than for NMO-IgG/AQP4-negative LETM. Hence, the scheme in Table 20.2 is expected to be of greater value for AQP4-negative LETM. Patients with recurrent AQP4-negative ON, particularly with mild relapses and good recovery, may not be necessarily part

of the NMO spectrum. However, patients with recurrent severe ON attacks and incomplete recovery might require similar treatment strategies as spatially limited NMO spectrum disorders.

NMO spectrum disorders associated with SLE/SS

Bearing in mind that further studies are required to support the NMSS Task Force decision about SLE/SS and NMO, the European panel suggests that NMO cases with clinical evidence of SLE or SS should be treated according to ACR and EULAR treatment protocols of neuropsychiatric lupus [153, 154].

Supportive and symptomatic treatment

Supportive and symptomatic treatment is an essential component of the overall management of NMO and aimed at control or reduction of symptoms impairing functional abilities and quality of life. Such symptoms include spasticity, tonic spasms, NMO-related pain syndromes, bladder symptoms, neurogenic bowel dysfunction, sexual dysfunction and cognitive impairment. Some patients with high cervical cord lesions will require long-term mechanical ventilation.

No trials specifically for symptomatic treatment of NMO have been performed, most evidence is derived from studies in MS and the readers are referred to recommendations for symptomatic treatment of MS for instance from the Multiple Sclerosis Therapy Consensus

Group (MSTCG) of the German Multiple Sclerosis Society [155].

Conflicts of interest

JS, MB, ZI and CM: no conflict of interest.

XM: Editorial/advisory board and speaker's fees from Almirall, Bayer Schering, Biogen Idec, Merck Serono, Sanofi-Aventis, Teva.

CP: Research grants from Bayer Schering, Biogen Idex, GSK, Merck Serono, Novartis, Teva, UCB. Consultant fees: Actelion, Bayer Schering, Biogen Idec, GSK, Merck Serono, Novartis, UCB, Roche, Teva.

RDP: Speaker's fees from Biogen Dompé, Biogen Idec, Merck Serono, Sanofi Aventis, GSK. Research grants from Bayer Schering, Biogen Dompé. Consultant fees from Biogen Dompé, Biogen Idec, Merck Serono. Travel grants from Bayer Schering, Biogen Dompé, Merck Serono.

RH: Research grants from Biogen Idex, Merck Serono, Novartis. Consultant fees from

Biogen Idec, Merck Serono.

PSS: Editorial/advisory board fees from Biogen Idec, Merck Serono, Teva. Speaker's fees from Bayer Schering, Biogen Idec, Merck Serono, Novartis, Teva. Unrestricted educational grant from Biogen Idec, Bayer Schering, Merck Serono, Novartis. Research grant from Biogen Idec, Merck Serono.

BH: Editorial/advisory board and speaker's fees from Bayer Schering, Biogen Idec, Merck Serono, Novartis, Teva. Travel grants from Bayer, Biogen Idec, Merck Serono. Research Grants: Bayer, BiogenIdec, MerckSerono, Novartis.

Abbreviations

ACR	American College of Rheumatology
AQP4	aquaporin-4
BAEP	brainstem acoustic-evoked potential
BON	bilateral optic neuritis
CIS	clinically isolated syndrome
CNS	central nervous system
CSF	cerebrospinal fluid
EDSS	expanded disability status scale
GFAP	glial fibrillary acid protein
HLA	human leukocyte antigen
IVIG	intravenous immunoglobulin
LETM	longitudinally extensive transverse myelitis
MRI	magnetic resonance imaging
MG	myasthenia gravis
MS	multiple sclerosis
NfH	neurofilament heavy chain
NMO	neuromyelitis optica
NMSS	National Multiple Sclerosis Society (USA)
OCB	oligoclonal bands
ON	optic neuritis
OSMS	opticospinal multiple sclerosis
PRES	posterior reversible encephalopathy syndrome
RION	recurrent isolated optic neuritis
SEP	somatosensory evoked potential
SLE	systemic lupus erythematosus
SS	Sjögren's syndrome
VEP	visual evoked potential

References

1. Zephir, H, Fajardy, I, Outteryck, O, et al. Is neuromyelitis optica associated with human leukocyte antigen? Mult Scler 2009; **15**:571–9.

2. O'Riordan, JI, Gallagher, HL, Thompson, AJ, et al. Clinical, CSF, and MRI findings in Devic's neuromyelitis optica. J Neurol Neurosurg Psychiatry 1996; **60**:382–7.

3. El Otmani, H, Rafai, MA, Moutaouakil, F, et al. La neuromyelite optique au Maroc. Etude de neuf cas. Rev Neurol (Paris) 2005; **161**:1191–6.

4. Bichuetti, DB, Oliveira, EM, Souza, NA, et al. Neuromyelitis optica in Brazil: a study on clinical and prognostic factors. Mult Scler 2009; **15**:613–19.

5. Wu, JS, Zhang, MN, Carroll, WM, et al. Characterisation of the spectrum of demyelinating disease in Western Australia. J Neurol Neurosurg Psychiatry 2008; **79**: 1022–6.

6. Rivera, VM, Cabrera, JA. Aboriginals with multiple sclerosis: HLA types and predominance of neuromyelitis optica. Neurology 2001; **57**:937–8.

7. Rivera, JF, Kurtzke, JF, Booth, VJ, et al. Characteristics of Devic's disease (neuromyelitis optica) in Mexico. J Neurol 2008; **255**:710–15.

8. Wingerchuk, DM, Hogancamp, WF, O'Brien, PC, et al. The clinical course of neuromyelitis optica (Devic's syndrome). Neurology 1999; **53**:1107–14.

9. Kira, J. Multiple sclerosis in the Japanese population. Lancet Neurol 2003; **2**:117–27.

10. Matsushita, T, Matsuoka, T, Isobe, N, et al. Association of the HLA-DPB1*0501 allele with anti-aquaporin-4 antibody positivity in Japanese patients with idiopathic central nervous system demyelinating disorders. Tissue Antigens 2009; **73**:171–6.

11. Das, A, Puvanendran, K. A retrospective review of patients with clinically definite multiple sclerosis. *Ann Acad Med Singapore* 1998; **27**:204–9.

12. Papais-Alvarenga, RM, Miranda-Santos, CM, Puccioni-Sohler, M, *et al*. Optic neuromyelitis syndrome in Brazilian patients. *J Neurol Neurosurg Psychiatry* 2002; **73**:429–35.

13. Chopra, JS, Radhakrishnan, K, Sawhney, BB, *et al*. Multiple sclerosis in North-West India. *Acta Neurol Scand* 1980; **62**:312–21.

14. Albutt, T. On the opthalmoscopic signs of spinal disease. *Lancet* 1870; **1**:76–8.

15. Devic, E. (1894) Myélite subaiguë compliquée de névrite optique. *Bull Med (Paris)* 1894; **8**:1033–4.

16. Gault, F. De la neuromyélite optique aiguë 1894; *Thèse Lyon, France*.

17. Lennon, VA, Wingerchuk, DM, Kryzer, TJ, *et al*. A serum autoantibody marker of neuromyelitis optica: distinction from multiple sclerosis. *Lancet* 2004; **364**:2106–12.

18. Matiello, M, Lennon, VA, Jacob, A, *et al*. NMO-IgG predicts the outcome of recurrent optic neuritis. *Neurology* 2008; **70**:2197–200.

19. Weinshenker, BG, Wingerchuk, DM, Vukusic, S, *et al*. Neuromyelitis optica IgG predicts relapse after longitudinally extensive transverse myelitis. *Ann Neurol* 2006; **59**:566–9.

20. Pittock, S.J., Lennon, V.A., de Seze, J. *et al*. Neuromyelitis optica and non organ-specific autoimmunity. *Arch Neurol* 2008; **65**:78–83.

21. McKeon, A, Lennon, VA, Jacob, A, *et al*. Coexistence of myasthenia gravis and serological markers of neurological autoimmunity in neuromyelitis optica. *Muscle Nerve* 2009; **39**:87–90.

22. Kira, J. Neuromyelitis optica and Asian phenotype of multiple sclerosis. *Ann N Y Acad Sci* 2008; **1142**:58–71.

23. Brainin, M, Barnes, M, Baron, JC, *et al*. Guidance for the preparation of neurological management guidelines by EFNS scientific task forces – revised recommendations 2004. *Eur J Neurol* 2004; **11**:577–81.

24. Yamakawa, K, Kuroda, H, Fujihara, K, *et al*. Familial neuromyelitis optica (Devic's syndrome) with late onset in Japan. *Neurology*2000; **5**: 318–20.

25. Braley, T, Mikol, DD. Neuromyelitis optica in a mother and daughter. *Arch Neurol* 2007; **64**:1189–92.

26. Wingerchuk, DM, Lennon, VA, Lucchinetti, CF, *et al*. The spectrum of neuromyelitis optica. *Lancet Neurol* 2007; **6**:805–15.

27. Wu, JS, Zhang, JM, Carroll, WM, *et al*. Characterisation of the spectrum of Demyelinating disease in Western Australia. *J Neurol Neurosurg Psychiatry* 2008; **79**: 1022–1026.

28. Cabre, P, Heinzlef, O, Merle, H, *et al*. MS and neuromyelitis optica in Martinique (French West Indies). *Neurology* 2001; **56**:507–14.

29. Misu, T, Fujihara, K, Nakashima, I, *et al*. Pure optic-spinal form of multiple sclerosis in Japan. *Brain* 2002; **125**:2460–8.

30. Bizzoco, E, Lolli, F, Repice, AM, *et al*. Prevalence of neuromyelitis optica spectrum disorder and phenotype distribution. *J Neurol* 2009; **256**:1891–8.

31. Weinshenker, BG, Wingerchuk, DM, Nakashima, I, *et al*. (2006) OSMS is NMO, but not MS: proven clinically and pathologically. *Lancet Neurol* 2006; **5**:110–11.

32. Yamasaki, K, Horiuchi, I, Minohara, M, *et al*. HLA-DPB1*0501-associated opticospinal multiple sclerosis: clinical, neuroimaging and immunogenetic studies. *Brain* 1999; **122**(**Pt 9**):1689–96.

33. Cabrera-Gomez, JA, Kurtzke, JF, Gonzalez-Quevedo, A, *et al*. An epidemiological study of neuromyelitis optica in Cuba. *J Neurol* 2009; **256**:35–44.

34. de Seze, J, Stojkovic, T, Ferriby, D, *et al*. Devic's neuromyelitis optica: clinical, laboratory, MRI and outcome profile. *J Neurol Sci* 2002; **197**:57–61.

35. Banwell, B, Tenembaum, S, Lennon, VA, *et al*. Neuromyelitis optica-IgG in childhood inflammatory demyelinating CNS disorders. *Neurology* 2008; **70**:344–52.

36. Filley, CM, Sternberg, PE, Norenberg, MD. Neuromyelitis optica in the elderly. *Arch Neurol* 1984; **41**:670–2.

37. Barbieri, F, Buscaino, GA. Neuromyelitis optica in the elderly. *Acta Neurol (Napoli)* 1989; **11**:247–51.

38. Lotze, TE, Northrop, JL, Hutton, GJ, *et al*. Spectrum of pediatric neuromyelitis optica. *Pediatrics* 2008; **122**:e1039–e1047.

39. Confavreux, C, Vukusic, S. The clinical epidemiology of multiple sclerosis. *Neuroimaging Clin N Am* 2008; **18**:589–622, ix–x.

40. Wingerchuk, DM, Weinshenker, BG. Neuromyelitis optica: clinical predictors of a relapsing course and survival. *Neurology* 2003; **60**:848–53.

41. Wingerchuk, DM, Pittock, SJ, Lucchinetti, CF, *et al*. A secondary progressive clinical course is uncommon in neuromyelitis optica. *Neurology* 2007; **68**:603–5.

42. Merle, H, Olindo, S, Bonnan, M, *et al*. Natural history of the visual impairment of relapsing neuromyelitis optica. *Ophthalmology* 2007; **114**:810–15.

43. Mandler, RN, Davis, LE, Jeffery, DR, *et al*. Devic's neuromyelitis optica: a clinicopathological study of 8 patients. *Ann Neurol* 1993; **34**:162–8.

44. Fardet, L, Genereau, T, Mikaeloff, Y, *et al*. Devic's neuromyelitis optica: study of nine cases. *Acta Neurol Scand* 2003; **108**:193–200.

45. de Seze, J, Blanc, F, Jeanjean, L, *et al*. Optical coherence tomography in neuromyelitis optica. *Arch Neurol* 2008; **65**:920–3.

46. Naismith, RT, Tutlam, NT, Xu, J, et al. Optical coherence tomography differs in neuromyelitis optica compared with multiple sclerosis. *Neurology* 2009; **72**:1077–82.

47. Nakamura, M, Miyazawa, I, Fujihara, K, et al. Preferential spinal central gray matter involvement in neuromyelitis optica. An MRI study. *J Neurol* 2008; **255**:163–70.

48. Sellner, J, Luthi, N, Buhler, R, et al. Acute partial transverse myelitis: risk factors for conversion to multiple sclerosis. *Eur J Neurol* 2008; **15**:398–405.

49. Cordonnier, C, de Seze, J, Breteau, G, et al. Prospective study of patients presenting with acute partial transverse myelopathy. *J Neurol* 2003; **250**:1447–52.

50. Misu, T, Fujihara, K, Nakashima, I, et al. Intractable hiccup and nausea with periaqueductal lesions in neuromyelitis optica. *Neurology* 2005; **65**:1479–82.

51. Pittock, SJ, Lennon, VA, Krecke, K, et al. Brain abnormalities in neuromyelitis optica. *Arch Neurol* 2006; **63**:390–6.

52. Wingerchuk, DM, Lennon, VA, Pittock, SJ, et al. Revised diagnostic criteria for neuromyelitis optica. *Neurology* 2006; **66**:1485–9.

53. Magana, SM, Matiello, M, Pittock, SJ, et al. Posterior reversible encephalopathy syndrome in neuromyelitis optica spectrum disorders. *Neurology* 2009; **72**:712–17.

54. Poppe, AY, Lapierre, Y, Melancon, D, et al. Neuromyelitis optica with hypothalamic involvement. *Mult Scler* 2005; **11**:617–21.

55. Blanc, F, Zephir, H, Lebrun, C, et al. Cognitive functions in neuromyelitis optica. *Arch Neurol* 2008; **65**:84–8.

56. Vernant, JC, Cabre, P, Smadja, D, et al. Recurrent optic neuromyelitis with endocrinopathies: a new syndrome. *Neurology* 1997; **48**:58–64.

57. Cabre, P, González-Quevedo, A, Bonnan, M, et al. Relapsing neuromyelitis optica: long term history and predictors of death. *J Neurol Neurosurg Psychiatry* 2009; **80**:1162–4.

58. Johnson, G, Miller, DH, MacManus, D, et al. STIR sequences in NMR imaging of the optic nerve. *Neuroradiology* 1987; **29**:238–45.

59. Kupersmith, MJ, Alban, T, Zeiffer, B, et al. Contrast-enhanced MRI in acute optic neuritis: relationship to visual performance. *Brain* 2002; **125**:812–22.

60. Cabrera-Gomez, JA, Quevedo-Sotolongo, L, Gonzalez-Quevedo, A, et al. Brain magnetic resonance imaging findings in relapsing neuromyelitis optica. *Mult Scler* 2007; **13**:186–92.

61. Krampla, W, Aboul-Enein, F, Jecel, J, et al. Spinal cord lesions in patients with neuromyelitis optica: a retrospective long-term MRI follow-up study. *Eur Radiol* 2009; **19**:2535–43.

62. Filippi, M, Rocca, MA, Moiola, L, et al. MRI and magnetization transfer imaging changes in the brain and cervical

63. Nakashima, I, Fujihara, K, Miyazawa, I, et al. Clinical and MRI features of Japanese patients with multiple sclerosis positive for NMO-IgG. *J Neurol Neurosurg Psychiatry* 2006; **77**:1073–5.

64. Sellner, J, Luthi, N, Schupbach, WM, et al. Diagnostic workup of patients with acute transverse myelitis: spectrum of clinical presentation, neuroimaging and laboratory findings. *Spinal Cord* 2009; **47**:312–17.

65. Pittock, SJ, Weinshenker, BG, Lucchinetti, CF, et al. Neuromyelitis optica brain lesions localized at sites of high aquaporin 4 expression. *Arch Neurol* 2006; **63**:964–8.

66. Cabrera-Gomez, J, Saiz-Hinarejos, A, Graus, F, et al. Brain magnetic resonance imaging findings in acute relapses of neuromyelitis optica spectrum disorders. *Mult Scler* 2008; **14**:248–51.

67. Li, Y, Xie, P, Lv, F, et al. Brain magnetic resonance imaging abnormalities in neuromyelitis optica. *Acta Neurol Scand* 2008; **118**:218–25.

68. McKeon, A, Lennon, VA, Lotze, T, et al. CNS aquaporin-4 autoimmunity in children. *Neurology* 2008; **71**:93–100.

69. Nakamura, M, Misu, T, Fujihara, K, et al. Occurrence of acute large and edematous callosal lesions in neuromyelitis optica. *Mult Scler* 2009; **15**:695–700.

70. Ito, S, Mori, M, Makino, T, et al. 'Cloud-like enhancement' is a magnetic resonance imaging abnormality specific to neuromyelitis optica. *Ann Neurol* 2009; **66**:425–8.

71. Correale, J, Fiol, M. Activation of humoral immunity and eosinophils in neuromyelitis optica. *Neurology* 2004; **63**:2363–70.

72. Bichuetti, DB, Rivero, RL, Oliveira, DM, et al. Neuromyelitis optica: brain abnormalities in a Brazilian cohort. *Arq Neuropsiquiatr* 2008; **66**:1–4.

73. Milano, E, Di Sapio, A, Malucchi, S, et al. Neuromyelitis optica: importance of cerebrospinal fluid examination during relapse. *Neurol Sci* 2003; **24**:130–3.

74. Bergamaschi, R, Tonietti, S, Franciotta, D, et al. Oligoclonal bands in Devic's neuromyelitis optica and multiple sclerosis: differences in repeated cerebrospinal fluid examinations. *Mult Scler* 2004; **10**:2–4.

75. Jarius, S, Franciotta, D, Bergamaschi, R, et al. Polyspecific, antiviral immune response distinguishes multiple sclerosis and neuromyelitis optica. *J Neurol Neurosurg Psychiatry* 2008; **79**:1134–6.

76. Miyazawa, I, Nakashima, I, Petzold, A, et al. High CSF neurofilament heavy chain levels in neuromyelitis optica. *Neurology* 2007; **68**:865–7.

77. Misu, T, Takano, R, Fujihara, K, et al. Marked increase in cerebrospinal fluid glial fibrillary acidic protein in neuromy-

elitis optica: an astrocytic damage marker. *J Neurol Neurosurg Psychiatry* 2009; **80**:575–7.

78. Kanzaki, M, Mochizuki, H, Ogawa, G, *et al.* Clinical features of opticospinal multiple sclerosis with anti-aquaporin 4 antibody. *Eur Neurol* 2008; **60**:37–42.

79. Graber, DJ, Levy, M, Kerr, D, *et al.* Neuromyelitis optica pathogenesis and aquaporin 4. *J Neuroinflammation* 2008; **5**:22.

80. Tait, MJ, Saadoun, S, Bell, BA, *et al.* Water movements in the brain: role of aquaporins. *Trends Neurosci* 2008; **31**:37–43.

81. Tani, T, Sakimura, K, Tsujita, M, *et al.* Identification of binding sites for anti-aquaporin 4 antibodies in patients with neuromyelitis optica. *J Neuroimmunol* 2009; **211**:110–13.

82. Kinoshita, M, Nakatsuji, Y, Moriya, M, *et al.* Astrocytic necrosis is induced by anti-aquaporin-4 antibody-positive serum. *Neuroreport* 2009; **20**:508–12.

83. Kinoshita, M, Nakatsuji, Y, Kimura, T, *et al.* Neuromyelitis optica: passive transfer to rats by human immunoglobulin. *Biochem Biophys Res Commun* 2009; **386**:623–7.

84. Bennett, L, Lam, C, Reddy Kalluri, S, *et al.* Intrathecal pathogenic anti-aquaporin-4 antibodies in early neuromyelitis optica. *Ann Neurol* 2009; **66**(5):617–29.

85. Fazio, R, Malosio, ML, Lampasona, V, *et al.* Antiacquaporin 4 antibodies detection by different techniques in neuromyelitis optica patients. *Mult Scler* 2009; **15**:1153–63.

86. Waters, P, Vincent, A. Detection of anti-aquaporin-4 antibodies in neuromyelitis optica: current status of the assays. *Int MS J* 2008; **15**:99–105.

87. Marignier, R, De Seze, J, Vukusic, S, *et al.* NMO-IgG and Devic's neuromyelitis optica: a French experience. *Mult Scler* 2008; **14**:440–5.

88. Takahashi, T, Fujihara, K, Nakashima, I, *et al.* Anti-aquaporin-4 antibody is involved in the pathogenesis of NMO: a study on antibody titre. *Brain* 2007; **130**:1235–43.

89. Paul, F, Jarius, S, Aktas, O, *et al.* Antibody to aquaporin 4 in the diagnosis of neuromyelitis optica. *PLoS Med* 2007; **4**:e133.

90. McKeon, A, Fryer, JP, Apiwattanakul, M, *et al.* Diagnosis of neuromyelitis spectrum disorders: comparative sensitivities and specificities of immunohistochemical and immunoprecipitation assays. *Arch Neurol* 2009; **66**:1134–8.

91. Saiz, A, Zuliani, L, Blanco, Y, *et al.* Revised diagnostic criteria for neuromyelitis optica (NMO). Application in a series of suspected patients. *J Neurol* 2007; **254**:1233–7.

92. Nishiyama, S, Ito, T, Misu, T, *et al.* A case of NMO seropositive for aquaporin-4 antibody more than 10 years before onset. *Neurology* 2009; **72**:1960–1.

93. Jarius, S, Aboul-Enein, F, Waters, P, *et al.* Antibody to aquaporin-4 in the long-term course of neuromyelitis optica. *Brain* 2008; **131**:3072–80.

94. Hinson, SR, McKeon, A, Fryer, JP, *et al.* Prediction of neuromyelitis optica attack severity by quantitation of complement-mediated injury to aquaporin-4-expressing cells. *Arch Neurol* 2009; **66**:1164–7.

95. Smith, CH, Waubant, E, Langer-Gould, A. Absence of neuromyelitis optica IgG antibody in an active relapsing-remitting multiple sclerosis population. *J Neuroophthalmol* 2009; **29**:104–6.

96. Scott, TF, Kassab, SL, Pittock, SJ. Neuromyelitis optica IgG status in acute partial transverse myelitis. *Arch Neurol* 2006; **63**:1398–400.

97. Ravaglia, S, Bastianello, S, Franciotta, D, *et al.* NMO-IgG-negative relapsing myelitis. *Spinal Cord* 2009; **47**:531–7.

98. Klawiter, EC, Alvarez, E, III, Xu, J, *et al.* NMO-IgG detected in CSF in seronegative neuromyelitis optica. *Neurology* 2009; **72**:1101–03.

99. Miller, DH, Weinshenker, BG, Filippi, M, *et al.* Differential diagnosis of suspected multiple sclerosis: a consensus approach. *Mult Scler* 2008; **14**:1157–74.

100. Pittock, SJ. Neuromyelitis optica: a new perspective. *Semin Neurol* 2008; **28**:95–104.

101. Furukawa, Y, Yoshikawa, H, Yachie, A, *et al.* Neuromyelitis optica associated with myasthenia gravis: characteristic phenotype in Japanese population. *Eur J Neurol* 2006; **13**:655–8.

102. Gold, R, Linington, C. Devic's disease: bridging the gap between laboratory and clinic. *Brain* 2002; **125**:1425–7.

103. Hui, AC, Wong, RS, Ma, R, *et al.* Recurrent optic neuromyelitis with multiple endocrinopathies and autoimmune disorders. *J Neurol* 2002; **249**:784–5.

104. Petravic, D, Habek, M, Supe, S, *et al.* Recurrent optic neuromyelitis with endocrinopathies: a new syndrome or just a coincidence? *Mult Scler* 2006; **12**:670–3.

105. Kira, J, Kawano, Y. Recurrent optic neuromyelitis with endocrinopathies. *Neurology* 1997; **49**:1475–6.

106. Komolafe, MA, Komolafe, EO, Sunmonu, TA, *et al.* New onset neuromyelitis optica in a young Nigerian woman with possible antiphospholipid syndrome: a case report. *J Med Case Reports* 2008; **2**:348.

107. Birnbaum, J, Kerr, D. Devic's syndrome in a woman with systemic lupus erythematosus: diagnostic and therapeutic implications of testing for the neuromyelitis optica IgG autoantibody. *Arthritis Rheum* 2007; **57**:347–51.

108. Ferreira, S, Marques, P, Carneiro, E, *et al.* Devic's syndrome in systemic lupus erythematosus and probable antiphospholipid syndrome. *Rheumatology (Oxford)* 2005; **44**:693–5.

109. Chan, AY, Liu, DT. Devic's syndrome in systemic lupus erythematosus and probable antiphospholipid syndrome. *Rheumatology (Oxford)* 2006; **45**:120–1; **author reply 121**.

110. Mehta, LR, Samuelsson, MK, Kleiner, AK, *et al.* Neuromyelitis optica spectrum disorder in a patient with systemic lupus erythematosus and anti-phospholipid antibody syndrome. *Mult Scler* 2008; **14**:425–7.

111. Mochizuki, A, Hayashi, A, Hisahara, S, *et al.* Steroid-responsive Devic's variant in Sjogren's syndrome. *Neurology* 2000; **54**:1391–2.

112. Lehnhardt, FG, Impekoven, P, Rubbert, A, *et al.* Recurrent longitudinal myelitis as primary manifestation of SLE. *Neurology* 2004; **63**:1976.

113. Jacob, A, Boggild, M. Neuromyelitis optica. *Pract Neurol* 2006; **6**:180–4.

114. Jacob, A, Matiello, M, Wingerchuk, DM, *et al.* Neuromyelitis optica: changing concepts. *J Neuroimmunol* 2007; **187**:126–38.

115. Rubiera, M, Rio, J, Tintore, M, *et al.* Neuromyelitis optica diagnosis in clinically isolated syndromes suggestive of multiple sclerosis. *Neurology* 2006; **66**:1568–70.

116. Weinshenker, BG, O'Brien, PC, Petterson, TM, *et al.* A randomized trial of plasma exchange in acute central nervous system inflammatory demyelinating disease. *Ann Neurol* 1999; **46**:878–86.

117. Keegan, M, Pineda, AA, McClelland, RL, *et al.* Plasma exchange for severe attacks of CNS demyelination: predictors of response. *Neurology* 2002; **58**:143–6.

118. Llufriu, S, Castillo, J, Blanco, Y, *et al.* Plasma exchange for acute attacks of CNS demyelination: Predictors of improvement at 6 months. *Neurology* 2009; **73**:949–53.

119. Watanabe, S, Nakashima, I, Misu, T, *et al.* Therapeutic efficacy of plasma exchange in NMO-IgG-positive patients with neuromyelitis optica. *Mult Scler* 2007; **13**:128–32.

120. Ruprecht, K, Klinker, E, Dintelmann, T, *et al.* Plasma exchange for severe optic neuritis: treatment of 10 patients. *Neurology* 2004; **63**:1081–3.

121. Bonnan, M, Valentino, R, Olindo, S, *et al.* Plasma exchange in severe spinal attacks associated with neuromyelitis optica spectrum disorder. *Mult Scler* 2009; **15**:487–92.

122. Miyamoto, K, Kusunoki, S. Intermittent plasmapheresis prevents recurrence in neuromyelitis optica. *Ther Apher Dial* 2009; **13**:505–8.

123. Nozaki, I, Hamaguchi, T, Komai, K, *et al.* Fulminant Devic disease successfully treated by lymphocytapheresis. *J Neurol Neurosurg Psychiatry* 2006; **77**:1094–5.

124. Wingerchuk, DM, Weinshenker, BG. Neuromyelitis optica. *Curr Treat Options Neurol* 2008; **10**:55–66.

125. Saida, T, Tashiro, K, Itoyama, Y, *et al.* Interferon beta-1b is effective in Japanese RRMS patients: a randomized, multi-center study. *Neurology* 2005; **64**:621–30.

126. Warabi, Y, Matsumoto, Y, Hayashi, H. Interferon beta-1b exacerbates multiple sclerosis with severe optic nerve and spinal cord demyelination. *J Neurol Sci* 2007; **252**: 57–61.

127. Tanaka, M, Tanaka, K, Komori, M. Interferon-beta(1b) treatment in neuromyelitis optica. *Eur Neurol* 2009; **62**:167–70.

128. Shimizu, Y, Yokoyama, K, Misu, T, *et al.* Development of extensive brain lesions following interferon beta therapy in relapsing neuromyelitis optica and longitudinally extensive myelitis. *J Neurol* 2008; **255**:305–7.

129. Papeix, C, Vidal, JS, de Seze, J, *et al.* Immunosuppressive therapy is more effective than interferon in neuromyelitis optica. *Mult Scler* 2007; **13**:256–9.

130. Gartzen, K, Limmroth, V, Putzki, N. Relapsing neuromyelitis optica responsive to glatiramer acetate treatment. *Eur J Neurol* 2007; **1**:e12–e13.

131. Bakker, J, Metz, L. Devic's neuromyelitis optica treated with intravenous gamma globulin (IVIG). *Can J Neurol Sci* 2004; **31**:265–7.

132. Magraner, MJ, Bosca, I, Simó-Castelló, M, *et al.* An open label study of the effects of intravenous immunoglobulin in neuromyelitis optica spectrum disorders. Manuscript.

133. Mandler, RN, Ahmed, W, Dencoff, JE. Devic's neuromyelitis optica: a prospective study of seven patients treated with prednisone and azathioprine. *Neurology* 1998; **51**:1219–20.

134. La Mantia, L, Mascoli, N, Milanese, C. Azathioprine. Safety profile in multiple sclerosis patients. *Neurol Sci* 2007; **28**:299–303.

135. Wingerchuk, DM, Weinshenker, BG. Neuromyelitis optica. *Curr Treat Options Neurol* 2005; **7**:173–82.

136. Killian, JM, Bressler, RB, Armstrong, RM, *et al.* Controlled pilot trial of monthly intravenous cyclophosphamide in multiple sclerosis. *Arch Neurol* 1988; **45**:27–30.

137. Bonnet, F, Mercie, P, Morlat, P, *et al.* Devic's neuromyelitis optica during pregnancy in a patient with systemic lupus erythematosus. *Lupus* 1999; **8**:244–7.

138. Arabshahi, B, Pollock, AN, Sherry, DD, *et al.* Devic disease in a child with primary Sjogren syndrome. *J Child Neurol* 2006; **21**:285–6.

139. Birnbaum, J, Kerr, D. Optic neuritis and recurrent myelitis in a woman with systemic lupus erythematosus. *Nat Clin Pract Rheumatol* 2008; **4**:381–6.

140. Mok, CC, To, CH, Mak, A, *et al.* Immunoablative cyclophosphamide for refractory lupus-related neuromyelitis optica. *J Rheumatol* 2008; **35**:172–4.

141. Stojanovich, L, Stojanovich, R, Kostich, V, *et al.* Neuropsychiatric lupus favourable response to low dose i.v. cyclophosphamide and prednisolone (pilot study). *Lupus* 2003; **12**:3–7.

142. La Mantia, L, Milanese, C, Mascoli, N, *et al.* Cyclophosphamide for multiple sclerosis. *Cochrane Database Syst Rev* 2007; 1, CD002819.

143. Minagar, A, Sheremata, WA. Treatment of Devic's disease with methotrexate and prednisone. *Int J MS Care* 2000; **2**:39–43.

144. Weinstock-Guttman, B, Ramanathan, M, Lincoff, N, *et al.* Study of mitoxantrone for the treatment of recurrent neuromyelitis optica (Devic disease). *Arch Neurol* 2006; **63**: 957–63.

145. Ellis, R, Boggild, M. Therapy-related acute leukaemia with mitoxantrone: what is the risk and can we minimise it? *Mult Scler* 2009; **15**:505–8.

146. Jacob, A, Matiello, M, Weinshenker, BG, *et al.* Treatment of neuromyelitis optica with mycophenolate mofetil: retrospective analysis of 24 patients. *Arch Neurol* 2009; **66**: 1128–33.

147. Falcini, F, Trapani, S, Ricci, L, *et al.* Sustained improvement of a girl affected with Devic's disease over 2 years of mycophenolate mofetil treatment. *Rheumatology (Oxford)* 2006; **45**:913–15.

148. Watanabe, S, Misu, T, Miyazawa, I, *et al.* Low-dose corticosteroids reduce relapses in neuromyelitis optica: a retrospective analysis. *Mult Scler* 2007; **13**:968–74.

149. Jacob, A, Weinshenker, BG, Violich, I, *et al.* Treatment of neuromyelitis optica with rituximab: retrospective analysis of 25 patients. *Arch Neurol* 2008; **65**:1443–8.

150. Cree, BA, Lamb, S, Morgan, K, *et al.* An open label study of the effects of rituximab in neuromyelitis optica. *Neurology* 2005; **64**:1270–2.

151. Kimby, E. Tolerability and safety of rituximab (MabThera). *Cancer Treat Rev* 2005; **31**:456–73.

152. Joseph, FG, Scolding, NJ. Neurolupus. *Pract Neurol* 2010; **10**:4–15.

153. Bertsias, G, Ioannidis, JP, Boletis, J, *et al.* EULAR recommendations for the management of systemic lupus erythematosus. Report of a Task Force of the EULAR Standing Committee for International Clinical Studies Including Therapeutics. *Ann Rheum Dis* 2008; **67**:195–205.

154. American College of Rheumatology Ad Hoc Committee on Systemic Lupus Erythematosus Guidelines. Guidelines for referral and management of systemic lupus erythematosus in adults. *Arthritis Rheum* 1999; **42**:1785–96.

155. Henze, T, Rieckmann, P, Toyka, KV. Symptomatic treatment of multiple sclerosis. Multiple Sclerosis Therapy Consensus Group (MSTCG) of the German Multiple Sclerosis Society. *Eur Neurol* 2006; **56**:78–105.

CHAPTER 21

Screening for tumours in paraneoplastic syndromes

M.J. Titulaer,[1] R. Soffietti,[2] J. Dalmau,[3,6] N.E. Gilhus,[4] B. Giometto,[5] F. Graus,[6] W. Grisold,[7] J. Honnorat,[8] P.A.E. Sillevis Smitt,[9] R. Tanasescu,[10] C.A. Vedeler,[4] R. Voltz[11] and J.J.G.M. Verschuuren[1]

[1]Leiden University Medical Centre, Leiden, The Netherlands; [2]University San Giovanni Battista, Turin, Italy; [3]University of Pennsylvania, Philadelphia, USA; [4]University of Bergen, Bergen, and Haukeland University Hospital, Bergen, Norway; [5]Ospedale Ca'Foncello, Treviso, Italy; [6]Hospital Clinic, Universitat de Barcelona, and Institut d'Investigació Biomèdica August Pi i Sunyer (IDIBAPS), Barcelona, Spain; [7]KFJ Hospital, Vienna, Austria; [8]Centre de référence Maladie Rare 'Syndromes neurologiques Paranéoplasiques', Hospices Civils de Lyon, and INSERM U842, Université Lyon 1, Lyon, France; [9]Erasmus University Medical Center, Rotterdam, the Netherlands; [10]Colentina Hospital, Carol Davila University of Medicine and Pharmacy, Bucharest, Romania; [11]University of Cologne, Cologne, Germany

Background

Paraneoplastic neurological syndromes (PNSs) are rare and occur as a remote effect of tumour, not directly caused by mass lesions, metastases, infections, nutritional factors or anti-tumour treatment. Among the tumours associated with PNSs, small cell lung cancer (SCLC) is the most frequent one [1]. Other tumours related to PNSs are thymoma, ovarian carcinoma and teratoma, breast carcinoma, testicular tumours and Hodgkin's disease. PNSs occur in 1–3% of SCLC patients [2, 3], which is far less common than other cancer complications [4]. However, recognition and diagnosis of PNS are important because neurological symptoms almost invariably predate direct symptoms of the primary tumour [5–8], and treatment at earlier stage provides better chance of good outcome. Proper treatment is also important because most PNSs cause severe disabilities. Criteria for diagnosis and management of PNSs have been published by the PNS Euronetwork [9], in a recent review by Dalmau [10] and by the European Federation of Neurological Societies

(EFNS) Task Force guideline of 2006 [11]. This chapter outlines screening recommendations for PNSs.

Methods

The Task Force decided to focus on screening of tumours in classic PNSs [9]: Lambert–Eaton myasthenic syndrome (LEMS), paraneoplastic limbic encephalitis (PLE), subacute sensory neuronopathy (SSN), subacute autonomic neuropathy (SAN), paraneoplastic cerebellar degeneration (PCD), paraneoplastic opsoclonus–myoclonus (POM), paraneoplastic peripheral nerve hyperexcitability (PPNH), myasthenia gravis (MG) and paraneoplastic retinopathy (CAR). Dermatomyositis is mentioned briefly, but paraproteinaemic neuropathies are not included.

The clinical characteristics of the syndromes are not described, but referred to in the text and tables. The tables point out the interrelationship of the clinical syndrome, antibodies and related tumours. Screening is described

European Handbook of Neurological Management: Volume 2, Second Edition. Edited by Nils Erik Gilhus, Michael P. Barnes, Michael Brainin.
© 2012 Blackwell Publishing Ltd. Published 2012 by Blackwell Publishing Ltd.

for the tumours according to available literature. If no description was available, recommendations were based on screening strategies for this tumour in the general population or high-risk patients. Search strategies included English literature from the Cochrane Database, MedLine and PubMed, using the keywords: 'Lambert–Eaton myasthenic syndrome', 'limbic encephalitis', 'sensory neuronopathy', 'autonomic neuropathy', 'cerebellar ataxia', opsoclonus-myoclonus', 'neuromyotonia', 'myasthenia gravis' and 'paraneoplastic retinopathy', in combination with 'investigation' or 'screening'. In addition, search strategies using 'small cell lung carcinoma', 'thymoma', 'breast carcinoma', 'ovarian teratoma', 'ovarian carcinoma', 'testicular' 'Hodgkin's' in combination with 'paraneoplastic' and 'screening' were used, and the words 'Hu', 'CV2' or 'CRMP5' or 'CRMP-5', 'Yo', 'Ri', 'Ma2', 'amphiphysin', 'recoverin', 'Tr', 'VGCC (voltage-gated calcium channels)', 'acetylcholine', 'VGKC (voltage-gated potassium channels)', 'NMDA (N-methyl-D-aspartic acid)', 'AMPA (α-amino-3-hydroxyl-5-methyl-4-isoxazole-pro-

prionate)', 'GAD (glutamic acid decarboxylase)' and 'GABAR (γ-aminobutyric acid receptor)' were used in combination with 'paraneoplastic' and 'screening'. Only one study reached level III evidence [7], whereas all other studies contained level IV evidence. No level A, B or C recommendations could be made. However, good practice points were agreed by consensus, according to the EFNS guidelines [12].

Screening for tumours in patients with PNSs and paraneoplastic antibodies

When the diagnosis of a PNS is made, detection of the associated paraneoplastic antibody is of great importance because the type of tumour and the chance of an underlying malignancy depend mostly on the associated antibody. The interrelationships of PNS, antibody and tumour are summarized in Tables 21.1 and 21.2. For a

Table 21.1 Paraneoplastic syndromes and their associated antibodies and tumours.

Neurological syndrome	Antibody	Tumour	References
Encephalomyelitis/Limbic encephalitis	**Anti-Hu, anti-Ma2**, anti-CV2/CRMP5, anti-VGKC, anti-Ri, anti-amphiphysin, anti-GABABR, anti-AMPAR, anti-GAD	**SCLC, testicular tumour,** thymoma, neuroblastoma, prostate carcinoma, breast cancer, Hodgkin's lymphoma	[6, 16–21]
Cerebellar degeneration	**Anti-Yo, anti-Hu**, anti-VGCC, anti-CV2/CRMP5, anti-Ma2, anti-Ri, anti-Tr, anti-GAD, anti-mGluR1-α	**SCLC, ovarian cancer, breast cancer, Hodgkin's lymphoma**, thymoma	[8, 22–25]
Brain-stem encephalitis/ Opsoclonus–myoclonus	**Anti-Ri, anti-Ma2**, anti-Hu, anti-amphiphysin	Breast cancer, ovarian cancer, testicular tumour, SCLC, neuroblastoma (children)	[16, 26]
Encephalitis with psychiatric manifestations, seizures, dyskinesias, dystonia and autonomic instability	**Anti-NMDAR**	**Ovarian teratoma**, testis teratoma, SCLC	[5, 27]
Neuromyotonia	**Anti-VGKC**	Thymoma, SCLC	[28]
LEMS	**Anti-VGCC**	**SCLC**	[29]
Myasthenia gravis	**Anti-AChR**	**Thymoma**	[30]
Subacute sensory neuronopathy	**Anti-Hu**, anti-CV2/CRMP5, anti-amphiphysin	**SCLC**, breast cancer, ovarian cancer	[6, 31]
Subacute autonomic neuropathy	Anti-gAChR, anti-Hu	**SCLC**, thymoma	[31]
Stiff person syndrome	**Anti-amphiphysin**, anti-GAD	**Breast cancer**, SCLC	[32–35]
Cancer-associated retinopathy	Anti-recoverin	**SCLC**, endometrium cancer	[36–38]

The most frequent antibodies and tumours are in bold type.
See text (and references) for abbreviations.

Table 21.2 Paraneoplastic antibodies in relation to the associated neurological syndromes and tumours.

Antibodies	Tumour present (%) [39]	Neurological syndrome	Tumour	References
Antibodies to non-surface antigens in PNSs				
Anti-Hu (ANNA-1)	98	Encephalomyelitis, limbic encephalitis, sensory neuropathy, cerebellar degeneration, autonomic neuropathy	**SCLC**, neuroblastoma, prostate cancer	[6, 23, 31, 40–43]
Anti-Yo (PCA1)	98	Cerebellar degeneration	**Ovarian carcinoma**, breast cancer	[8, 22, 25, 40, 44]
Anti-CV2/CRMP5	96	Cerebellar degeneration, sensory (motor) neuropathy, chorea, limbic encephalitis, encephalomyelitis, optic neuritis	**SCLC, thymoma**	[40, 43, 45, 46]
Anti-Ma2 (anti-Ta)	96	Limbic encephalitis, brainstem encephalitis, cerebellar degeneration	**Testicular tumour (males <50 years)**, lung cancer, breast cancer	[16, 18, 47]
Anti-Ri (ANNA-2)	97	Opsoclonus–myoclonus, brain-stem encephalitis, cerebellar degeneration	**Breast cancer, SCLC**, gynaecological tumours	[25, 26, 48, 49]
Anti-amphiphysin	95	Stiff person syndrome, encephalomyelitis, sensory (motor) neuropathy	**Breast cancer**, SCLC, ovarian cancer	[32–34, 49]
Anti-recoverin	99	Cancer-associated retinopathy	**SCLC**, endometrium cancer, thymoma, prostate cancer	[36–38]
Anti-Tr	89	Cerebellar degeneration	**Hodgkin's lymphoma**	[24, 41, 50, 51]
Anti-GAD	8[a]	Cerebellar degeneration, limbic encephalitis, stiff person syndrome	SCLC, lung cancer, thymic cancer, pancreatic cancer, renal cell cancer	[21, 35]
Antibodies to surface antigens in PNSs				
Anti-VGCC	55	Lambert–Eaton myasthenic syndrome Cerebellar degeneration	**SCLC**	[23, 29, 52]
Anti-AChR	15[b]	Myasthenia gravis	**Thymoma**	[30]
Anti-gAChR	15	Autonomic neuropathy	**SCLC**, thymoma	[53, 54]
Anti-NMDAR	9–56	Encephalitis with psychiatric manifestations, seizures, dyskinesias, dystonia and autonomic instability	**Ovarian teratoma**, testicular teratoma	[5, 27]
Anti-VGKC-related proteins (LGI1, CASPR2)	25–31	Limbic encephalitis Neuromyotonia Morvan's syndrome	Thymoma, SCLC	[28, 55, 56]
Anti-GABABR	47	Limbic encephalitis	**SCLC**, lung tumour	[17]
Anti-AMPAR	70	Limbic encephalitis	Thymoma, lung cancer, breast cancer	[20]
Antibodies, reported in case reports				
Anti-mGluR1-α		Cerebellar degeneration	Hodgkin's lymphoma	[57]
ANNA-3		Encephalomyelitis, sensory neuropathy	SCLC	[58]
PCA-2		Encephalomyelitis, cerebellar degeneration	SCLC	[59]
Anti-Zic4		Cerebellar degeneration	SCLC	[60]

The most frequently associated tumour type are in bold types.
[a]Possible anti-GABABR related,
[b]Almost invariably with tumour.
See text (and references) for abbreviations.

clinical description of the PNS, the reader is referred to the references in the tables, to extensive reviews [10, 13–15] and to the EFNS Task Force Guideline 'Management of paraneoplastic syndromes' [11]. Screening is described by tumour.

A thorough history to determine risk factors and (sub)clinical complaints and examination, including examination of the pelvic region (rectal for prostate carcinoma in men, testicular in search for testicular tumours in men and gynaecological examination in women for ovarian tumours) and examination of the breast, are a requirement. As tumours can arise in many organs or body parts, thorough screening requires a multidisciplinary approach.

SCLC

SCLC was detected in 96% of patients with SCLC LEMS within 1 year [7]. Incidental reports of more than 2 years between onset of PNS symptoms and detection of SCLC are available, but most are reports published before the widespread use of standard screening protocols and using inferior quality computed tomography (CT) scans [7, 28, 61–63]. One patient with an interval of 54 months is described whereas [^{18}F]fluorodeoxyglucose positron emission tomography (FDG-PET) scanning was available [40], but this patient received chemotherapy at diagnosis of his paraneoplastic encephalomyelitis (PEM) after the initial CT scan was negative. Screening by thoracic radiograph is insufficient because the sensitivity is only 43%. A CT scan of the thorax showed a sensitivity of 83% at primary screening and 92% overall in LEMS patients [7].

In a French study, conventional screening by radiograph and CT of the thorax detected 71 of 85 SCLCs (84%) in patients with PNSs [40]. For 15 patients with an anti-Hu syndrome, described previously, sensitivity of the same investigations was 80% [64]. In a German study of eight anti-Hu patients, CT of the thorax detected only three of six tumours [41]. As one patient had a neuroblastoma, one developed the PNS on recurrence of the SCLC and the number of patients was small, we think it appropriate to estimate sensitivity of CT of the thorax for SCLC in PNSs to 80–85%. FDG-PET has shown additional value in case series in comparison to CT of the thorax. As FDG-PET has only recently become widely available, it has not been compared in large studies. Studies representing 19 patients with LEMS [7] and 13 patients with different PNSs [41] directly compared CT

of the thorax with FDG-PET. Other studies investigated use of FDG-PET after the initial CT of the thorax was negative in patients with different PNSs [40, 65, 66]. All results showed an additive effect of FDG-PET scans. Delay between initial CT of the thorax and FDG-PET makes it impossible to determine accuracy of this combination in initial screening.

Combined FDG-PET/CT scanners might pose new opportunities, but data to support this are lacking. Bronchoscopy provided no additional information in LEMS patients if imaging revealed no abnormalities [7]. Often, the only abnormalities are in the mediastinal lymph nodes, so special focus should be aimed towards this region. Minimal invasive techniques, such as endoscopic ultrasound-guided fine needle aspiration (EUS-FNA), reduce the need for mediastinoscopies and thoracotomies in SCLC (without PNSs) in 70% [67]. Mediastinoscopy (and eventually thoracotomy) may be necessary sometimes to obtain a histological or cytological diagnosis. The additional value of EUS-FNA, if imaging techniques are negative, is unknown.

Recommendation

Screen for SCLC by CT of the thorax, followed by FDG-PET or integrated FDG-PET/CT (good practice point).

Thymoma

CT of the thorax is currently considered first choice to screen for a thymoma. A chest radiograph will merely show broadening of the mediastinum and is not as sensitive [68]. One retrospective study, directly comparing CT and magnetic resonance imaging (MRI) of the thorax, showed sensitivity of CT to be at least equal to MRI [69]. CT of the thorax showed moderate sensitivity (75–88%), but less specificity (42–81%), most problems arising in distinguishing thymic hyperplasia (associated with early onset myasthenia gravis) from thymoma [70]. Reliability in this study was lower than expected, most probably due to the long study period (1989–2003), because CT techniques developed rapidly during the study period. Difficulties in distinguishing hyperplasia from thymoma were also detected in a Canadian study [71]. FDG-PET was helpful in distinguishing thymic hyperplasia, thymoma and thymic carcinoma [72, 73], as well as FDG-PET/CT [74].

Recommendation

Screen for thymoma by CT of the thorax (followed by
FDG-PET) or integrated FDG-PET/CT (good practice point).

Breast cancer

Mammography revealed breast cancer or infiltrated
lymph nodes in 83% of patients with paraneoplastic cerebellar degeneration, anti-Yo antibodies and breast
cancer [8]. CT of the thorax showed metastatic lymph
nodes in the other two patients. Additional value of FDG-
PET over mammography, ultrasonography, CT and MRI
has been described in patients with PNSs in case reports
and case series [40, 75–77]. In one patient, diagnosis of
breast cancer was made only 5 years after diagnosis of
PCD, despite adequate repeated screening by CT of the
chest/abdomen and FDG-PET [76]. Much research has
focused on screening strategies in patients at high risk for
breast cancer, but the subgroup with PNSs has not been
evaluated specifically.

A Dutch prospective cohort study showed superior
sensitivity of MRI (80%) versus mammography (33%) in
1909 patients with a familial or genetic predisposition for
breast cancer [78]. An American cohort study of 609
patients (asymptomatic, high-risk women with a negative mammogram before) compared mammography,
ultrasonography and MRI over the next 2 years. Breast
cancer was found in 18 patients, and the sensitivity was
44%, 17% and 71% respectively [79]. Five other prospective cohort studies comparing MRI with mammography
and ultrasonography in women with a lifetime risk for
breast cancer of more than 20–25% showed similar
results: sensitivity was 77–100% for MRI, 16–40% for
mammography and 16–40% for ultrasonography [80].
Recent American guidelines for breast screening recommended MRI breast screening as an adjunct to mammography in women with a lifetime risk of more than
25% [80, 81].

Recommendation

Screen for breast cancer by mammography, followed by MRI of
the breast. If negative follow by FDG-PET/CT (good practice
point).

Ovarian teratoma and carcinoma

The optimal modality for screening the ovaries will
depend on the expected tumour: carcinoma in anti-Yo-,
anti-Ri- and anti-amphiphysin-related PNS and teratoma in anti-NMDAR related PNS.

Teratoma

Most teratomas are mature cystic teratomas (MCTs).
Immature teratomas (ITs), constituting 1% of all teratomas, were present in 29% of anti-N-methyl-D-aspartate
receptor (NMDAR)-related cases [5]. Bilateral teratomas
were present in 14% [5], comparable to 12% described
in general [82]. Ultrasonography showed an MCT with a
highly variable sensitivity of 58–94% [82]. ITs are more
difficult to differentiate by ultrasonography [82]. Most
studies have used transvaginal ultrasonography (TVUS),
but a direct comparison of TV and transabdominal ultrasonography (TAUS) has not been performed. CT showed
a very good sensitivity of 93% [83] to 98% [84]. The only
direct comparison of TVUS and CT showed a better sensitivity for CT: 93 versus 79% [83]. MRI also has a very
good sensitivity of 93–96% [85]. FDG-PET has not been
studied in teratomas, but MCTs have no or little uptake
of FDG. FDG-PET is not expected to be sensitive for
teratomas. An advantage of CT over ultrasonography is
that extrapelvic teratomas (occasionally described as
anti-NMDAR-related teratomas) can also be detected [5].
TVUS, followed by CT or MRI, is the investigation of
choice [10]. In young patients, MRI may be first choice
to avoid radiation by repeated CT.

Recommendation

Screen for ovarian teratoma by TVUS, followed by CT/MRI of
the pelvis/abdomen. If negative, follow by CT of the thorax
(good practice point).

Ovarian carcinoma

Ultrasonography is the investigation of first choice to
detect ovarian carcinomas. TVUS is a more sensitive
investigation than TAUS [86]. Sensitivity for ovarian carcinoma was 85% in medium- to high-risk patients [87].
A meta-analysis by Liu et al. [88] compared ultrasonography, CT and MRI showing similar results with sensitivities of 89%, 85% and 89%, respectively. The current
National Comprehensive Cancer Network (NCCN)

Clinical Practice Guidelines in Oncology recommend TVUS, combined with cancer antigen 125 (CA-125) each 6 months in patients with a genetic/familial high risk for ovarian carcinoma [81]. Integrated FDG-PET/CT has been studied only to detect recurrence of ovarian carcinoma or in patients selected by abnormal ultrasonography or markedly raised CA-125. A few case reports describe an additional value of FDG-PET in such patients [40, 41, 44, 75]. Even if screening revealed no malignancy, surgical exploration and removal of ovaries have been suggested in patients with anti-Yo cerebellar degeneration and worsening neurological status, especially in postmenopausal women [22]. Although the neurological condition does not ameliorate with surgery, diagnosis and treatment of the primary tumour may improve survival. In addition, the neurological symptoms can stabilize, especially in moderately affected patients [89].

Recommendation

Screen for ovarian carcinoma by TV US, followed by CT-pelvis/abdomen or integrated FDG-PET/CT (good practice point).

Testicular tumours

Ultrasound investigation of the testicular region detected 18 (72%) of 25 testicular tumours [16]. CT scan of the pelvic region added one patient. FDG-PET scanning had no additional value in the two patients tested. This study showed that it has additional value when obtaining tissue (biopsy or orchiectomy, unilateral or even bilateral) in young male patients (<50 years) with anti-Ma2 antibodies, deteriorating neurological disease and microcalcifications on ultrasonography.

Recommendation

Screen for testicular tumour by ultrasonography, followed by CT of the pelvic region (good practice point).

Other tumours

Other tumours such as Hodgkin's lymphoma, small cell prostate carcinoma and neuroblastoma (in children) have been described in relation to paraneoplastic disorders. All reports describe single cases or small series, with little relevance for screening recommendations.

Screening for tumours in possible PNSs without identified paraneoplastic antibodies

The recommendations for screening for tumours in patients with a possible PNS, but with no detectable antibodies are less clear. Mason et al.[23] described 57 cases with PCDs and SCLCs. This study concluded that almost half the patients had 'no antibodies', but only anti-Hu and anti-VGCC antibodies were examined. As listed in Table 21.1, other antibodies can also be found in PCDs. Two studies report the use of FDG-PET in PNSs with and without known antibodies. Rees et al. [66] found only 46% of patients to have anti-Hu or anti-Yo antibodies. As most patients presented with non-classic PNSs or syndromes related to other antibodies (e.g. brain-stem encephalitis and LEMS), this percentage is not useful for routine clinical practice. Hadjivassiliou et al. [65] described FDG-PET in 80 patients with a negative whole-body CT scan. They found four patients with a classic PNS, no antibodies and a pathologically proven tumour. One patient had clinical LEMS, in which a screening is warranted. In three other patients, it is not clear if all relevant antibodies had been tested. As whole-body CT was negative, it was a highly selected group and percentages of antibody negativity cannot be extrapolated to clinical practice.

Recommendation

If no antibodies are found, the patient has a classic PNS and the neurological condition is deteriorating, screening according to the most likely site, guided by the type of PNS with conventional methods, and if negative by total-body FDG-PET, is recommended (good practice point).

Dermatomyositis

The reported frequency of malignancy in dermatomyositis varies from 6% to 60%, but large population-based cohort studies report a frequency of 20–25% [90]. No particular paraneoplastic antibodies have been described for dermatomyositis. Several cancer types show this association. The most common are ovarian, lung, pancreatic, stomach and colorectal cancers and lymphomas [91]. The risk for lymphoma was raised only the first year after diagnosis of dermatomyositis. For the other tumours, the risk is the highest within the first year of follow-up dropping substantially thereafter. The risk for ovarian, pancreatic and lung cancer remains above average even after 5 years [91]. At diagnosis, thorough examination is requested. In children, specific attention should be paid to splenomegaly or lymphadenopathy [92]. In adults, abnormalities should guide screening tactics, but lack of abnormalities does not imply that no screening is needed. Although the risk rises with age, all adult patients should be screened. Women should be screened by ultrasonography of the pelvic region and mammography and by CT of the thorax/abdomen. Men should be tested by CT of the thorax/abdomen. Men under the age of 50 years should have an ultrasound of the testes. All patients aged >50 years (men and women) should have a colonoscopy. Screening is to be repeated annually for 3 years. Afterwards, screening is performed only if new symptoms or findings give the alert [90, 93]. Evidence about any additional value of FDG-PET is lacking.

Recommendation

Screen all adult patients with dermatomyositis by CT of the thorax/abdomen. Women are tested also by ultrasonography of the pelvic region and mammography. Male patients aged <50 years should have ultrasonography of the testes. Patients aged >50 years should have a colonoscopy (good practice point).

Use of clinical information and laboratory investigations in screening

The combination of a clinical syndrome and an associated antibody is the most powerful predictor for an underlying tumour and its possible location. As most syndromes and tumours are related to more than one antibody, screening for a panel of antibodies is more fruitful than focusing on one specific target [94]. Within the clinical syndromes, no specific predicting factor can be assigned to discriminate between tumour and non-

tumour forms. A more severe clinical picture has been described in patients with SCLC and LEMS [95, 96], but the specificity is not high enough to be helpful in individual patients.

Recommendation

As most clinical PNS are not specifically related to one antibody, testing for several paraneoplastic antibodies simultaneously will improve the yield, avoiding loss of time before a malignancy is detected (good practice point).

Biomarkers

Paraneoplastic antibodies are related to different PNSs (see Table 21.2). The individual antibodies are referred to in the table, but are not described in detail in the chapter. Other antibodies are not related clinically to specific PNSs, but have been described as specific biomarkers, such as SOX1 antibodies for SCLC. SOX1 antibodies were present in 22–32% of SCLC patients without PNSs [97–99]. In patients with SCLC of LEMS and SCLC of PCD (with VGCC antibodies), SOX1 antibodies were present in 65% and 67%, respectively. In patients with SCLC and anti-Hu syndrome, antibodies were present in 32–40% of sera [97, 98]. Only two patients with LEMS without SCLC were positive, whereas none of 80 controls was.

Although sensitivity is low to moderate, specificity is high and seropositivity indicates a very high suspicion of an underlying tumour. Case series described two patients with PLE, SCLC and VGKC antibodies positive for SOX1, whereas seven patients with SCLC and PLE without VGKC antibodies and seven with a non-tumour PLE with VGKC antibodies were SOX1 negative [100]. One patient with PLE, SCLC and antibodies for receptor B for γ-aminobutyric acid (GABABR) had SOX1 antibodies, whereas six other patients with GABABR antibodies, PLE and a tumour and eight patients without tumour were SOX1 negative [17]. No data are available for other syndromes or other tumours related to PNSs.

Anti-titin antibodies are a sensitive marker for thymoma (69–95%) [101–103], but not specific. Although only 8–10% of early onset MG patients are positive for anti-titin antibodies, 58–78% of late-onset MG patients are positive [101, 102]. RyR antibodies are more specific (95%), but a less sensitive marker (70%), in direct comparison to anti-titin antibodies [102].

Neuron specific enolase (NSE) has been the tumour marker of choice in SCLC. Sensitivity was 65% in a cohort of 175 SCLC patients (without PNSs), but depended on tumour stage [104]. Sensitivity was only 54% in limited disease SCLC patients (versus 74% in patients with extended disease). Awareness of a tumour is better in patients with PNSs, which are found to have more limited disease [7], limiting the value of NSE.

Progastrin-releasing peptide (ProGRP) is another, relatively new, marker for SCLC. Sensitivity is better than for NSE (77%) and does not differ between patients with limited or extended disease (74% versus 78%) [104]. Unfortunately, ProGRP is not yet routinely available. Both markers have not been investigated in PNSs. CA-125 is a marker for ovarian cancer. Although serial serum values detect up to 86% of ovarian carcinomas in postmenopausal women [105], a single CA-125 value has a sensitivity of only 62% [105]. In mature cystic teratomas, CA-125, cancer antigen 19-9 (CA19-9), α-fetoprotein (AFP) and carcinoembryonic antigen (CEA) were elevated in 23%, 39%, 0.6% and 16% of cases, respectively [106]. In immature teratomas, AFP is raised in up to 50% of cases [82]. The β subunit of the human chorionic gonadotrophin (βhCG) and AFP are elevated in about 80% of non-seminomatous testicular cancers [107]. It is recommended to determine βhCG and AFP in patients with suspected testicular tumours [108]. In the limited number of paraneoplastic cases in which ultrasonography was unreliable, βhCG and AFP were also negative [16].

> ### Recommendation
> Positive tumour markers raise suspicion of a tumour, but normal values do not exclude malignancy as sensitivity is low to moderate (good practice point).

Repetition of screening if initial screening is negative

The current recommendation is to repeat screening regularly every 6 months up to 4 years in patients with PNSs and paraneoplastic antibodies [11]. The first repetition of screening should be done after 3 or 4 months if suspicion of a malignancy remains high. In patients with LEMS, a large cohort study shows that 2 years of screen-

ing is sufficient [7]. Screening by thoracic radiograph or tumour markers is not reliable.

> ### Recommendation
> If initial screening is negative in a patient with a PNS and paraneoplastic antibodies, a second screening should be repeated after 3–6 months, followed by regular screening every 6 months for 4 years. In LEMS patients 2 years is sufficient. Radiograph or blood sampling is not reliable (good practice point).

Recommendations/Good practice points

• Nature of antibody, and to a lesser extent the clinical syndrome, determines the risk and type of underlying malignancy.

• As most PNSs are not specifically related to one antibody, testing for several paraneoplastic antibodies simultaneously will improve the yield, avoiding loss of time before a malignancy is detected.

• Screen for SCLC by CT of the thorax, followed by FDG-PET or integrated FDG-PET/CT.

• Screen for thymoma by CT of the thorax (followed by FDG-PET) or integrated FDG-PET/CT.

• Screen for breast cancer by mammography, followed by MRI of the breast. If negative follow by FDG-PET/CT.

• Screen for ovarian teratoma by TVUS, followed by CT/MRI of the pelvis/abdomen. If negative, follow by CT of the thorax.

• Screen for ovarian carcinoma by TVUS and CA-125, followed by CT of the pelvis/abdomen or integrated FDG-PET/CT.

• Screen for testicular tumour by ultrasonography, βhCG and AFP, followed by CT of the pelvic region. Biopsy is recommended in males under the age of 50 with classic PNSs and microcalcifications on ultrasonography.

• If tumour screening is negative and the neurological condition is worsening, exploratory surgery and eventually preventive removal of the ovaries is warranted in postmenopausal women with an anti-Yo-associated PNSs.

• Additional laboratory investigations have extra value if the antibody and the associated PNS are related to both a paraneoplastic and a non-paraneoplastic subtype (such as LEMS and myasthenia gravis). Positive markers raise suspicion of a tumour, but normal values do not exclude malignancy because sensitivity is low to moderate.

• If no paraneoplastic antibodies are found, the patient has a classic PNS and the neurological condition is deteriorating, screening according to the most likely site, guided by the type of PNS with conventional methods, and if negative by total-body FDG-PET, is recommended.

• Screen all adult patients with dermatomyositis by CT of the thorax/abdomen. Women should also be tested by ultrasonography of the pelvic region and mammography. Male patients aged <50 years should have ultrasonography of the testes. Patients aged >50 years should have a colonoscopy.

• If initial screening is negative in a patient with a PNS and paraneoplastic antibodies, screening should be repeated after 3–6 months, followed by regular screening every 6 months for 4 years. In LEMS patients 2 years is sufficient. Radiograph and tumour markers are not reliable.

References

1. Darnell, RB, Posner, JB Paraneoplastic syndromes affecting the nervous system. *Semin Oncol* 2006; **33**:270–98.

2. Maddison, P, Lang, B Paraneoplastic neurological autoimmunity and survival in small cell lung cancer. *J Neuroimmunol* 2008; **201–202**:159–62.

3. Wirtz, PW, Lang, B, Graus, F, et al. P/Q-type calcium channel antibodies, Lambert-Eaton myasthenic syndrome and survival in small cell lung cancer. *J Neuroimmunol* 2005; **164**:161–5.

4. DeAngelis, LM, Posner, JB *Neurologic Complications of Cancer*, 2nd edn, New York: Oxford University Press, 2008.

5. Dalmau, J, Gleichman, AJ, Hughes, EG, et al. Anti-NMDA-receptor encephalitis: case series and analysis of the effects of antibodies. *Lancet Neurol* 2008; **7**:1091–8.

6. Graus, F, Keime-Guibert, F, Rene, R, et al. Anti-Hu-associated paraneoplastic encephalomyelitis: analysis of 200 patients. *Brain* 2001; **124**:1138–48.

7. Titulaer, MJ, Wirtz, PW, Willems, LN, et al. Screening for small-cell lung cancer: a follow-up study of patients with Lambert–Eaton myasthenic syndrome. *J Clin Oncol* 2008; **26**:4276–81.

8. Rojas, I, Graus, F, Keime-Guibert, F, et al. Long-term clinical outcome of paraneoplastic cerebellar degeneration and anti-Yo antibodies. *Neurology* 2000; **55**:713–15.

9. Graus, F, Delattre, JY, Antoine, JC, et al. Recommended diagnostic criteria for paraneoplastic neurological syndromes. *J Neurol Neurosurg Psychiatry* 2004; **75**: 1135–40.

10. Dalmau, J, Rosenfeld, MR Paraneoplastic syndromes of the CNS. *Lancet Neurol* 2008; **7**:327–40.

11. Vedeler, CA, Antoine, JC, Giometto, B, et al. Management of paraneoplastic neurological syndromes: report of an EFNS Task Force. *Eur J Neurol* 2006; **13**:682–90.

12. Brainin, M, Barnes, M, Baron, JC, et al. Guidance for the preparation of neurological management guidelines by EFNS scientific task forces – revised recommendations 2004. *Eur J Neurol* 2004; **11**:577–81.

13. Darnell, RB, Posner, JB Paraneoplastic syndromes involving the nervous system. *N Engl J Med* 2003; **349**: 1543–54.

14. Antoine, JC, Camdessanche, JP Peripheral nervous system involvement in patients with cancer. *Lancet Neurol* 2007; **6**:75–86.

15. Didelot, A, Honnorat, J Update on paraneoplastic neurological syndromes. *Curr Opin Oncol* 2009; **21**:566–72.

16. Mathew, RM, Vandenberghe, R, Garcia-Merino, A, et al. Orchiectomy for suspected microscopic tumor in patients with anti-Ma2-associated encephalitis. *Neurology* 2007; **68**:900–5.

17. Lancaster, E, Lai, M, Peng, X, et al. Antibodies to the GABA(B) receptor in limbic encephalitis with seizures: case series and characterisation of the antigen. *Lancet Neurol* 2010; **9**:67–76.

18. Dalmau, J, Graus, F, Villarejo, A, et al. Clinical analysis of anti-Ma2-associated encephalitis. *Brain* 2004; **127**: 1831–44.

19. Gultekin, SH, Rosenfeld, MR, Voltz, R, et al. Paraneoplastic limbic encephalitis: neurological symptoms, immunological findings and tumour association in 50 patients. *Brain* 2000; **123**(Pt 7):1481–94.

20. Lai, M, Hughes, EG, Peng, X, et al. AMPA receptor antibodies in limbic encephalitis alter synaptic receptor location. *Ann Neurol* 2009; **65**:424–34.

21. Saiz, A, Blanco, Y, Sabater, L, et al. Spectrum of neurological syndromes associated with glutamic acid decarboxylase antibodies: diagnostic clues for this association. *Brain* 2008; **131**:2553–63.

22. Peterson, K, Rosenblum, MK, Kotanides, H, Posner, JB Paraneoplastic cerebellar degeneration. I. A clinical analysis of 55 anti-Yo antibody-positive patients. *Neurology* 1992; **42**:1931–7.

23. Mason, WP, Graus, F, Lang, B, et al. Small-cell lung cancer, paraneoplastic cerebellar degeneration and the Lambert-Eaton myasthenic syndrome. *Brain* 1997; **120**(Pt 8): 1279–300.

24. Bernal, F, Shams'ili, S, Rojas, I, et al. Anti-Tr antibodies as markers of paraneoplastic cerebellar degeneration and Hodgkin's disease. *Neurology* 2003; **60**:230–4.

25. Shams'ili, S, Grefkens, J, de Leeuw, B, et al. Paraneoplastic cerebellar degeneration associated with antineuronal antibodies: analysis of 50 patients. *Brain* 2003; **126**:1409–18.

26. Bataller, L, Graus, F, Saiz, A, Vilchez, JJ Clinical outcome in adult onset idiopathic or paraneoplastic opsoclonus-myoclonus. *Brain* 2001; **124**:437–43.

27. Dalmau, J, Tuzun, E, Wu, HY, et al. Paraneoplastic anti-*N*-methyl-D-aspartate receptor encephalitis associated with ovarian teratoma. *Ann Neurol* 2007; **61**:25–36.

28. Hart, IK, Maddison, P, Newsom-Davis, J, Vincent, A, Mills, KR Phenotypic variants of autoimmune peripheral nerve hyperexcitability. *Brain* 2002; **125**:1887–95.

29. Titulaer, MJ, Verschuuren, JJ Lambert-Eaton myasthenic syndrome: tumor versus nontumor forms. *Ann N Y Acad Sci* 2008; **1132**:129–34.

30. Oosterhuis, HJ The natural course of myasthenia gravis: a long term follow up study. *J Neurol Neurosurg Psychiatry* 1989; **52**:1121–7.

31. Sillevis, SP, Grefkens, J, de Leeuw, B, et al. Survival and outcome in 73 anti-Hu positive patients with paraneoplastic encephalomyelitis/sensory neuronopathy. *J Neurol* 2002; **249**:745–53.

32. Antoine, JC, Absi, L, Honnorat, J, et al. Antiamphiphysin antibodies are associated with various paraneoplastic neurological syndromes and tumors. *Arch Neurol* 1999; **56**: 172–7.

33. Murinson, BB, Guarnaccia, JB Stiff-person syndrome with amphiphysin antibodies: distinctive features of a rare disease. *Neurology* 2008; **71**:1955–8.

34. Nguyen-Huu, BK, Urban, PP, Schreckenberger, M, Dieterich, M, Werhahn, KJ Antiamphiphysin-positive stiff-person syndrome associated with small cell lung cancer. *Mov Disord* 2006; **21**:1285–7.

35. McHugh, JC, Murray, B, Renganathan, R, Connolly, S, Lynch, T GAD antibody positive paraneoplastic stiff person syndrome in a patient with renal cell carcinoma. *Mov Disord* 2007; **22**:1343–6.

36. Adamus, G, Ren, G, Weleber, RG Autoantibodies against retinal proteins in paraneoplastic and autoimmune retinopathy. *BMC Ophthalmol* 2004; **4**:5.

37. Keltner, JL, Thirkill, CE Cancer-associated retinopathy vs recoverin-associated retinopathy. *Am J Ophthalmol* 1998; **126**:296–302.

38. Ohguro, H, Yokoi, Y, Ohguro, I, et al. Clinical and immunologic aspects of cancer-associated retinopathy. *Am J Ophthalmol* 2004; **137**:1117–19.

39. Graus, F, Saiz, A, Dalmau, J Antibodies and neuronal autoimmune disorders of the CNS. *J Neurol* 2010; **257**: 509–17.

40. Younes-Mhenni, S, Janier, MF, Cinotti, L, et al. FDG-PET improves tumour detection in patients with paraneoplastic neurological syndromes. *Brain* 2004; **127**:2331–8.

41. Linke, R, Schroeder, M, Helmberger, T, Voltz, R Antibody-positive paraneoplastic neurologic syndromes – value of CT and PET for tumor diagnosis. *Neurology* 2004; **63**: 282–6.

42. Dalmau, J, Graus, F, Rosenblum, MK, Posner, JB Anti-Hu-associated paraneoplastic encephalomyelitis/sensory neuronopathy. A clinical study of 71 patients. *Medicine (Baltimore)* 1992; **71**:59–72.

43. Honnorat, J, Cartalat-Carel, S, Ricard, D, et al. Onco-neural antibodies and tumour type determine survival and neurological symptoms in paraneoplastic neurological syndromes with Hu or CV2/CRMP5 antibodies. *J Neurol Neurosurg Psychiatry* 2009; **80**:412–16.

44. Marchand, V, Graveleau, J, Lanctin-Garcia, C, et al. A rare gynecological case of paraneoplastic cerebellar degeneration discovered by FDG-PET. *Gynecol Oncol* 2007; **105**: 545–7.

45. Vernino, S, Tuite, P, Adler, CH, et al. Paraneoplastic chorea associated with CRMP-5 neuronal antibody and lung carcinoma. *Ann Neurol* 2002; **51**:625–30.

46. Yu, ZY, Kryzer, TJ, Griesmann, GE, et al. CRMP-5 neuronal autoantibody: marker of lung cancer and thymoma-related autoimmunity. *Ann Neurol* 2001; **49**:146–54.

47. Sahashi, K, Sakai, K, Mano, K, Hirose, G Anti-Ma2 antibody related paraneoplastic limbic/brain stem encephalitis associated with breast cancer expressing Ma1, Ma2, and Ma3 mRNAs. *J Neurol Neurosurg Psychiatry* 2003; **74**: 1332–5.

48. Luque, FA, Furneaux, HM, Ferziger, R, et al. Anti-Ri – an antibody associated with paraneoplastic opsoclonus and breast-cancer. *Ann Neurol* 1991; **29**:241–51.

49. Pittock, SJ, Lucchinetti, CF, Lennon, VA Anti-neuronal nuclear autoantibody type 2: paraneoplastic accompaniments. *Ann Neurol* 2003; **53**:580–7.

50. Graus, F, Dalmau, J, Valldeoriola, F, et al. Immunological characterization of a neuronal antibody (anti-Tr) associated with paraneoplastic cerebellar degeneration and Hodgkin's disease. *J Neuroimmunol* 1997; **74**:55–61.

51. Hammack, J, Kotanides, H, Rosenblum, MK, Posner, JB Paraneoplastic cerebellar degeneration. II. Clinical and immunologic findings in 21 patients with Hodgkin's disease. *Neurology* 1992; **42**:1938–43.

52. Graus, F, Lang, B, Pozo-Rosich, P, et al. P/Q type calcium-channel antibodies in paraneoplastic cerebellar degeneration with lung cancer. *Neurology* 2002; **59**:764–6.

53. Vernino, S, Adamski, J, Kryzer, TJ, Fealey, RD, Lennon, VA Neuronal nicotinic Ach receptor antibody in subacute autonomic neuropathy and cancer-related syndromes. *Neurology* 1998; **50**:1806–13.

54. Vernino, S Autoimmune and paraneoplastic channelopa- thies. *Neurotherapeutics* 2007; **4**:305–14.

55. Lai, M, Huijbers, MGM, Lancaster, E, et al. Investigation of LGI1 as the antigen in limbic encephalitis previously attributed to potassium channels: a case series. *Lancet Neurol* 2010; **9**:776–85.

56. Irani, SR, Alexander, S, Waters, P, et al. Antibodies to Kv1 potassium channel complex proteins leucine-rich, glioma inactivated 1 protein and contactin-associated prtoein-2 in limbic encephalitis, Morvan's syndrome and acquired neu- romyotonia. *Brain* 2010; **133**:2734–48.

57. Sillevis, SP, Kinoshita, A, de Leeuw, B, et al. Paraneoplastic cerebellar ataxia due to autoantibodies against a glutamate receptor. *N Engl J Med* 2000; **342**:21–7.

58. Chan, KH, Vernino, S, Lennon, VA ANNA-3 anti-neuronal nuclear antibody: marker of lung cancer-related autoim- munity. *Ann Neurol* 2001; **50**:301–11.

59. Vernino, S, Lennon, VA New Purkinje cell antibody (PCA- 2): marker of lung cancer-related neurological autoimmu- nity. *Ann Neurol* 2000; **47**:297–305.

60. Bataller, L, Wade, DF, Graus, F, et al. Antibodies to Zic4 in paraneoplastic neurologic disorders and small-cell lung cancer. *Neurology* 2004; **62**:778–82.

61. Dongradi, G, Poisson, M, Beuve-Mery, P, et al. [Association of a lung cancer and several paraneoplastic syndromes (Lambert-Eaton syndrome, polymyositis and Schwartz- Bartter syndrome)]. *Ann Med Interne (Paris)* 1971; **122**:959–64.

62. O'Neill, JH, Murray, NMF, Newsom-Davis, J The Lambert– Eaton myasthenic syndrome – a review of 50 cases. *Brain* 1988; **111**:577–96.

63. Ramos-Yeo, YL, Reyes, CV Myasthenic syndrome (Eaton– Lambert syndrome) associated with pulmonary adenocar- cinoma. *J Surg Oncol* 1987; **34**:239–42.

64. Antoine, JC, Cinotti, L, Tilikete, C, et al. [¹⁸F] Fluorodeoxyglucose positron emission tomography in the diagnosis of cancer in patients with paraneoplastic neuro- logical syndrome and anti-Hu antibodies. *Ann Neurol* 2000; **48**:105–8.

65. Hadjivassiliou, M, Alder, SJ, Van Beek, EJ, et al. PET scan in clinically suspected paraneoplastic neurological syn- dromes: a 6-year prospective study in a regional neuro- science unit. *Acta Neurol Scand* 2009; **119**:186–93.

66. Rees, JH, Hain, SF, Johnson, MR, et al. The role of [¹⁸F] fluoro-2-deoxyglucose-PET scanning in the diagnosis of paraneoplastic neurological disorders. *Brain* 2001; **124**: 2223–31.

67. Annema, JT, Versteegh, MI, Veselic, M, Voigt, P, Rabe, KF Endoscopic ultrasound-guided fine-needle aspira- tion in the diagnosis and staging of lung cancer and its impact on surgical staging. *J Clin Oncol* 2005; **23**: 8357–61.

68. Tomaszek, S, Wigle, DA, Keshavjee, S, Fischer, S Thymomas: review of current clinical practice. *Ann Thorac Surg* 2009; **87**:1973–80.

69. Tomiyama, N, Honda, O, Tsubamoto, M, et al. Anterior mediastinal tumors: diagnostic accuracy of CT and MRI. *Eur J Radiol* 2009; **69**:280–8.

70. de Kraker, M, Kluin, J, Renken, N, Maat, AP, Bogers, AJ CT and myasthenia gravis: correlation between mediastinal imaging and histopathological findings. *Interact Cardiovasc Thorac Surg* 2005; **4**:267–71.

71. Nicolaou, S., Dubec, JJ, Munk, PL, Oger JJ. Thymus in myasthenia gravis: comparison of CT and pathologic find- ings and clinical outcome after thymectomy. *Radiology* 1996; **201**:471–4.

72. El-Bawab, H, Al-Sugair, AA, Rafay, M, et al. Role of flourine-18 fluorodeoxyglucose positron emission tomog- raphy in thymic pathology. *Eur J Cardiothorac Surg* 2007; **31**:731–6.

73. Liu, RS, Yeh, SH, Huang, MH, et al. Use of fluorine-18 fluorodeoxyglucose positron emission tomography in the detection of thymoma: a preliminary report. *Eur J Nucl Med* 1995; **22**:1402–7.

74. Kumar, A, Regmi, SK, Dutta, R, et al. Characterization of thymic masses using (18)FFDG PET-CT. *Ann Nucl Med* 2009; **23**:569–77.

75. Frings, M, Antoch, G, Knorn, P, et al. Strategies in detection of the primary tumour in anti-Yo associated paraneoplas- tic cerebellar degeneration. *J Neurol* 2005; **252**:197–201.

76. Mathew, RM, Cohen, AB, Galetta, SL, Alavi, A, Dalmau, J Paraneoplastic cerebellar degeneration: Yo-expressing tumor revealed after a 5-year follow-up with FDG-PET. *J Neurol Sci* 2006; **250**:153–5.

77. Brieva-Ruiz, L, Diaz-Hurtado, M, Matias-Guiu, X, et al. Anti-Ri-associated paraneoplastic cerebellar degeneration and breast cancer: an autopsy case study. *Clin Neurol Neurosurg* 2008; **110**:1044–6.

78. Kriege, M, Brekelmans, CT, Boetes, C, et al. Efficacy of MRI and mammography for breast-cancer screening in women with a familial or genetic predisposition. *N Engl J Med* 2004; **351**:427–37.

79. Weinstein, SP, Localio, AR, Conant, EF, et al. Multimodality screening of high-risk women: a prospective cohort study. *J Clin Oncol* 2009; **27**:6124–8.

80. Saslow, D, Boetes, C, Burke, W, et al. American Cancer Society guidelines for breast screening with MRI as an adjunct to mammography. *CA Cancer J Clin* 2007; **57**:75–89.

81. Daly, MB, Axilbund, JE, Buys, S, et al. Genetic/familial high-risk assessment: breast and ovarian. *J Natl Compr Canc Netw* 2010; **8**:562–94.

82. Saba, L, Guerriero, S, Sulcis, R, et al. Mature and immature ovarian teratomas: CT, US and MR imaging characteristics. *Eur J Radiol* 2009; **72**:454–63.

83. Guerriero, S, Mallarini, G, Ajossa, S, et al. Transvaginal ultrasound and computed tomography combined with clinical parameters and CA-125 determinations in the differential diagnosis of persistent ovarian cysts in premenopausal women. *Ultrasound Obstet Gynecol* 1997; **9**:339–43.

84. Buy, JN, Ghossain, MA, Moss, AA, et al. Cystic teratoma of the ovary: CT detection. *Radiology* 1989; **171**:697–701.

85. Yamashita, Y, Hatanaka, Y, Torashima, M, et al. Mature cystic teratomas of the ovary without fat in the cystic cavity: MR features in 12 cases. *AJR Am J Roentgenol* 1994; **163**:613–16.

86. Clarke-Pearson, DL Clinical practice. Screening for ovarian cancer. *N Engl J Med* 2009; **361**:170–7.

87. van Nagell, JRJ, Depriest, PD, Ueland, FR, et al. Ovarian cancer screening with annual transvaginal sonography: findings of 25,000 women screened. *Cancer* 2007; **109**:1887–96.

88. Liu, J, Xu, Y, Wang, J Ultrasonography, computed tomography and magnetic resonance imaging for diagnosis of ovarian carcinoma. *Eur J Radiol* 2007; **62**:328–34.

89. Keime-Guibert, F, Graus, F, Fleury, A, et al. Treatment of paraneoplastic neurological syndromes with antineuronal antibodies (anti-Hu, anti-Yo) with a combination of immunoglobulins, cyclophosphamide, and methylprednisolone. *J Neurol Neurosurg Psychiatry* 2000; **68**:479–82.

90. Callen, JP, Wortmann, RL Dermatomyositis. *Clin Dermatol* 2006; **24**:363–73.

91. Callen, JP Relation between dermatomyositis and polymyositis and cancer. *Lancet* 2001; **357**:85–6.

92. Morris, P, Dare, J Juvenile dermatomyositis as a paraneoplastic phenomenon: an update. *J Pediatr Hematol Oncol* 2010; **32**:189–91.

93. Callen, JP When and how should the patient with dermatomyositis or amyopathic dermatomyositis be assessed for possible cancer? *Arch Dermatol* 2002; **138**:969–71.

94. Monstad, SE, Knudsen, A, Salvesen, HB, Aarseth, JH, Vedeler, CA Onconeural antibodies in sera from patients with various types of tumours. *Cancer Immunol Immunother* 2009; **58**:1795–800.

95. Wirtz, PW, Wintzen, AR, Verschuuren, JJ Lambert–Eaton myasthenic syndrome has a more progressive course in patients with lung cancer. *Muscle Nerve* 2005; **32**:226–9.

96. Titulaer, MJ, Wirtz, PW, Kuks, JB, et al. The Lambert–Eaton myasthenic syndrome 1988–2008: a clinical picture in 97 patients. *J Neuroimmunol* 2008; **201–202**:153–8.

97. Sabater, L, Titulaer, M, Saiz, A, et al. SOX1 antibodies are markers of paraneoplastic Lambert-Eaton myasthenic syndrome. *Neurology* 2008; **70**:924–8.

98. Titulaer, MJ, Klooster, R, Potman, M, et al. SOX antibodies in small-cell lung cancer and Lambert-Eaton myasthenic syndrome: frequency and relation with survival. *J Clin Oncol* 2009; **27**:4260–7.

99. Vural, B, Chen, LC, Saip, P, et al. Frequency of SOX group B (SOX1, 2, 3) and ZIC2 antibodies in Turkish patients with small cell lung carcinoma and their correlation with clinical parameters. *Cancer* 2005; **103**:2575–83.

100. Zuliani, L, Saiz, A, Tavolato, B, et al. Paraneoplastic limbic encephalitis associated with potassium channel antibodies: value of anti-glial nuclear antibodies in identifying the tumour. *J Neurol Neurosurg Psychiatry* 2007; **78**:204–5.

101. Buckley, C, Newsom-Davis, J, Willcox, N, Vincent, A Do titin and cytokine antibodies in MG patients predict thymoma or thymoma recurrence? *Neurology* 2001; **57**:1579–82.

102. Romi, F, Skeie, GO, Aarli, JA, Gilhus, NE Muscle autoantibodies in subgroups of myasthenia gravis patients. *J Neurol* 2000; **247**:369–75.

103. Voltz, RD, Albrich, WC, Nagele, A, et al. Paraneoplastic myasthenia gravis: detection of anti-MGT30 (titin) antibodies predicts thymic epithelial tumor. *Neurology* 1997; **49**:1454–7.

104. Molina, R, Auge, JM, Bosch, X, et al. Usefulness of serum tumor markers, including progastrin-releasing peptide, in patients with lung cancer: correlation with histology. *Tumour Biol* 2009; **30**:121–9.

105. Skates, SJ, Menon, U, Macdonald, N, et al. Calculation of the risk of ovarian cancer from serial CA-125 values for preclinical detection in postmenopausal women. *J Clin Oncol* 2003; **21**:206S–10S.

106. Emin, U, Tayfun, G, Cantekin, I, et al. Tumor markers in mature cystic teratomas of the ovary. *Arch Gynecol Obstet* 2009; **279**:145–7.

107. Fizazi, K, Culine, S, Kramar, A, et al. Early predicted time to normalization of tumor markers predicts outcome in poor-prognosis nonseminomatous germ cell tumors. *J Clin Oncol* 2004; **22**:3868–76.

108. Motzer, RJ, Agarwal, N, Beard, C, et al. NCCN clinical practice guidelines in oncology: kidney cancer. *J Natl Compr Canc Netw* 2009; **7**:618–30.

CHAPTER 22

Treatment of miscellaneous idiopathic headache disorders[*]

S. Evers,[1][†] P. Goadsby,[2] R. Jensen,[3] A. May,[4] J. Pascual[5] and G. Sixt[6]

[1]University of Münster, Münster, Germany; [2]University of California, San Francisco CA, USA and UCL, Institute of Neurology, Queen Square, London, UK; [3]Glostrup Hospital, University of Copenhagen, Denmark; [4]University of Hamburg, Hamburg, Germany; [5]University Hospital 'Central de Asturias', Oviedo, Spain; [6]Regional Hospital, Bolzano, Italy

Objectives

These guidelines aim to make recommendations for the treatment of headache disorders classified as the so-called group 4 headaches in the second edition of the *International Classification of Headache Disorders* (ICHD-II) [1]. Due to the assumed low prevalence and poor awareness of these headache disorders, placebo-controlled double-blind trials are almost completely missing. Therefore, these guidelines are based largely on publications with a low level of evidence and on expert consensus. A brief clinical description of the headache disorders is included. The definitions follow the diagnostic criteria of the ICHD-II.

Background

The ICHD-II allocated a group of headache disorders considered relatively rare idiopathic entities as group 4. These conditions seemed to stand apart from the more common primary headache disorders: migraine, tension-type headache and the trigeminal autonomic

cephalalgias. The group was thus heterogeneous and may be underdiagnosed. In the first edition of the IHS classification, facial pain syndromes with specific triggers were also classified in this group [2]. In the present classification, only headache types with pain localized predominantly in the first trigeminal branch are listed [1].

The purpose of this chapter is to give drug and non-drug treatment recommendations for these headache disorders for both acute and prophylactic treatment. The recommendations are based on the scientific evidence from clinical trials and case reports, and on the expert consensus by the respective Task Force of the EFNS. The legal aspects of drug prescription and drug availability in the different European countries will not be considered. The definitions of the recommendation levels follow the EFNS criteria [3].

Search strategy

A literature search was performed using the reference databases MedLine, Science Citation Index and the Cochrane Library; the key words used were 'headache' together with the respective description of the eight different headache types (last search April 2010). All papers published in English, German or French were considered

---

[*] Group 4 of the IHS classification.
[†] Chair and corresponding author.

European Handbook of Neurological Management: Volume 2, Second Edition. Edited by Nils Erik Gilhus, Michael P. Barnes, Michael Brainin.

when they described a controlled trial or a case report or series on the treatment of one of these headache disorders. In addition, a review book [4] and the German treatment recommendations for these headache disorders [5] were considered.

Method for reaching consensus

The first draft of the manuscript was written by the chair of the Task Force. All other members of the Task Force read this draft and discussed changes by email. A second draft was then written by the chair, which was again discussed by email. All recommendations had to be agreed by all members of the Task Force. The background of the research strategy and of reaching consensus and the definitions of the recommendation levels used in this chapter have been described in the EFNS recommendations [3].

Common principles in diagnosis and therapy

The headache disorders in group 4 of the ICHD-II are classified nearly exclusively according to their clinical features as reported by the patient. The criteria are presented in Table 22.1. There are no apparative procedures proving

Table 22.1 Diagnostic criteria of the headache disorders of group 4 of the IHS classification.

4.1 Primary stabbing headache
   A. Head pain occurring as a single stab or a series of stabs and fulfilling criteria B–D
     1. Exclusively or predominantly felt in the distribution of the first division of the trigeminal nerve (orbit, temple and parietal area)
     2. Stabs last for up to a few seconds and recur with irregular frequency ranging from one to many per day
   B. No accompanying symptoms
   C. Not attributed to another disorder
4.2 Primary cough headache
   A. Headache fulfilling criteria B and C
   B. Sudden onset, lasting from one second to 30 minutes
   A. Brought on by and occurring only in association with coughing, straining and/or Valsalva manoeuvre
   C. Not attributed to another disorder
4.3 Primary exertional headache
   A. Pulsating headache fulfilling criteria B and C
   B. Lasting 5 minutes–48 hours
   C. Brought on by and occurring only during or after physical exertion
   D. Not attributed to another disorder
4.4 Primary headache associated with sexual activity
   4.4.1 Preorgasmic headache
     A. Dull ache in the head and neck associated with awareness of neck and/or jaw muscle contraction and meeting criterion B
     B. Occurs during sexual activity and increases with sexual excitement
     C. Not attributed to another disorder
   4.4.2 Orgasmic headache
     A. Sudden severe ('explosive') headache meeting criterion B
     B. Occurs at orgasm
     C. Not attributed to another disorder
4.5 Hypnic headache
   A. Dull headache fulfilling criteria B–D
   B. Develops only during sleep, and awakens patient
   C. At least two of the following characteristics:
     1. occurs >15 times per month
     2. lasts >15 minutes after waking
     3. first occurs after age of 50 years
   D. No autonomic symptoms and no more than one of nausea, photophobia or phonophobia
   E. Not attributed to another disorder

Table 22.1 continued

4.6 Primary thunderclap headache
  A. Severe head pain fulfilling criteria B and C
  B. Both of the following characteristics:
      1. sudden onset, reaching maximum intensity in <1 minute
      2. lasts 1 hour–10 days
  C. Does not recur regularly over subsequent weeks or months
  D. Not attributed to another disorder

4.7 Hemicrania continua
  A. Headache for >3 months fulfilling criteria B–D
  B. All of the following characteristics:
      1. unilateral pain without side-shift
      2. daily and continuous, without pain-free periods
      3. moderate intensity, but with exacerbations of severe pain
  C. At least one of the following autonomic features occurs during exacerbations and ipsilateral to the side of pain:
      1. conjunctival injection and/or lacrimation
      2. nasal congestion and/or rhinorrhoea
      3. ptosis and/or miosis
  D. Complete response to therapeutic doses of indomethacin
  E. Not attributed to another disorder

4.8 New daily-persistent headache
  A. Headache that, within 3 days of onset, fulfils criteria B–D
  B. Unremitting headache present daily for >3 months
  C. At least two of the following pain characteristics:
      1. bilateral location
      2. pressing/tightening (non-pulsating) quality
      3. mild or moderate intensity
      4. not aggravated by routine physical activity such as walking or climbing
  D. Both the following:
      1. no more than one of photophobia, phonophobia or mild nausea
      2. neither moderate or severe nausea nor vomiting
  E. Not attributed to another disorder

a diagnosis. Whether or not apparative procedures are necessary other than the patient's history and the neurological examination must be decided in each case. An obligatory indication for brain scanning by MRI and for other diagnostic investigations (e.g., lumbar puncture) is given if the clinical examination was abnormal and in the headache types 4.2 (primary cough headache), 4.4 (headache associated with sexual activity) and 4.5 (primary thunderclap headache).

Primary stabbing headache (IHS 4.1)

Clinical picture

The primary stabbing headache must be distinguished from the trigeminal autonomic headaches in group 3 of ICHD-II. In this entity, the patients experience paroxysmal, very short (often <1 second) pain attacks, which occur as single or repetitive pain stabs. They affect a circumscribed area of the head (maximum size about 20 mm). These areas can be found predominantly in the distribution of the first trigeminal branch (frontal, orbital, parietal, temporal). The character of the pain is stabbing and mild to moderate in intensity. The frequency is between once a year to more than 100 times a day. The attacks can occur in bouts or over several years. Patients with another idiopathic headache disorder such as migraine, cluster headache, tension-type and hemicrania continua headache are more liable to this headache type. The attacks can occur spontaneously or can be triggered (e.g., by ice and cold drinks). This headache disorder also includes the jabs-and-jolts syndrome (randomized, clearly located, stabbing head-ache), the icepick-like pain (induced by coldness) and the ophthalmodynia (lancinating pains lasting for seconds in the inner angle of the eye). An important clinical point is that there are no cranial autonomic symptoms, such as are seen in trigeminal autonomic headaches, associated with the stabs of pain. The patho-physiology is unknown.

Epidemiology

The headache is often diagnosed in patients with pre-existing migraine, tension-type headache or cluster head-ache. The prevalence in these patients has been reported to be between 2% and 35% [6, 7, 8]. It can occur in children, but is less often recorded in this age group [9]. When it is seen in children it can be very disabling for of weeks to months. Women are more affected than men with a ratio of 1.5:1 [7] to 6:1 [10]. All ages can be affected, however the incidence is positively correlated with age [10].

Treatment

Normally, this headache type does not require treatment. In patients with high attack frequency and severe inten-sity of pain and with impairment of their quality of life, treatment with indomethacin is recommended. This leads to a sufficient attack reduction in more than 65% of all patients [10–13]. Indomethacin should be given in a dose of 25–50 mg b.i.d., and gastric-protecting agents may be required (e.g., antacid drugs, H_2-antagonists or proton pump inhibitors). There are reports that nifed-ipine 90 mg [14], melatonin 3–12 mg [15], gabapentin 800 mg [16], or etoricoxib 60 mg [17] may be efficacious if indomethacin does not work or is not tolerated. However, this has still to be confirmed.

Primary cough headache (IHS 4.2)

Clinical picture

Primary cough headache starts suddenly and lasts between 1 second and 30 minutes. It is exclusively trig-gered by coughing, pressing or other types of Valsalva manoeuvre. In 11– > 50% of the cases, the headache trig-gered by coughing is a symptomatic headache [18–21]. The most frequent cause of a symptomatic cough head-ache is an Arnold-Chiari malformation type I. Other symptomatic types can be caused by mass lesions in the posterior intracranial fossa, craniocervical anomalies such as basilary impression or platybasia, non-ruptured cerebral aneurysms and by pathologies in the carotid or vertebrobasilary arteries [22, 23].

The aetiology of the primary cough headache is unclear. Coughing induces an increase of the intrathoracic/intra-abdominal pressure and subsequently an increase of the central venous pressure and thus also an increase of intracranial pressure. A link between cough headache and an increase of intracranial pressure seems plausible [24, 25]. In one study, patients with primary cough head-ache had an increased volume of cerebrospinal fluid (CSF) [26]. This lead to an increased pressure gradient directly after coughing (the CSF pressure in the basal cisterns was higher for a short time than the lumbar CSF pressure), and this lead to a compression of the dura mater. This mechanism would also explain the efficacy of indomethacin, which induces a reduction of CSF pres-sure [27], the efficacy of acetazolamide, which decreases the production of CSF [28] and the efficacy of a lumbar puncture, although it is complex to explain the continu-ing improvement of patients after a single lumbar punc-ture [24, 29]. An inherited crowdedness of the posterior intracranial fossa in a patient with primary cough head-ache but without Arnold-Chiari malformation has also been reported [30]. Finally, spontaneous or orthostatic low cerebrospinal fluid pressure syndrome can mimic primary cough headache [31, 32].

Epidemiology

The prevalence of primary cough headache has been reported to be 1% for 25–64 years [6] or 1.2% of all patients referred to a headache clinic [18, 19]. The mean age at onset is between 55 and 65 years. Men seem to be affected 3–5 times more often than women. More than half (57%) of all patients with cough headache have a symptomatic type with an earlier age at onset (39 ± 14 years). The course of this headache disorder often shows spontaneous remission. In most of the patients the pain persists between 2 months and 2 years, however patients with a disease duration of 12 years and more have been described [29].

Treatment

Since most of the attacks are of short duration, there is normally no need for acute treatment. If possible, the cough headache should be prevented by effective treatment of disorders of the upper airway and pulmonary system in order to avoid coughing.

In the case of frequent cough headache attacks, prophylactic medication is possible. In a small, double-blind, placebo-controlled crossover study with indomethacin in a dose of 50 mg t.i.d., the efficacy of this drug in primary cough headache was shown [33]. This has been confirmed in open studies [19, 24, 30, 34] with a response rate of 73% in primary and 38% in symptomatic cough headache [19]. The daily effective dose ranged from 25 mg to 200 mg (mean 78 mg). The duration of drug treatment was between 6 months and 4 years. In some patients, agents to protect the stomach are required (e.g., antacid drugs, H_2-antagonists or proton pump inhibitors).

An alternative to indomethacin is the carboanhydrase inhibitor acetazolamide. In an open study ($n = 5$) this drug was effective in primary cough headache [26]. The patients received acetazolamide for at least 4 weeks, starting with 125 mg t.i.d. and in a mean continuing dose of 625 mg (maximum dose 2,000 mg). Two of these patients were completely headache-free, two had only headache after strong coughing and one showed no effect. Further, there are two case reports on patients who responded to a treatment with methysergide (2 mg per day) [35, 36], and a small case-series on the efficacy of topiramate 50–75 mg [37].

Finally, there are case reports that patients with primary or symptomatic cough headache responded to a lumbar puncture (removal of about 40 ml CSF) [29]. Of 14 patients, six were completely pain-free after lumbar puncture. The other eight patients were treated with indomethacin, which led to no further headache in six [24]. Other case reports suggested the efficacy of naproxen 550 mg, ergonovin, 1 mg dihydroergotamine i.v. and phenelzine [24, 38, 39]. Propranolol has been reported to be without efficacy [36].

Primary exertional headache (IHS 4.3)

Clinical picture
This headache is triggered by different types of physical exertion. Typical situations are sports such as weightlifting, swimming and running [40, 41, 42]. The character

of this headache is pulsating and the duration can be between 5 minutes and 48 hours, however the headache does not fulfil the criteria of migraine [43]. The headache is exclusively induced by physical activity and occurs during or after this activity. There are secondary types of exertional headache which are responsible for about 22–43% of all cases and require adequate diagnostic work-up, in particular after the first occurrence of exertional headache [20, 44]. Important differential diagnoses are subarachnoid haemorrhage, cervical artery dissection, Arnold-Chiari malformation, cranio-cervical anomalies, mass lesions in the posterior intracranial fossa and sinusitis [18, 20, 44, 45]. In particular, intracranial venous anomalies or stenoses have been assumed to be a cause of symptomatic exertional headache [46, 47]. In those cases with older age at first occurrence and with vascular risk factors, coronary heart disease has to be excluded as a cause of a symptomatic exertional headache – so-called cardiac cephalgia [48, 49, 50, 51, 52]. The exact mechanisms of this primary headache type are unknown. An intermittent increase of intracranial pressure by the Valsalva manoeuvre has been postulated, however there are patients who have exertional headache but no cough headache or headache associated with sexual activity [36].

Epidemiology
The lifetime prevalence has been estimated to be between 1% and 35% [6, 53, 54]. The sex ratio is unknown and has been estimated between a male preponderance (4–7 times higher) [20, 55] and a female preponderance (2 times higher) [53, 54]. The age at onset is mostly in early adulthood [20] but can also occur during adolescence [54]. There is a reported comorbidity with primary headache associated with sexual activity in about 40%. About 46% of the sufferers have comorbidity with migraine [43, 54]. Spontaneous remissions are normal, symptomatic episodes can last some days up to several years [20, 56].

Treatment
As non-pharmacological treatment, the avoidance or a slow increase of physical activity, in particular during heat or at high altitude, is recommended [57]. Regular physical activity and normal body mass index are also assumed to be helpful. Drugs of first choice are indomethacin, which has shown efficacy in some case reports [20, 58, 59, 60], and propranolol. If a patient is doing sports

or other physical activity rarely, a short-term prophylaxis with 25–50 mg indomethacin about 1 hour before the activity can be sufficient. In the case of regular physical activity and regular exertional headache, a prophylactic intake of 25–50 mg t.i.d. of indomethacin is recommended. In some cases, medication to protect the stomach (e.g., antacid drugs, H_2-antagonists or a proton pump inhibitor) may be required.

Small case-series suggest the efficacy of beta-blockers, flunarizine and ergotamine in some patients [18, 20, 56, 61], most often propranolol in a dose of 20–80 mg t.i.d. is recommended. Flunarizine in a dose of 5–10 mg per day can be used as a prophylactic agent, whereas ergotamine in a dose of 2 mg is recommended as short-term prophylaxis directly before physical activity. Since spontaneous remissions of exertional headache regularly occur, a trial of stopping the medication should be commenced after about 6–8 weeks.

Primary headache associated with sexual activity (4.4)

Clinical picture

This headache exclusively occurs during sexual activity and so is also called sexual or sex headache. It is not associated with other types of physical activity *per se*, but patients may have exertional or cough headache too. According to ICHD-II, an orgasmic and preorgasmic subtype are differentiated. The preorgasmic headache is a dull pain in the neck and head slowly increasing during sexual activity, with sufferers experiencing contractions of the neck and the masticatory muscles. The orgasmic headache occurs suddenly with or just before the orgasm as an abrupt pain like an explosion. The pain is mostly bilateral and diffuse or occipital. The median duration is about 30 minutes and the maximal duration is 24 h. Sometimes, a milder pain can remain for up to 72 h [62]. The headache occurs independently of the kind of sexual practice [62]. For the appropriate first diagnosis, the exclusion of a secondary headache is obligatory. For instance, subarachnoid haemorrhages occur in up to 11% during sexual activity and have to be ruled out by additional procedures such as CT scan, lumbar puncture or angiography [63]. Also, arterial dissection can mimic primary orgasmic headache [64].

The exact mechanisms of this headache disorder are unknown. Early studies postulated a link between preorgasmic headache and tension-type headache and between orgasmic headache and migraine [65]. Recent studies may demonstrate a dysfunction of the cerebrovascular autoregulation in patients suffering from orgasmic headache [66]. Cognitive dishabituation as measured by evoked potentials has been shown for the orgasmic headache. This phenomenon is very similar to that observed in migraine patients and supports a pathophysiological link between these two headache types [67]. Recently, reversible vasospam of intracranial arteries have been observed in this headache type [68, 69].

Epidemiology

The lifetime prevalence has been estimated to be ~1% [6, 70]. Men are 3–4 times more frequently affected than women [20, 56, 62, 65]. The age at onset has two peaks, with a maximum between 20 and 24 and 35 and 44 years [62]; the youngest patient reported to date was 12 years old [71]. The orgasmic headache subtype is 3–4 times more frequent than the preorgasmic subtype [62, 72]. In 19–47% of sufferers there is comorbidity with migraine, in 29–40% comorbidity with primary exertional headache, and in 45% comorbidity with tension-type headache [20, 56, 62, 65, 70]. Spontaneous remissions are the rule, though symptomatic episodes can last for a few days to several years and can also be relapsing [56, 73].

Treatment

As non-drug treatment, a more passive role during sexual activity is recommended [62]. Stopping sexual activity after onset of the first symptoms may prevent a further increase of headache in about 40% and is particularly successful in the preorgasmic subtype [62]. As long as a mild headache continues, the risk of a new attack of sexual headache is particularly high; therefore, patients should remain inactive during this time [62, 65].

Patients with long-lasting headache episodes with recurrent sexual headache attacks often need drug therapy. This treatment is the same for both subtypes. The primary aim of drug treatment is the prevention of attacks, particularly because analgesics such as paracetamol, ibuprofen, acetylsalicylic acid and diclofenac have been shown to be ineffective in the treatment of acute attacks in 90% of the sufferers [73]. Sometimes, triptans can abort the headache after orgasm [74]. If the sexual activity can be planned, a short-term prophylaxis with indomethacin is possible. The recommended dose is 50–75 mg taken about 1 hour before sexual activity. The responder rate is >80% [73, 75]. Case reports also showed efficacy of naratriptan 2.5 mg [76] or of other triptans [74] as short-term prophylaxis. For diazepam and ergotamine as short-term prophylaxis, both positive and negative case reports are available [20, 56, 77–81]. In some patients, continuous prophylaxis is necessary. Propranolol is the drug of first choice and has shown efficacy in several larger case-series [20, 56, 61, 72, 73, 81]. The recommended dose is 20–80 mg t.i.d., the responder rate is > 80%. The beta-blockers metoprolol and atenolol seem to be effective as well, but experience with them is low [56, 73, 82]. A positive case report has been published for diltiazem and a negative one for verapamil; therefore, calcium channel blockers are not recommended [76, 83]. Prophylactic medication should end about 6–8 weeks after spontaneous remissions in sexual headache.

As an experimental procedure, injection of a steroid and local anaesthetic combination to the greater occipital nerve of the symptomatic site has been described [84].

Hypnic headache (4.5)

Clinical picture

Hypnic headache was first described in 1988 [85] and has been integrated into the ICHD-II. In this entity, almost every night (at least every week) a headache attack occurs during sleep. These attacks typically begin at the same time after sleep onset. This is why this headache has also been called clockwise headache. For all published cases of hypnic headache, a meta-analysis has been performed [86]. Recent case-series confirmed these findings [87, 88]. According to this meta-analysis, the headache is typically bilateral and frontotemporal or diffuse, it can be pulsating or dull, it is of moderate intensity and lasts 30 minutes to 3 h. There are no accompanying autonomous or vegetative symptoms. Rarely, a second headache attack can occur in the same night. This headache normally starts after the age of 50, the mean age at onset is 63 with a broad range of 36–83. The course is mostly chronic or relapsing-remitting, and about 20% of the patients show spontaneous remission. The most severe problem is the impaired quality of life due to disturbed sleep.

The exact pathophysiology is unknown. Polysomnographic studies could show that the headache frequently occurs during the first REM-sleep phase [89, 90, 91]. An association between REM sleep and the onset of attacks is also known for cluster headache [92, 93, 94] and – less impressive – for migraine [95]. Probably, these headache types result from a dysfunction of the central pain-controlling systems in the brain stem during REM sleep. However, a minority of patients also had hypnic headache attacks during non-REM sleep [87, 96]. An important secondary cause of hypnic headache is nocturnal hypertension, which if treated controls headache [97].

Epidemiology

The population-based prevalence of this headache is unknown. In two case series, hypnic headache represented about 0.1% of all patients in a tertiary headache clinic [90, 98]. Women are about twice as likely to be affected as men. There is no known comorbidity with other idiopathic headaches or with psychiatric or internal diseases.

Treatment

Hypnic headache often requires no treatment if it occurs rarely (i.e., <3 times a week) and if there is no impairment in quality of life. Often, it is sufficient to inform the patients about the harmless nature of the headache. Controlled studies for drug treatment are not available. According to a meta-analysis, the first step should be a trial of strong coffee or oral caffeine [86]. About 50% of the sufferers show remission of the nightly attack if they drink strong coffee before going to sleep.

If caffeine is not effective, a preventive treatment can be given. The drug of first choice is lithium in a dose of 150–600 mg per day. Lithium should be dosed according to the plasma level (0.6–1.2 mmol/l). Control of the thyroid and renal function is necessary. About 75% of the patients taking lithium report good or very good efficacy. Drugs of second choice are indomethacin (100–150 mg per day), flunarizine (10 mg in the evening) and verapamil (80 mg t.i.d.). Prophylactic inhalation of oxygen during the night, beta-blockers and antidepressants are ineffective in the majority of cases. In recent reports, the efficacy of topiramate up to 100 mg [99, 100], botulinum-toxin [101] and pregabalin [102] has been described.

There are very few reports on the acute treatment of hypnic headache attacks. A moderate efficacy in aborting the attacks has only been reported for acetylsalicylic acid.

Primary thunderclap headache (4.6)

Clinical picture

Primary thunderclap headache is a sudden headache of maximal intensity which is similar to the headache due to a rupture of an intracranial aneurysm. By definition, cerebral CT and MRI scans as well as lumbar puncture are completely normal. In the acute headache phase, diffuse, segmental or multifocal vasospasms in all vessel territories without evidence of an aneurysm or bleed have been shown in cerebral panangiography of some but not all patients [103–105]. These vasospasms were completely reversible in control examinations 2–5 weeks later. In recent years, the term reversible cerebral vasoconstriction syndrome has been suggested for this type of thunderclap headache [106, 107]. It remains to be determined whether primary thunderclap headache and this syndrome are the same entity [108].

Typically, primary thunderclap headache occurs only once in a life. It can be triggered by heat [109]. In up to 44% of patients, one or more relapses can occur in irregular frequency without any evidence of a secondary subarachnoid haemorrhage [105, 110, 11, 12, 113].

Different life-threatening disorders can co-occur with a sudden headache of maximal intensity [108]. Therefore, the following disorders have to be ruled out by an appropriate diagnostic work-up: subarachnoid haemorrhage, intracerebral haematoma, sinus thrombosis, non-ruptured vessel malformations, arterial dissection, isolated CNS vasculitis, apoplexy of the pituitary gland, colloid cyst of the third ventricle, spontaneous intracranial hypotension, acute sinusitis and hypertensive crisis (e.g., due to phaeochromocytoma).

Epidemiology

There are no data on the prevalence of primary thunderclap headache. Women seem to be affected twice as much as men, the mean age at the first thunderclap headache attack is 45 years, with a range of 25–67 years [48, 111]; 30–46% of sufferers have migraine or tension-type headache in their prior history [111, 112, 113].

Treatment

Since the intensity of thunderclap headache is severe in the first hours, analgesic treatment should be initiated immediately in the emergency room. Even after appropriate diagnostic work-up with exclusion of subarachnoid haemorrhage in the acute phase, several life-threatening differential diagnoses remain which require an MRI scan and other procedures in the following days [108, 110]. Therefore, it is strongly advised to avoid vasoconstrictive agents such as ergotamine or triptans and platelet inhibitors such as acetylsalicylic acid or NSAIDs. In this phase, analgesic treatment with paracetamol, metamizole or an opioid is recommended. Normally, the very severe intensity of this headache lasts a few hours only and as it occurs only once in a life, further treatment is often not required.

Based on the observation that nimodipine is effective in the treatment of vasospams due to subarachnoid haemorrhage, 11 patients with primary thunderclap headache were treated in an open (i.e., not placebo-controlled) trial with nimodipine. After initiation of 30–60 mg oral nimodipine every 4 h, 10 patient experienced complete remission of the headache within 24 h [114]. However, all these patients unusually had recurrent attacks. The same group found that oral nimodipine effectively aborted further attacks on 83% of 52 treated patients [115]. In a case of thunderclap headache due to reversible vasoconstriction syndrome, intravenous nimodipine was helpful [116]. Another case reported efficacy of gabapentin [117].

Hemicrania continua (4.7)

Clinical picture

Hemicrania continua was first described in 1984 [118] and shares some similarities with so-called trigeminal autonomic headaches. It was classified into group 4 based on the relatively few systematic descriptions and the lack of any substantial pathophysiological data to understand the condition more fully. In contrast to cluster headache, patients with hemicrania continua complain of a continuous pain which increases in severity in attacks of different duration. These attacks may be accompanied by mild cranial autonomic features [119, 120]. About 50% of the patients report an increase in intensity at night. More than 50% of the patients with hemicrania continua have a chronic course from the beginning. Only a minority (less than 15%) experience an exclusively episodic course with alternating active and inactive episodes. Secondary types have been described [121]. In the patient's history, a careful evaluation of analgesic intake is necessary, since the clinical picture sometimes can be similar to that of a headache due to medication overuse.

Epidemiology

The prevalence is unknown and the disorder is under-diagnosed. In contrast to cluster headache, women are about 1.5 times more affected than men [122]. Hemicrania continua usually starts between the age of 20 and 30. However, there have been reports of onset between 11 and 58 years.

Treatment

A response to indomethacin is a diagnostic criterion for hemicrania continua in the ICHD-II. The onset of efficacy is usually prompt, although some patients have a delayed response. The treatment should be started with 25 mg t.i.d. of indomethacin and, if this is not effective, the dose should be increased to up to 225 mg a day [123]. A so-called indo test with an intramuscular injection of 50 mg indomethacin has been used and gives relief of the headache within 30 minutes [124]. Recently, a placebo-controlled indomethacin test has been described to refine the diagnosis and thus clinical features [122]. If high doses of indomethacin are ineffective, the diagnosis must be questioned. In some cases, medication to protect the stomach (e.g., antacids, H_2-antagonist sor proton pump inhibitors) may be required.

In the literature, single case reports on the efficacy of verapamil, naproxen, caffeine, lamotrigine, gabapentin, methysergide, topiramate, melatonin and steroids exist [120, 125, 126, 127, 128, 129, 130].

Recently, stimulation of the greater occipital nerve was efficacious in hemicrania continua in a crossover study and in case series [131, 132].

New daily-persistent headache (4.8)

Clinical picture

This headache type first appeared in the ICHD-II in 2004. The differentiation from a chronic tension-type headache is very difficult and still debated, as indeed is the single entity. New daily-persistent headache has an acute or subacute onset within 3 days, and is present from this time on, continuously. The semiology of this headache resembles that of chronic tension-type headache and may have migrainous features. This means that this headache is bilateral, mostly not pulsating, duller and of mild to moderate intensity; mild phonophobia, photophobia and/or nausea can accompany symptoms, with up to 60% of the patients reporting these symptoms [133, 134, 135, 136].

An obligatory predisposition is that patients remember the acute or subacute onset of the headache and that no episodic headache with increasing frequency had been present before the onset of the new chronic headache. Other disorders with a subacute onset of continuous headache, such as idiopathic intracranial hypertension (also called pseudotumour cerebri), sinus thrombosis, spontaneous intracranial hypotension or chronic meningitis, have to be excluded. Overuse of analgesics or anti-migraine drugs should be considered before the diagnosis is made.

Experimental studies or models of this headache type are not available. Some authors report a post-infection occurrence. In the first description of this headache disorder, an association with viral infection was reported [137]. Later case reports and small case-series have repeatedly presented patients with this headache type and a positive and high titre for Epstein-Barr virus antibodies [134, 138, 139, 140]. In a large case-series on children with chronic headache ($n = 175$), 40 children with an acute onset have been identified. Of these, 43% showed an onset of headache during an infection, which was in half of the sufferers an Epstein-Barr virus infection [140]. Elevated levels of tumour necrosis factor have also been described [141].

Epidemiology

According to population-based studies, about 3–5% of the population suffer from chronic headache (i.e., more than 15 days/month). The majority (2–3% of the total population) suffer from chronic tension-type headache most of whom are female (female:male ratio 2:1). About 1–2% have a chronic migraine and about 0.2% have a new daily-persistent headache or, very rarely, a hemicrania continua [142, 143]. In an Indian study of 2003, 1.5% of all patients with chronic headache had a new daily-persistent headache [144]. In a population-based study from Norway, the 1-year prevalence was 0.03% [145].

Table 22.2 Pragmatic recommendations for the treatment of headache disorders group 4 of the IHS classification.

Level A: established as effective, ineffective, or harmful by at least one convincing Class I study or at least two consistent, convincing Class II studies
Level B: probably effective, ineffective, or harmful by at least one convincing Class II study or overwhelming Class III evidence
Level C: possibly effective, ineffective, or harmful by at least two convincing Class III studies

4.1 Primary stabbing headache
Indomethacin 25–50 mg b.i.d. (B)
2. choice: melatonin 3–12 mg in the evening or gabapentin 400 mg b.i.d. (C)

4.2 Primary cough headache
Indomethacin 25–200 mg per day (B)
Acetazolamide 125 mg t.i.d. (up to 200 t.i.d) (B)
Lumbar puncture with decrease of CSF pressure (B)
Methysergide 2 mg, naproxen 550 mg per day (C)

4.3 Primary exertional headache
Avoidance of physical activity during heat or in high altitude
Regular training and slow increase of activity in sports
Normal body mass index
Indomethacin 50–100 mg as short-term prophylaxis long-term prophylaxis (C)
1. choice: indomethacin 25–50 mg t.i.d. (B)
2. choice: propranolol 20–80 mg t.i.d., flunarizine 10 mg per day (C)

4.4 Primary headache associated with sexual activity
Avoidance of strong physical activity during sexual activity
Indomethacin 50–75 mg as short-term prophylaxis (B)
Propranolol 20–80 mg t.i.d. as long-term prophylaxis (B)

4.5 Hypnic headache
Caffeine before sleeping (B)
1. choice: lithium 300–600 mg per day (B)
2. choice: indomethacin 100–150 mg per day, flunarizine 10 mg per day (C)

4.6 Primary thunderclap headache
Acute phase: exclusion of subarachnoid haemorrhage and dissection by CT/MRI/MRA scan and lumbar puncture
In the acute phase pain treatment with 500 mg paracetamol t.i.d., metamizole 500 mg t.i.d. or tramadol 200 mg t.i.d. (or similar opioid)
After the acute phase in relapsing cases treatment with nimodipine 30–60 mg every 4 hours over 14 days (C)

4.7 Hemicrania continua
Indomethacin 25 mg t.i.d. up to 200 mg per day (A)

4.8 New daily-persistent headache
Valproic acid 600–900 mg per day
Amitriptyline up to 150 mg per day

For this chronic headache type, an equal sex ratio [146] or a slight preponderance of women has been described [134, 139]. The age at onset shows two peaks: between 10 and 30 years and between 50 and 60 years. Other primary headaches are reported by 30–40% of the patients in their prior history [134, 146]. It is probable that another peak of the age at onset lies in childhood before the age of 10 [140, 147].

Treatment

Evidence-based treatment recommendations have not been published for this headache type. According to expert consensus, treatment is problematic [133, 146, 148]. The basic therapy of this headache disorder should be decided according to the primary features. If the headache is more migraine-like, treatment with valproic acid (900 mg per day) has been recommended; if the headache is more like a tension-type headache, tricyclic antidepressants (e.g., amitriptyline up to 150 mg a day) should be given [133]. A specific treatment strategy with an initial centrally acting muscles relaxation drug, a tricyclic antidepressant, then a selective serotonin-reuptake inhibitor and finally an antiepileptic drug resulted in a relief of more than 50% of headache days in about 25% of the patients [146]. There are no observations on the long-term course of this headache disorder. In an earlier study, it was assumed that about 30% of the patients are free of headache after three months and about 80% after 24 months [149], but this observation has not been confirmed [133, 146, 148]. Normally, this headache disorder has a refractory course with a duration of at least 40 months in more than 50% of the sufferers [146].

In a case-series on patients with new daily-persistent headache and viral infection, intravenous methylprednisolone was effective in aborting the headache [150].

Perspectives

The headache disorders described in these treatment recommendations are diagnosed very infrequently, although they may not be rare. With increasing recognition it can be expected that they will be diagnosed more often. The diagnosis itself can be established very easily according to the ICHD-II (Table 22.1). Importantly, the treatment is often very easy and does not require expertise (overview in Table 22.2). The treatment recommendations presented in this chapter are not based on controlled trials but on case reports or series and on expert consensus. Therefore, this Task Force urgently suggests controlled trials for these headache disorders (even with a low number of patients) in order to base their treatment on a higher scientific level.

Need of update

These recommendations should be updated within 5 years and should then be structured according to the third edition of the International Headache Society.

Conflicts of interest

The present guidelines were developed without external financial support. The authors report the following financial support:

SE: Salary from the University of Münster; honoraria and research grants from Addex Pharm, AGA Medical, Allergan, Almirall, AstraZeneca, Berlin Chemie, Boehringer, CoLucid, Desitin, Eisai, GlaxoSmithKline, Ipsen Pharma, Janssen Cilag, MSD, Novartis, Pfizer, Pharm Allergan, Pierre Fabre, Reckitt-Benckiser, UCB.

PJG: Salary from the University of California, San Francisco. The author has no relationships that are relevant to this review.

RJ: Salary from the University of Copenhagen and Glostrup Hospital; honoraria and research grants from Berlin Chemie, Allergan Norden, Medotech, Norpharma, MSD.

AM: Salary from the University of Hamburg; research grants from DFG and BMBF; grants and honoraria from several pharmaceutical companies.

JP: Salary from the Spanish Health Service; honoraria from Allergan, Almirall, Janssen-Cilag, Juste, MSD.

GS: none

References

1. Headache Classification Subcommittee of the International Headache Society. The international classification of headache disorders, 2nd edition. *Cephalalgia* 2004; **24**(Suppl. 1):1–151.

2. Headache Classification Committee of the International Headache Society. Classification and diagnostic criteria for headache disorders, cranial neuralgias and facial pain. *Cephalalgia* 1988; **8**(Suppl. 7):1–96.

3. Brainin, M, Barnes, M, Baron, JC, *et al*. Guidance for the preparation of neurological management guidelines by EFNS scientific Task Forces – revised recommendations 2004. *Eur J Neurol* 2004; **11**:577–81.

4. Olesen, J, Goadsby, PJ, Ramadan, NM, *et al*. (eds). *The Headaches*, 3rd edn, 2006; Lippincott, Williams & Wilkins, Philadelphia.

5. Evers, S, Frese, A, May, A, *et al*. Therapie seltener idiopathischer Kopfschmerzerkrankungen. *Nervenheilkunde* 2005; **24**:217–226.

6. Rasmussen, BK, Olesen, J. Symptomatic and nonsymptomatic headaches in a general population. *Neurology* 1992; **42**:1225–31.

7. Sjaastad O, Pettersen, H, Bakketeig, LS. The Vaga study: epidemiology of headache I: the prevalence of ultrashort paroxysms. *Cephalalgia* 2001; **21**:207–15.

8. Sjaastad, O, Pettersen, H, Bakketeig, LS. The Vaga study of headache epidemiology II. Jabs: clinical manifestations. *Acta Neurol Scand* 2002; **105**:25–31.

9. Fusco, C, Pisani, F, Faienza, C. Idiopathic stabbing headache: clinical characteristics of children and adolescents. *Brain Dev* 2003; **25**:237–40.

10. Pareja, JA, Ruiz, J, de Isla, C, *et al*. Idiopathic stabbing hedache (jabs and jolts syndrome). *Cephalalgia* 1996; **16**:93–6.

11. Dodick, DW. Indomethacin-responsive headache syndromes. *Curr Pain Headache Rep* 2004; **8**:19–26.

12. Rozen, TD. Short-lasting headache syndromes and treatment options. *Curr Pain Headache Rep* 2004; **8**:268–73.

13. Fuh, JL, Kuo, KH, Wang, SJ. Primary stabbing headache in a headache clinic. *Cephalalgia* 2007; **27**:1005–9.

14. Jacome, DE. Exploding head syndrome and idiopathic stabbing headache relieved by nifedipine. *Cephalalgia* 2001; **21**:617–18.

15. Rozen, TD. Melatonin as treatment for idiopathic stabbing headache. *Neurology* 2003; **61**:865–6.

16. Franca, MC, Costa, ALC, Maciel, JA. Gabapentin-responsive idiopathic stabbing headache. *Cephalalgia* 2004; **24**: 993–6.

17. O'Connor, MB, Murphy, E, Phelan, MJ, Regan, MJ. Primary stabbing headache can be responsive to etoricoxib, a selective COX-2 inhibitor. *Eur J Neurol* 2008; **15**:e1.

18. Pascual, J, González-Mandly, A, Martín, R, Oterino, A. Headaches precipitated by cough, prolonged exercise or sexual activity: a prospective etiological and clinical study. *J Headache Pain* 2008; **9**:259–66.

19. Chen, PK, Fuh, JL, Wang, SJ. Cough headache: a study of 83 consecutive patients. *Cephalalgia* 2009; **29**:1079–85.

20. Pascual, J, Iglesias, F, Oterino, A, *et al.* Cough, exertional, and sexual headache. *Neurology* 1996; **46**:1520–4.

21. Ozge, C, Atiş, S, Ozge, A, *et al.* Cough headache: frequency, characteristics and the relationship with the characteristics of cough. *Eur J Pain* 2005; **9**:383–8.

22. Britton, TC, Guiloff, RJ. Carotid artery disease presenting as cough headache. *Lancet* 1988; **i**:1406–7.

23. Smith, WS, Messing, RO. Cerebral aneurysm presenting as cough headache. *Headache* 1993; **33**:203–4.

24. Raskin, NH. The cough headache syndrome: treatment. *Neurology* 1995; **45**:1784.

25. Williams, B. Cerebrospinal fluid pressure changes in response to coughing. *Brain* 1976; **99**:331–46.

26. Wang, SJ, Fuh, JL, Lu, SR. Benign cough headache is responsive to acetazolamide. *Neurology* 2000; **55**:149–50.

27. Slavik, RS, Rhoney, DH. Indomethacin: a review of its cerebral blood flow effects and potential use for controlling intracranial pressure in traumatic brain injury patients. *Neurol Res* 1999; **21**:491–9.

28. Maren, TH. Carbonic anhydrase: chemistry, physiology and inhibition. *Physiol Rev* 1967; **47**:597–781.

29. Symonds, C. Cough headache. *Brain* 1956; **79**:557–68.

30. Chen, Y, Lirg, J, Fuh, J, *et al.* Primary cough headache is associated with posterior fossa crowdedness: a morphometric MRI study. *Cephalalgia* 2004; **24**:694–9.

31. Evans, RW, Boes, CJ. Spontaneous low cerebrospinal fluid pressure syndrome can mimic primary cough headache. *Headache* 2005; **45**:374–437.

32. Bono, F, Giliberto, C, Lavano, A, Quattrone, A. Posture-related cough headache and orthostatic drop in lumbar CSF pressure. *J Neurol* 2005; **252**:237–8.

33. Mathew, NT. Indomethacin responsive headache syndromes. *Headache* 1981; **21**:147–50.

34. Boes, CJ, Matharu, MS, Goadsby, PJ. Benign cough headache. *Cephalagia* 2002; **22**:772–9.

35. Bahra, A, Goadsby, PJ. Cough headache responsive to methysergide. *Cephalalgia* 1998; **18**:495–6.

36. Calandre, L, Hernadez-Lain, A, Lopez-Valdez, E. Benign Valsalva maneuver-related headache: an MRI study of six cases. *Headache* 1996; **36**:251–3.

37. Medrano, V, Mallada, J, Sempere, AP, *et al.* Primary cough headache responsive to topiramate. *Cephalalgia* 2005; **25**:627–8.

38. Hazelrigg, RL. IV DHE-45 relieves exertional cephalalgia. *Headache* 1986; **26**:52.

39. Mateo, I, Pascual, J. Coexistence of chronic paroxysmal emicrania and benign cough headache. *Headache* 1999; **39**:437–8.

40. Indo, T, Takahashi, A. Swimmer's migraine. *Headache* 1990; **30**:485–7.

41. Massey, EW. Effort headaches in runners. *Headache* 1982; **22**:99–100.

42. Paulson, GW. Weightlifter's headache. *Headache* 1983; **23**:193–4.

43. Sjaastad, O, Bakketeig, LS. Exertional headache – II. Clinical features Vaga study of headache epidemiology. *Cephalalgia* 2003; **23**:803–7.

44. Sands, GH, Newman, L, Lipton, R. Cough, exertional, and other miscellaneous headaches. *Med Clin North Am* 1991; **75**:733–47.

45. Maggioni, F, Marchese-Ragona, R, Mampreso, E, *et al.* Exertional headache as unusual presentation of the syndrome of an elongated styloid process. *Headache* 2009; **49**:776–9.

46. Donnet, A, Dufour, H, Levrier, O, Metellus, P. Exertional headache: a new venous disease. *Cephalalgia* 2008; **28**:1201–3.

47. Doepp, F, Valdueza, JM, Schreiber, SJ. Incompetence of internal jugular valve in patients with primary exertional headache: a risk factor? *Cephalalgia* 2008; **28**:182–5.

48. Lipton, RB, Lowenkopf, T, Bajwa, ZH, *et al.* Cardiac cephalgia: a treatable form of exertional headache. *Neurology* 1997; **49**:813–16.

49. Lance, JW, Lambros, J. Headache associated with cardiac ischemia. *Headache* 1998; **38**:315–16.

50. Sathirapanya, P. Anginal cephalgia: a serious form of exertional headache. *Cephalalgia* 2004; **24**:231–4.

51. Cutrer, FM, Huerter, K. Exertional headache and coronary ischemia despite normal electrocardiographic stress testing. *Headache* 2006; **46**:165–7.

52. Wei, JH, Wang, HF. Cardiac cephalalgia: case reports and review. *Cephalalgia* 2008; **28**:892–6.

53. Sjaastad, O, Bakketeig, LS. Exertional headache – I. The Vaga study of headache epidemiology. *Cephalalgia* 2002; **22**:784–90.

54. Chen, SP, Fuh, JL, Lu, SR, Wang, SJ. Exertional headache – a survey of 1963 adolescents. *Cephalalgia* 2009; **29**: 401–7.

55. Rooke, ED. Benign exertional headache. *Med Clin North Am* 1968; **52**:801–8.

56. Silbert, PL, Edis, RH, Stewart-Wynne, EG, Gubbay, SS. Benign vascular sexual headache and exertional headache: interrelationship and long term prognosis. *J Neurol Neurosurg Psychiatry* 1991; **54**:417–21.

57. Lambert, RW, Jr, Burnet, DL. Prevention of exercise induced migraine by quantitative warm-up. *Headache* 1985; **25**:317–19.

58. Diamond, S, Medina, JL. Benign exertional headache: successful treatment with indomethacin. *Headache* 1979; **19**:249.

59. Diamond, S. Prolonged benign exertional headache: its clinical characteristics and response to indomethacin. *Headache* 1982; **22**:96–8.

60. Moorjani, B, Rothner, AD. Indomethacin-responsive headaches in children and adolescents. *Semin Pediatr Neurol* 2001; **8**:40–5.

61. Kim, JS. Swimming headache followed by exertional and coital headaches. *J Korean Med Sci* 1992; **7**:276–9.

62. Frese, A, Eikermann, A, Frese, K, *et al.* Headache associated with sexual activity. Demography, clinical futures, and comorbidity. *Neurology* 2003; **61**:796–800.

63. Lundberg, PO, Osterman, PO. The benign and malignant forms of orgasmic cephalgia. *Headache* 1974; **14**:164–5.

64. Delasobera, BE, Osborn, SR, Davis, JE. Thunderclap headache with orgasm: a case of basilar artery dissection associated with sexual intercourse. *J Emerg Med* 2009; [Epub ahead of print].

65. Lance, JW. Headaches related to sexual activity. *J Neurol Neurosurg Psychiatry* 1976; **39**:1226–30.

66. Evers, S, Schmidt, O, Frese, A, *et al.* The cerebral hemodynamics of headache associated with sexual activity. *Pain* 2003; **102**:73–8.

67. Frese, A, Frese, K, Ringelstein, EB, *et al.* Cognitive processing in headache associated with sexual activity. *Cephalalgia* 2003; **23**:545–51.

68. Valença, MM, Valença, LP, Bordini, CA, *et al.* Cerebral vasospasm and headache during sexual intercourse and masturbatory orgasms. *Headache* 2004; **44**:244–8.

69. Theeler, BJ, Krasnokutsky, MV, Scott, BR. Exertional reversible cerebral vasoconstriction responsive to verapamil. *Neurol Sci* 2010; **31**:773–5.

70. Biehl, K, Evers, S, Frese, A. Comorbidity of migraine and headache associated with sexual activity. *Cephalalgia* 2007; **27**:1271–3.

71. Evers, S, Peikert, A, Frese, A. Sexual headache in young adolescence: a case report. *Headache* 2009; **49**,:1234–5.

72. Johns, DR. Benign sexual headache within one family. *Arch Neurol* 1986; **43**: 1158–60.

73. Frese, A, Rahmann, A, Gregor, N, *et al.* Headache associated with sexual activity: prognosis and treatment options. *Cephalalgia* 2007; **27**:1265–70.

74. Frese, A, Gantenbein, A, Marziniak, M, *et al.* Triptans in orgasmic headache. *Cephalalgia* 2006; **26**:1458–61.

75. Raskin, NH. Short-lived head pains. *Neurol Clin* 1997; **15**:143–52.

76. Evans, RW, Pascual, J. Orgasmic headaches: clinical features, diagnosis, and management. *Headache* 2000; **40**: 491–4.

77. Kraft, M. Benign koital cefalalgi. *Ugeskr Laeger* 1979; **141**:2454–5.

78. Lewis, GN. Orgasm headaches. *J Indiana State Med Assoc* 1976; **69**:785–8.

79. Nutt, NR. Sexually induced headaches. *Br Med J* 1977; **i**:1664.

80. Paulson, GW, Klawans, HL. Benign orgasmic cephalgia. *Headache* 1974; **13**: 181–7.

81. Porter, M, Jankovic, J. Benign coital cephalalgia. *Arch Neurol* 1981; **38**:710–12.

82. Vincent, FM. Benign masturbatory cephalalgia. *Arch Neurol* 1982; **39**:673.

83. Akpunonu, BE, Ahrens, J. Sexual headaches: case report, review, and treatment with calcium blocker. *Headache* 1991; **31**:141–5.

84. Selekler, M, Kutlu, A, Dundar, G. Orgasmic headache responsive to greater occipital nerve blockade. *Headache* 2009; **49**:130–1.

85. Raskin, NH. The hypnic headache syndrome. *Headache* 1988; **28**:534–6.

86. Evers, S, Goadsby, PJ. Hypnic headache. Clinical features, pathophysiology, and treatment. *Neurology* 2003; **60**: 905–10.

87. Liang, JF, Fuh, JL, Yu, HY, *et al.* Clinical features, polysomnography and outcome in patients with hypnic headache. *Cephalalgia* 2008; **28**:209–15.

88. Donnet, A, Lantéri-Minet, M. A consecutive series of 22 cases of hypnic headache in France. *Cephalalgia* 2009; **29**:928–34.

89. Dodick, DW. Polysomnography in hypnic headache syndrome. *Headache* 2000; **40**:748–52.

90. Evers, S, Rahmann, A, Schwaag, S, *et al.* Hypnic headache – the first German cases including polysomnography. *Cephalalgia* 2003; **23**:20–3.

91. Pinessi, L, Rainero, I, Cicolin, A, *et al.* Hypnic headache syndrome: association of the attacks with REM sleep. *Cephalalgia* 2003; **23**:150–4.

92. Dexter, JD, Weitzman, ED. The relationship of nocturnal headaches to sleep stage patterns. *Neurology* 1970; **20**:513–18.

93. Nobre, ME, Filho, PF, Dominici, M. Cluster headache associated with sleep apnoea. *Cephalalgia* 2003; **23**:276–9.

94. Pfaffenrath, V, Pollmann, W, Ruther, E, *et al.* Onset of nocturnal attacks of chronic cluster headache in relation to sleep stages. *Acta Neurol Scand* 1986; **73**:403–7.

95. Dodick, DW, Eross, E, Parish, JM. Clinical, anatomical, and physiological relationship between sleep and headache. *Headache* 2003; **43**:282–92.

96. Dolso, P, Merlino, G, Fratticci, L, *et al.* Non-REM hypnic headache: a circadian disorder? A clinical and polysomnographic study. *Cephalalgia* 2007; **27**:83–6.

97. Gil-Gouveia, R, Goadsby, PJ. Secondary 'hypnic headache'. *J Neurol* 2007; **254**:646–54.

98. Dodick, DW, Mosek, AC, Campbell, JK. The hypnic ('alarm clock') headache syndrome. *Cephalalgia* 1998; **18**:152–6.

99. Autunno, M, Messina, C, Blandino, A, Rodolico, C. Hypnic headache responsive to low-dose topiramate: a case report. *Headache* 2008; **48**:292–4.

100. Guido, M, Specchio, LM. Successful treatment of hypnic headache with topiramate: a case report. *Headache* 2006; **46**:1205–6.

101. Marziniak, M, Voss, J, Evers, S. Hypnic headache successfully treated with botulinum toxin type A. *Cephalalgia* 2007; **27**:1082–4.

102. Ulrich, K, Gunreben, B, Lang, E, *et al.* Pregabalin in the therapy of hypnic headache. *Cephalalgia* 2006; **26**:1031–2.

103. Dodick, DW, Brown, RD, Britton, JW, Huston, J. Nonaneurysmal thunderclap headache with diffuse, multifocal, segmental, and reversible vasospasm. *Cephalalgia* 1999; **19**:118–23.

104. Slivka, A, Philbrook, B. Clinical and angiographic features of thunderclap headache. *Headache* 1995; **35**:1–6.

105. Sturm, JW, Macdonell, RA. Recurrent thunderclap headache associated with reversible intracerebral vasospasm causing stroke. *Cephalalgia* 2000; **20**:132–5.

106. Gerretsen, P, Kern, RZ. Reversible cerebral vasoconstriction syndrome: a thunderclap headache-associated condition. *Curr Neurol Neurosci Rep* 2009; **9**:108–14.

107. Liu, HY, Fuh, JL, Lirng, JF, *et al.* Three paediatric patients with reversible cerebral vasoconstriction syndromes. *Cephalalgia* 2010; **30**:354–9.

108. Schwedt, TJ, Matharu, MS, Dodick, DW. Thunderclap headache. *Lancet Neurol* 2006; **5**:621–31.

109. Liao, YC, Fuh, JL, Lirng, JF, *et al.* Bathing headache: a variant of idiopathic thunderclap headache. *Cephalalgia* 2003; **23**:854–9.

110. Dodick, DW. Thunderclap headache. *J Neurol Neurosurg Psychiatry* 2002; **72**:6–11.

111. Linn, FHH, Rinkel, GJE, Algra, A, van Gijn, J. Follow-up of idiopathic thunderclap headache in general practice. *J Neurol* 1999; **246**:946–8.

112. Markus, H. A prospective follow up of thunderclap headache mimicking subarachnoid haemorrhage. *J Neurol Neurosurg Psychiatry* 1991; **54**:1117–18.

113. Wijdicks, EFM, Kerkhoff, H, van Gijn, J. Long term follow up of 71 patients with thunderclap headache mimicking subarachnoid hemorrhage. *Lancet* 1988; **ii**:68–70.

114. Lu, SR, Liao, YC, Fuh, JL, *et al.* Nimodipine for treatment of primary thunderclap headache. *Neurology* 2004; **62**:1414–16.

115. Chen, SP, Fuh, JL, Lirng, JF, *et al.* Recurrent primary thunderclap headache and benign CNS angiopathy: spectra of the same disorder? *Neurology* 2006; **67**:2164–9.

116. Elstner, M, Linn, J, Müller-Schunk, S, Straube, A. Reversible cerebral vasoconstriction syndrome: a complicated clinical course treated with intra-arterial application of nimodipine. *Cephalalgia* 2009; **29**:677–82.

117. Garza, I, Black, DF. Persistent primary thunderclap headache responsive to gabapentin. *J Headache Pain* 2006; **7**:419–21.

118. Sjaastad, O. *Cluster Headache Syndrome*, 1992; Saunders, London. 118.

119. Matharu, MS, Boes, CJ, Goadsby, PJ. Management of trigeminal autonomic cephalgias and hemicrania continua. *Drugs* 2003; **63**:1637–77.

120. Rapoport, AM, Bigal, ME. Hemicrania continua: clinical and nosographic update. *Neurol Sci* 2003; **24**(Suppl. 2):S118–S121.

121. Trucco, M, Mainardi, F, Maggioni, F, *et al.* Chronic paroxysmal hemicrania, hemicrania continua and SUNCT syndrome in association with other pathologies: a review. *Cephalalgia* 2004; **24**:173–84.

122. Cittadini, E, Goadsby, PJ Hemicrania continua: a clinical study of 39 patients with diagnostic implications. *Brain* 2010; **133**:1973–86.

123. Sjaastad, O., Stovner, L.J., Stolt Nielsen, A., *et al.* CPH and hemicrania continua: requirements of high indomethacin dosages – an ominous sign? *Headache* 1995; **35**:363–7.

124. Antonaci, F, Pareja, JA, Caminero, AB, Sjaastad, O. Chronic paroxysmal hemicrania and hemicrania continua. Parenteral indomethacin: the 'indotest'. *Headache* 1998; **38**:122–8.

125. Spears, RC. Hemicrania continua: a case in which a patient experienced complete relief on melatonin. *Headache* 2006; **46**:524–7.

126. Spears, RC. Is gabapentin an effective treatment choice for hemicrania continua? *J Headache Pain* 2009; **10**:271–5.

127. Prakash, S, Brahmbhatt, KJ, Chawda, NT, Tandon, N. Hemicrania continua responsive to intravenous methyl prednisolone. *Headache* 2009; **49**:604–7.

128. Camarda, C, Camarda, R, Monastero, R. Chronic paroxysmal hemicrania and hemicrania continua responding to topiramate: two case reports. *Clin Neurol Neurosurg* 2008; **110**:88–91.

129. Brighina, F, Palermo, A, Cosentino, G, Fierro, B. Prophylaxis of hemicrania continua: two new cases effectively treated with topiramate. *Headache* 2007; **47**:441–3.

130. Rajabally, YA, Jacob, S. Hemicrania continua responsive to verapamil. *Headache* 2005; **45**:1082–3.

131. Schwedt, TJ, Dodick, DW, Hentz, J, *et al.* Occipital nerve stimulation for chronic headache – long-term safety and efficacy. *Cephalalgia* 2007; **27**:153–7.

132. Burns, B, Watkins, L, Goadsby, PJ. Treatment of hemicrania continua by occipital nerve stimulation with a bion device: long-term follow-up of a crossover study. *Lancet Neurol* 2008; **7**:1001–12.

133. Goadsby, PJ, Boes, C. New daily persistent headache. *J Neurol Neurosurg Psychiatry* 2002; **72**(Suppl. 2):ii6–ii9.

134. Li, D, Rozen, TD. The clinical characterisation of new daily persistent headache. *Cephalalgia* 2002; **22**:66–9.

135. Silberstein, SD, Lipton, RB, Solomon, S, Mathew, NT. Classification of daily and near daily headaches: proposed revisions to the IHS-criteria. *Headache* 1994; **34**:1–7.

136. Robbins, MS, Grosberg, BM, Napchan, U, *et al.* Clinical and prognostic subforms of new daily-persistent headache. *Neurology* 2010; **74**:1358–64.

137. Vanast, WJ, Diaz-Mitoma, F, Tyrrell, DL. Hypothesis: chronic benign daily headache is an immune disorder with a viral trigger. *Headache* 1987; **27**:138–42.

138. Diaz-Mitoma, F, Vanast, WJ, Tyrrell, DL. Increased frequency of Epstein-Barr virus excretion in patients with new daily persistent headaches. *Lancet* 1987; **i**: 411–15.

139. Evans, RW. New daily persistent headache. *Curr Pain Headache Rep* 2003; **7**, 303–7.

140. Mack, KJ. What incites new daily persistent headache in children? *Pediatr Neurol* 2004; **31**:122–5.

141. Rozen, T, Swidan, SZ. Elevation of CSF tumor necrosis factor alpha levels in new daily persistent headache and treatment refractory chronic migraine. *Headache* 2007; **47**:1050–5.

142. Láinez, MJ, Monzon, MJ. Chronic daily headache. *Curr Neurol Neurosci Rep* 2001; **1**:118–24.

143. Lanteri-Minet, M, Auray, JP, El Hasnaoui, A, *et al.* Prevalence and description of chronic daily headache in the general population in France. *Pain* 2003; **102**:143–9.

144. Chakravarty, A. Chronic daily headaches: clinical profile in Indian patients. *Cephalalgia* 2003; **23**:348–53.

145. Grande, RB, Aaseth, K, Lundqvist, C, Russell, MB. Prevalence of new daily persistent headache in the general population. The Akershus study of chronic headache. *Cephalalgia* 2009; **29**:1149–55.

146. Takase, Y, Nakano, M, Tatsumi, C, Matsuyama, T. Clinical features, effectiveness of drug-based treatment, and prognosis of new daily persistent headache (NDPH): 30 cases in Japan. *Cephalalgia* 2004; **24**:955–9.

147. Baron, EP, Rothner, AD. New daily persistent headache in children and adolescents. *Curr Neurol Neurosci Rep* 2010; **10**:127–32.

148. Evans, RW, Rozen, TD. Etiology and treatment of new daily persistent headache. *Headache* 2001; **41**:830–2.

149. Vanast, WJ. New daily persistent headaches definition of a benign syndrome. *Headache* 1986; **26**:318.

150. Prakash, S, Shah, ND. Post-infectious new daily persistent headache may respond to intravenous methylprednisolone. *J Headache Pain* 2010; **11**:59–66.

CHAPTER 23

Treatment of medication overuse headache

S. Evers[1] and R. Jensen[2]

[1]University of Münster, Münster, Germany; [2]Glostrup Hospital, University of Copenhagen, Denmark

Objectives

This guideline aims to give recommendations for the treatment of medication overuse headache (MOH) as classified by the International Headache Society (IHS) [1]. Although this headache disorder is frequent and a major problem in the treatment of chronic headache patients, placebo- or sham-controlled double-blind trials for a specific treatment of this condition are almost completely absent. Nearly all published trials are underpowered or have a high number of drop-outs. Therefore, these guidelines are based on publications with a low level of evidence and on expert consensus. A brief clinical description of this potentially preventable and treatable type of headache disorder is included.

Background

The classification of the IHS provides diagnostic criteria for chronic headache which is accompanied by the overuse of acute headache drugs such as analgesics, triptans and opioids (Table 23.1). In the first edition of the IHS classification, this headache disorder was defined as drug-induced headache, implying that the frequent drug intake itself is the cause of the headache [2]. In the present classification, medication overuse with all its somatic and psychological implications is regarded as an association and possibly not the only cause of chronic headache [1]. However, it has become apparent that some subtypes were missing and that headache features of

MOH cannot be defined in general. Therefore, a revision of these diagnostic criteria was published in 2005 [3]. These criteria remain valid, although a further revision developed for research purposes was published in 2006 [4].

The purpose of this chapter is to give recommendations for the specific management of MOH, including treatment of withdrawal headache. The recommendations are based on the scientific evidence from clinical trials and on the expert consensus by the respective Task Force of the EFNS. The definitions of the recommendation levels follow EFNS criteria [5].

Search strategy

A literature search was performed using the reference databases in Medline, Science Citation Index and the Cochrane Library; the key words used were 'headache' together with the term 'medication overuse' or 'drug-induced' (last search January 2011). All papers published in English, German or French were considered when they described a controlled trial or a case report or series on the treatment of one of these headache disorders. In addition, a review book [6] was considered.

Clinical aspects

The development of MOH is mainly reported in patients with a primary headache disorder such as migraine and

European Handbook of Neurological Management: Volume 2, Second Edition. Edited by Nils Erik Gilhus, Michael P. Barnes, Michael Brainin.
© 2012 Blackwell Publishing Ltd. Published 2012 by Blackwell Publishing Ltd.

Table 23.1 Current diagnostic criteria of the International Headache Society for medication overuse headache.

8.2 Medication overuse headache

Diagnostic criteria:

    A. Headache[1] present on ≥15 days/month fulfilling criteria C and D

    B. Regular overuse[2] for ≥3 months of one or more drugs that can be taken for acute and/or symptomatic treatment of headache[3]

    C. Headache has developed or markedly worsened during medication overuse

    D. Headache resolves or reverts to its previous pattern within 2 months after discontinuation of overused medication[4]

Subtypes of medication overuse headache

8.2.1 Ergotamine-overuse headache

Ergotamine intake on ≥10 days/month on a regular basis for >3 months

8.2.2 Triptan-overuse headache

Triptan intake (any formulation) on ≥10 days/month on a regular basis for >3 months

8.2.3 Analgesic-overuse headache

Intake of simple analgesics on ≥15 days/month on a regular basis for >3 months

8.2.4 Opioid-overuse headache

Opioid intake on ≥10 days/month on a regular basis for >3 months

8.2.5 Combination analgesic-overuse headache

Intake of combination analgesic medications[1] on ≥10 days/month on a regular basis for >3 months

8.2.6 Medication-overuse headache attributed to the combination of acute medications

Intake of any combination of ergotamine, triptans, analgesics and/or opioids on ≥10 days/month on a regular basis for >3 months without overuse of any single class alone[1]

8.2.7 Headache attributed to other medication overuse

Regular overuse[1] for >3 months of a medication other than those described above

8.2.8 Probable medication-overuse headache

    A. Headache fulfilling criteria A, C and D for 8.2 **Medication-overuse headache**

    B. Medication overuse fulfilling criterion B for any one of the subforms 8.2.1–8.2.7

    C. One of the following:

        1. overused medication has not yet been withdrawn

        2. medication overuse has ceased within the last 2 months but headache has not so far resolved or reverted to its previous pattern

1The headache associated with medication overuse is variable and often has a peculiar pattern with characteristics shifting, even within the same day, from migraine-like to tension-type headache.

2Overuse is defined in terms of duration and treatment days per week. What is crucial is that treatment occurs both frequently and regularly (i.e., 2 or more days a week). Bunching of treatment days with long periods without medication intake, practised by some patients, is much less likely to cause medication-overuse headache and does not fulfil criterion B.

3MOH can occur in headache-prone patients when acute headache medications are taken for other indications.

4A period of 2 months after cessation of overuse is stipulated in which improvement (resolution of headache or reversion to its previous pattern) must occur if the diagnosis is to be definite. Prior to cessation, or pending improvement within 2 months after cessation, the diagnosis of 8.2.8 **Probable medication-overuse headache** should be applied. If such improvement does not then occur within 2 months, this diagnosis must be discarded.

1Combination typically implicated are those containing simple analgesics combined with opioids, butalbital and/or caffeine.

1The specific subform(s) 8.2.1–8.2.5 should be diagnosed if criterion B is fulfilled in respect of any one or more single class(es) of these medications.

1The definition of overuse in terms of treatment days per week is likely to vary with the nature of the medication.

tension-type headache, but has also been reported in smaller series of secondary headaches [7, 8, 9, 10, 11]. For cluster headache, studies have been published showing that these patients can also fulfil the criteria for MOH [12, 13]. However, most of these patients had migraine as a comorbid headache or migraine in their family history, and many cluster headache patients take analgesics, ergotamine derivatives or triptans daily without MOH. Patients with other pain conditions, such as rheumatic diseases and no headache disorder, do not develop chronic headache de novo when taking analgesics for their pain condition [14, 15, 16, 17].

The population-based one-year prevalence of MOH in different countries ranges from 0.7% to 1.7% with a female preponderance between 62% and 92% [18]. The incidence of MOH has not been studied in specific population-based studies. In a study on episodic migraineurs, the 1-year incidence of chronic headache including MOH was 14% [19]. Among all patients in headache clinics or centres of tertiary care, MOH patients are one of the largest patient groups. In Europe up to 30% and in the USA more than 50% of patients in such centres present with MOH [18, 20]. In India, for example, only 3.1% of the patients in a headache clinic fulfil the criteria for MOH [21].

In principle, all acute drugs for the treatment of headache have been described to cause MOH (i.e., ergotamine derivatives, barbiturates, triptans, analgesics – simple and combined – opioids, benzodiazepines; possibly also caffeine). Currently, simple analgesics and triptans are the most frequent drugs taken by patients with MOH [20, 22].

Withdrawal treatment

There is evidence, although neither overwhelming nor unanimously shown in prospective trials, that withdrawal therapy is the best treatment for MOH. However, all experts and headache centres agree that withdrawal therapy should be offered to patients with MOH. The goal is not only to detoxify the patients and stop the chronic headache but also, probably, to improve responsiveness to acute or prophylactic drugs [23].

Withdrawal procedure

The recommended procedures for withdrawal of patients with MOH vary and no study has compared abrupt withdrawal treatment, with tapered withdrawal in prospective randomized trials. Most headache specialists favour the abrupt discontinuation of pain medication under the impression that abrupt withdrawal is associated with faster resolution of the drug-induced pain-coping behaviour [24]. However, tapered withdrawal seems to be advisable for opioids, barbiturates and benzodiazepines. The main withdrawal symptoms are worsening of the headache, nausea, vomiting, arterial hypotension, tachycardia, sleep disturbance, restlessness, anxiety and nervousness. These symptoms normally last 2–10 days, but

can persist for up to 4 weeks. The withdrawal headache was shorter in patients taking triptans (mean 4.1 days) than ergotamine derivatives (mean 6.7 days) or NSAIDs (mean 9.5 days) [25].

The outcome of withdrawal therapy in patients with MOH followed up by a neurologist as compared to a primary care physician did not differ significantly for calculated mean headache and improvement of headache days [26]. Therefore, it is suggested that a primary care physician can follow these patients after detoxification, which was made in this study in hospital, as well as a neurologist or a pain specialist.

With regard to non-pharmacological approaches, combined short-term psychodynamic psychotherapy and pharmacological therapy improved headache in MOH, and the combination of both was superior to pharmacological therapy alone for reducing long-term relapses and the reduction of quality of life in a non-randomized study [27]. In another study, 120 uncomplicated MOH patients were treated with three different modalities: 1) strong advice to withdraw overused medication; 2) a standard outpatient detoxification programme (rapid withdrawal of overused medication plus oral prednisolone for 8 days and personalized prophylactic drugs); 3) inpatient treatment (rapid withdrawal of overused medication plus oral prednisolone for 8 days and personalized prophylactic drugs with parenteral fluid and antiemetics; close observation for 8 days). The percentages of patients achieving successful withdrawal and the headache frequency were not different between the groups during the follow-up period of 60 days [28].

A direct comparison between inpatient withdrawal and outpatient withdrawal treatment showed that both methods revealed a significant decrease of headache days per month after 12 months and a reduction of the scores of migraine disability. Neither was superior [29]. Although outpatient withdrawal is less expensive and as successful in a motivated patient group than inpatient withdrawal, the advantages of inpatient withdrawal are the close monitoring of medication intake and the clinical state, professional psychological support, immediate treatment of withdrawal symptoms and if necessary the administration of intravenous drugs. The overuse of opioids, barbiturates or benzodiazepines, psychological problems, severe medical comorbidities, severe withdrawal symptoms (e.g., vomiting, status migrainosus), or previous medication withdrawal failure are reasons for inpatient treatment according to expert consensus or national guidelines [30, 31, 32]. However, this recommendation is not supported by randomized prospective trials.

A recent prospective, multicentre study investigated three relatively small groups: 1) only personalized preventive medication from day 1 ($n = 17$); 2) abrupt withdrawal plus rescue medication ($n = 20$); 3) no preventive medication plus no advice to stop overused drugs ($n = 19$) [33]. The primary endpoint – change in headache days – did not differ significantly between the three groups. Due to the more pronounced reduction of the headache index of the first group in comparison to the second group, there might be an advantage for a personalized preventive medication without abrupt withdrawal. In another study, advice alone was successful as withdrawal therapy in nearly all patients with simple MOH but significantly less successful in patients with complicated MOH [34]. More, larger prospective trials are therefore necessary.

Studies on a specific preventive therapy for MOH have not been undertaken. Therefore the choice of the preventive agent in MOH should be based on the primary headache (e.g., migraine vs. tension-type headache), the possible side-effects of the drugs, the comorbidities and the patient's preference and previous therapeutic experience. Several open-label trials showed positive effects of different substances such as valproic acid and topiramate in the prophylactic treatment of chronic daily headache with excessive medication intake. A double-blind trial in patients with a specific diagnosis of chronic migraine and medication overuse showed a significant reduction in the mean number of migraine days per month by topiramate (range 50–200 mg per day) in comparison to placebo ($-3.5 +/-6.3$ vs. $-0.2 +/-4.7$; $P < 0.05$). However, side-effects were reported by 75% of the patients in the topiramate group compared to 37% in the placebo group [35]. The headache reduction was nevertheless not big enough to change the chronic headache into an episodic form. In a similar study on chronic migraine, topiramate achieved a significant reduction of migrainous days per month by 6.4 as compared to placebo which achieved a reduction of 4.7 days per month [36]. In a large-scale study of 335 MOH patients from the Danish Headache Centre, where abrupt detoxification was initiated, the headache frequency was reduced by 67% in migraine patients and by

37% in those with combined migraine and tension-type headache after a 2-month observation period without prophylactic medication [37]. In a recent project with two large studies on the efficacy of onabotulinum toxin A in the treatment of chronic migraine, patients with medication overuse were also treated [38]. Although no specific data on the efficacy of onabotulinum toxin in this specific group of patients (between 63% and 69% of all patients in the different treatment arms) is given, the studies show evidence that onabotulinum toxin A is efficacious in the reduction of headache days in MOH. In summary, it is suggested that detoxification prior to initiating prophylactic therapy may not be required in all patients with MOH [39], whereas other studies support the importance of initial detoxification [23 and 20].

Treatment of withdrawal headache

Since most drugs helpful for the treatment of withdrawal headache can cause MOH, corticosteroids were regarded as an option for the treatment of withdrawal headache [40, 41]. The only controlled, randomized, double-blind study that investigated oral prednisolone during the first 6 days after medication withdrawal revealed no effect on a combined primary endpoint. Out of total 97 patients, 49 received prednisolone (60 mg on days 1 and 2, 40 mg on days 3 and 4, and 20 mg on days 5 and 6) and 48 placebo [42]. Conversely, a large open-label trial on patients with chronic daily headache and medication overuse showed that treatment with 60 mg prednisone for 2 days tapering by 20 mg every other day effectively reduced rebound-headache and withdrawal symptoms [43]. Recently, in a small proof-of-concept study, nine patients with MOH received either placebo or 100 mg prednisone for 5 days [44]. The duration of withdrawal headache was significantly lower in the prednisone group as compared to the placebo group. Thus corticosteroids might be efficacious in withdrawal symptoms in MOH patients, but high quality placebo-controlled trials are needed.

There are no other controlled trials on the specific treatment of withdrawal headache or of other symptoms during withdrawal therapy. One open study suggested the combination of intravenous hydration, dexamethasone, metoclopramide and benzodiazepines for 7–15 days [41]. Very early studies suggested that subcutaneous sumatriptan, naproxen (500 mg) and amitriptyline (10–50 mg) were effective in mitigating withdrawal headache [40, 45, 46]. However, none of these studies was placebo-controlled. Therefore, by expert consensus, headache drugs and analgesics are not recommended for the treatment of headache during withdrawal therapy, except a single intravenous administration in very severe cases.

Prognosis of withdrawal therapy

The relapse rate of MOH is about 30% (range 14–41%) after 1 year, regardless of whether inpatient, outpatient or advice alone treatment was applied [18]. Further, the relapse rates do not differ significantly when a short or a long observation period is used and most studies indicate that the eventual relapse occurs at an early stage (i.e., within a few months) after detoxification. In one study, for example, the relapse rate was 23% after 2 months and after 1 year in the same sample [47]; in another example, the relapse rate was 41% after 1 year and 44% after 4 years [48]. Overall, detoxification is fairly successful in most patients and all MOH patients should be informed and encouraged to discontinue their overuse. In the general population, simple advice regarding MOH was sufficient to result in a successful treatment of MOH in 76% of all patients after 1.5 years [49].

In an Italian study on different withdrawal therapies, a long duration of migraine before medication overuse, a higher frequency of migraine after withdrawal therapy and a greater number of previous preventive treatments were associated with a higher risk for relapse of MOH [50]. In other studies, predictors of relapse were male sex, intake of combination analgesics after withdrawal therapy, nicotine and alcohol consumption, and taking the former medication again after withdrawal therapy [51, 52]. Recently, use of codeine-containing drugs, low self-reported sleep quality and high self-reported bodily pain as measured by the quality of life tool SF-36 were predictors for a poor outcome [53]. In some studies, the prognosis was better for patients with migraine as the underlying primary headache disorder than for patients with tension-type headache and for ergotamine or triptan withdrawal than for analgesic withdrawal [37, 48]. It is likely that the results in these studies with respect to predictors of relapse are due to different study designs and different background populations.

Specific pattern in children and adolescents

Several studies showed that MOH is observed in children and adolescents [18]. Population-based epidemiological studies detected a 1-year prevalence of 0.3–0.5% in

Table 23.2 Recommendations for the treatment of medication overuse headache.

The level of recommendation is classified as follows:
Level A: established as effective, ineffective or harmful by at least one convincing class I study or at least two consistent convincing class II studies
Level B: probably effective, ineffective or harmful by at least one convincing class II study or overwhelming class III evidence
Level C: possibly effective, ineffective or harmful by at least two convincing class III studies
Good practice point: lack of evidence but consensus within the Task Force

1. Patients with medication overuse headache should be offered advice and taught to encourage withdrawal treatment. (Level B)
2. There is no general evidence whether abrupt or tapering withdrawal treatment is preferred. For the overuse of analgesics, ergotamine derivatives or triptans, abrupt withdrawal is recommended. For the overuse of opioids, benzodiazepines or barbiturates, tapering of the medication should be offered. (Good practice point)
3. The type of withdrawal treatment (inpatient, outpatient, advice alone) has no influence on the success of the treatment and the relapse rate in general. (Level A)
4. In patients with opioid, benzodiazepine or barbiturate overuse, with severe psychiatric or medical comorbidity, or with failure of a previous outpatient withdrawal treatment, inpatient withdrawal treatment should be offered. (Good practice point)
5. Individualized preventive medication should be started on the first day of withdrawal treatment or earlier if applicable. (Level C)
6. Topiramate 100 mg (up to 200 mg maximum) per day may be effective in the treatment of medication overuse headache. (Level B)
7. Corticosteroids (at least 60 mg prednisone or prednisolone) and amitriptyline (up to 50 mg) may be effective in the treatment of withdrawal symptoms. (Good practice point)
8. After withdrawal therapy patients should be followed up regularly to prevent relapse. (Good practice point)

adolescents, all of them overusing OTC analgesics (mainly combined analgesics) [54, 55].

Children also benefit from withdrawal therapy [56]. However, very few data are available on the best treatment in this age group. One month after withdrawal therapy, about 53% of all children had a reduction of headache frequency by more than 90% regardless of whether they were on preventive medication or not; the only predictor for a poor outcome after withdrawal therapy was a duration of MOH longer than 2 years [57].

Conclusion

As described above, very few controlled and/or randomized trials are available to give evidence-based recommendations for the treatment of MOH. Therefore, the conclusions of this guideline are of low evidence or are good practice points as agreed by expert consensus. A summary of our clinical recommendations are presented in Table 23.2.

References

1. Headache Classification Subcommittee. The international classification of headache disorders. *Cephalalgia* 2004; **24**(Suppl. 1):1–160.
2. Headache Classification Committee. Classification and diagnostic criteria for headache disorders, cranial neuralgias and facial pain. *Cephalagia* 1988; **8**(Suppl. 7):1–96.
3. Silberstein, SD, Olesen, J, Bousser, MG, *et al*. International Headache Society. The International Classification of Headache Disorders, 2nd edition (ICHD-II)–revision of criteria for 8.2 Medication-overuse headache. *Cephalalgia* 2005; **25**:460–5.
4. Headache Classification Committee. New appendix criteria open for a broader concept of chronic migraine. *Cephalalgia* 2006; **26**:742–6.
5. Brainin, M, Barnes, M, Baron, JC, et al. Guidance for the preparation of neurological management guidelines by EFNS scientific task forces – revised recommendations 2004. *Eur J Neurol* 2004; **11**:577–81.
6. Olesen, J, Goadsby, PJ, Ramadan, NM, *et al*. (eds). *The Headaches*, 3rd edn, 2006; Lippincott, Williams & Wilkins, Philadelphia.
7. Bauer, B, Evers, S, Lindörfer, HW, *et al*. Headache caused by a sphenoid mucocele but presenting as an ergotamine-induced headache. *Headache* 1997; **376**:460–2.
8. Baandrup, L, Jensen, R. Chronic post-traumatic headache – a clinical analysis in relation to the International Headache Classification 2nd edition. *Cephalalgia* 2005; **25**: 132–8.
9. Wolfe, S, Van Stavern, G. Characteristics of patients presenting with ocular pain. *Can J Ophthalmol* 2008; **43**:432–4.
10. Cady, RK, Schreiber, CP. Sinus problems as a cause of headache refractoriness and migraine chronification. *Curr Pain Headache Rep* 2009; **13**:319–25.
11. Willer, L, Jensen, R, Juhler, M. Medication overuse as a cause of chronic headache in shunted hydrocephalus patients. *J Neurol Neurosurg Psychiatry* 2010; **81**:1261–4.
12. Evers, S, Bauer, B, Suhr, S. Ergotamine-induced headache associated with cluster headache. *Neurology* 1996; **46**: 291.
13. Paemeleire, K, Bahra, A, Evers, S, *et al*. Medication-overuse headache in patients with cluster headache. *Neurology* 2006; **67**:109–13.
14. Lance, F, Parkes, C, Wilkinson, M. Does analgesic abuse cause headaches de novo? *Headache* 1988; **28**:61–2.
15. Wilkinson, SM, Becker, WJ, Heine, JA. Opiate use to control bowel motility may induce chronic daily headache in patients with migraine. *Headache* 2001; **41**:303–9.
16. Bahra, A, Walsh, M, Menon, S, Goadsby, PJ. Does chronic daily headache arise de novo in association with regular use of analgesics? *Headache* 2003; **43**:179–90 .
17. Zwart, JA, Dyb, G, Hagen, K, *et al*. Analgesic overuse among subjects with headache, neck, and low-back pain. *Neurology* 2004; **62**:1540–4.
18. Evers, S, Marziniak, M. Clinical features, pathophysiology, and treatment of medication-overuse headache. *Lancet Neurol* 2010; **9**:391–401.
19. Katsarava, Z, Schneeweiss, S, Kurth, T, *et al*. Incidence and predictors for chronicity of headache in patients with episodic migraine. *Neurology* 2004; **62**:788–90.
20. Jensen, R, Zeeberg, P, Dehlendorff, C, Olesen, J. Predictors of outcome of the treatment programme in a multidisciplinary headache centre. *Cephalalgia* 2010; **30**:1214–24.
21. Ravishankar, K. Medication overuse headache in India. *Cephalalgia* 2008; **28**:1223–6.
22. Bigal, ME, Serrano, D, Buse, D, *et al*. Acute migraine medications and evolution from episodic to chronic migraine: a longitudinal population-based study. *Headache* 2008; **48**: 1157–68.
23. Zeeberg, P, Olesen, J, Jensen, R. Discontinuation of medication overuse in headache patients: recovery of therapeutic responsiveness. *Cephalalgia* 2006; **26**:1192–8.
24. Rossi, P, Jensen, R, Nappi, G, *et al*. A narrative review on the management of medication overuse headache: the steep road from experience to evidence. *J Headache Pain* 2009; **10**:407–17.

25. Katsarava, Z, Fritsche, G, Muessig, M, et al. Clinical features of withdrawal headache following overuse of triptans and other headache drugs. Neurology 2001; 57:1694–8.

26. Bøe, MG, Salvesen, R, Mygland, A. Chronic daily headache with medication overuse: predictors of outcome 1 year after withdrawal therapy. Eur J Neurol 2009; 16:705–12.

27. Altieri, M, Di Giambattista, R, Di Clemente, L, et al. Combined pharmacological and short-term psychodynamic psychotherapy for probable medication overuse headache: a pilot study. Cephalalgia 2009; 29:293–9.

28. Rossi, P, Di Lorenzo, C, Faroni, J, et al. Advice alone vs. structured detoxification programmes for medication overuse headache: a prospective, randomized, open-label trial in transformed migraine patients with low medical needs. Cephalalgia 2006; 26:1097–105.

29. Grazzi, L, Andrasik, F, Usai, S, Bussone, G. In-patient vs. day-hospital withdrawal treatment for chronic migraine with medication overuse and disability assessment: results at one-year follow-up. Neurol Sci 2008; 29(Suppl. 1): 161–3.

30. Paemelaire, K, Crevitis, L, Goadsby, PH, Kaube, H. Practical management of medication overuse headache. Acta Neurol Belg 2006; 106:43–51.

31. Obermann, M, Katsarava, Z. Management of medication overuse headache. Expert Rev Neurother 2007; 7:1145–55.

32. Straube, A, May, A, Kropp, P, et al. Therapie primärer chronischer Kopfschmerzen: Chronische Migräne, chronischer Kopfschmerz vom Spannungstyp und andere chronische tägliche Kopfschmerzen. Nervenheilkunde 2007; 26:186–99.

33. Hagen, K, Albretsen, C, Vilming, ST, et al. Management of medication overuse headache: 1-year randomized multicentre open-label trial. Cephalalgia 2009; 29:221–32.

34. Rossi, P, Faroni, JV, Nappi, G. Short-term effectiveness of simple advice as a withdrawal strategy in simple and complicated medication overuse headache. Eur J Neurol 2011; 18:396–401.

35. Diener, HC, Bussone, G, Van Oene, JC, et al. Topiramate reduces headache days in chronic migraine: a randomized, double-blind, placebo-controlled study. Cephalalgia 2007; 27:814–23.

36. Silberstein, SD, Lipton, RB, Dodick, DW, et al. Efficacy and safety of topiramate for the treatment of chronic migraine: a randomized, double-blind, placebo-controlled trial. Headache 2007; 47:170–80.

37. Zeeberg, P, Olesen, J, Jensen, R. Probable medication-overuse headache: the effect of a 2-month drug-free period. Neurology 2006; 66:1894–8.

38. Dodick, DW, Turkel, CC, DeGryse, RE, et al. Onabotulinumtoxin A for treatment of chronic migraine: pooled results from the double-blind, randomized, placebo-controlled phases of the PREEMPT clinical program. Headache 2010; 50:921–36.

39. Diener, HC, Dodick, DW, Goadsby, PJ, et al. Utility of topiramate for the treatment of patients with chronic migraine in the presence or absence of acute medication overuse. Cephalalgia 2009; 29:1021–7.

40. Bonuccelli, U, Nuti, A, Lucetti, C, et al. Amitriptyline and dexamethasone combined treatment in drug-induced headache. Cephalalgia 1996; 16:198–200.

41. Trucco, M, Meineri, P, Ruiz, L, et al. Medication overuse headache: withdrawal and prophylactic therapeutic regimen. Headache 2010; 50:989–97.

42. Bøe, MG, Mygland, A, Salvesen, R. Prednisolone does not reduce withdrawal headache: a randomized, double-blind study. Neurology 2007; 69:26–31.

43. Krymchantowski, AV, Barbosa, JS. Prednisone as initial treatment of analgesic-induced daily headache. Cephalalgia 2000; 20:107–13.

44. Pageler, L, Katsarava, Z, Diener, HC, Limmroth, V. Prednisone vs. placebo in withdrawal therapy following medication overuse headache. Cephalalgia 2008; 28: 152–6.

45. Diener, HC, Haab, J, Peters, C, et al. Subcutaneous sumatriptan in the treatment of headache during withdrawal from drug-induced headache. Headache 1991; 31: 205–9.

46. Hering, R, Steiner, TJ. Abrupt outpatient withdrawal of medication in analgesic-abusing migraineurs. Lancet 1991; 337:1442–3.

47. Ghiotto, N, Sances, G, Galli, F, et al. Medication overuse headache and applicability of the ICHD-II diagnostic criteria: 1-year follow-up study (CARE I protocol). Cephalalgia 2009; 29:233–43.

48. Katsarava, Z, Muessig, M, Dzagnidze, A, et al. Medication overuse headache: rates and predictors for relapse in a 4-year prospective study. Cephalalgia 2005; 25:12–15.

49. Grande, RB, Aaseth, K, Benth, JŠ, et al. Reduction in medication-overuse headache after short information. The Akershus study of chronic headache. Eur J Neurol 2011; 18: 129–37.

50. Rossi, P, Faroni, JV, Nappi, G. Medication overuse headache: predictors and rates of relapse in migraine patients with low medical needs. A 1-year prospective study. Cephalalgia 2008; 28:1196–200.

51. Suhr, B, Evers, S, Bauer, B, et al. Drug-induced headache: long-term results of stationary versus ambulatory withdrawal therapy. Cephalalgia 1999; 19:44–9.

52. Sances, G, Ghiotto, N, Galli, F, et al. Risk factors in medication-overuse headache: a 1-year follow-up study (care II protocol). Cephalalgia 2010; 30:329–36.

53. Bøe, MG, Salvesen, R, Mygland, A. Chronic daily headache with medication overuse: a randomized follow-up by neurologist or PCP. Cephalalgia 2009; 29:855–63.

54. Wang, SJ, Fuh, JL, Lu, SR, Juang, KD. Chronic daily headache in adolescents: prevalence, impact, and medication overuse. *Neurology* 2006; **66**:193–7.

55. Dyb, G, Holmen, TL, Zwart, JA. Analgesic overuse among adolescents with headache: the Head-HUNT-Youth Study. *Neurology* 2006; **66**:198–201.

56. Hershey, AD Chronic daily headache in children. *Expert Opin Pharmacother* 2003; **4**:485–91.

57. Kossoff, EH, Mankad, DN. Medication-overuse headache in children: is initial preventive therapy necessary? *J Child Neurol* 2006; **21**:45–8.

Index

Figures in **bold** refer to Tables
Figures in *italics* refer to Figures

14-3-3 protein 175, 176, 178, 188

abeta-lipoproteinaemia (ABL) **77**, 79
acetaminophen 299
acetazolamide 78, 88, 89, 136
  headache disorders 324, 325, **330**
acetylcholine receptor (AChR) 116–17
acetylsalicylic acid 326, 328
actigraphy **135**
acupuncture **231**, 232–3
acupuncture-like 12, 13, **14–15**, 26
acute bacterial meningitis (ABM) 145–57
  comparison of CSF **149**
  complications 155
  differential diagnosis **147**
  emergency management **150**
  investigations 148, **149**, 149, **150**, 151
  time line **146**
acute disseminated encephalomyelitis
  (ADEM) 119, 292, 296
adenylate deaminase **283**
AIDS-dementia complex (ADC) **177**, **185**,
  187
alcohol 256, 269–70, 341
  injections 41
  WE 239, **240**, 241, **242–3**, 243, 245,
    246–7, 248–9
allodynia 13
Alpers–Huttenlocher syndrome (AHS) 67,
  70
Alzheimer's disease (AD) 90, 92–3, **93**, 94,
  95
  CSF investigations 176, 178, **182**, **184**,
    187, 188
  sleep disorders 130, 132
ε-aminocaproic acid 266
aminoglycosides 152
amitriptyline 330, **330**, 341
  TTHs 229–30, **230**, 231, 232

amitriptylinoxide 230
amoxicillin 151, 152, 164, **166**, 168
amphetamines 256
ampicillin 151, 152
ampicillin–chloramphenicol 148, 152
amputation and phantom limb pain **15**, 16,
  19, 22, 24, **25**
  deep brain stimulation 20, **21**, 27
amyloid angiopathies 90
amyloid β peptide 175, 176, **177**, 178, 187,
  188
amyotrophic lateral sclerosis (ALS) 98, **99**,
  101, 280
  CSF investigations **177**, 181, **182–3**, 187
  neuroimaging 199, 200, 201–6
  sleep disorders 130, 133, 136, 137
amyotrophic lateral sclerosis-FTD 98, **99**,
  201–2
analgesics 326, 328, 329
  MOH 337, **338**, 338–9, **341**, 341–2
  TTHs 226–7, **228**, 228–30
ancillary protein mutations 65, 66
Andersen–Tawil syndrome (ATS) 88, **89**
aneurysm 255, 258, 263–4, 266, 328
angiography 326
angiotensin-converting enzyme (ACE)
  inhibitor 270
anterolateral cordotomy 22
anti-amphiphysin antibodies **310**
antibiotics 265
  ABM 145, 146–8, **150**, 151–4, 156
  LNB 159, 164, **165–6**, 167, 168
anticoagulants 256, 22, 267-, **268**, 269
anticonvulsants 155, 229
antidepressants 229, 230, 231
antiepileptic drugs (AEDs) 216, 218, 219,
  330–1
  ICH 260, 263, **264**
antigen detection 162
antihistamines 299
anti-Hu syndrome **310**, 312, 314
antiplatelet agents 256, 270

anti-psychotic drugs **280**
anti-titin antibodies 315
anti-VGCC antibodies **310**, 314, 315
anti-Yo antibodies **310**, 313, 314, 316
apoptosis 68–9
apparently sporadic spastic paraplegia 83
aprotinin 266
aquaporin 4 (AQP4) 287–8, 291, 292–4,
  295, 295–6, **296**, 297, 300–1
Arnold–Chiari malformation 324, 325
arteriovenous malformations (AVMs) 255,
  256, 258, 265–6, 267
Asian opticospinal MS 288, 296
aspirin 227, 228, **228**, 256, 270
astrocytic brain tumours 181
astrocytomas 214, 215, 216, 218, 219
ataxia 73, 74, **75–7**, 78–9
  autosomal dominant cerebellar 74, 78
  autosomal recessive cerebellar 74,
    78–9
  X-linked 74, 79
ataxia oculomotor apraxia (AOA) **77**, 78–9,
  206
ataxia telangiectasia (AT) 74, **77**, 78, 79
ataxia telangiectasia-like disorder **77**
ataxia with Vitamin E deficiency **77**, 79
atenolol 327
autosomal dominant cerebellar ataxias 74,
  78
autosomal dominant hereditary neuropathy
  101
autosomal dominant HSPs 80, **81–2**,
  83
autosomal dominant optic atrophy (ADOA)
  64, 70
autosomal dominant PEO **64**, 66–7, 70
autosomal recessive cerebellar ataxia 74,
  78–9
autosomal recessive hereditary neuropathy
  101
autosomal recessive HSPs 80, **81–2**, 83
autosomal recessive PEO **64**, 66–7, 70

autosomal recessive spastic ataxia of
    Charlevoix–Saguenay (ARSACS) **82**,
    83
azathioprine 293, 298, 299, 300, **300**

baclofen **38**, 40–1, 45, 120
bacterial meningitis 145–57
    CSF investigations 180, 181, **182**
balloon compression (BC) 41, **42**, 43
Balo's concentric sclerosis 119
Bannwarth's syndrome 160, 164, 168
barbiturates 260, **262**, 339, **341**
Barth's syndrome 68, 70
Becker muscular dystrophy (BMD) 104
benign familial neonatal-infantile seizure
    89, 90
benign infantile neonatal epilepsy 89–90
benign neonatal epilepsy (BNE) **89**
benzodiazepines 40, 137, **264**
    MOH 339, 340, **341**
benzyl penicillin 151, 152, 156
beri-beri 239, 243
beta-blockers **280**, 326, 327
beta trace protein (βTP) 176, **180**, 180–1
beta-2 transferrin (β₂-transferrin) 175, 176,
    179–80
bilateral optic neuritis (BON) 288, 294,
    295, 296, **301**, 300
bilevel-PAP (bi-PAP) 134, 136, 138
Binswanger's disease **186**
biomarkers 315–16
body mass index (BMI) 256, 270, 325, **330**
Borrelia afzelii 161
Borrelia burgdorferi (*Bb*) 159–61, 162–4
botulinum toxin 229, 230, 327
brachial plexus damage 16, **19**, 21, 22, 24,
    25
brain atlas co-registration 16
brain atrophy 201–2, 205, 206
brain-derived neurotrophic factor 203
brain lesions 291, 293, 294, *295*, 295, 298
brain parenchymal fraction (BPF) 201
brain-stem encephalitis **310**, **311**, 314
breast cancer 309, **310**, **311**, 312, 313, 316
bronchoscopy 312
bruxism 132
bulbospinal muscular atrophy 280
buspirone 230

caffeine 327, 329, **330**, 339
    TTHs **228**, 229, 231
calcium antagonists 259–60
calcium channel blockers 327
calpainopathy **281**, **283**
cancer-associated retinopathy **310**, **311**
capsaicin 40
captopril 260, 263
carbamazepine (CBZ) 89, 216, 218
    TN 31, 36, **38**, **39**, 40, 45, 46
cardiac arrest **186**
cardiac cephalgia 325
cataplexy 132, 175, 178–9, **179**, 188
catathrenia 131

caveolinopathy **281**, **283**
cavernous angiomas 258, 266
cefixime 164
cefotaxime 164, **165**, 168
    ABM 148, 151, 15
ceftriaxone 164, **165**, **166**, 167, 168
    ABM 148, 151, 152, 156
central nervous system (CNS) 160, 164,
    168, 187
    gliomas 181, **182**
    NMO 287, 290, 292, 297
central core disease (CCD) 108
central pain of brain origin 16, **19**
central pain of spinal cord origin **19**, 21
central post-stroke pain (CPSP) 20, **21**,
    24–5, **25**, 27
    MCS 22, **23**, 27
central sleep apnoea 137
central sleep apnoea – hypopnoea
    syndrome (CSAHS) 130, 136
cephalagia 21
cephalosporins 146, 148, 151, 152, 156, 164,
    165–6
cerebellar degeneration **310**, **311**, 313, 314
cerebellar non-aneurysmal ICH 264
cerebral amyloid angiopathy (CAA) 90, **91**,
    92, 255
    Dutch type 90, **91**
    Icelandic type 90, **91**
cerebral autosomal dominant arteriopathy
    with subcortical infarcts and
    leukencephalopathy (CADASIL) 90, **91**,
    92
cerebral cavernous malformations (CCM)
    90–1, **91**
cerebral computed tomography (CCT) 255,
    263
cerebral palsy (CP) 58
cerebral perfusion pressure (CCP) 259,
    260, **262**, 264
cerebrospinal fluid (CSF) 62, 69, 175–97
    ABM 145, **146**, 147–9, **149–50**, 151–2,
    154, 156
    headache disorders 324, 325, **330**
    ICH 256, 257, 265
    leaks *41*, 43, *44*, 179–81
    LNB 159, 161, 162, 163–4, **165–6**, 167
    neurofilaments 176, 181, **183–6**, 188
    NMO 291, 292, 293, 294
cerebrovascular diseases 90, **91**, 91–2
cervical radiculopathy 13
channelopathies 87, 88–9, **89**
    muscular 88–9, **89**
    neuronal 88, **89**, 89–90
Charcot–Marie–Tooth (CMT) disease 68,
    101, **102**, 102–4
    axonal (CMT2) 101, **102**, 102, 103–4
    demyelinating (CMT1) 101, **102**, 102,
    103–4
    X-linked (CMTX) **102**, 102
chemokine CXCL13 162
chemoprophylaxis 155–6
chemotherapy 215, 216, **217**, 217–19, 312

Cheyne–Stokes breathing syndrome (CSBS)
    131, 136
childhood absence epilepsy 89, 90
chloramphenicol 148, 151, 152
chloride potassium salts 88
choline 202, 215
chorea **311**
chronic inflammatory demyelinating
    polyradiculoneuropathy (CIDP) 111,
    113–15
chronic meningitis 145, 149, **149**
chronic neuroborreliosis (late LNB) 160
chronic progressive external
    ophthalmoplegia (mtPEO) **64**, 69, 69
chronic tension-type headache 225, **226**,
    226–7, 230–1, 233
circadian rhythm sleep disorders 130, 131,
    132, 137
ciprofloxacin 155, 156
citalopram 230
classical trigeminal neuralgia (CTN) 31, 46
    diagnosis 33, **34**, *35*, 35, **35–6**, 36, **37**
    pharmacology 36, 40, 45
clockwise headache 327
clomipramine 230, **230**, 231
clonazepam 40, 137, **264**
clonidine 260
clopidogrel 256, 270
cluster headaches 65, 323–4, 327–9, 338
cocaine 256
codeine 229, 341
coenzyme Q₀ (CoQ) 68, 70
cognitive behavioural therapy **231**, 232, 233
colchicines **280**
collection of scientific data 8–9
colonoscopy 315, 317
colorectal cancer 315
community-acquired acute bacterial
    meningitis *see* acute bacterial
    meningitis
complex regional pain syndromes (CRPS)
    22, 24, **25**
    SCS 13, 16, **18**, 26
compound muscle action potentials
    (CMAPs) 101
computed tomography (CT) 31, **32**, 33,
    180, 218, 245
    ABM 147, **148**, **150**, 153, 155
    headache disorders 326, 328, **330**
    ICH 257, 258
    PNSs 312–14, 315, 316, 317
computed tomography angiography (CTA)
    257–8
confidentiality 53
congenital hypomyelinating neuropathy
    (CHN) 101–2
congenital insensitivity to pain with
    anhidrosis (CIPA) 103, 104
congenital muscular dystrophies **105**, 107,
    108
congenital myasthenia 88
congenital myasthenia syndrome (CMS)
    89

congenital myopathy **106**, 107–8, **283**
continuous positive airway pressure (CPAP) 133, 134, 136, 137, 138
controlled hyperventilation 260, **262**, 263
corticobasal degeneration (CBD) 130, 132, **177**
corticobasal syndrome (CBS) 94
corticospinal tract (CST) hyperintensities 200–6
corticosteroids 113, 116, 260, 340, **341**
    ABM 151, 153
    NMO 297, 298, 300
cotrimoxazole 151
CPT 2 deficiency **283**
craniotomy 264, 267
creatine 202
creatine kinase (CK) 279, **280**, 280–2, **283**, 284
Creutzfeld–Jakob disease (CJD) **93**, 94, 176, 178, 188
cryotherapy 41
cryptococcal meningitis **182**
cyclophosphamide 216, 293, 298–9, 300, **301**
cyst formation 163

dabigatran 269
deafness–dystonia syndrome (DDS) 68
deep brain stimulation (DBS) 11, 16, 20, **20**, **21**, 26, 26–7
deep vein thrombosis (DVT) prevention 262
Déjerine–Sottas neuropathy 102
dementia 87, 90, 92–5, 137, 218
    CSF investigations 176, **177**, 178, 187, 188
    inherited 92–5
    see also Alzheimer's disease
dementia with Lewy bodies (DLB) 130, 131–2, 176, **177**, **185**
denato-rubro-pallidoluysian atrophy (DRPLA) **54**, 55, 74, **76**
dermatomyositis (DM) 111, 115–16, 309, 314–15, 317
desminopathy **281**, **283**
detoxification 339, 340, 341
developmental arteriovenous malformations (DAVMs) 266
developmental venous anomalies (DVAs) 266
Devic's disease (neuromuelitis optica) 119, 287–307
    CSF investigations 186, 187
dexamethasone 340
    ABM 145, 148, **150**, 151, 153–4
diabetic neuropathy **14**, 16, **18**
diagnosis
    ABM 145–7, **147**, 148, **149**, 151, 153, 155
    ataxias and spastic paraplegias 73–85
    CFS investigations 175, 179, 181, 187–8
    channelopathies 87–96
    headache disorders 321, 322, **322–3**, 323, 325, 328–9, 331

hyperCKemia 280, 281–2, **283**, 284–5
ICH 257, 270
LGGs 214, 219
LNB 159, 160, 161–4
mitochondrial disorders 61–70
MND 199
MOH 337, **338**
neurogenetic 51–60, 97–109
neuromyelitis optica 287, 288–90, 292, 294–6
PNSs 309, 310, 312–15
sleep disorders 130, 131, 132, 134, 137–8
STN **32**, 33, **34**, 35, **35–6**, 36
TN **32**, 33, **34**, 35, **35–6**, 35–6, 37
TTHs 225, **226**, 227
WE 239, 241, 243, **244**, 245
diazepam 120, **264**, 327
diclofenac 228, **228**, 326
diffuse astrocytomas 214
diffusion tensor imaging (DTI) 199, 203–4, 205, 206
diffusion-weighted images (DWIs) 245, **247**
digital subtraction angiography (DSA) 257–8, 266
dihydroergotamine 325
diltiazem 327
diphenylhydantoin 89
dipyridamole 270
distal hereditary motor neuropathy (HMN) 98, 101
distal myopathies **106**, 108
diuretics 260, **261**, 270
donepezil 137
dopamine agonists 137
dopaminergic drugs 132, 134, 137
dopa-responsive dystonia (DRD) **56**, 58
doxycycline 164, **165**, **166**, 167, 168
driving 7
drug-resistant infantile epilepsy (DRIE) 120
Duchenne/Becker muscular dystrophy (DMD/BMD) 104
Duchenne muscular dystrophy (DMD) 104
dynamic contrast enhanced MRI (DCE-MRI) 215, 219
dynamic susceptibility contrast MRI (DSC-MRI) 215
dysferlinopathy **281**, **283**
dystonia 11, 51, **56**, 57–8
dystonia-plus syndromes 57–8
dystrophinopathy **281**, **283**, 284

eating disorders 131
EFNS guidelines 5–10
Ehlers–Danlos syndrome 92
electro-acupuncture 12, 13
electromyography (EMG) 88–9, 131, 132, 282, 284
    biofeedback **231**, 232, 233
electro-oculography 132
electrophysiology 292

elevated level of serum homocysteine **91**, 91–2
Emery–Drelfuss-type muscular dystrophy 107
enalapril 260
enalaprilat **261**
encephalitis **310**
encephalomyelitis **310**, **311**, 312
encephalomyopathic depletion syndrome (DPS) 67
endometrium cancer **310**, **311**
endoscopic ultrasound-guided fine needle aspiration (EUG-FNA) 312
endovascular embolization 266
Enterobacter 146
enuresis 131
eosinophilic meningitis **182**
epilepsy 6, 11, 36, 40, 87–9, **89**
    ABM **148**, 153, 155
    ICH 260, 262, **264**
    IVIG 120
    LGGs 215, 216, 217, 218, 219
    sleep disorders 131
episodic ataxia 74, **76**, 78, 88, 89
Epstein–Barr virus 329
ergonovin 325
ergotamine 326, 327, 328
    MOH **338**, 338, 339, **341**, 341
Escherichia coli 146
esmolol **261**
essential tremor 58
ethnicity **54**, 55, 57, 83, 88
    ataxias 74, 79
    ICH 253, 256
    hyperCKemia 279, **280**
    LNB 160–1
    NMO 287, 291, 292
etoricoxib 324
evidence classification 6–7, **254**
excessive daytime sleepiness (EDS) 129, 131, 132–4, 137
exercise 279, **280**, 284
exploding head syndrome 131

Fabry's disease 91, 92
Facial pain **19**, 20, 21, 22, 24, 27
facloscapulohumeral muscular dystrophy (FSHD) 104, 108
failed back surgery syndrome (FBSS) 16, **17**, 21, 26
failed neck surgery syndrome (FNSS) **17**
familial Creutzfeld–Jakob disease (CJD) **93**, 94
familial hemiplegic migraine (FHM) 78, **91**, 92
fenoldopam **261**
fibrates **280**
fibrillary astrocytomas 214
fingolimod 299
flucloxacillin 152
fluconazole 164

fluid-attenuated inversion recovery (FLAIR) imaging 200–1
   LGGs 215, 216, 218
   WE 245, **247**
flunarizine 326, 327, **330**
fluorodeoxyglucose (FDG) 215, 219
fluorodeoxyglucose positron emission tomography (FDG-PET) 312–17
folic acid 92
fosphenytoin 40, 155
fractional anisotropy (FA) 203–4, 206
fragile X tremor/ataxia syndrome (FXTAS) **77**, 79
frequent episodic tension-type headache 225, **226**, 226–7, 229–31, 233
fresh frozen plasma (FFP) 268, **268**, 269
Friedreich ataxia (FRDA) 74, **77**, 78, 79
frontotemporal dementia (FTD) 98, **99**, 201, 205
   CSF investigations 176, **177**
frontotemporal dementia with parkinsonism (FTDP) **93**
frontotemporal dementia with ubiquitinated lesions (FTD-U) **93**, 94
frontotemporal lobar degeneration (FTLD) 93–4, 95, **99**, 199–201
   CSF investigations **185**, 187
fukutin-related protein (FKRP) **281**, **283**
functional magnetic resonance imaging (fMRI) 199, 204–5, 219
fungal meningitis 149
furosemide **261**

gabapentin 40–1, 203, 216, 218
   headache disorders 324, 328, 329, **330**
gadolinium enhancement 290, 291
gamma-aminobutyric acid (GABABR) **310**, **311**, 315
gamma knife surgery (GKS) 32, **41**, **42**, 43–4, 46
Gasserian ganglion 12, 32, 41
gate-control therapy 12, 13, 16
Gaucher's disease 57
gemistocytic astrocytomas 214
gender 227, 339, 341
   headache disorders 324–30
   hyperCKemia 279, **280**, 284, 285
   NMO 289, 297
generalized epilepsy with febrile seizure-plus (GEFS+) **89**, 90
genetic counselling 52, 53, 54, 57, 73, 101
   dementias 92, 94, 95
genetic testing 51–3, 54, 54–5, 57, 58, 103
   Alzheimer's disease 93, 95
   ataxias 73–4, 78, 79
   channelopathies 88, 90
   MIDs 62, 69
   motorneuron disorders 98, 101
   spastic paraplegias 73–4
gentamicin 151, 152
glatiramer acetate 297

glial fibrillary acidic protein (GFAP) 292
gliomas 181, **182**, 213–23
glucocorticoid treatment 178
glucosidase deficiency **283**
glycerol 41, 43, 263
glycogenoses 282, **283**, 284
GR surgery technique **42**
gram-negative bacilli 146, 151, 152, 153
grey matter (GM) 201–2, 206, 291
Guillain–Barré syndrome (GBS) 111, 112–13, 296
   CSF investigations **177**, **186**
gynaecological cancer **311**, 312

Haemophilus influenzae 146–7, 151–2, 155–6
haemostatic therapy 266–7
headache 5, 256–7, 321–35
   classification of disorders **322–3**
   medication overuse 337–44
   tension type 225–38
   treatment **330**
heart failure with lactic acidosis 243
hemicrania continua **323**, 323, 328–9, **330**
heparin 155, 262, 263, **268**
hepatocerebral depletion syndrome (DPS) 67
hereditary episodic neuropathies 101, **102**
hereditary motor neuropathy (HMN) 98, 101, 103–4
hereditary motor and sensory neuropathy (HMSN) 101
hereditary neuralgic amyotrophy (HNA) 103, 104
hereditary neuropathy with susceptibility to pressure palsies (HNPP) 103, 104
hereditary sensory-autonomic neuropathy (HSAN) 101, 103, 104
hereditary spastic paraplegias (HSPs) 73, 80, **81–2**, 83
   X-linked HSPs 80, **81–2**, 83
herpes simplex virus (HSV) encephalitis **186**
Hib meningitis 146, 153, 154, 156
high-performance liquid chromatography (HPLC) 245
HIV 154, **182**
Hodgkin's disease 309, **310**, **311**, 314
homocystinuria 91–2
Huntington's disease (HD) 51–5, **54**, 55, 58, 134
Huntington's disease-like (HDL) disorders **54**, 55
hydralazine **261**
hydrocephalus 148, 153, 255, 264–5, 267
hyperCKemia 279–82, **283**, 284–6
   asymptomatic 280–2, **283**, 284
   causes **280**
   pauci-symptomatic 280–2, **283**, 284
hyperemesis gravidarum 241
HyperHAES **262**, 263

hyperkalaemic periodic paralysis (HYPP) 88, **89**
hyperphosphorylated tau (P-tau) 176, **177**, 188
hypersomnia 130, 131, 178
hypertension 327, 329
   ICH 255–60, **261**, 263, 269–70
   management 259–60, **261**
hypnagogic hallucinations 178
hypnic headache **322**, 327–8, **330**
hypocretin 175, 178–9, **179**, 188
hypocretin deficiency 132
hypokalaemic periodic paralysis (HOKPP) 88, **89**, 89
hypoxaemia 133

ibuprofen 228, **228**, 229, 230, 326
idiopathic hypersomnia 131
immune complex tests 162–3
immunomodulatory treatment 297
immunosuppressive treatment 298–299, **300**
implanted pulse generator (IPG) 13, 16, 22
inclusion body myositis (IBM) 116, **283**
indapamide 269
indomethacin 324, 325–6, 327, 329, **330**
inflammatory myopathy 115–16, **283**
informed consent 52, 53, 54, 92
infrequent episodic tension-type headache 225, **226**, 226–7, 229, 231, 233
insomnia 129, 130, 132–4, 137
intercostal neuralgia **19**, **21**
interferon-β 297
intergenomic signalling defects 65, 66
internal capsule **21**
interstitial cystitis 13, **15**
intracerebral haemorrhage (ICH) 253–77
   antihypertensive drugs **261**
   evidence classification **254**
   prevention 269–70
intracranial pressure (ICP) 324, 325
   ICH 259, 260, **261**, **262**, 263–4
intravenous immunoglobulin (IVIG) 111–27
   NMO 296, 297, **300**, 300
   side effects 120
intraventricular haemorrhage (IVH) 255, 256, 264
irinotecan 216
isoniazid 164
isoretinoin **280**

juvenile myoclonic epilepsy **89**, 90

Kearns–Sayre syndrome (KSS) 62–3, **64**, 65, 69, 69–70
Kennedy disease **100**, 101
ketoprofen 228, **228**, 229
ketorolac 228
Klebsiella 146
Korsakoff's amnestic syndrome 239

labetalol 260, **261**, 263
Lambert–Eaton myasthenic syndrome
   (LEMS) 115, 309, **310**, **311**, 312,
   314–17
lamotrigine **38**, 40–1, 45, 216, 218, 329
Landau–Kleffner syndrome (LKS) 120
laryngeal stridor 132, 134, 137
Leber's hereditary optic neuropathy
   (LHON) 62, **64**, 65, 69, 69–70
leg cramps 132
Leigh's syndrome (LS) **64**, 65, 66
Lennox–Gastaut syndrome 120
leptomeningeal metastases 181, **181**,
   188
levetiracetam 218
levodopa 58
lidocaine 41, 43
light therapy 137
limb-girdle muscular dystrophy (LGMD)
   107, 108
   hyperCKemia **281**, **283**, 284
limbic encephalitis 115, **310**, **311**
linezolid 151–2
Listeria monocytogenes 146, 151
Listerial meningitis 145, 148–9, 151–3
lithium 327, **330**
lobulated fibre myopathy **283**
longitudinally extensive transverse myelitis
   (LETM) 288, 290–5, *295*, **301**,
   296–301
lorazepam **264**
low grade gliomas (LGGs) 213–23
low-molecular weight heparin (LMWH)
   262, 263
lower motor neurons (LMNs) 199, 204
lumbar puncture (LP)
   AMB 145, 147, 148, **150**
   contraindications 147, **148**
   headache disorders 324–6, 328, **330**
lung cancer **311**, 315
lyme neuroborreliosis (LNB) 159–73
   case definitions **163**
   early 160–2, 164, 178
   laboratory tests 161–4
   late 160–2, 164, 167
   treatment 164, **165–6**
lymphocyte apheresis 297
lymphocyte transformation test (LTT)
   163
lymphocytic meningitis 160, 161
lymphomas 315
   Hodgkin's disease 309, **310**, **311**, 314

Machado–Joseph disease (MJD) 131, 134
macrophagic myositis **283**
magnesium deficiency 245
magnetic resonance angiography (MRA)
   257–8, 266, **330**
magnetic resonance imaging (MRI) 80, 91,
   118
   ABM **148**, 148–9, **150**, 153, 155
   DBS 16, 20

headache disorders 323, 328, **330**
   ICH 255, 257–8, 263
   Leigh's syndrome 66
   LGGs 214, 215, 216–17, 218–19
   MCS 22
   MND 200–1, 203, 204, 205, 206
   NMO 290–1, 293–4, *295*, 295–6, 299
   PNSs 312, 313, 316
   TN **28**, 31, **32**, 33, 35–6, **37**, 43, 46
   WE 243, 245, **247**, 248
magnetization transfer (MT) MRI 204
maintenance of wakefulness test (MWT)
   134, **135**
malignancy pain **21**
malignant hyperthermia (MH) myopathy
   283, 284
malignant hyperthermia susceptibility
   (MHS) 108
mammography 313, 315, 316, 317
mannitol 154, 260, **262**, 263
maprotiline 230, **230**, 231
Marchiafava–Bignami syndrome 243
massage 232–3
maternally inherited diabetes and deafness
   (MIDD) 65
maternally inherited Leigh's syndrome
   (MILS) **64**, 65
maternally inherited PEO 65
mature cystic teratomas (MCTs) 313
mean diffusivity (MD) 203–4
Meckel's cave 12, 41
medication overuse headache (MOH) 3,
   329, 337–44
   diagnostic criteria **338**
   tension-type 226–7, **228**, 229, 230, 338,
     340–1
   treatment **341**
   withdrawal procedure 339–41, **341**,
     342
melatonin 137, 324, 329, **330**
memantine 230
meninges 164, 168
meningitis 145–57
   CSF investigations 180, 181, **182**
   LNB 159–92
meningococcal meningitis 151, 152, 153,
   156
meningococcemia 148, **150**, 154
meningo-encephalitis **149**
meningoradiculitis 160
meropenem 151, 152
metabolic myopathies **283**
metamizole 228, 328, **330**
11C-methionine (MET) 215, 216, 219
methotrexate 298, **300**, 301
methylphenidate 137
methylprednisolone 119, 187, 331
   Guillain–Barré syndrome 112, 113
   NMO 291, 293, 296–7
methysergide 325, 329, **330**
metoclopramide 340
metoprolol 327

metronidazole 164
mexiletine 89
mianserin 230, **230**, 231
micro-sleep episodes 132
microvascular decompression (MVD) 32,
   35–6, **41**, 41, **42**, 43–4, 46
midazolam **264**
migraine 5, 11, 87–9, 90, **91**, 92, 321,
   323–30
   compared with TTH 227, 228
   MOH 337, 339, 340, 341
Miller–Fisher syndrome 113
minocycline 155
mirtazapine 230, **230**, 231
misoprostol 40
mitochondrial biogenesis defects
   68
mitochondrial depletion syndrome (DPS)
   64
mitochondrial disorders (MIDs) 61–3, *63*,
   64, 65–9, 69, 70
   classification 63, *63*
mitochondrial DNA (mtDNA) 62, 63, *63*,
   64, 65–70
   breakage syndromes 66–7
   depletion syndromes 67, 70
mitochondrial encephalopathy, lactic
   acidosis and stroke-like episodes
   (MELAS) 63, **64**, 65, 69, 69–70
mitochondrial lipid milieu defects 68
mitochondrial myopathy **283**
mitochondrial protein synthesis machinery
   67–8, 70
mitochondrial transport machinery defects
   68
mitoxantrone 298, 299, 301, **300**
modafinil 137
Mohr–Tranebjaerg syndrome 68, 70
monoclonal gammopathy 114
monoclonal gammopathy of undetermined
   significance (MGUS) 114–15
Morvan's syndrome **311**
motor cortex stimulation (MCS) 11, 20, 22,
   23–4, 25–6, *26*, 27
motor end-plate disease 133–4
motor neuron degeneration (MND)
   94
motor neuron disorders 97–8, **99**–100, 101,
   199–211
   sleep 130, 133–4
moxifloxacin 152
multifocal motor neuropathy (MMN) 111,
   114
multiple sclerosis (MS) **21**, 111, 118–19,
   132
   compared with NMO 287–92, 294,
     296–9, 301–2
   CSF investigations 177, 178, **184**,
     187
   TN 31, 32, 40, **42**, 43–4
multiple sleep latency test (MSLT) 134,
   135

multiple system atrophy (MSA) **177, 183,** 187
  sleep disorders 130, 131, 132–3, 134, 136
multiplex ligation-dependent probe amplification (MLPA) 83
muscle biopsy 280, 281–2, 284–5, **285**
muscle disorders 97–8, 133–4
muscle relaxants 229, 230
muscle-specific tyrosin kinase (MuSK) 116–17
muscular dystrophies 104, **105–6,** 107–8, 133
  hyperCKemia 279–82, **282, 283,** 284–5
myasthenia gravis (MG) 116–17, 130, 133
  NMO 295, 296, 298, 300
  PNSs 309, **310, 311,** 312, 315, 317
mycophenolate mofetil 299, **300,** 301
myelin basic protein (MBP) 175, 176, 187
myelitis 289, 290, 293, 294, 296
myoclonic epilepsy 120
myoclonus–dystonia (M–D) **56,** 58
myoclonus epilepsy with ragged red fibres (MERRF) 63, **64,** 65, 69, 69–70
myofibrillar myopathy **106,** 108, **283**
myo-inositol (mI) 203
myoneurogastrointestinal encephalomyopathy (MNGIE) **64,** 67, 70
myopathic depletion syndrome (DPS) 67
myopathies 97–8, 104, **105–6,** 107–8
myophosphorylase deficiency 282, **283**
myotonia 88–9, **89,** 90
myotonia congenita **89**
myotonia fluctuans **283**
myotonic dystrophy 90, 104, **105–6,** 107, 108
  hyperCKemia **281, 283,** 284
  sleep disorders 130, 133

N-acetylaspartate (NAA) 202–3, 205, 215
naproxen 228, **228,** 229, 341
  headache disorders 325, 329, **330**
naratripan 327
narcolepsy 131, 132, 134, 137
  CSF investigations 175, 178–9, **179,** 188
narcolepsy with cataplexy 132
nasal continuous positive airway pressure (nCPAP) 136
nasal intermittent positive pressure ventilation (NIPPV) 136, 138
natalizumab 299
Neisseria meningitidis 146, 151, 155, 156
nerve block 233
nerve conduction velocity (NCV) 101
nerve root stimulation (NRS) 11, 12–13, **14–15**
neurectomies 41
neuroacanthocytosis 55
neuroblastoma **310, 311,** 312, 314
neurocognitive defects 218

neurodegenerative disorders 65, 66, 94, 129–38, 296
  ataxias 78, 80
  CSF investigations 176, **182,** 187, 188
neuroferritinopathy 55
neurofilaments (Nf) 292
  CSF investigations 176, 181, **183–6,** 188
neurogenetic disorders 51–60, 73–4, 97–109
neurogenic myopathy 280, **283**
neurogenic weakness, ataxia and retinitis pigmentosa (NARP) 63, **64,** 65, 69, 69–70
neuroimaging 199–211
  ICH 255, 257–8, 263
  LGGs 215, 216, 219
  NMO 287, 290, 291
  TTHs 227
  see also computed tomography, magnetic resonance imaging
neuroleptic malignant syndrome **280**
neuromuscular disease **177**
  hyperCKemia 280–1, **281, 282, 283,** 284–5
neuromyelitis optica (NMO) 119, 187, 287–307
  comorbidities 295
  differential diagnosis 296
  prevention 297–300
  spectrum disorders 294–6, 301
neuromyelitis optica–immunoglobulin G (NMO–IgC) 287–8, 292–4, *295,* 295–6, **300,** 297, 300–1
neuromyotonia **310, 311**
neuron specific enolase (NSE) 316
neuropathic pain 11–27
neurostimulation therapy 11–27
new daily persistent headache **323,** 329, **330,** 330–31
new variant CJD 176, 178
nicardipine **261**
nifedipine 263, 324
nightmare disorder 131, 132
nimodipine 328, **330,** 330
nitroglycerin 263
nitrosureas 216, 218
nitroprussidea **261**
nociceptive pain 13, 20
nocturia 132
nocturnal oxygen desaturations 133
nocturnal seizures 129
non-dystrophic myotonia 88
non-rapid eye movement (NREM) sleep 131, 133, 327
non-steroidal anti-inflammatory drugs (NSAIDs) 227, 228, 229, 328, 339
noradrenaline 230
normal pressure hydrocephalus (NPH) **177, 186**
nuclear DNA (nDNA) 62, *63,* **64,** 65

obsessive compulsive disorder 11
obstructive sleep apnoea syndrome (OSAS) 130, 132–3, 134, 136–8
oligoastrocytomas 214–15, 216, 219
oligoclonal band (OCB) 291
oligodendroglioma 214–19
onabotulinum toxin 340
ophthalmoscopy 289
optic coherence tomography 289
optic nerve 290
optic neuritis (ON) 187, **311**
  NMO 287, 289–90, 292, 294–7, 301
opticospinal MS (OSMS) 288, 294, 296, 297
opioids 40, 229, 328
  MOH 337, **338,** 339, **341**
orexin 175, 178–9, **179,** 188
otorrhea 175, 176, 180, **180**
ovarian carcinoma 309, **310, 311,** 312–16
ovarian teratoma 30, **310, 311,** 313, 316
oxcarbazepine (OXC) 36, **39,** 40, 45, 216
oxidative phosphorylation (OXPHOS) defects 62, 65, 83
oximetry 133–4, **135,** 137

paclitaxel 216
Paget's disease 94
painful diabetic neuropathy **14**
pancreatic cancer **311,** 315
pancreatitis 65
paracetamol 326, 328, **330**
  TTHs 227, 228, **228,** 229
paramyotonia congenita (PMC) 88–9, **89**
paraneoplastic antibodies 310, **310, 311,** 314–17
paraneoplastic cerebellar degeneration (PCD) 115, 309, **310, 311,** 313–15
paraneoplastic encephomyelitis (PEM) 312
paraneoplastic limbic encephalitis (PLE) 309, 315
paraneoplastic neurological syndromes (PNSs) 115, 309–10, **310–11,** 312–20
paraneoplastic neuromyotonia 115
paraneoplastic opsoclonus–myoclonus (POM) 309, **310, 311**
paraneoplastic opsoclonusataxia syndrome 115
paraneoplastic peripheral nerve hyperexcitability (PPNH) 309
paraneoplastic retinopathy 309
paraproteinaemic demyelinating neuropathy 114–15
parasomnia 130, 131–2
Parkinson's disease and parkinsonism 5, 11, 51, 55, **56,** 57, 58
  CSF investigations **177, 183,** 187
  sleep disorders 130, 131–2, 137
paroxysmal dystonias **56,** 58
partial spinal cord injury 16

Pearson's syndrome (PS) 62–3, **64**, *69*, 69–70
Pelizaeus–Merzbacher disease (PMD) 80
pelvic pain 13, **15**
penicillin
    ABM 146–8, 151–3, 156
    LNB 164, **165**, 167, 168
pentobarbital 260
percutaneous electrical nerve stimulation (PENS) **14–15**
percutaneous gasserian lesions (PGLs) 32, *41*, 41, 46
percutaneous procedures on Gasserian ganglion 41, 43, 44, 46
percutaneous rhizotomies 41
perindopril 269
periodic limb movements (PLMs) 129, 132, 133–4, 137
periodic paralysis 88, 90
peripheral acupuncture 41
peripheral nerve injury 16, **18**, *21*, 24, *26*
peripheral nerve stimulation (PNS) 11, 12–13, **14–15**
peripheral nervous system (PNS) 160, 164
peripheral neuropathy **18**, 20, 97, 101, **102**, 102–4
periventricular grey matter (PVG) 16, 20, **21**
pharmacotherapy 11, 36, 40
    TN 31–2, 36, **38**, **39**, 40–1, 43–6
    TTHs 225–6, 227, **228**, 228–30, **230**, 231
phenobarbital 264
phenobarbitone 218
phenol injection 41
phenoxymethyl penicillin 156
phenprocoumon 268
phenytoin 155, **264**
    LGGs 216, 218
    TN 31, 36, 40
phosphofructokinase deficiency 282, **283**
phosphorylase-b kinase **283**
physical therapy **231**, 232–3
physiotherapy 232–3
Pick's disease 94
pimozide **39**, 40–1
plasma exchange 112–13, 114, 116–17, 119, 120
    NMO 297, **301**, 301
plasmapheresis 297, 300
pleocytosis 291–2
plexopathies 20
pneumococcal meningitis 147–8, 151–6, **182**
POEMS syndrome 181, **182**
polygraphy 134, **135**
polymerase chain reaction (PCR) 52, 53, 159, 161, 163
polymyositis 115, 116, **283**
polyneuropathies 97
polysomnography (PSG) 132, 133–4, **135**, 137
poor sleep hygiene 131

positron emission tomography (PET) 22, 255
    fluorodeoxyglucose (FDG-PET) 312–17
    LGGs 215–16, 219
    MND 199, 200, 204–5
    PNSs 312, 313
posterior reversible encephalopathy syndrome (PRES) 290, 291, 295
post-herpetic neuralgia (PHN) 13, **15**, 16, **19**, 21
post-lyme disease syndrome (PLDS) 167–8
post-polio syndrome (PPS) 111, 117–18, 133, 280
potassium 88, 90
potassium-aggravated myotonia **89**
prednisolone (prednisone) 116, 299
    MOH 339, 340, **341**
    NMO 298–9, 300, **301**
pre-eclampsia **182**
pregabalin 41, 327
pregnancy 117
presymptomatic diagnosis 53
primary cough headache **322**, 323, 324–5, 326, **330**
primary dystonia **56**, 57
primary exertional headache **322**, 325–6, **330**
primary headache associated with sexual activity **322**, 323, 325, 326–7, **330**
    orgasmic **322**, 326–7
    preorgasmic **322**, 326
primary lateral sclerosis (PLS) 199–204
primary non-fluent aphasia 94
primary stabbing headache **322**, 323–4, **330**
primary thunderclap headache **323**, 323, 328, **330**
prion diseases 55, 94
procarbazine, CCNU and vincristine (PCV) 217, 218
progastrin-releasing peptide (PROGRP) 316
progressive muscular atrophy (PMA) 199, 200, 203, 204
progressive supranuclear palsy (PSP) 94, 130, 132, **177**, **183**
proparacaine **38**
propofol **264**
proposing, planning and writing guidelines 9–10
propranolol 325–6, 327, **330**
prostaglandin D synthase (PGDS) 176, 180–1
prostate carcinoma 310, **311**, 312, 314
protamine sulphate **268**
proteolipid protein (PLP) 80
prothrombin complex (PCC) 267–8, **268**, 269
proton density (PD)-weighted imaging 200–1, 257, 258
proton magnetic resonance spectroscopic imaging (^{1}H-MRSI) 199, 202–3, 205
proton magnetic resonance spectroscopy (MRS) 215

protoplasmic astrocytomas 214
proximal spinal muscular atrophy (SMA) 98
pseudomonal meningitis 152, 153
Pseudomonas aeruginosa 146, 152, 153
psychobehavioural treatment **231**, 232
psychotherapy 339
pulmonary embolism (PE) prevention 262

radicellectomy 22
radiculopathy 13, **14–15**, 20
radiofrequency thermocoagulation (RFT) 41, **42**, 43
radiography 312, 316, 317
radiosurgery 266
radiotherapy (RT) 215, **217**, 217–18, 219
ragged red fibres 62, 63, 65
rapid eye movement (REM) sleep 129, 131, 133, 134, 327
rapid eye movement (REM) sleep behaviour disorder (RBD) 131–2, 133, 134, 137
rapid onset dystonia-parkinsonism **56**, 58
Rasmussen's encephalitis (RE) 111, 120
recombinant activated factor VIIa (rFVIIa) 266–7, 268–9
recurrent focal neuropathies 103
recurrent isolated optic neuritis (RION) 288, 293–4, **295**, 296, **301**, 299–300
recurrent isolated sleep paralysis 131
refractory pain 11
relapsing-remitting multiple sclerosis (RRMS) 118–19
relaxation training **231**, 232, 233
renal cell cancer **311**
repetitive transcranial magnetic stimulation (rTMS) 11, 22, 24–5, **25**, *26*, 27
    MCS 22, 24, 25, 27
respiratory chain complexes 63, 65–8, 70
respiratory chain defects 62–3
respiratory chain subunits mutations 65
respiratory polygraphy (RP) 134, **135**, 137
restless leg syndrome (RLS) 58, 129, 132, 134, 137
rhinorrhoea 175, 176, 180, **180**
rhythmic movement disorders 132
rifampicin 151, 152, 155, 156
riluzole 203
rituximab 299–**300**, 301
RyR antibodies 315

S-100 176
salt intake 270
sarcoglycanopathy **281**, **283**
sarcoid myopathy **283**
seizures
    ICH 258–9, 260, 262–3, **264**
    LGGs 215, 216, 217, 218
    see also epilepsy
selective serotonin reuptake inhibitors (SSRIs) 230, 330
semantic dementia (SD) 94, **177**

sensory ataxic neuropathy dysarthria
    ophthalmoplegia (SANDO) 67, 70
sensory neuropathy 115
sensory thalamus (ST) 16, 20, **21**, 22
serotonin 230
serotonin-noradrenaline reuptake inhibitors
    41
sertraline 230
serum creatine kinase (sCK) 279, **280**, 280,
    284
severe myoclonic epilepsy of infancy
    (SMEI) **89**, 90
short-tau inversion recovery (STIR) 290
Sjögren's syndrome (SS) 294, 295, 298, 302
skull abnormalities 31
sleep 129–43, 327
    CSF investigations 175, 178–9, 188
sleep apnoea 133, 134, 137–8
sleep-disordered breathing (SDB) 129,
    130–1
sleep fragmentation 129, 131, 132
sleep insufficiency syndrome 131
sleep paralysis 178
sleep-related breathing disorders (SBD)
    130, 131–4, 136–8
sleep-related groaning (catathrenia) 131
sleep-related hallucinations 131, 132
sleep-related hypoventilation/hypoxaemic
    syndromes (SHVSs) 131, 133–4, 136
sleep-related movement disorders 130, 132
sleep terror 131
sleep–wake disturbance 132
sleep walking 131
small cell lung cancer (SCLC) 309, **310**,
    311, 312, 314–16
smoking 256, 270, 341
sodium 88, 90
sodium channel myotonia 88, **89**
sodium nitroprusside 260, 263
sodium oxybate 137
somatosensory-evoked potentials (SEPs)
    16, 22
SOX1 antibodies 315
spastic paraplegias 52, 80, **81**, 83
spatially limited NMO spectrum disorders
    294–5, 295, **301**, 296, 300–1
SPAX1 **82**
spectroscopy 215
spinal and bulbar muscular atrophy
    (SBMA) **100**, 101
spinal cord lesions 22, 24, **25**
    NMO 290–1, 293, 294, 295, 296
spinal cord stimulation (SCS) 11, 12, 13,
    16, **17–19**, 26, 26–7
    DBS 20
    MCS 22
spinal muscular atrophy (SMA) 98, **100**,
    101, 280
spinal muscular atrophy with respiratory
    distress (SMARD) 98, **100**, 101
spinocerebellar ataxia (SCA) 54, 55, 74,
    75–6, 78, 92
    sleep disorders 130

spinocerebellar ataxia and epilepsy (SCAE)
    67, 70
spongiform encephalopathies 94, 178
sporadic inclusion body myositis (S-IBM)
    115–16
sporadic progressive external
    ophthalmoplegia (PEO) 62–3
staphylococcal meningitis 151, 152
staphylococci 146
statins 256, 279, **280**, 284
status epilepticus 260, 262, **264**
stereotactic computerized tomography 16
stereotaxic aspiration 264, 267
steroids 114, 116, 119, 120, 164
    ABM 153–4
    headache disorders 327, 329
    NMO 296–7, 298, 300
    see also corticosteroids
stiff person syndrome (SPS) 111, 119–20,
    310, **311**
stomach cancer 315
Streptococcus pneumonia 145–6, 151, 153–4
Streptococcus suis 154
streptomycin 41, 43
stroke 5, 7–8, 87, 90, **91**, 91–2, 253–77
    CSF investigations 176, **177**
    haemorrhagic 90–1
    ischaemic 90, 92, 133, 253, 256–60, **261**,
        263, 269–70
    prevention 269–70
    sleep disorders 129–32, 133, 134, 137
    thromboembolic 91
stroke-like episodes (SLEs) 63
subacute autonomic neuropathy (SAN)
    309, **310**, **311**
subacute sensory neuropathy (SSN) 309,
    310, **311**
subarachnoid haemorrhage (SAH) 253,
    258, 265, 266, 270
    CFS investigations 181, **182**, **186**, 187
    headache disorders 325, 326, 328, **330**
sulfamethoxazole 152
sulfatid 176
sulphonamide 155
sumatriptan 341
sundowning psychosis 132
supratentorial non-aneurysmal ICH 163–4,
    265
surgery 136
    complications *41*, 43, **44–5**
    ICH 257–8, 263–4, *265*, 265–6, 267
    LGGs 216–17, 218, 219
    TN 32, 40, *41*, 41, **42**
    WE 241, 249
symptomatic trigeminal neuralgia (STN)
    31–2, 40, **42**, 46
    diagnosis 32, 33, **34**, *35*, **35–6**, 36
synucleinopathies 130, 132–3
systemic lupus erythematosus (SLE) 294,
    295, 298, 301

T1-weighted imaging 215, 257
    NMO 290–1, 294

T2-weighted imaging 257–8, 266
    LGGs 215, 216, 218
    MNDS 200–1, 203
    NMO 290–1, 294
tau protein 175, 176, **177**, 178, 187, 188
tauopathies 130, 132
temozolomide 216, 218
tension type headaches (TTHs) 225–38,
    321, 323–4, 326, 328–30
    MOH 226–7, **228**, 229, 230, 338, 340–1
    non-pharmacological treatment 231–2
teratomas 313, 316
    ovarian 30, **310**, **311**, 313, 316
testicular tumours 309, **310**, **311**, 312,
    314–17
tetracyclic antidepressants 230–1
theophylline 136
therapy-related acute leukaemia (TRAL)
    299
thiamine 239, 241, 243, 245, 248–9
thin corpus callosum 206
thiopental **262**, **264**
thiotepa 216
thromboembolism 262, 263, 267, 269
thymectomy 117
thymoma 309, **310**, **311**, 312–13, 316
tizanidine **38**, 40, 230
TMZ 218
tocainide **39**, 40
topiramate 40, 230, 340, **341**
    headache disorders 325, 327, 329
    LGGs 216, 218
topotecan 216
tracheostomy 136–7
tramadol **330**
tranexamic acid 266
transcutaneous electrical nerve stimulation
    (TENS) 11, 12–13, **14–15**, 16, 26,
    27
transient ischaemic attacks (TIAs) 256,
    269
transitoric ischaemic attacks (TIAs) 90, 92
transverse myelitis 178
trauma **14–15**, 21
    CSF investigations 176, **177**, **185**
tricyclic antidepressants (TCAs) 40, 41, 330
    TTHs 229, 230, 231, 232
trigeminal autonomic cephalagias 321
trigeminal autonomic headache 323–4,
    328
trigeminal nerve 22, 24, **25**, 27
trigeminal neuralgia (TN) 31–49
    diagnosis 32, 33, **34**, *35*, **35–6**, 35–6, 37
    pharmacology 36, **38**, **39**, 40–1, 45–6
    surgery 40, *41*, 41, **42**, 43–4, **44–5**, 45–6
trigeminopathic pain **19**, 21
trimethoprim 152
trimethoprim-sulfamethoxazole 164
triptans 227, 229
    headache disorders 326–7, 328
    MOH 337, **338**, 338–9, 341, **341**
tuberculous meningitis 145, 149, **149**, **182**
tubular aggregates **283**